# ANNUAL REVIEW OF
# NUTRITION

# ANNUAL REVIEW OF NUTRITION

## VOLUME 21, 2001

DONALD B. McCORMICK, *Editor*
Emory University

DENNIS M. BIER, *Associate Editor*
Children's Nutrition Research Center, Houston

ROBERT J. COUSINS, *Associate Editor*
University of Florida

www.AnnualReviews.org    science@AnnualReviews.org    650-493-4400

ANNUAL REVIEWS
4139 El Camino Way • P.O. BOX 10139 • Palo Alto, California 94303-0139

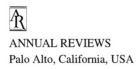

ANNUAL REVIEWS
Palo Alto, California, USA

*International Standard Serial Number: 0199-9885*
*International Standard Book Number: 0-8243-2821-3*

Annual Review and publication titles are registered trademarks of Annual Reviews.
♾ The paper used in this publication meets the minimum requirements of American National Standards for Information Sciences—Permanence of Paper for Printed Library Materials, ANSI Z39.48-1992.

Annual Reviews and the Editors of its publications assume no responsibility for the statements expressed by the contributors to this *Annual Review*.

TYPESET BY TECHBOOKS, FAIRFAX, VA
PRINTED AND BOUND IN THE UNITED STATES OF AMERICA

# PREFACE

In prefaces to previous volumes of the *Annual Review of Nutrition*, the attempt has been made to point out that the topics range from updated findings at the basic science end of our discipline to those extensions that may be considered applied. Given the unwarranted trepidation of some to use such terms as "basic" and "applied," I can offer the two sides of this argument by quoting well-known earlier scientists: Louis Pasteur wrote in 1871 that "... there does not exist a category of science to which one can give the name applied science. There are science and the applications of science ..." (translated by I. B. Cohen from *Revue Scientifique*). Somewhat later Albert Einstein wrote in 1931 that "... you should understand about applied science in order that your work may increase man's blessings." (Address at the California Institute of Technology.)

As seen in previous volumes and in numerous discourses on what is a nutritionist, it is satisfying to most of us that we can fit our expertise and interest somewhere in the broad span from the molecular-oriented sciences of life to the preventive and corrective measures that carry into public health and clinical practice. Again the topics of chapters in the present volume offer some of this diverse menu. Much of what has been discovered at the basic level, as in the past, will surely lead to useful applied outcome. With regard to the mix of basic and applied topics of nutrition to be found in this volume, one can read updates of a basic, molecular nature that are found in the chapter on catabolism of folate by J. Suh, A. K. Herbig, & P. Stover or on mammalian selenium-containing proteins by D. Behne and A. Kyriakopoulos. Subjects that bridge from basic to applied are represented by such a chapter as by M. Hambidge and N. Krebs that deals with key variables of human zinc homeostasis as relate to dietary requirements or by C. Stephensen on vitamin A and its impact on immune function. Clearly there are other extrapolations that a careful reader may draw from chapters dealing with findings from basic science, just as all of us should be pleased by those applications that guide us toward better health. At the applied and clinical level is a chapter by M. Serdula et al that reviews dietary assessment of preschool children, and the problems with present nutritional management of maintenance dialysis patients are considered by R. Mehrotra and J. Kopple in their chapter. L. Hallberg has provided us in the prefatory chapter with his scholarly perspectives on nutritional iron deficiency. Though our species of major consideration is the human, there are some interesting findings of a comparative nature with chapters by P. Trotter on genetics of fatty acid metabolism in yeast and by M. Wells and his colleagues on fat metabolism in insects.

My thanks as always to our Associate Editors (Drs. Bier and Cousins), the Editorial Committee and guests (listed in the front), and to Lisa Dean, the production editor, Roberta Parmer, the copyeditor, and Dr. Sam Gubins as president of Annual Reviews.

Donald B. McCormick
Editor

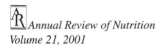

*Annual Review of Nutrition*
*Volume 21, 2001*

# CONTENTS

ERRATA
An online log of corrections *The Annual Review of Nutrition* chapters (if any have yet been occasioned, 1997 to the present) may be found at http://nutr.AnnualReviews.org/

# RELATED ARTICLES

From the *Annual Review of Biochemistry*, Volume 70 (2001)

*DNA Primases*, David N. Frick and Charles C. Richardson

*Channeling of Substrates and Intermediates in Enzyme-Catalyzed Reactions*, Xinyi Huang, Hazel M. Holden, and Frank M. Raushel

*Replisome-Mediated DNA Replication*, Stephen J. Benkovic, Ann M. Valentine, and Frank Salinas

*Synthesis and Function of 3-Phosphorylated Inositol Lipids*, Bart Vanhaesebroeck, Sally J. Leevers, Khatereh Ahmadi, John Timms, Roy Katso, Paul C. Driscoll, Rudiger Woscholski, Peter J. Parker, and Michael D. Waterfield

*Mechanisms Underlying Ubiquitination*, Cecile M. Pickart

*Transcriptional Coactivator Complexes*, Anders M. Näär, Bryan D. Lemon, and Robert Tjian

*DNA Topoisomerases: Structure, Function, and Mechanism*, James J. Champoux

*Function, Structure, and Mechanism of Intracellular Copper Trafficking Proteins*, David L. Huffman and Thomas V. O'Halloran

*Fidelity of Aminoacyl-tRNA Selection on the Ribosome: Kinetic and Structural Mechanisms*, Marina V. Rodnina and Wolfgang Wintermeyer

*Analysis of Proteins and Proteomes by Mass Spectrometry*, Matthias Mann, Ronald C. Hendrickson, and Akhilesh Pandey

*Folding of Newly Translated Proteins in Vivo: the Role of Molecular Chaperones*, Judith Frydman

From the *Annual Review of Cell and Developmental Biology*, Volume 17 (2001)

*Boundaries in Development: Formation and Function*, Kenneth D. Irvine and Cordelia Rauskolb

*Molecular Bases of Circadian Rhythms*, Stacey L. Harmer, Satchidananda Panda, and Steve A. Kay

From the *Annual Review of Genomics and Human Genetics*, Volume 2 (2001)

*Odorant Receptors and Other Chemosensory Receptors*, Peter Mombaerts

From the *Annual Review of Medicine*, Volume 52 (2001)

*New Oral Therapies for Type 2 Diabetes Mellitus: The Glitazones or Insulin Sensitizers*, Sunder Mudaliar and Robert R. Henry

*Evolving Treatment Strategies for Inflammatory Bowel Disease*, Stephen B. Hanauer and Themistocles Dassopoulos

*Effects of Neuropeptides and Leptin on Nutrient Partitioning: Dysregulations in Obesity*, Bernard Jeanrenaud and Francoise Rohner-Jeanrenaud

From the ***Annual Review of Physiology***, Volume 63 (2001)

$^{13}C$ *NMR of Intermediary Metabolism: Implications for Systemic Physiology,* Robert G. Shulman and Douglas L. Rothman

*The Gastrins: Their Production and Biological Activities*, G. J. Dockray, A. Varro, R. Dimaline, and T. Wang

*Cellular Mechanisms of Oxygen Sensing*, Jose Lopez-Barneo, Ricardo Pardal, and Patricia Ortega-Saenz

*Resurgence of Sodium Channel Research*, Alan L. Goldin

From the ***Annual Review of Public Health***, Volume 22 (2001)

*Selected Statistical Issues in Group Randomized Trials*, Ziding Feng, Paula Diehr, Arthur Peterson, and Dale McLerran

*Preventing Obesity in Children and Adolescents*, William H. Dietz and Steven L. Gortmaker

*Environmental Influences on Eating and Physical Activity*, Simone A. French, Mary Story, and Robert W. Jeffery

*Minisymposium on Obesity: Overview and Some Strategic Considerations*, Shiriki K. Kumanyika

*The Public Health Impact of Obesity*, Tommy L. S. Visscher and Jacob C. Seidell

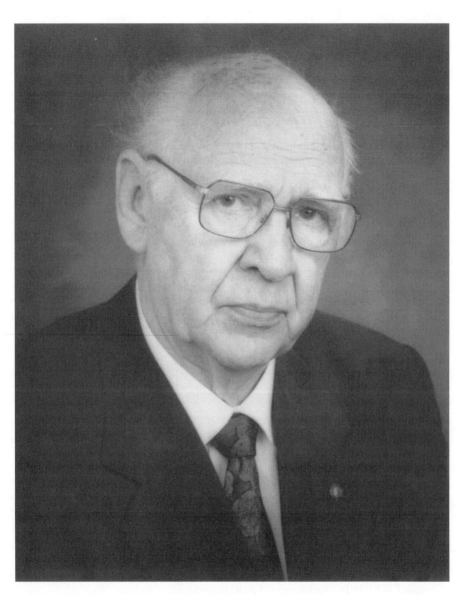

Annu. Rev. Nutr. 2001. 21:1–21

# PERSPECTIVES ON NUTRITIONAL IRON DEFICIENCY

## Leif Hallberg

*Department of Clinical Nutrition, Göteborg University, Sahlgrenska, University Hospital, Annedalsklinikerna, SE-413 45 Göteborg, Sweden; e-mail: hallberg@medtak.qu.se*

**Key Words** iron absorption, iron requirements, bioavailability, iron absorption regulation, liabilities of iron deficiency

■ **Abstract** Nutritional iron deficiency (ID) is caused by an intake of dietary iron insufficient to cover physiological iron requirements. Studies on iron absorption from whole diets have examined relationships between dietary iron bioavailability/absorption, iron losses, and amounts of stored iron. New insights have been obtained into regulation of iron absorption and expected rates of changes of iron stores or hemoglobin iron deficits when bioavailability or iron content of the diet has been modified and when losses of iron occur. Negative effects of ID are probably related to age, up to about 20 years, explaining some of earlier controversies. Difficulties in establishing the prevalence of mild ID are outlined. The degree of underestimation of the prevalence of mild ID when using multiple diagnostic criteria is discussed. It is suggested that current low-energy lifestyles are a common denominator for the current high prevalence not only of ID but also of obesity, diabetes, and osteoporosis.

## CONTENTS

0199-9885/01/0715-0001$14.00

**1**

## INTRODUCTION

Iron deficiency (ID), the most common deficiency disorder in the world, affects millions of people (26). ID develops when absorption of dietary iron cannot cover the physiological losses and requirements of iron. This review deals with nutritional ID and focuses on new information, new approaches, and new interpretations of available information.

## PATHOGENESIS OF NUTRITIONAL IRON DEFICIENCY

Iron metabolism is unique in several aspects. The body is economical in its handling of iron in the body. When a red cell dies, its iron is reutilized. Iron absorption is in some ways controlled by the requirements of the body. Extra iron can be stored by a specially designed protein (ferritin), which is utilized at times of increased iron requirements. The highly reactive properties of iron are balanced by unique control and transport systems. In spite of these ingenious mechanisms, ID is the most common deficiency disorder in the world and the main remaining deficiency in the industrialized, developed world. To understand this paradox, and to find effective ways to combat the deficiency, it is necessary to examine incomes (absorption) and expenditures (requirements) of iron, as well as current knowledge of the various control systems in the body responsible for maintenance of iron balance. An important observation was made by McCance & Widdowson in 1937 (70). In their studies, they found that iron was not excreted from the body, which implies that iron balance was maintained by a regulation of iron absorption.

## PHYSIOLOGICAL IRON REQUIREMENTS

Basal iron losses from the exterior and internal surfaces of the body, menstrual iron losses, and iron needed for growth, including pregnancy, determine physiological iron requirements.

### Basal Iron Losses

Iron lost from exterior and interior surfaces of the body constitute basal iron losses. A collaborative study showed that basal iron losses in men were of a magnitude of 14 $\mu$g/kg of body weight/day (38). The study was based on the rate of decrease of the specific activity of the long-lived radioisotope $^{55}$Fe administered intravenously. The dilution of the tracer by the absorption of iron to cover these losses was followed for several years. This ingenious principle was developed in 1959 by Finch (30). Further studies indicated that about half of these losses represented "physiological" blood losses (12).

Loss of iron from sweating was once considered marked, especially in the tropics (33). However, indirect studies comparing total iron losses in those living in hot and humid environments with those living in nontropical environments showed no differences (38). Direct studies of the iron content of sweat under controlled conditions showed that sweat iron losses are negligible (15).

## Menstrual Iron Losses

An early study showed that menstrual iron losses varied between 6 and 179 milliliters in 100 healthy women (8). The intraindividual variation was examined in 13 women and was considered marked. This finding was in contrast to later observations that for each individual, iron losses were almost constant (54). A probable reason for the different results was the great care taken in the latter studies to ensure a complete sampling of the menstrual blood. These unexpected observations had important consequences for understanding iron balance in menstruating women. By studying a random sample of women at a time before the introduction of contraceptive pills and intrauterine devices, the basal variation in iron requirements in women could be established (47). Later studies in a random sample of Swedish women confirmed the distribution of iron requirements, and the effect of contraceptive pills could be examined (55). Studies in nonidentical and identical twins (83) indicated that menstrual blood losses were genetically controlled and that this control was mediated by the contents of plasminogen activators in the uterine mucosa (82). Several studies in geographically widely separated countries strongly suggest that menstrual iron losses are the same worldwide and, thus, that iron requirements have been the same for very long time, probably many thousands of years. It could thus be concluded that differences in prevalence of ID is mainly related to differences in absorption of dietary iron, disregarding differences in iron losses related to parity and birth spacing and degree of infestation with, mainly, hookworm.

## Growth Requirements

***The Newborn, Full-Term Infant***     Iron requirements during the first 4–6 months of life are negligible, especially if late clamping of the umbilical cord has occurred. This unique situation for iron is explained by the excess of circulating hemoglobin (Hb) the infant is born with. This is due to the high affinity of fetal Hb for oxygen. The fetus thus "wins" over the mother in the struggle for oxygen at the placental interface. However, as a direct consequence, the delivery of oxygen from fetal Hb to tissues is lowered. The fetus thus needs more Hb to deliver a certain amount of oxygen to its tissues (regulated by erythropoietin). At delivery, the production of fetal Hb is exchanged for the production of normal Hb A, and oxygen is more readily available from the lungs. Successively, much iron is thus released to build up iron stores of the infant. This extra iron covers iron needs for the infant during the first 4–6 months of life. After about 6 months, when iron stores are exhausted, the iron requirements are very high, especially during the following 18 months, the weaning period. Iron requirements may amount to about 100 $\mu$g/kg/day, which is about four times more than for an average adult menstruating woman. After about the age of 2 years, iron requirements per unit of body weight are reduced.

*Adolescence*    The growth spurt during adolescence is another period of high iron requirements. For boys, puberty is associated with both considerable growth and a marked increase in Hb concentration and mass. Iron requirements for boys are about 20% higher than average iron requirements for menstruating women. For girls, growth is not completed at menarche and thus total iron requirements are high. For 14-year-old girls, for example, median iron requirements can be about 30% higher than for their mothers (79).

## Pregnancy

Iron requirements in pregnancy are very high, as discussed in previous reviews (41, 42). A main problem is the uneven distribution of the requirements over the duration of pregnancy. Because of the absence of menstrual iron losses and the negligible needs of the fetus, iron requirements in the first trimester are very low. They get successively higher as the pregnancy continues, reaching a maximum in the third trimester. The ability to absorb dietary iron increases as the iron requirement increases. Despite the increased propensity to absorb iron, however, even with a highly bioavailable diet, iron needs during pregnancy cannot be met by diet alone, especially during the second half of pregnancy. In addition, during the second half of pregnancy, when requirements are high, the actual absorption of iron from the diet is far below the need. This is true also for a highly bioavailable Western-type diet. Thus, to a great extent, iron balance during pregnancy is dependent on the amount of stored iron. It may be the main physiological role of iron stores. The problem is the low iron stores in present-day women in both developed and developing countries. It can be estimated that in our early ancestors, who consumed high-meat diets, iron stores may have amounted to about 500 mg, which is approximately the amount of stored iron needed to cover iron requirements during pregnancy. This is the reason for the paradoxical, unphysiological necessity of supplying pregnant women with iron supplements during the later half of pregnancy. The very high iron requirement of pregnancy is a special problem in teenage pregnancies because girls in their teens may not have reached their full growth. The anemia that is seen in early pregnancy (the physiological anemia of pregnancy) (41) is due primarily not to ID but to an increased plasma volume combined with the increased capacity of red blood cells to deliver oxygen to the placenta, which is probably mainly due to an increased concentration in red blood cells of 2,3-diglycerophosphate (41). This is a mechanism similar to that seen in "sports anemia," where the change is less well adapted to its purpose. (53).

## DIETARY IRON ABSORPTION

The first studies to estimate the absorption of dietary iron were chemical balance studies. Some of these early, meticulous studies gave good information about the magnitude of iron absorption from the diet. No information was obtained, however, about the variation in iron absorption related to different meal compositions or about the variation between subjects.

When radioiron isotopes became available, they were added to several "standard meals" of different composition to assess the variation in iron absorption between iron-deficient and iron-replete subjects. A detailed review of this early phase of iron absorption studies was published by Moore (74). It was known early on (45, 57, 58, 96) that heme and nonheme iron were absorbed differently. The iron porphyrin ring of heme iron is absorbed by utilization of a special receptor on the mucosal cell surface (37, 94). Heme iron is then degraded within the mucosal cell by heme oxygenase (77) and then enters the same iron pool in the intestinal mucosal cells as the absorbed nonheme iron.

In 1951, the technique of using biosynthetically radioiron-labeled foods to study nonheme iron absorption was introduced by Moore & Dubach (75). Several studies of labeled single-food items were made by several investigators and summarized by Moore in 1968 (74) and later by Martinez-Torres & Layrisse (69). There was a marked variation in nonheme iron absorption from different foods and more iron was absorbed by iron-deficient subjects. Another important observation was that there was an interaction between foods in the absorption of iron, e.g. meat enhanced the absorption of nonheme iron (66). The results of these new studies on iron absorption from single, biosynthetically labeled foods did not, however, allow estimations of iron absorption from the total diet. To be able to understand the paradoxical relationship between dietary iron intakes, which were often quite high, and iron status in different populations, which was often low, there was an obvious need for this knowledge.

At this time it was known that there were two kinds of dietary iron—heme iron, found mainly in meat and constituting up to 15% of the dietary iron, and nonheme iron, found in cereals fruits, roots, vegetables, etc, and constituting the remaining part and sometimes all of the dietary iron. At a 1969 joint meeting of the International Atomic Energy Agency and the World Health Organization, four participating groups agreed to examine the validity of measuring iron absorption from an inorganic iron salt with radiolabeled iron and taken as a drink with a specific food radiolabeled with another iron tracer. This became the starting point for the development of the extrinsic tag method, which made it possible to measure iron absorption not only from single foods but from different meals simply by adding a radio-labeled iron tracer to a food or a meal. This methodological development then suddenly made it possible to identify various dietary factors that enhanced or inhibited iron absorption. It also allowed quantitative studies on interactions between different foods. The currently recognized factors are outlined in Table 1.

The information about these factors was reviewed in the first volume of this series 20 years ago (40). The main new factors that have been identified since then deal with the strongly inhibiting iron-binding polyphenols and their widespread occurrence in nature (14, 16), and with the inhibition of both heme and nonheme iron by calcium, which probably acts within the mucosal cells (46, 56). Contradictory results about the effect of calcium on iron absorption have been obtained by different groups. The reasons for the discrepancies have been discussed (43).

**TABLE 1**  Factors influencing dietary iron absorption

| Determinant | Factors |
|---|---|
| Absorption | |
| Heme iron | Iron status of subject |
| | Amount of heme iron as meat |
| | Calcium content |
| | Food preparation (time, temperature) |
| Nonheme iron | Iron status of subject |
| | Amount of potentially available nonheme iron (adjustment for fortification and contamination iron, which may be only partially available) |
| Dietary factors | |
| Enhancing | Ascorbic acid |
| | Meat, chicken, fish and other seafood |
| | Fermented vegetables and soy sauces (not all items) |
| Inhibiting | Phytate and other inositol phosphates |
| | Iron-binding phenolic compounds |
| | Calcium |
| | Soy proteins |

Several attempts have been made to develop an algorithm to predict the absorption of dietary iron (21, 72, 73, 95). One algorithm was recently published based on only three dietary factors: meat, ascorbic acid, and phytate (78). Recently, a more comprehensive algorithm was developed to predict the absorption of iron from composite meals based on the content of eight dietary factors known to influence iron absorption (48). The algorithm is based on analyses of "dose-response" relationships between these factors influencing iron absorption and the interaction between the factors. The validity of the algorithm to predict iron absorption from single meals was examined by direct comparisons of observed and predicted absorption of iron from several meals. It was also shown that the algorithm could also be used to predict iron absorption from a whole varied diet over several days.[1]

It has been suggested that the iron absorption from a single meal given in a fasting state does not correctly describe the effect of various factors in a meal when given as part of the whole diet (21). The variation in iron absorption between different single meals is more marked than the variation between diets composed of

[1]In Equation 2 in the published algorithm (78), two parentheses were incorrectly inserted. The correct Equation 2 should be as follows: absorption ratio $= 1 + 0.01\,AA + \log(P+1)^* 0.01^*10^{0.8875^*\log(AA + 1)}$, where AA is ascorbic acid (in milligrams) and P is phytate phosphorus (in milligrams).

many different meals. It might be possible, for example, that the absorption from one single meal is influenced by the absorption of iron from preceding meals. However, in direct studies, this was not observed (36, 93). Moreover, the fact that the sum of the absorption of iron from many single meals (48) was the same as the total absorption from the diet over several days strongly contradicts such a supposition.

## CONTROL OF DIETARY IRON ABSORPTION

Iron status is determined by the balance between iron requirements and iron absorption. The total amounts of iron in the body cannot be controlled by excretion of iron but only by a regulation of the absorption, as mentioned in the introduction. Two factors have been considered to control the absorption of dietary iron: the amount of iron in stores, and the erythropoietic activity (13, 29). The erythroid regulator mainly responds to acute marrow iron needs whereas, by influencing the absorption of dietary iron, the store regulator would be mainly responsible for the maintenance of iron balance. Nothing is known, however, about the nature of these regulators, as outlined in a critical review by Finch (29).

Recently, interest has been focused on molecular biological structures and components in the intestinal mucosal cells that seem to control the absorption of iron to meet bodily needs at the mucosal level. What is not known, however, is how and where actual information about iron status and iron requirements of the body are evaluated and mediated to the intestinal mucosal cells, wherein reside the physiological mechanisms involved in preventing ID and iron overload. In other words, how is the absorption of iron controlled? Recently, new observations about the relationships between iron absorption, iron requirements, and iron stores have thrown new light on the capacity and ability of this control (50, 51).

Several studies in humans have shown a straight-line relationship between log iron absorption from reference doses of inorganic iron (3 mg of $Fe^{2+}$) and log serum ferritin (SF) (11, 22, 88, 92). Similar relationships between log iron absorption from whole diets and log SF (35, 52, 60) have been shown and have provided a possible new interpretation of the relationship between log total daily dietary iron absorption and log SF. Furthermore, a reevaluation and recalculation of the relationship between log SF and iron stores (50) has made it possible to validly estimate iron stores from log SF.

We found straight-line relationships between log daily iron absorption per unit of body weight (micrograms of Fe per kilogram of body weight per day) and iron stores (micrograms of Fe per kilogram of body weight) for different diets. Moreover, diets with different iron bioavailability formed parallel regression lines (50). Corresponding parallel regression lines were actually observed previously between log SF and log iron absorption from single meals with different bioavailability, including the reference dose (92).

A diagram showing the linear relationship between log dietary iron absorption and iron stores is shown in Figure 1 to illustrate the new principle for analyzing the

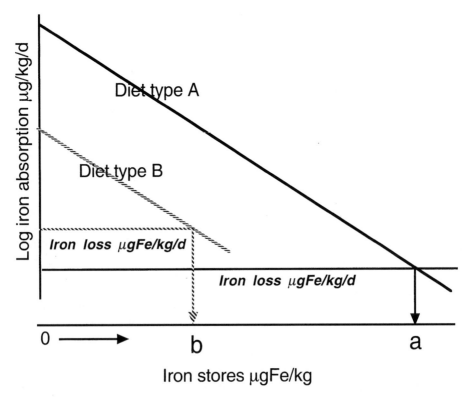

**Figure 1**    The relationship between iron absorption, iron stores, and iron losses—two examples with two diets (*A* and *B*) with different bioavailabilities and with two different iron losses. For a subject consuming a diet of type *A* and having the low daily iron loss (the lowest horizontal line), the balance point where absorption equals losses is projected to point *a* on the iron store scale. A subject consuming a diet of type *B* with a lower bioavailability shows a lower, parallel regression line (log iron absorption vs iron stores). The balance point, point of intersection between absorption, and loss lines corresponds to an iron store of point *b*.

relationship between total daily iron absorption, iron stores, and total daily iron requirements (50). A horizontal line, corresponding to the actual iron losses (iron requirements—micrograms of Fe per kilogram of body weight per day), is inserted. At the point of intersection between these two lines, absorption equals losses and corresponds to the maximal amount of stored iron that can be present under the conditions prevailing. Figure 1 shows two examples with different bioavailability, different iron losses, and different resulting iron stores.

These relationships can be described mathematically with no model assumptions in an exponential equation.

$$dM/dt = k_1 e^{Mk_2} - L,  \hspace{2cm} 1.$$

where $k_1$ is absorption at zero iron stores (micrograms of Fe per kilogram of body weight per day), $M$ is the amount of stored iron (micrograms of Fe per kilogram of body weight), and $k_2$ a constant (see below). Steady states for iron stores can be calculated for different amounts of absorbed and lost iron by setting $dM/dt = 0$. The constant $k_2$ describing the slope of the relationship between absorption and iron stores is calculated from actual absorption studies (35, 52, 60). The constant $k_2$ was found to be 0.00024 in three separate studies. The absolute value of the constant $k_2$ depends on the units used. It is probable that the constant is an expression for a biological, fundamental property describing the control of iron absorption in relation to iron stores that may also be found in other animals besides humans.

By integrating the exponential equation, describing the relationship between absorption, losses, and iron stores, the rates of change in iron stores over time can also be calculated, e.g. the time needed to reach a certain iron store when changing iron losses or changing the bioavailability of the dietary iron.

Unexpectedly, it was observed that when modifying losses or absorption of iron, a main part (about 90%) of the changes in iron stores occurred within 1 year, approaching asymptotically a new steady state after about 2–3 years. In practice, this means that the main effects on iron status by iron fortification or by improvements in dietary bioavailability are expected to be observed after about 1 year. Inversely, it can be concluded that the main changes in iron status (e.g. in SF) observed in a population sample at a later date can not be ascribed to dietary modifications made. A later increase in SF may, for example, be due to a higher prevalence of infections. The strict control of iron absorption is only valid for dietary iron and is not valid for iron taken as supplements.

The basis for the calculations is that at any steady-state absorption equals losses. The recently described inertia or adaptation in absorption (62) when changing the diet to a lower or higher bioavailability does not contradict this fact. The current observations and calculations have other important implications. With increasing iron stores, the absorption of iron is reduced to the level needed to cover the daily iron requirements. This explains the observations that SF remained unchanged in men after 2 years of iron fortification with 7.5 mg of highly available iron given daily (7), and that the same was seen when 10 mg of iron as ferrous sulphate was given to an iron-replete man for 500 days (85). Another example of the effective control of iron stores is the observation in iron-replete men that 2 g of ascorbic acid given with meals for 2 years had no effect on SF. It may seem paradoxical that in that study, ascorbic acid given with meals still had an effect on the absorption of small iron doses. The amounts of iron absorbed, however, were well within the range of iron absorption required to cover the basal iron losses (20). All these observations are consistent with the observations that iron stores remain constant in men after about the age of 20–25 years, as illustrated by rather constant median SF values in the N-HANES II studies (76). The unchanged iron content in iron stores with age was also observed in US autopsy studies of liver iron content in subjects who suffered traumatic deaths (91). An important implication of the effective control of iron absorption is that it would be impossible to induce iron overload by consuming diets with even very high iron contents due to, for example, high intake of red meat, or excessive iron fortification in iron-replete men. Exceptions would be the few subjects who are homozygotes for hereditary hemochromatosis and those who have thalassemia major.

In the N-HANES II studies in the United States (76), higher SF values were observed with increasing age, especially at ages above 45 years, not only in post-menopausal women but also in men. The autopsy studies mentioned above (91) directly measuring iron stores showed no corresponding increase in iron stores with age. Observations of a very effective control of iron absorption preventing iron overload are also inconsistent with any "physiological growth" of iron stores with age (50). Because SF is a sensitive, acute-phase reactant increasing, for example, after simple infections (61) or with regular use of alcohol (67, 71, 90), it is possible that some unknown external factor may increase with age—a kind of an unknown aging factor? No sufficiently valid explanation has been found. One implication of these observations is that great care must be taken in simple translations of SF into iron stores, especially in middle-aged or older people. It has been suggested that high iron stores (SF > 200 $\mu$g/liter) are associated with coronary artery disease (84) and cancer (89). A more obvious explanation, that a high SF may be the effect of different pathological conditions related to the development of coronary heart disease and not a cause of it, seems not to have been carefully considered, especially because other studies have not confirmed such a hypothesis (2–4, 87).

In an extensive study of 203 women, all aged 38 years, the relationships between iron absorption, iron requirements, and various parameters of iron status, including examination of bone marrow smears, were studied (49). It was evident that SF and transferrin saturation showed a continuous decrease with increasing iron requirements, based on measurements of menstrual iron losses and body weight, indicating successively lower iron stores. Iron absorption increased with increasing iron requirements, but it could only balance the increasing iron losses up to a certain point when the stainable iron in the bone marrow suddenly disappeared at the same time as Hb dropped and transferrin concentration in plasma increased. These comprehensive observations fit well with the predicted changes using the new equations (50). It is thus evident that menstruating women with high iron requirements, and/or consuming diets with low iron bioavailability, will be iron deficient (have no iron stores) and may even develop an ID anemia (IDA). It is also evident that the average woman with average menstrual iron losses and consuming a "typical" Western diet with low-to-moderate meat intake will have iron stores rather below than above 100 mg. This implies that it is impossible for the present-day Western woman, even those consuming a good diet, to build up iron stores of the magnitude needed (about 500 mg) to fully cover the extra iron requirements for pregnancy. It is interesting, however, that according to the new algorithm presented above (48), and information about a probable composition of the diet in early women (27), iron stores of such a magnitude (about 500 mg) were probably present in early women, who had a very high intake of meat and ascorbic acid. This fact probably also balanced the estimated high intakes of phytate and calcium in the diets of early man (50).

## HOW IS THE IRON BALANCE COMMUNICATED TO THE INTESTINAL MUCOSA?

When iron requirements increase and iron balance becomes negative, for example due to hookworm infestation, the body tries to prevent the development of ID by increasing the absorption of iron. Studies with both humans and animals indicate that the up-regulation of iron absorption in some way, as mentioned above, is related to the amount of iron present in iron stores (13, 29, 51). When studying the relationship between iron absorption and SF as a measure of iron stores, Hallberg et al (51) unexpectedly observed that the relationship between iron absorption and iron stores (SF), noted in iron-replete subjects, was also valid in subjects with ID—with "negative iron stores," suggested by SF < 15 $\mu$g/liter, and with subnormal Hb (51). This implied that it is not only the empty iron stores per se but also a Hb iron deficit that in some way controls the absorption of dietary iron. Analyzing more closely the relationships between iron absorption on the one hand and the iron stores on the other, and the relationship between iron absorption and Hb deficit, it was evident that the two relationships formed a continuum. As discussed in a recent paper (51) on the physiological control of iron absorption, including the effect of various hematological disorders, the balance of evidence including the observed continuum suggest that the hepatocyte may be a probable cell that registers both the amounts of stored iron and a deficit of Hb iron. This interpretation is also supported by observations from rat liver transplantation studies, which suggest that the hepatocyte iron stores are a major determining factor controlling iron absorption (1). How the hepatocyte mediates the iron status to the intestinal mucosa is still, however, unknown.

## WHAT IS IRON DEFICIENCY AND WHAT IS IRON DEFICIENCY ANEMIA?

How is the internal transport of iron to tissues controlled? The observation that transferrin was a specific transport protein for iron in the body was an important discovery (65). The extremely strong binding of iron to transferrin at physiological pH was required to prevent the toxic effect of iron ions. It remained a mystery, however, how iron could be released and delivered from transferrin to tissues. The existence of specific cell membrane receptors for transferrin was suggested about 40 years ago by Jandl & Katz (63). Intense research resulted in the isolation and characterization of the receptor [for a review, see Baker & Morgan (5)]. The important discovery that all cells had specific receptors on their surface, to bind the transferrin-iron, explained the mystery. The entire complex of transferrin-iron and transferrin receptor was shown to be taken up by the cells by invagination of a part of the cell wall to form a vacuole, thus transferring the entire complex from the exterior to the interior of the cell. Iron is then released in the vacuole by lowering the pH within the vacuole. Each cell expresses its actual need for iron by the number of receptors on the cell surface. This ingenious system controls the transport of iron within the body from plasma to the cells in different tissues requiring iron, thus also preventing the presence of free iron extracellularly. Within the cells, other mechanisms prevent the formation of free iron radicals. The chemical structure of the transferrin receptor is well known and is the same for cells in different tissues. This implies that if the transfer of iron to one kind of cell needing iron is shown to be insufficient, for example, to produce Hb in red blood cells in the erythron, then it can be predicted that the transfer of iron to all cells in other tissues needing iron at the same time would also be insufficient. In practice, it means that if erythropoiesis is observed to be limited because of a lack of iron, then it can be deduced that the transfer of iron to such tissues as brain and muscle is also insufficient. A demonstration of an iron-deficient erythropoiesis thus implies that a true, functionally important ID is present even if it may be technically difficult to demonstrate symptoms from various organs.

## LIABILITIES OF IRON DEFICIENCY

Negative effects of ID are not directly related to a reduction in Hb because the body has several effective mechanisms to compensate for an insufficient supply of oxygen to tissues caused by a lowered Hb. The most immediate compensatory step is an increased cardiac output delivering more oxygen per unit of time to tissues. The next step is an increase in the concentration of 2,3-diglycerophosphate in red blood cells causing a shift in the form of the Hb-oxygen dissociation curve, thus facilitating oxygen delivery to tissues. This latter change needs about 2–3 days to be fully effective. With more longstanding problems in oxygen delivery, there will be an increased production of erythropoietin to increase the concentration of Hb if possible. There are thus a series of consecutive mechanisms to ensure an adequate supply of oxygen to tissues. It follows that symptoms of ID are probably directly caused not by a lowered Hb level but by an insufficient supply of iron to the tissues. During the development of a negative iron balance and when iron stores are exhausted, the supply of iron to all tissues, including the erythron in the bone marrow, will be compromised. The concentration of Hb will then start to decrease. This stage is the beginning of an iron deficient erythropoiesis. Theoretically, there is no intermediate stage between normality and ID. Sometimes the term iron depletion has been used with other laboratory criteria of ID. This concept might be a paraphrase of ID that is still not detectable with current laboratory methods. The distribution of the Hb in healthy, iron-replete subjects is very wide, e.g. in adult women, roughly between 120 and 160 g/liter. This variation is due mainly to a variation in Hb between subjects and only to a small extent to the day-to-day variation within each individual because each subject has a markedly constant Hb. This means that a woman with no iron stores, who normally has her homeostatic Hb level set at 160 g/liter, can lose about 25% of her Hb mass and still have a Hb remaining within the normal range of a population of healthy women. ID anemia (IDA), usually defined as an ID combined with a Hb < 120 g/liter (a Hb value below the mean minus two standard deviations of the population), is thus a statistical cutoff value in a population with no specific biological meaning. The main use of IDA is to compare iron status in different populations and not in different subjects, not even in clinical practice except when Hb < 120 g/liter.

During a negative iron balance in an iron-replete subject, iron stores will at first be successively depleted. At a certain point, when the rate of release of iron from stores is lower than the amount of iron needed for all tissues, including the erythron, a functional ID is reached—the delivery of iron to all tissues is then compromised (is insufficient). The first thing easily noted is a successive decrease in Hb concentration. With a continued negative iron balance, the decrease in Hb will continue and may pass below the mean Hb minus two standard deviations of the distribution of Hb of the population. This is the established statistical concept of IDA in a population. Negative effects of ID in different tissues may be expected to occur before the Hb in an individual has passed below the lowest normal level of the population. The severity of symptoms related to ID may of course be expected to be more pronounced the more severe the deficiency and the longer the time the deficiency has existed. Symptoms of ID from various tissues may thus be expected to be more severe if the deficiency has led to a reduction in Hb below the subnormal level of the population. IDA is sometimes a practical level in both clinical and epidemiological work.

Including the presence of anemia in the definition of ID, however, will underestimate the true prevalence of ID. In clinical practice, knowledge of previous Hb levels of a patient is extremely valuable in the diagnosis of ID, for example, in patients with pathological gastrointestinal bleedings due to cancer in the gastrointestinal tract and may lead to early detection of a bleeding cancer.

The nestor in hematology, Maxwell M. Wintrobe, once chairing an expert WHO meeting on nutritional anemias, defined ID, didactically, as a state (a) when an otherwise healthy individual has a Hb below the optimal value for that specific individual, (b) when there is no infection or other disorder present, (c) when there is no lack of other nutrients required for an optimal hematopoiesis, and (d) when laboratory signs are compatible with ID. These considerations are important for understanding that ID without anemia, in its classical definition, has been shown to have various negative effects (see below). Another factor to consider when evaluating negative effects of ID is related to the fact that symptoms of nutritional ID probably have developed over a long period of time and therefore might be considered as a normal state in most subjects. This is a well-established clinical fact in many patients with various disorders having symptoms that have developed over a long period of time. General symptoms that may be related to ID, such as lowered physical work capacity or mental changes, must therefore be analyzed according to changes in symptoms after double-blind treatments with iron and placebo over a sufficiently long time period.

There are many conflicting reports about symptoms of ID without anemia [for a review, see Beutler et al (10)]. Other important reviews about negative effects of ID can be found elsewhere (9, 24, 86).

Studies on negative effects of ID are often more easily studied in animals. A real breakthrough in the understanding of effects of ID on rats on work performance was made by Edgerton et al in 1972 (28) and Finch et al in 1976 (31). In the latter study, for example, it was shown that the reduced working performance in iron-deficient rats was due not to the induced anemia but to tissue ID and probably to lack in the muscles of certain enzymes related to phosphorylation. Several studies were made confirming these results. The studies were all made using growing, iron-deficient rats. One study, however, was made using adult rats where, contrary to previous findings in weanling rats, there was no decrease in muscle enzymes in spite of a moderate anemia (64). These data strongly suggest that the age when ID is induced is important for its effect on muscle enzymes. In a detailed study of nine healthy adult men with a mean age of 29 years, an IDA induced by repeated venesections and maintained for 9 weeks was not associated with a reduction in maximal muscle enzyme activities. After retransfusion, normal endurance was reestablished (18). In contrast, maximal muscle enzyme activities in 17 Indonesian subjects, both normal and iron deficient, and studied by the same group, showed significantly lower maximal muscle enzyme activities unrelated to their present iron status (19). These observations might suggest that the significantly reduced maximal muscle enzyme activities in this sample were an effect of ID earlier in life, as a parallel to the different findings in weanling and adult rats. These results suggest that it may be difficult to induce negative effects of ID in adult subjects and possibly that it may be impossible to treat potential symptoms of ID induced when young.

Most negative effects of ID are thus expected in growing individuals from infancy and childhood up through adolescence. The three tissues that are early on finally differentiated and developed in the body are brain, muscle, and the eye lens. The brain develops up to the age of about 20 years and the brain iron content also increases up to this age (59). Animal experiments indicate that to ensure an adequate supply when different structures are being formed, it is important that the iron be delivered to the brain in sufficient amounts and at the correct time (25). The huge number of studies made on effects of ID on mental performance was extensively reviewed by the British Nutrition Foundation (13a). Studies of infants and animals suggest that it may be difficult to repair negative effects of ID that had developed earlier. Therefore, it may be assumed that iron adequacy should be optimal at least during the first 20 years of life. It should be remembered that there are several well-designed studies, all of adolescent girls, showing that there are negative effects of ID related to both mental symptoms and physical activity that are unrelated to anemia (6, 17, 80, 98).

# HOW TO ESTABLISH A DIAGNOSIS OF IRON DEFICIENCY?

The wide variation in the concentration of Hb in healthy, iron-replete subjects makes it difficult to establish whether a specific person has a normal or a subnormal level of Hb. The traditional indicators of iron status, e.g. mean cell Hb (MCH), mean cell volume (MCV), and transferrin saturation, have the same problem with wide interindividual variations in both iron-replete and iron-deficient subjects. Thus, very marked overlaps are observed in the distributions of all these parameters in normal and iron-deficient subjects. Thus, any cut-off value chosen will have either a low specificity or a low sensitivity. The use of technically perfect, stained bone marrow smears is still the gold standard to evaluate iron status and thus also to examine the validity of different laboratory methods. In this way, the sensitivity and specificity of different laboratory methods has been evaluated (44). So far, SF seems to best discriminate between iron-deficient and iron-replete subjects. A SF $\leq$ 15 $\mu$g/liter always means ID. Also, above this limit ID may be present, especially in subjects with even a simple, recent infection (61). In the actual study (44), however, this information was unfortunately not available. There are reasons to believe that even a regular moderate use of alcohol may induce an increase in SF (67, 71). Because SF seems to be a very sensitive acute-phase reactant, associations between high SF and other diseases must be interpreted with great caution, e.g. iron overload, coronary heart disease, and cancer. The concentration of transferrin receptors in serum has also been used to establish a diagnosis of ID (23, 88). The main advantages are that it allows separation between ID and chronic anemia and that it is not influenced by infections. Its disadvantages are the lower sensitivity to detect mild ID and the fact that there is still no material available to standardize the different methods used. All these facts imply that it is difficult to establish a diagnosis of mild ID, especially in epidemiological studies, where, for example, the interpretation of a therapeutic trial with iron supplements and placebo is impossible in mild ID due to the "regression toward the mean" using repeated Hb measurements.

In some studies, therefore, combined diagnostic criteria have been used, for example in the N-HANES II studies in the United States. In all kind of studies and for all diseases, use of combined criteria will improve the specificity but decrease the sensitivity. This will automatically lead to an underestimation of the true prevalence of ID. This was demonstrated in a study of 203 women, where iron-stained bone marrow smears were used as a gold standard (44) and different criteria could be validly tested. In the N-HANES II studies, performed between 1976 and 1980 and using the multiple criteria, the prevalence of ID in women aged 20–49 years, for example, was estimated at about 10% (39) (calculated 95% confidence limits were 8%–12%) and at 11% in the more recent N-HANES III studies (68). As stated elsewhere (39), these cut-off values were arbitrarily chosen. It is of great interest, however, that at about the same time as the N-HANES II studies were made, there was a more direct, but much smaller, study on iron status in the United States based on measurements of the content of iron in liver samples in 259 subjects who died traumatic deaths (91). Very low iron contents in the liver was used as an indicator of ID and was found in 10 out of 28 women aged 20–50 years. The observed prevalence of ID in the autopsy material had a 95% confidence interval of 18%–56%.

In a random sample of 38-year-old women in Sweden studied at about the same time, the prevalence of ID, based on absence of stainable iron in bone marrow smears, was observed in 90 out of 286 women (32%) in the original sample (81). The 95% confidence range was 26%–37%. It should be mentioned that the distribution of SF in women at this age was almost identical in the N-HANES II 1976–1980 study in the United States (76), in the 1976 Nutrition Canada National Survey (97), and in the study in Sweden (44). When calculating the prevalence expected in this Swedish sample, using combined criteria similar to that used in the N-HANES II study, the prevalence was likewise reduced from about 32% to around 10% (44). This latter study was made in a subsample of 203 women out of the total 286, where all measurements needed were available.

Although the amount of autopsy material was small compared with the N-HANES II material, using Fisher's exact test, the difference for the two prevalences representing the United States was significant ($p < 0.001$). This important observation suggests that the use of multiple criteria in the N-HANES II study probably led to a considerable underestimation of the true prevalence of ID in the United States, and to the same extent as was noted in the Swedish studies using combined criteria. The balance of evidence would suggest that the 10% prevalence of ID in 20- to 44-year-old women reported in the United States is probably much too low and would be about two to three times higher had not the combined criteria been used.

## CONCLUDING COMMENTS

The balance of current evidence strongly indicates that to ensure optimal health and development, it is important to prevent and treat even mild ID in growing individuals, at least up to the age of around 20 years, and in pregnancy. Considering the ingenious systems available that control the absorption and metabolism of iron, it is paradoxical that ID is the most common deficiency disorder in the world and the main remaining deficiency in the developed world. A reasonable explanation may be the marked changes that have occurred in human nutrition. Before about 10,000 years ago, humans lived as nomads and a main part of the diet was obtained by hunting and fishing (27, 34). The introduction of cereals at about this time, first wheat and later on rice and maize, formed the basis for formation of societies, but it was also associated with a diminution in body size. The diet was thus radically changed. Another factor influencing human nutrition was the rapid growth of populations during the past millenium and especially during the past few centuries. Industrialization, automation, and other developments have successively reduced energy requirements and thus the need for food. The current low-energy lifestyle and the dramatic increase in the number of cars and in the number of hours spent watching television and using computers have further led to a situation where the risk of nutrient deficiencies, especially ID, has increased. At the same time, the risk of obesity, diabetes, coronary heart disease, and osteoporosis have also increased. It is important to prevent ID in infants, children, adolescents, and women of childbearing age, especially those who are pregnant, to ensure optimal development of muscles and brain. The weaning period in infants is especially critical because of the extremely high iron requirements and the importance of adequate iron nutrition during this crucial period of development.

## ACKNOWLEDGMENTS

These studies were supported in part by the Swedish Medical Research Council (project B96-19X-04721-21A), the Swedish Council for Forestry and Agriculture Research (50.0120/95 and 997/881, 113:3), the Swedish Dairy Association, and the Danone International Prize for Nutrition 1999.

**Visit the Annual Reviews home page at www.AnnualReviews.org**

## LITERATURE CITED

1. Adams PC, Reece AS, Powell LW, Halliday JW. 1989. Hepatic iron in the control of iron absorption in a rat liver transplantation model. *Transplantation* 48:19–21

2. Ascherio A, Willett WC. 1996. Epidemiological studies relating iron status to coronary heart disease and cancer. See Ref. 43a, pp. 303–11

3. Ascherio A, Willett WC, Rimm EB, Giovanucci EL, Stampfer MJ. 1994. Dietary iron intake and risk of coronary heart disease among men. *Circulation* 89:969–74

4. Baer DM, Tekawa IS, Hurley LB. 1994. Iron stores are not associated with myocardial infarction. *Circulation* 89:2915–18

5. Baker E, Morgan EH. 1994. Iron transport. In *Iron Metabolism in Health and Disease*, ed. JH Brock, JW Halliday, MJ Pippard, LW Powell, pp. 63–95. London: Saunders

6. Ballin A, Berar M, Rubinstein U, Yeshyadu K, Herchkovitz A, Meytes D. 1992. Iron state in female adolescents. *Am. J. Dis. Child.* 146:803–5

7. Ballot DE, MacPhail AP, Bothwell TH, Gillooly M, Mayet F. 1989. Fortification of curry powder with NaFe(III)EDTA in an iron deficient population: report of a controlled iron-fortification trial. *Am. J. Clin. Nutr.* 49:162–69

8. Barer AP, Fowler WM. 1936. The blood loss during normal menstruation. *Am. J. Obstet. Gynecol.* 31:979–86

9. Baynes RD, Bothwell TH. 1990. Iron deficiency. *Annu. Rev. Nutr.* 10:133–48

10. Beutler E, Fairbanks VF, Fahey JL. 1963. *Clinical Disorders of Iron Metabolism.* New York: Grune & Statton

11. Bezwoda W, Bothwell TH, Torrance JD, MacPhail AP, Charlton RW, et al. 1979. The relationship between marrow iron stores, plasma ferritin concentrations and iron absorption. *Scand. J. Haematol.* 22:113–20

12. Bothwell TH. 1970. Total iron loss and relative importance of different sources. In *Iron Deficiency, Pathogenesis, Clinical*

*Aspects, Therapy*, ed. L Hallberg, H-G Harwerth, A Vanotti, pp. 151–61. London: Academic

13. Bothwell TH, Charlton RW, Cook JD, Finch CA. 1979. *Iron Metabolism in Man*. Oxford, UK: Blackwell Sci.

13a. Br. Nutr. Found. 1995. *Iron—Nutritional and Physiological Significance*. London: Chapman & Hall

14. Brune M, Hallberg L, Skånberg A-B. 1991. Determination of iron-binding phenolic groups in foods. *J. Food Sci.* 56:131–67

15. Brune M, Magnusson B, Persson H, Hallberg L. 1986. Iron losses in sweat. *Am. J. Clin. Nutr.* 43:438–43

16. Brune M, Rossander L, Hallberg L. 1989. Iron absorption and phenolic compounds: importance of different phenolic structures. *Eur. J. Clin. Nutr.* 43:547–58

17. Bruner AB, Joffe A, Duggan AK, Casella JF, Brandt J. 1996. Randomised study of cognitive effects of iron supplementation in nonanaemic iron-deficient adolescent girls. *Lancet* 348:992–96

18. Celsing F, Blomstrand E, Werner B, Pihlstedt P, Ekblom B. 1986. Effect of iron deficiency on endurance and muscle enzyme activity in man. *Med. Sci. Sports Exerc.* 18:156–61

19. Celsing F, Ekblom B, Sylvén C, Everett J, Åstrand P-O. 1988. Effect of chronic iron deficiency anaemia on myoglobin content, enzyme activity, and capillary density in the human skeletal muscle. *Acta Med. Scand.* 223:451–57

20. Cook J, Watsson SS, Simpson KM, Lipschitz DA, Skikne BS. 1984. The effect of high ascorbic acid supplementation on body iron stores. *Blood* 64:721–26

21. Cook JD, Dassenko SA, Lynch SR. 1991. Assessment of the role of non heme-iron availability in iron balance. *Am. J. Clin. Nutr.* 54:717–22

22. Cook JD, Lipschitz DA, Miles LEM, Finch CA. 1974. Serum ferritin as a mea-

sure of iron stores in normal subjects. *Am. J. Clin. Nutr.* 27:681–87

23. Cook JD, Skikne B, Baynes R. 1996. The use of transferrin receptor for the assessment of iron status. See Ref. 43a, pp. 49–58

24. Dallman PR. 1986. Biochemical basis for the manifestations of iron deficiency. *Annu. Rev. Nutr.* 6:13–40

25. Dallman PR, Siimes MA, Mauies EC. 1975. Brain iron: persistent deficiency following short-term iron deprivation in the young rat. *Br. J. Haematol.* 31:209–15

26. DeMaeyer E, Adiels-Tegman M, Raystone E. 1985. The prevalence of anemia in the world. *World Health Stat. Q.* 38:302–16

27. Eaton SB, Eaton SB III, Konner M. 1997. Paleolithic nutrition revisited: a twelve year retrospective on its nature and implications. *Eur. J. Clin. Nutr.* 51:207–16

28. Edgerton VR, Bryant SL, Gillespie CA, Gardner GW. 1972. Iron deficiency anemia and physical performance and activity of rats. *J. Nutr.* 102:381–400

29. Finch C. 1994. Regulators of iron balance in humans. *Blood* 84:1697–702

30. Finch CA. 1959. Body iron exchange in man. *J. Clin. Invest.* 38:392–96

31. Finch CA, Miller LR, Inamdar AR, Person R, Seiler K, Mackler B. 1976. Iron deficiency in the rat. Physiological and biochemical studies of muscle dysfunction. *J. Clin. Invest.* 58:447–53

32. Deleted in proof

33. Foy H, Kondi A. 1957. Anaemia of the tropics. Relation to iron intake, absorption and losses during growth, pregnancy and lactation. *J. Trop. Med. Hyg.* 60:105–16

34. Garn SM, Leonard WR. 1989. What did our ancestors eat? *Nutr. Rev.* 47:337–45

35. Gleerup A, Rossander-Hultén L, Gramatkowski E, Hallberg L. 1995. Iron absorption from the whole diet: comparison of the effect of two different distributions of daily calcium intake. *Am. J. Clin. Nutr.* 61:97–104

36. Gleerup A, Rossander-Hultén L, Hallberg L. 1993. Duration of the inhibitory effect of calcium on nonhaem iron absorption in man. *Eur. J. Clin. Nutr.* 47:875–79

37. Grasbeck R, Kouvonen I, Lundberg M, Tenhunen R. 1979. An intestinal receptor for heme. *Scand. J. Haematol.* 23:5–9

38. Green R, Charlton RW, Seftel H, Bothwell TH, Mayet F, et al. 1968. Body iron excretion in man. A colloborative study. *Am. J. Med.* 45:336–53

39. Group ESW. 1985. Summary of a report on assessment of the iron nutritional status of the United States population. *Am. J. Clin. Nutr.* 42:1318–30

40. Hallberg L. 1981. Bioavailability of dietary iron in man. *Annu. Rev. Nutr.* 1:123–47

41. Hallberg L. 1988. Iron balance in pregnancy. In *Vitamins and Minerals in Pregnancy and Lactation, Nestlé Nutr. Workshop Ser.*, ed. H Berger, 16:115–27. New York: Raven

42. Hallberg L. 1992. Iron balance in pregnancy and lactation. In *Nutritional Anemias*, ed. SJ Fomon, S Zlotkin, pp. 13–25. New York: Raven

43. Hallberg L. 1998. Does calcium interfere with iron absorption? *Am. J. Clin. Nutr.* 68:3–4

43a. Hallberg L, Asp N-G, eds. 1996. *Iron Nutrition in Health and Disease.* London: Libbey

44. Hallberg L, Bengtsson C, Lapidus L, Lundberg P-A, Hulthén L. 1993. Screening for iron deficiency: an analysis based on bone-marrow examinations and serum ferritin determinations in a population sample of women. *Br. J. Haematol.* 85:787–98

45. Hallberg L, Björn-Rasmussen E, Howard L, Rossander L. 1979. Dietary haem iron absorption. A discussion of possible mechanisms for the absorption-promoting effect of meat and for the regulation of iron absorption. *Scand. J. Gastroenterol.* 14:769–79

46. Hallberg L, Brune M, Erlandsson M, Sandberg A-S, Rossander-Hulthén L. 1991. Calcium: effect of different amounts on nonheme- and heme-iron absorption in man. *Am. J. Clin. Nutr.* 53:112–19

47. Hallberg L, Högdahl A-M, Nilson L, Rybo G. 1966. Menstrual blood loss: a population study. Variation at different ages and attempts to define normality. *Acta Obstet. Gynaecol. Scand.* 45:320–51

48. Hallberg L, Hulthén L. 2000. Prediction of dietary iron absorption. An algorithm to calculate absorption and bioavailability of dietary iron. *Am. J. Clin. Nutr.* 71:1147–60

49. Hallberg L, Hulthén L, Bengtsson C, Lapidus L, Lindstedt G. 1995. Iron balance in menstruating women. *Eur. J. Clin. Nutr.* 49:200–7

50. Hallberg L, Hulthén L, Garby L. 1998. Iron stores in man in relation to diet and iron requirements. *Eur. J. Clin. Nutr.* 52:623–31

51. Hallberg L, Hulthén L, Garby L. 2000. Iron stores and haemoglobin iron deficits in menstruating women. Calculations based on variations in iron requirements and bioavailability of dietary iron. *Eur. J. Clin. Nutr.* 54:650–57

52. Hallberg L, Hulthén L, Gramatkovski E. 1997. Iron absorption from the whole diet in men: How effective is the regulation of iron absorption? *Am. J. Clin. Nutr.* 66:347–56

53. Hallberg L, Magnusson B. 1984. The etiology of "sports anemia." *Acta Med. Scand.* 216:145–48

54. Hallberg L, Nilsson L. 1964. Constancy of individual menstrual blood loss. *Acta Obstet. Gynaecol. Scand.* 43:352–59

55. Hallberg L, Rossander-Hulthén L. 1991. Iron requirements in menstruating women. *Am. J. Clin. Nutr.* 54:1047–58

56. Hallberg L, Rossander-Hulthén L, Brune M, Gleerup A. 1992. Calcium and iron absorption: mechanism of action and nutritional importance. *Eur. J. Clin. Nutr.* 46:317–27

57. Hallberg L, Sölvell L. 1964. Absorption of

hemoglobin iron in man. *Am. J. Digest. Dis.* 9:787–88

58. Hallberg L, Sölvell L. 1967. Absorption of hemoglobin iron in man. *Acta Med. Scand.* 181:335–54

59. Hallgren B, Sourander P. 1958. The effect of age on the nonhaemin iron in the human brain. *J. Neurochem.* 34:41–51

60. Hulthén L, Gramatkovski E, Gleerup A, Hallberg L. 1995. Iron absorption from the whole diet. Relation to meal composition, iron requirements and iron stores. *Eur. J. Clin. Nutr.* 49:794–808

61. Hulthén L, Lindstedt G, Lundberg P-A, Hallberg L. 1998. Effect of a mild infection on serum ferritin concentration— clinical and epidemiological implications. *Eur. J. Clin. Nutr.* 52:376–79

62. Hunt JR, Roughhead ZK. 2000. Adaptation of iron absorption in men consuming diets with high or low bioavailability. *Am. J. Clin. Nutr.* 71:94–102

63. Jandl JH, Katz JH. 1963. The plasma-to-cell cycle of transferrin. *J. Clin. Invest.* 42:314–26

64. Koziol BJ, Ohira Y, Simpson DR, Edgerton VR. 1978. Biochemical skeletal muscle and hematological profiles of moderate and severely iron deficient and anemic adult rats. *J. Nutr.* 108:1306–14

65. Laurell CB. 1947. Studies on the transportation and metabolism of iron in the body. *Acta Physiol. Scand.* 14(Suppl. 46):1–129

66. Layrisse M, Martinez-Torres C, Roche M. 1968. The effect of interaction of various foods on iron absorption. *Am. J. Clin. Nutr.* 21:1175–83

67. Leggett BA, Brown NN, Bryant SJ, Duplock L, Powell LW, Halliday JW. 1990. Factors affecting the concentrations of ferritin in serum in a healthy Australian population. *Clin. Chem.* 36:1350–555

68. Looker AC, Dallman PR, Carrol MD, Gunter EW, Johnson CL. 1997. Prevalence of iron deficiency in the United States. *JAMA* 277:973–76

69. Martinez-Torres C, Layrisse M. 1973. Nutritional factors in iron deficiency: food iron absorption. In *Clinics in Haematology*, ed. ST Callender, pp. 339–52. London: Saunders

70. McCance RA, Widdowson EM. 1937. Absorption and excretion of iron. *Lancet* 2:680–84

71. Milman N, Kirchhoff M. 1996. Relations between serum ferritin, alcohol intake and social status in 2235 Danish men and women. *Ann. Haematol.* 72:145–51

72. Monsen ER, Balintfy JL. 1982. Calculating dietary iron bioavailability: refinement and computerization. *J. Am. Diet. Assoc.* 80:307–11

73. Monsen ER, Hallberg L, Layrisse M, Hegsted DM, Cook JD, et al. 1978. Estimation of available dietary iron. *Am. J. Clin. Nutr.* 31:134–41

74. Moore CV. 1968. The absorption of iron from foods. In *Occurrence, Causes and Prevention of Nutritional Anaemias*, ed. G Blix, pp. 92–102. Uppsala, Sweden: Almquist Wiksells

75. Moore CV, Dubach R. 1951. Observations on the absorption of iron from foods tagged with radioiron. *Trans. Assoc. Am. Physicians* 64:245–46

76. Pilch SM, Senti FRE. 1984. *Assessment of the Iron Nutritional Status of the US Population Based on Data Collected in the Second National Health and Nutrition Examination Survey, 1976–1980.* Bethesda, MD: Life Sci. Res. Off., Fed. Am. Soc. Exp. Biol.

77. Raffin SB, Woo CH, Roost KT, Price DC, Schmid R. 1974. Intestinal absorption of hemoglobin iron—heme clevage by mucosal heme oxygenase. *J. Clin. Invest.* 54:1344–52

78. Reddy MB, Hurrell RF, Cook JD. 2000. Estimation of nonheme-iron bioavailability from meal composition. *Am. J. Clin. Nutr.* 71:937–43

79. Rossander-Hulthén L, Hallberg L. 1996.

Prevalence of iron deficiency in adolescents. See Ref. 43a, pp. 149–56

80. Rowland TW, Deisroth MB, Green GM, Kelleher JF. 1988. The effect of iron therapy on the exercise capacity of nonanemic iron-deficient adolescent runners. *Am. J. Dis. Child.* 142:165–69

81. Rybo E, Bengtsson C, Hallberg L. 1985. Iron status of 38-year-old women in Gothenburg, Sweden. *Scand. J. Haematol.* 34(Suppl. 43):41–56

82. Rybo G. 1966. Plasminogen activators in the endometrium. I. Methodological aspects. II. Clinical aspects. *Acta Obstet. Gynaecol. Scand.* 45:411–28

83. Rybo G, Hallberg L. 1966. Influence of heredity and environment on normal menstrual blood loss. *Acta Obstet. Gynaecol. Scand.* 45:389–410

84. Salonen JT, Nyyssönen K, Korpela H, Tuomilehto J, Seppänen R, Salonen R. 1992. High stored iron levels are associated with excess risk of myocardial infarction in eastern Finnish men. *Circulation* 86:803–11

85. Sayers MH, English G, Finch CA. 1994. Capacity of the store-regulator in maintaining iron balance. *Am. J. Hematol.* 47:194–97

86. Scrimshaw NS. 1984. Functional consequences of iron deficiency in human populations. *J. Nutr. Sci. Vitaminol.* 30:47–63

87. Sempos CT, Looker AC, Gillum RF, Makue DM. 1994. Body iron stores and the risk of coronary heart disease. *N. Engl. J. Med.* 330:1119–24

88. Skikne BS, Flowers CH, Cook JD. 1990. Serum transferrin receptor: a quantitative measure of tissue iron deficiency. *Blood* 75:1870–76

89. Stevens RG, Jones DY, Micozzi MS, Taylor PR. 1988. Body iron stores and the risk of cancer. *N. Engl. J. Med.* 319:1047–52

90. Strain JJ, Thompson KA. 1991. Elevated estimates of iron status and calculated iron stores in regular alcohol drinkers in the Northern Ireland population. *Trace Elem. Med.* 8:65–69

91. Sturgeon P, Shoden A. 1971. Total liver storage iron in normal populations of the USA. *Am. J. Clin. Nutr.* 24:469–74

92. Taylor P, Martinez-Torres C, Leets I, Ramirez J, Garcia-Casal MN, Layrisse M. 1988. Relationships among iron absorption, percent saturation of plasma transferrin and serum ferritin concentration in humans. *J. Nutr.* 118:1110–15

93. Taylor PG, Méndez-Castellanos H, Jaffe W, Lopez de Blanco M, Landaeta-Jiménez M, et al. 1995. Iron bioavailability from diets consumed by different socioeconomic strata of the Venezuelan population. *J. Nutr.* 125:1860–68

94. Tenhunen R, Gräsbeck R, Kouvonen I, Lundberg M. 1980. An intestinal receptor for heme: its partial characterisation. *Int. J. Biochem.* 12:713–16

95. Tseng M, Chakraborty H, Robinson DT, Mendez M, Kohlmeyer L. 1997. Adjustment for iron intake for dietary enhancers and inhibitors in population studies: bioavailable iron in rural and urban residing Russian women and children. *J. Nutr.* 127:1456–68

96. Turnbull AL, Cleton F, Finch CA. 1962. Iron absorption. IV. The absorption of hemoglobin iron. *J. Clin. Invest.* 41:1898–907

97. Valberg LS, Sorbie J, Ludwig J, Pelletier O. 1976. Serum ferritin and the iron status of Canadians. *Can. Med. Assoc. J.* 114:417–21

98. Zhu YI, Haas JD. 1997. Iron depletion without anemia and physical performance in young women. *Am. J. Clin. Nutr.* 66:334–41

Annu. Rev. Nutr. 2001. 21:23–46

# FAT METABOLISM IN INSECTS

Lilián E Canavoso, Zeina E Jouni, K Joy Karnas, James E Pennington, and Michael A Wells

*Department of Biochemistry and Molecular Biophysics, and Center for Insect Science, University of Arizona, Tucson, Arizona 85721; e-mail: lcanavoso@email.arizona.edu, eljouniz@email.arizona.edu, karnas@email.arizona.edu, penningj@email.arizona.edu, mawells@email.arizona.edu*

**Key Words** lipophorin, fat body, midgut, hemolymph, flight muscle, oocyte

■ **Abstract** The study of fat metabolism in insects has received considerable attention over the years. Although by no means complete, there is a growing body of information about dietary lipid requirements, and the absolute requirement for sterol is of particular note. In this review we (*a*) summarize the state of understanding of the dietary requirements for the major lipids and (*b*) describe in detail the insect lipid transport system. Insects digest and absorb lipids similarly to vertebrates, but with some important differences. The hallmark of fat metabolism in insects centers on the lipid transport system. The major lipid transported is diacylglycerol, and it is carried by a high-density lipoprotein called lipophorin. Lipophorin is a reusable shuttle that picks up lipid from the gut and delivers it to tissues for storage or utilization without using the endocytic processes common to vertebrate cells. The mechanisms by which this occurs are not completely understood and offer fruitful areas for future research.

## CONTENTS

# INTRODUCTION

Insects are the most abundant form of animal life on the planet, with perhaps a million species and at least a billion individuals for each of the approximately 5 billion humans. Insects have evolved to utilize every conceivable type of available nutrient and are obviously well established and successful. Humans most often think of insects as pests that transmit diseases or consume agricultural products. In fact, life as we know it would not be possible without insects. Insects pollinate plants, produce useful products such as honey and silk, and play a critical role in removing dead material from the biosphere—without insects we would soon be buried in debris. Except in Eurocentric cultures, insects are also an important supplement to human nutrition (43).

Insects and vertebrates share many common metabolic pathways. In many areas of research, insects are useful models that can facilitate our general understanding of biology. This review, however, focuses on several insect-specific processes in fat metabolism. Understanding fat metabolism in insects increases our knowledge of insect metabolism and expands our appreciation of the ways in which different organisms have solved common biochemical problems. In many ways, fat metabolism in insects is less complex than in vertebrates, so insects can serve as a viable model system for understanding fundamental aspects of fat metabolism.

Most of the results reported in the literature and reviewed here are based on the study of only a few insect species, usually those that are easy to rear in the laboratory. Thus, caution should be exercised in drawing general conclusions, particularly when examining dietary lipid requirements. To obtain unequivocal results, such studies often require raising insects for several generations on artificial diets. As is understandable, this arduous task has not been undertaken often. In this review, we take a broad view, which we hope will inform those readers who are interested in nutrition but who have just a passing curiosity about insects. Because of the breadth of the topic and space limitations, we rely heavily on review articles rather than original literature. We apologize to our insect science colleagues for this necessity.

We first summarize the state of understanding of the requirements for the major lipids in the diet and then describe in detail the insect lipid transport system.

## LIPID NUTRITIONAL REQUIREMENTS

Three classical approaches have been used to assess the essentiality of lipid nutrients (35): (*a*) the deletion method, which measures the effect of eliminating one specific component from a chemically defined diet on which the insect can develop under sterile conditions; (*b*) substitution of an essential nutrient by analogues; and (*c*) the use of radiolabeled precursors to measure endogenous biosynthesis (54). The complexity of establishing nutritional requirements for insects can be appreciated by considering the case of aphids. Aphids derive their food from plant phloem, a carbohydrate-rich and amino acid–poor food. Aphids derive their essential amino acids from intracellular symbionts (46). It has been reported that aphids can be reared on fat-free diets for many generations (46). Some interpret this to mean that aphids either do not require essential fatty acids and sterols or that bacterial symbionts provide them. The lack of a requirement for essential fatty acids is due to the fact that aphids, unlike vertebrates, are able to make linoleic acid (44). Linoleic acid biosynthesis has been found in 8 of 32 insect species tested, representing 4 of 13 orders, meaning that most insects probably cannot make it. When some aphids, containing their obligate symbionts, were grown on media containing labeled mevalonate, no incorporation of label was found in any sterols (20). In this case, neither the aphid nor its symbionts can make sterol, so the question of the origin of this aphid's sterol remains unanswered.

### Sterols

***Dietary Requirements***    All insects require sterol in their diets (36, 129). The dietary need for sterols was first established in the blowfly *Lucilla sericata* (61), and has been extended to all orders studied, including Hymenoptera (ants, wasps, bees), Coleoptera (beetles), Diptera (flies), Hemiptera (bugs), Lepidoptera (moths and butterflies), Orthoptera (grasshoppers and crickets), and Homoptera (aphids and cicadas) (117). In a few specific cases, such as cigarette beetles, *Laspoderma serrlione*, microbial symbionts provide sufficient sterol for the insects (36).

Cholesterol is the major sterol found in insects. It serves as a structural component of cell membranes and as the precursor of the insect molting hormones, ecdysteroids (58, 117). Cholesterol has been shown to support normal development in most insects (36, 54). Most species have adapted to transform a wide range of dietary sterols into cholesterol (117, 118). However, there are some exceptions to this generalization. Both the fruit fly *Drosophila pachea* (60) and the beetle *Xyleborus ferrugineous* (32) require dietary $\Delta^7$-sterols (where $\Delta$ refers to the position of the double bond). On the other hand, grasshoppers develop most efficiently to the adult stage on diets containing $\Delta^5$-sterols (e.g. cholesterol and sitosterol) and fail to develop on diets that contain $\Delta^7$ and/or $\Delta^{22}$-sterols (e.g. stigmasterol) (15). It is interesting that these $\Delta^7$- and/or $\Delta^{22}$-sterols can prevent development in the desert locusts *Schistocerca americana*, even when a suitable sterol (e.g. sitosterol) is present (14). In the corn earworm *Heliothis zea*, cholesterol also supports normal growth of larvae, which die when reared on ergosterol or lanosterol (83). A diet containing a high concentration of cholesterol (5%) was mildly toxic to larvae of the tobacco hornworm *Manduca sexta*, whereas the presence of comparable amounts of sitosterol in the diet was toxic (ZE Jouni, MA Wells, unpublished data). The replacement of cholesterol or campesterol by $\beta$-sitosterol in the diet of the housefly *Musca domestica* produced adults that failed to produce viable eggs (67).

***Metabolic Transformations***    Most omnivorous and hematophagous (blood feeding) insects are able to obtain sufficient cholesterol from their diets (118). However, cholesterol itself is not a normal dietary sterol for phytophagous (plant feeding) insects that consume a wide variety of phytosterols, $C_{28}$ or $C_{29}$ sterols with a double bond at position 5 or 7 and a methyl or ethyl group at position $C_{24}$. In plants, phytosterols are usually esterified to fatty acids. Utilization of sterol esters depends on the rate of hydrolysis in the intestinal lumen, as demonstrated in the beetle *Trogoderma granarium* (82). As in vertebrates, cholesterol and other lipids present in the diet may affect phytosterol absorption. Absorbed phytosterols may be unchanged or converted to cholesterol or other sterols in the midgut cells. Then they are released to lipophorin, the major lipoprotein circulating in the hemolymph (blood), and distributed to different tissues for utilization or storage in free or esterified forms.

Dealkylation at $C_{24}$ is the most common metabolic pathway for the conversion of $C_{28}$ and $C_{29}$ dietary sterols into cholesterol. Dealkylation, prevalent in most phytophagous and omnivorous insects, is preceded by oxidation and epoxidation steps (118). Demosterol has been identified as the dealkylation intermediate of phytosterols in several insect species (126).

Cholesterol is not always the end product of the dealkylation reactions. 7-Dehydrocholesterol was produced in the confused flour beetle *Tribolium confusum* (121) and the phytophagous sawfly *Xiphydria maculata* (117). In the Mexican bean beetle *Epilachna varivestis*, saturation of the $\Delta^5$-bond precedes $C_{24}$ dealkylation of phytosterols, resulting in the saturated sterol, cholestanol, instead of cholesterol (117).

***Synthesis of Insect Steroid Hormones***    The major steroid hormones in insects are the molting hormones, ecdysone or 20-hydroxyecdysone. These steroids are made from cholesterol in the prothoracic glands and other steroidogenic organs, such as ovaries, testes, and epidermis. In this pathway, an endoplasmic reticulum (ER) cytochrome P-450 catalyzes the conversion of cholesterol to 7-dehydrocholesterol (58, 152), followed by rapid conversion to ecdysone by the action of a 3-ketosteroid reductase, a hemolymph enzyme (98). The metabolism of ecdysone to 20-hydroxyecdysone occurs in several tissues, e.g. fat body, Malpighian tubules (insect kidney), and midgut (80). This step is catalyzed by ecdysone 20-monooxygenase (126, 156). Both the honeybee *Apis mellifera* (119) and the solitary bee *Megachile rotundata* (120) lack the ability to dealkylate phytosterols. Hence, both have 24-methylcholesterol as their major sterol and the $C_{28}$ ecdysteroid, makisterone A, as their molting hormone.

A number of other steroid hormones, including estrogens, androgens, and the mineralcorticoids, are produced by insects (58). The function of these steroid hormones in insects is unknown.

## Essential Fatty Acids

*Nutritional Requirements*   In addition to sterols, most insects have a dietary requirement for polyunsaturated fatty acids, and many studies have shown that either linoleic or linolenic acids adequately satisfy this nutritional need (36). This is an area that generated some controversy in the past because the concentration of linoleic and linolenic acid in tissue phospholipids is quite low, and many early analyses failed to detect them. Even lower concentrations of arachidonic acid and other polyunsaturated fatty acids went undetected until special efforts were made to measure them (113).

The requirement for essential fatty acids may differ substantially between species. One clear-cut example of essential fatty acid deficiency in insects is found in Lepidoptera and Hymenoptera, where there is a failure of the adult insect to form properly during metamorphosis; however, there are no effects during larval development (36). This deficiency is alleviated by linolenic acid, not linoleic acid. The function of linolenic acid in metamorphosis has yet to be established. Some members of the Orthoptera order express fatty acid deficiency by a markedly retarded nymph growth and the emergence of deformed adults (36). In contrast, the cockroach *Blatella germanica* shows no ill effect from deficiency imposed through larval development, but females develop deformed oothecae (a structure that covers the egg after laying), or a second generation of weak, short-lived nymphs (57). Coleoptera show a requirement for essential polyunsaturated fatty acids mainly by slow larval growth and decreased adult fecundity (36).

With the exception of mosquitoes, polyunsaturated fatty acids have not been found to be essential for any of the several species of Diptera (79). Larval mosquitoes require arachidonic acid or related 20- and 22-carbon polyunsaturated fatty acids to survive to adulthood. Neither linoleic nor linolenic acid satisfies that requirement (37).

*Prostaglandins*   Prostaglandins (PGs) have been extensively studied in vertebrates, where they cause myriad physiological and pharmacological reactions. By comparison, relatively few studies have been carried out using insects (62, 115). One well-defined system is the requirement of $PGE_2$ for egg-laying behavior in the cricket *Acheta domesticus* (45). PGs have been shown to mediate egg-laying behavior in a few other insects, but in most they have no obvious effects. PGs may play other undetermined roles in reproduction because they are found in the reproductive tracts of insect species in which they do not affect egg laying. Another well-studied system involves control of fluid secretion by the salivary glands of the blowfly *Calliphora erythrocephala*, where $PGE_1$ inhibits adenyl cyclase, a critical component of the fluid secretion signaling system (38, 39).

Other possible roles of PGs have been inferred based on the use of PG biosynthesis inhibitors. Among these are reports that PG may regulate fluid secretion in the Malpighian tubules of the mosquito *Aedes aegypti* (88) and the forest ant *Formica polyctena* (146), and that it may modulate insect immunity (114).

## Carotenoids

Carotenoids are lipid-soluble pigments made up of two diterpenoid units joined tail to tail. There are two types of carotenoids: the carotenes (hydrocarbons), which are unsubstituted terpenes, and the xanthophylls, which are oxidized derivatives of carotenes (70). Only plants and microorganisms synthesize carotenoids, so insects, like all animals, must obtain them from their diets. In some insects, absorption of carotenoids is selective, with some preferentially absorbing carotenes and others preferentially absorbing xanthophylls (50). Carotenoids contribute to the body colors of insects. Although the functions of carotenoids in coloration are not well understood, color has evolved as part of a strategy to avoid predators. It acts as a camouflage or as an advertisement of distastefulness (48).

The participation of carotenoids in vision is well characterized in both vertebrates and invertebrates. In insects, retinal and 3-hydroxyretinal are used as chromophores of visual pigments (101). The name xanthopsin is used for the visual pigments based on 3-hydroxyretinal, which is derived from such xanthophylls as lutein and zeaxanthin (149–151). The visual pigment in Diptera is 11-*cis* 3-hydroxyretinal (100, 149, 150). In *Drosophila melanogaster*, both retinoids and carotenoids serve as precursors of the chromophore. When carotenoids are the precursors, the insect can form 11-*cis* 3-hydroxyretinal in the dark. When retinoids are the precursors, the presence of light is obligatory for the isomerization of all-*trans* to 11-*cis* 3-hydroxyretinal (101).

## Fat-Soluble Vitamins

The few studies reported to date indicate that with the exception of vitamin D, the fat-soluble vitamins A, E, and K have some beneficial effect on the physiology of insects (36, 78). A deficiency in vitamin A or carotenes retards growth and causes anomalous color and behavior in the second generation of the migratory locust *Locusta migratoria* and the desert locust *Schistocerca gregaria* (36). A specific nutritional requirement for vitamin E ($\alpha$-tocopherol) has been demonstrated in a few species, mainly in connection with adult reproductive function. Vitamin E improves fecundity in moths and beetles. Its effect in *A. domesticus* is most clear in males, where larvae reared on diets without tocopherol failed to develop viable sperm (36, 78). Because of its function as an antioxidant, vitamin E is included in the formulation of most synthetic diets that incorporate polyunsaturated fatty acids (54). Vitamin K is required in vertebrates for its role in the synthesis of the clotting factor prothrombin and consequently is not expected to be necessary for insects. When vitamin K was tested in crickets as a substitute for vitamin E, it showed a growth-stimulatory effect, but it had no effect on male sterility (54, 77).

# LIPOPHORIN

## Properties

Most of the lipid in hemolymph is associated with a single lipoprotein particle, and although there is considerable variation in lipid composition between insects, the common name lipophorin is used for all insect lipoproteins (29). Under most physiological conditions, lipophorin exists as high-density lipophorin (HDLp) (D $\sim$ 1.15 g/ml). Every HDLp particle contains one molecule each of two apolipoproteins: apolipophorin-I (apoLp-I) ($M_r \sim 250$ kDa) and apolipophorin-II (apoLp-II) ($M_r \sim 70$ kDa) (31, 95). Several studies suggest that apoLp-I is located on the surface of HDLp and that apoLp-II is sequestered away from the surface (108). A third exchangeable apolipoprotein, apolipophorin-III (apoLp-III) ($M_r \sim 18$ kDa), is found free in the hemolymph or associated with low-density lipophorin (LDLp) (D $\sim$ 1.03 g/ml), which are discussed below.

Lipophorin contains a phospholipid-protein surface and a neutral lipid core (66). The core lipid composition varies with physiological status and across insect species (Table 1). The neutral lipid most commonly carried by lipophorin is sn-1,2-diacylglycerol (DAG) (31, 108). However, some Diptera belonging to the family Culicomorpha (mosquitoes, black flies, midges) transport neutral lipid in the form of triacylglycerol (TAG) (53; JE Pennington, MA Wells, unpublished data). Small amounts of sterols, free fatty acids, carotenoids, and monoacylglycerols are also transported by lipophorin, but sterol-esters are never found in any significant amount (108).

**TABLE 1**    Representative lipid compositions of lipophorins from several insect species[a]

| Insect lipophorin (Reference) | Density (g/ml) | %PL | %DAG | %ST | %TAG | %HC |
|---|---|---|---|---|---|---|
| *Manduca sexta* HDLp (89) | 1.151 | 16.7 | 15.7 | 1.2 | 1.1 | 2.8 |
| *M. sexta* LDLp (94) | 1.030 | 14.0 | 25.0 | 1.3 | 2.5 | 3.5 |
| *Aedes aegypti* HDLp (53) | 1.113 | 15.7 | 4.0 | 6.9 | 15.7 | ND |
| *Locusta migratoria* HDLp (31) | 1.120 | 14.8 | 13.4 | 3.2 | 0.7 | 8.7 |
| *L. migratoria* LDLp (28) | 1.065 | 10.9 | 26.1 | 2.4 | 0.5 | 6.4 |
| *Periplaneta americana* HDLp (30) | 1.120 | 22.8 | 8.0 | 2.7 | 1.0 | 15.0 |

[a]Lipid percentages are expressed as a percentage of total weight of the particle: HDLp, high-density lipophorin; LDLp, low-density lipophorin; PL, phospholipid; DAG, diacylglycerol; ST, sterol; TAG, triacylglycerol; HC, hydrocarbon; ND, not determined.

Other neutral lipids transported by lipophorin include long-chain hydrocarbons that make up a considerable portion of the neutral lipid content in some insects (30). Hydrocarbons (*a*) are synthesized in cells associated with the epidermis, (*b*) serve as sex attractants, and (*c*) are essential components of the insect cuticle, preventing loss of water and subsequent dehydration (18, 99). Methyl-branched hydrocarbons are a unique feature of insects and these compounds are made from the corresponding fatty acids by decarboxylation. The methyl branches are introduced using methylmalonyl-CoA in place of malonyl-CoA at specific points during fatty acid biosynthesis.

## Biosynthesis

*Apolipoproteins*    Labeling studies have demonstrated that apoLp-I and -II are synthesized in the fat body as a single precursor protein (140, 143, 153). The precursor protein is encoded by a single ~10-kb mRNA that has been sequenced fully for *M. sexta* (116) and *D. melanogaster* (72) and sequenced partially for *L. migratoria* (140) and *A. aegypti* (143). The cDNA sequences showed proapolipophorin is arranged with apoLp-II at its N-terminus and apoLp-I at its C-terminus (72, 116). A single consensus convertase cleavage site, RXRR, is present in between apoLp-II and apoLp-I in the precursor protein (72, 116). Thus, the 1:1 apolipoprotein stoichiometry in all lipophorins is accomplished by the proteolytic cleavage of proapolipophorin into its subunits.

Comparison of the entire deduced amino acid sequences of *M. sexta* and *D. melanogaster* precursor proteins shows an identity of approximately 21% (143). A higher percent identity (40%–70%) is found for some regions, which suggests that there are portions of these proteins that are more highly conserved (72, 143). Comparisons of sequences from *L. migratoria*, *M. sexta*, and *D. melanogaster* proapolipophorin with human apolipoprotein B (apoB), invertebrate and vertebrate vitellogenins, and the large subunit of mammalian microsomal triglyceride transfer protein revealed contiguous conserved sequence motifs, which the authors interpreted to mean that the genes coding for these proteins are members of the same multigene superfamily (9).

*Lipidation*    Lipidation refers to those processes whereby the apolipoproteins and the transported lipid are packaged together to form a soluble lipoprotein particle. Most of the work in the field of lipoprotein biosynthesis has involved studies on the lipidation of apoB. Its association with lipids to form very-low-density lipoproteins (VLDL) is a multistep process that begins with cotranslational translocation of apoB across the ER (92, 103). Lipid availability and the proper folding of apoB, particularly the formation of disulfide bonds, are required for lipidation (19, 127). Small amounts of core lipids are added to the membrane-bound apoB, leading to the formation of a high-density apoB-containing particle. One hypothesis for how this occurs is that apoB is actually inserted into the inner leaflet of the ER during translocation (34, 87, 110). It has been suggested (1, 33) that in apoB, pause transfer sequences cause a pause in translocation (1, 33), which allows addition of lipids to the protein.

The exact mechanism for lipidation of apolipophorins is unknown; however, the insolubility of apoLp-II (108), as well as the rapid (approximately 35 min) synthesis, processing, assembly, and secretion of apoLp-I and apoLp-II as HDLp (154), suggests that lipidation occurs during or closely following the translation of the precursor protein. The extent to which the nascent particle is lipidated prior to its release from the fat body is a controversial topic and may differ between insect species. The nascent HDLp described for *L. migratoria*, *Diatraea grandiosella* (the Colorado potato beetle), and *M. domestica* is similar in lipid composition and lipid load to that of circulating HDLp, which suggests it is fully loaded with lipid prior to its secretion from the fat body (25, 148, 154). Alternatively, in larval *M. sexta*, HDLp is secreted as a very high-density phospholipid-protein complex that is loaded with core lipid at the midgut (73, 89).

Two major differences exist between insect and human lipogenesis. First, the assembly of human lipoproteins requires the presence of the microsomal triglyceride transfer protein. This protein, not believed to be present in insects, is located in the lumen of the ER and is required for the proper assembly of apoB-containing lipoproteins (91). A second major difference is that VLDL production is regulated by lipid availability and not apoB translation. In lipid-poor conditions, cytosolic degradation of apoB occurs (157). In lipid-rich conditions, more apoB is translocated into the ER, where a second proteolytic pathway degrades any apoB that is not efficiently transferred to the Golgi. This second proteolysis step is designed presumably to eliminate any misfolded apoB (16). In contrast, the rate of lipophorin biosynthesis in larval *M. sexta* is independent of the amount of lipid in the diet. There is a direct correlation between the lipid content of lipophorin and the amount of lipid in the diet (51).

## Role as a Reusable Shuttle in Lipid Transport

There are several types of lipoproteins in vertebrate systems, most delivering their neutral lipid load to target tissues by a combination of lipoprotein lipase-mediated lipolysis (chylomicrons and VLDL) or endocytosis and degradation of the whole particle (LDL and chylomicron remnants). The insect system is more versatile than the vertebrate system in that in different insects, the same basic lipophorin particle can carry a wide variety of lipids. Additionally, lipophorin has the unique ability to selectively deliver specific lipids to specific tissues, e.g. hydrocarbons to the cuticle, carotenoids to the cuticle or the silk gland, etc (3, 73). The insect system is more efficient because lipid is delivered to tissues, for the most part, without internalization and destruction of lipophorin (3, 26, 96, 108). This observation led to the idea that lipophorin functions as a reusable shuttle moving lipid from sites of absorption or storage to sites of utilization (3, 26, 66, 108, 138).

## LIPOLYSIS, ABSORPTION, AND EXPORT

### Lipolysis

Midgut cells produce lipases that hydrolyze dietary TAGs, forming monoacyl-glycerols and free fatty acids. However, in some species, especially Lepidoptera, which have a high pH in the midgut lumen, acyl migration and subsequent hydrolysis leads to free glycerol and fatty acids (2, 3, 13, 47, 130, 133). Digestion of phospholipids and glycolipids has been examined in Lepidoptera, Coleoptera, and Diptera (133). Phospholipases $A_1$ and $A_2$ were found in the midgut of some Lepidoptera and are probably widespread among insects (125). Phospholipases C and/or D have also been found in the midgut of some insects (131). Galacto-lipids are hydrolyzed by $\alpha$- and $\beta$-galactosidases yielding galactose and DAG (74, 81, 123, 124). As noted above, utilization of sterol esters may be dependent on the rate of the hydrolysis in the midgut lumen (71, 133).

### Absorption

Insects do not have bile salts and have developed other strategies to facilitate lipid solubilization. These strategies include the use of lumenal glycolipids and the formation of fatty acyl–amino acid complexes, fatty acid micelles in the highly alkaline environment of Lepidopteran gut, and lysophospholipid micelles (133).

Absorbed fatty acids and partial acylglycerols, if present, are converted into intestinal DAG, TAG, and phospholipids. Synthesis could involve acylation of 2-monoacylglycerol (the monoacylglycerol pathway) or the de novo pathway that involves acylation of sn-glycerol-3-phosphate (the phosphatidic acid pathway) (22, 47, 77, 133). The relative contribution of the two pathways has only been established in larval M. sexta, where it was shown that the fatty acids arising from complete lumenal hydrolysis of TAG are transformed into DAG using the phosphatidic pathway (22). In the same insect, DAG is rapidly converted to TAG, which serves as a reservoir for absorbed fatty acids, or the DAG can be exported to the hemolymph (22). This mechanism assures maximal absorption of fatty acids from the midgut lumen while maintaining a low intracellular concentration of both fatty acids and DAG, which can be toxic at high concentrations. It has been proposed (22) that the uptake of fatty acids by the midgut cell is the rate-limiting step, which suggests the presence of a fatty acid transporter in the lumenal membrane (63, 112). Within midgut cells, fatty acids and other absorbed lipids are targeted to their metabolic pathways by unknown mechanisms. It is possible that cytosolic lipid-binding proteins are involved. Two fatty acid–binding proteins have been isolated from the midgut of M. sexta (104) and a lutein-binding protein was isolated from the midgut of the silkworm Bombyx mori (65).

Phospholipid and glycolipid absorption have received less attention and have been studied only in Lepidoptera (131). Lysophosphatidylcholine is readily absorbed by the midgut cells, where it is reacylated to phosphatidylcholine (133).

Sugars and DAG from glycolipid hydrolysis are also absorbed, and then DAG is exported to the hemolymph or converted to TAG (133). The midgut is the main site for absorption of cholesterol, although in some omnivorous and carnivorous insects, its absorption has been reported to take place in the foregut or the crop (64). Free cholesterol and cholesterol ester may be absorbed, but free cholesterol is subjected to some intracellular esterification (71, 132). In *M. sexta*, dietary free cholesterol is absorbed in a concentration-dependent manner and is stored in the midgut mainly in the free form (ZE Jouni, MA Wells, unpublished data). In phytophagous insects, the midgut is also the major tissue where nonmetabolized plant sterols are accumulated (15).

## Export

Unlike in vertebrates, which synthesize intestinal lipoproteins to carry dietary lipids through the blood, lipid export from the enterocytes in insects does not involve de novo synthesis of a lipoprotein particle. Rather, the lipids are added directly to the existing lipophorin in the hemolymph (26, 89, 93, 102, 108). Lipophorin cycles between the midgut, where it picks up lipids, and the fat body, where the lipids are delivered and stored. It is important to note that lipophorin does not enter the midgut cell or the fat body cell during this process (108, 128).

In vivo and in vitro studies using several insect orders showed DAG is the main lipid in the hemolymph after lipid digestion (10, 22, 90, 128, 155). In *M. sexta* it was demonstrated that dietary lipid is the source of lipophorin DAG because insects raised on a fat-free diet contained a circulating lipophorin essentially depleted of DAG (51). In the same insect, nearly 90% of fatty acid–labeled triolein was absorbed after 4 h, and of that absorbed, more than 70% was found in fat body as TAG (128). In the hemolymph, more than 90% of the label was in DAG and all the DAG was associated with lipophorin. Also, in *M. sexta* larvae, a kinetic model for DAG export showed that its release from the midgut occurs at a rate consistent with the intracellular lipolysis of the TAG pool (22; ER Rubiolo, MA Wells, unpublished data).

Little is known about the mechanisms involved in the transfer of lipids from the midgut to lipophorin in the hemolymph. Two factors proposed to be critical in this transfer are a lipophorin receptor and the lipid transfer particle (LTP). It is generally accepted that lipophorin interacts with tissues through specific binding sites (3, 8, 129, 136) and that the transfer process occurs at the surface of the cell without particle internalization (3, 10, 108, 128). Recently, lipophorin binding to the midgut of *M. sexta* larvae was characterized using membrane preparations (56). In *Aeschna cyanea* larvae, biochemical and immunocytochemical approaches showed that lipid loading and unloading of lipophorin both occur at the midgut without lipophorin internalization (10).

LTP is a very-high-density lipoprotein (VHDL) isolated from the hemolymph of several species (17, 94, 96, 97). The physiological function of LTP is not completely understood, but studies indicate that it serves to redistribute lipids between lipophorins and between lipophorins and membranes (3, 96). In vitro studies show

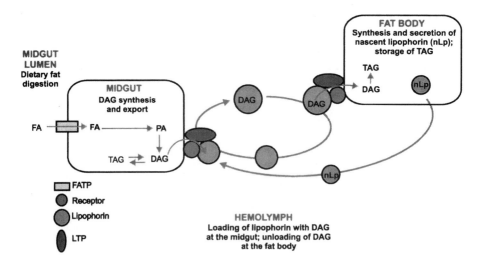

**Figure 1**  A scheme showing the absorption of fatty acid (FA) into the midgut enterocyte, the synthesis of diacylglycerol (DAG) in the midgut cell, and the transport of DAG to the fat body for storage. It has been proposed that a fatty acid transporter (FATP) is involved in the absorption of FA. The synthesis of DAG in the midgut cell involves the phosphatidic acid (PA) pathway. The export of DAG from the midgut cell requires a lipophorin receptor and lipid transfer particle (LTP). Central to this scheme is the biosynthesis of lipophorin in the fat body and its function as a reusable shuttle. TAG, triacylglycerol.

that DAG transfer from labeled *M. sexta* midgut sacs to lipophorin is completely blocked by pretreatment with anti-LTP antibody and is restored when LTP is added to the incubation medium (LE Canavoso, MA Wells, unpublished data). Therefore, it seems likely that LTP is necessary to facilitate DAG transfer from the midgut. A model for fatty acid absorption, DAG synthesis, and export to lipophorin is presented in Figure 1 (3).

## FAT STORAGE AND MOBILIZATION

### Storage in Fat Body

In insects, the majority of stored lipids are found in the fat body, an organ analogous to vertebrate adipose tissue and liver. It is also the site of synthesis of hemolymph proteins, the major organ involved in metabolism and the major storage site for glycogen (13, 23). More than 90% of the lipid stored in the fat body is TAG (7, 13, 21, 47). TAG storage is mainly the result of transfer of dietary fat from the midgut to the fat body during the feeding period (Figure 1). In addition, lipid storage can result from de novo lipid synthesis in the fat body from carbohydrates (13, 47).

During the transfer of lipids from lipophorin to the fat body, it has been proposed that lipophorin binds to a receptor (3, 96). A candidate receptor is a HDLp-binding

protein that has been characterized in the fat body of larval *M. sexta* (129). This protein requires $Ca^{2+}$ for HDLp binding (129). In contrast, another HDLp-binding
protein found in both intact fat body tissue and isolated membranes of nymph and
adult *L. migratoria* did not require divalent cations. The *L. migratoria* protein has a
broader specificity than the *M. sexta* protein, as it can bind human lipoproteins. Additionally, it was found that unlike the *M. sexta* protein (129), the *L. migratoria*
protein is involved in the endocytic internalization of lipophorin (40–42). Endocytosis of HDLp by fat body cells has also been shown in *A. cyanea* (11). The
function of this receptor-mediated endocytosis remains unclear because inhibition
of endocytosis did not reduce the transfer of the two main lipophorin lipid cargos,
diacylglycerol and cholesterol, to the fat body (3, 41, 96). The role of LTP in the
transfer of lipid from lipophorin to the fat body is also unclear. Anti-LTP antibodies
reversibly reduce DAG transfer by only 50% in in vivo and in vitro experiments
with larval *M. sexta* (LE Canavoso, MA Wells, unpublished data), which suggests
more than one pathway for DAG transfer from lipophorin to fat body.

## Mobilization from Fat Body

***Hormones***     Lipids are mobilized from the fat body as DAG, not free fatty acids
as in vertebrates. Mobilization is induced by two types of hormones: adipokinetic
hormone (AKH) (13) and octopamine (49). AKHs are a large family of 8– to
10–amino acid peptides secreted into hemolymph by the neurosecretory cells of the
corpora cardiaca (55). Injection of AKH into adult *L. migratoria* (76) and *M. sexta*
(5) stimulates the formation of lipophorin-associated *sn*-1,2-DAG. The most likely
mechanism for the production of *sn*-1,2-DAG is the direct stereospecific hydrolysis
of TAG catalyzed by a TAG-lipase (6, 7). A TAG-lipase has been purified from
the fat body of adult *M. sexta* (6). Like the vertebrate hormone-sensitive lipase,
which catalyzes the rate-limiting step in mobilization of adipose tissue fatty acid,
the *M. sexta* lipase is a phosphorylatable enzyme. In adult *M. sexta*, the activation
of the fat body TAG-lipase precedes the appearance of the *sn*-1,2-DAG in the
hemolymph, which suggests that AKH stimulates DAG secretion by activating the
fat body TAG-lipase (5).

AKH exerts its effects on lipid mobilization via signal transduction. Binding
of AKH to its receptor results in the induction of several events that activate key
enzymes in lipid and carbohydrate mobilization in the fat body. Receptor binding
both activates adenylate cyclase and mediates a rapid and sustained increase in
$Ca^{2+}$ influx, giving rise to two intracellular messengers, $Ca^{2+}$ and cAMP (4, 139).
In the fat body of two locusts, *S. gregaria* (111) and *L. migratoria* (147), AKH
increases the levels of $Ca^{2+}$, cAMP, and inositol (1,4,5)-triphosphate. Beyond
activation of TAG-lipase by phosphorylation (5), other roles of these intracellular
messages have not been characterized. Figure 2 presents a model for activation of
DAG production in response to AKH.

Octopamine, an analog of the vertebrate catecholamine noradrenaline, acts as
a neurotransmitter, modulating the release of AKH from the corpus cardiacum
(86). In addition, it acts as a neurohormone with direct energy store mobilizing

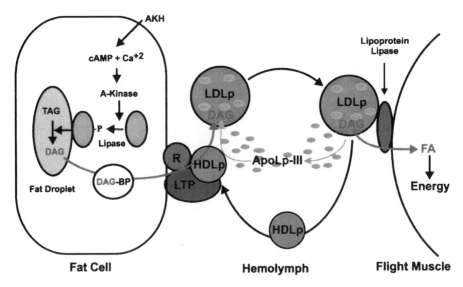

**Figure 2**  A model for low-density lipophorin (LDLp) production by the fat body and delivery of lipid to the flight muscle.  Adipokinetic hormone (AKH) stimulates diacylglycerol (DAG) production and secretion from the fat body.  DAG is produced by the action of a lipase acting on the stored triacylglycerol (TAG) and is transported to the plasma membrane via a DAG-binding protein (DAG-BP). Once in the membrane, the DAG leaves the cell and is added to high-density lipophorin (HDLp) with the assistance of lipid transfer particle (LTP) to produce LDLp. LDLp is stabilized by binding apolipophorin-III (apoLp-III). LDLp moves to the muscle cell where the DAG is hydrolyzed by a lipophorin lipase.  After delipidation, apoLp-III dissociates and LDLp is converted back to HDLp.  HDLp then cycles back to the fat body to pick additional DAG and apoLp-III. FA, Fatty acid; R, receptor.

activity (52, 84, 85). In *L. migratoria* and *A. domesticus*, an increase in hemolymph octopamine levels is a general response to different forms of stress, such as handling or starvation (47).

***Low-Density Lipophorin Synthesis***    Once DAG has been produced from the TAG stores in the fat body, it must be exported to the hemolymph for transport to tissues. As is the case in the midgut, DAG export from the fat body does not involve synthesis of new lipophorin particles; instead, DAG is added to preexisting HDLp in the hemolymph (27, 59, 108). The mechanism by which DAG traverses the fat body membrane and is added to HDLp is not completely understood, but LTP is required (142). As DAG is added to HDLp, the particle increases in diameter, leading to a particle whose surface is destabilized by DAG. ApoLp-III binds to the DAG-destabilized surface of lipophorin, stabilizing it and allowing the uptake of additional DAG (105–107). The end product of DAG and apoLp-III addition to HDLp is LDLp, whose mass is about twice that of HDLp. This increase in mass is due to the addition of approximately equal amounts of apoLp-III and DAG (Figure 2).

Why do insects go to the trouble of making DAG from stored TAG and repackaging it into LDLp for transport to tissues when the release of free fatty acids would seem a simpler solution? The reason probably lies in the fact that insects have an open circulatory system. If free fatty acids were released from the fat body they would not be carried away by blood flow. They would be rapidly taken back into the fat body and made into TAG (109). The synthesis of LDLp provides a lipid carrier that can be directed to specific tissues, such as flight muscle and oocytes (see below).

## LIPID DELIVERY TO TISSUES

### Flight Muscle

Insect flight muscle is the most metabolically active tissue known. On activation, oxygen consumption of flight muscle increases 50- to 100-fold, whereas in vertebrate muscle, the increase is only 7- to 14-fold. At maximum output, a locust flight muscle hydrolyzes ATP at a rate of 18 $\mu$mol/s, which means the entire energy-rich phosphate pool (ATP and phosphoarginine) of the muscle can sustain flight for 1 s. Hence, there must be prodigious ATP synthesis during flight, which can last several hours (12, 24, 27). Flight muscle has the capacity to use several fuel sources. Trehalose, proline, and ketone bodies have been described as sources of energy for flight muscle, but probably the most efficient source of energy is fatty acid (24).

Insect flight muscle is incapable of storing significant amounts of lipid, and the source of fatty acid is the DAG of LDLp. In keeping with the reusable shuttle model, LDLp is not internalized and degraded at any point in lipid delivery to the flight muscle (145). Based on immunofluorescence and immunogold studies, LDLp was found to be associated with the extracellular matrix and basement membranes of both resting and flying flight muscles (135). A muscle-specific lipophorin lipase hydrolyzes the DAG carried by LDLp, releasing free fatty acid and glycerol, which are taken up by the flight muscle. Membrane-associated flight muscle lipophorin lipases have been described in *L. migratoria* and *M. sexta* (141, 144, 145, 156). As DAG is removed from LDLp, apoLp-III dissociates from the particle and HDLp is regenerated in the hemolymph. Both HDLp and apoLp-III can then be used to reform LDLp at the fat body (Figure 2).

### Oocyte

In *M. sexta*, the most thoroughly studied system for lipid delivery to the oocyte, up to 40% of the dry weight of the mature egg is lipid (68). Biosynthesis accounts for about 1% of the lipid in the egg, and another 5% of the lipid is delivered by the yolk protein vitellogenin (68). LDLp and HDLp deliver the rest of the lipid to the oocyte. Of the total lipid, 90% is delivered by a lipophorin lipase-mediated process similar to that described for flight muscle (68, 137). The oocyte lipophorin lipase

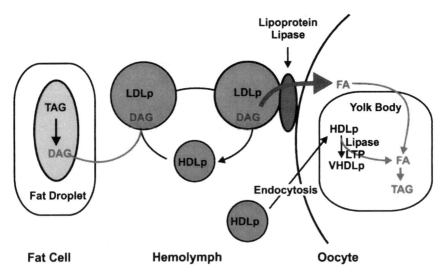

**Figure 3**  Lipid delivery to the oocyte. Lipid is delivered to the oocyte primarily by low-density lipophorin (LDLp) and requires the activity of a lipophorin lipase. In this case, lipophorin shuttles between the oocyte and the fat body. A minor pathway involves endocytosis of high-density lipophorin (HDLp), which is delipidated intracellularly and stored in the egg as VHDLp. TAG, triacylglycerol; DAG, *sn*-1,2-diacylglycerol; FA, fatty acids; LTP, lipid transfer particle; VHDLp, very-high-density lipophorin.

displays specificity for LDLp over HDLp, and a putative lipase responsible for this activity has been partially purified from follicle cell membranes (68, 137). The final mechanism involved in the delivery of lipid to the egg is selective endocytosis of HDLp. This is the only significant exception to the reusable shuttle model described so far. The lipid of HDLp is processed by a lipase and LTP, producing a very-high-density lipophorin (VHDLp) (D = 1.238 g/ml), which is stored in yolk bodies (69, 75, 134). During this processing, the protein subunits of HDLp are not degraded. A model for lipid delivery to the oocyte is shown in Figure 3.

## CONCLUSION

We have presented a broad overview of fat metabolism in insects. In doing so, we have tried to summarize the current state of knowledge and point out some of the many fruitful areas for future research. Indeed, there are many exciting questions begging to be investigated—from a thorough understanding of the requirements of lipids in insect nutrition to the elucidation of the detailed mechanisms of lipophorin biosynthesis and the mechanisms whereby lipophorin serves as a reusable shuttle. We hope some of the readers will become as fascinated as we are by this amazing group of animals and join the fun.

## ACKNOWLEDGMENTS

We thank Drs. G Bloomquist, C Schal, and D Stanley for helpful suggestions and Dr. G Bindford and A Stonehouse for providing editorial feedback. Work in our laboratory is supported by NIH grant GM 50008.

**Visit the Annual Reviews home page at www.AnnualReviews.org**

## LITERATURE CITED

1. Andrews DW, Johnson AE. 1996. The translocon: more than a hole in the ER membrane? *Trends Biochem. Sci.* 21:365–69
2. Applebaum SW. 1985. Biochemistry of digestion. See Ref. 70a, 10:279–311
3. Aresse EL, Canavoso LE, Jouni ZE, Pennington JE, Tsuchida K, Wells MA. 2001. Lipoprotein metabolism in insects: current status and future directions. *Insect Biochem. Mol. Biol.* 31:7–17
4. Arrese EL, Flowers MT, Gazard JL, Wells MA. 1999. Calcium and cAMP are second messengers in the adipokinetic hormone-induced lipolysis of triacylglycerols in *Manduca sexta* fat body. *J. Lipid Res.* 40:555–64
5. Arrese EL, Rojas-Rivas BI, Wells MA. 1996. The use of decapitated insects to study lipid mobilization in adult *Manduca sexta*, effects of adipokinetic hormone and trehalose on fat body lipase activity. *Insect Biochem. Mol. Biol.* 26:775–82
6. Arrese EL, Wells MA. 1994. Purification and properties of a phosphorylatable triacylglycerol lipase from the fat body of an insect, *Manduca sexta. J. Lipid Res.* 35:1652–59
7. Arrese EL, Wells MA. 1997. Adipokinetic hormone-induced lipolysis in the fat body of an insect, *Manduca sexta*, synthesis of sn-1,2-diacylglycerols. *J. Lipid Res.* 38:68–76
8. Atella GC, Gondim KC, Masuda H. 1995. Loading of lipophorin particles with phospholipids at the midgut of *Rhodnius prolixus. Arch. Insect Biochem. Physiol.* 30:337–50
9. Babin PJ, Bogerd J, Kooiman FP, Van Marrewijk WJ, Van der Horst DJ. 1999. Apolipophorin II/I, apolipoprotein B, vitellogenin, and microsomal triglyceride transfer protein genes are derived from a common ancestor. *J. Mol. Evol.* 49:150–60
10. Bauerfeind R, Komnick H. 1992. Lipid-loading and unloading of lipophorin in the midgut epithelium of dragonfly larvae, *Aeshna cyanea. J. Insect Physiol.* 38:147–60
11. Bauerfeind R, Komnick H. 1992. Immunocytochemical localization of lipophorin in the fat body of dragonfly larvae, *Aeshna cyanea. J. Insect Physiol.* 38:185–98
12. Beenakkers AMT, Van der Horst DJ, Van Marrewijk JA. 1984. Insect flight muscle metabolism. *Insect Biochem.* 14:243–60
13. Beenakkers AMT, Van der Horst DJ, Van Marrewijk WJA. 1985. Insect lipids and their role in physiological processes. *Prog. Lipid Res.* 24:19–67
14. Behmer ST, Elias DO. 1999. The nutritional significance of sterol metabolic constraints in the generalist grasshopper *Schistocerca americana. J. Insect Physiol.* 45:339–48
15. Behmer ST, Elias DO, Grebenok RJ. 1999. Phytosterol metabolism and absorption in the generalist grasshopper, *Schistocerca americana* (Orthoptera: Acriidae). *Arch. Insect Biochem. Physiol.* 42:13–25
16. Benoist F, Grand-Perret T. 1997. Co-translational degradation of apolipoprotein B100 by the proteasome is prevented by microsomal triglyceride transfer protein. *J. Biol. Chem.* 272:20435–42
17. Blacklock BJ, Ryan RO. 1994. Hemo-

lymph lipid transport. *Insect Biochem. Mol. Biol.* 24:855–73

18. Blomquist GJ, Tillman JA, Mpuru S, Seybold SJ. 1998. The cuticle and cuticular hydrocarbons of insects: structure, function and biochemistry. In *Pheromone Communication in Social Insects: Ants, Wasps, Bees and Termites,* ed. RK Vander Meer, MD Breed, ML Winston, KE Espelid, pp. 34–54. Boulder, CO: Westview

19. Burch WL, Herscovitz H. 2000. Disulfide bonds are required for folding and secretion of apolipoprotein B regardless of its lipidation state. *J. Biol. Chem.* 275:16267–74

20. Campbell BC, Nes WD. 1983. A reappraisal of sterol biosynthesis and metabolism in aphids. *J. Insect Physiol.* 29:149–56

21. Canavoso LE, Bertello LE, de Lederkremer RM, Rubiolo ER. 1998. Effect of fasting on the composition of the fat body lipid of *Dipetalogaster maximus, Triatoma infestans* and *Panstrongylus megistus* (Hemiptera: Reduviidae). *J. Comp. Physiol. B* 168:549–54

22. Canavoso LE, Wells MA. 2000. Metabolic pathways for diacylglycerol biosynthesis and release in the midgut of larval *Manduca sexta. Insect Biochem. Mol. Biol.* 30:1173–80

23. Candy DJ. 1985. Intermediary metabolism. See Ref. 70a, 10:1–41

24. Candy DJ, Becker A, Wegener G. 1997. Coordination and integration of metabolism in insect flight. *Comp. Biochem. Physiol.* 117B:475–82

25. Capurro M deL, de Bianchi AG. 1990. Larval *Musca domestica* lipophorin biosynthesis. *Comp. Biochem. Physiol.* 97B:655–59

26. Chino H. 1985. Lipid transport: biochemistry of hemolymph lipophorin. See Ref. 70a, 10:115–35

27. Chino H. 1997. Physiological significance of lipid transport by lipophorin for long-distance flight in insects. *Comp. Biochem. Physiol.* 117B:475–82

28. Chino H, Downer RG, Takahashi K. 1986. Effect of adipokinetic hormone on the structure and properties of lipophorin in locusts. *J. Lipid Res.* 27:21–29

29. Chino H, Downer RG, Wyatt GR, Gilbert LI. 1981. Lipophorins, a major class of lipoprotein in insect hemolymph. *Insect Biochem.* 11:491

30. Chino H, Katase H, Downer RGH, Takahashi K. 1981. Diacylglycerol-carrying lipoprotein of hemolymph of the American cockroach: purification, characterization, and function. *J. Lipid. Res.* 22:7–15

31. Chino H, Kitazawa K. 1981. Diacylglycerol-carrying lipoprotein of hemolymph of the locust and some insects. *J. Lipid Res.* 22:1042–52

32. Chu HM, Norris DM, Kok LT. 1970. Pupation requirement of the beetle, *Xyleborus ferrugineus*: sterols other than cholesterol. *J. Insect Physiol.* 16:1379–87

33. Chuck SL, Lingappa VR. 1992. Pause transfer: a topogenic sequence in apolipoprotein B mediates stopping and restarting of translocation. *Cell* 68:9–21

34. Chuck SL, Yao Z, Blackhart BD, McCarthy BJ, Lingappa VR. 1990. New variation on the translocation of proteins during early biogenesis of apolipoprotein B. *Nature* 346:282–85

35. Dadd RH. 1977. Qualitative requirements and utilization of nutrients: insects. In *CRC Handbook Series in Nutrition and Food*, ed. M Rechcigl Jr, pp. 305–46. Cleveland, OH: CRC

36. Dadd RH. 1985. Nutrition: organisms. See Ref. 70a, 4:313–90

37. Dadd RH, Kleinjan JE, Stanley-Samuelson DW. 1987. Polyunsaturated fatty acids on mosquitoes reared with single dietary polyunsaturated. *Insect Biochem.* 17:7–16

38. Dalton T. 1977. Threshold and receptor reserve in the action of 5-hydroxytryptamine on the salivary glands of *Calliphora erythrocephala. J. Insect Physiol.* 23:625–31

39. Dalton T. 1977. The effect of prostaglandin $E_1$ on cyclic AMP production in the

salivary glands of *Calliphora erythrocephala*. *Experientia* 33:1320–30

40. Dantuma NP, Pijnenburg MAP, Diederen JHB, Van der Horst DJ. 1997. Developmental down-regulation of receptor-mediated endocytosis of an insect lipoprotein. *J. Lipid Res.* 38:254–65

41. Dantuma NP, Potters M, De Winther MPJ, Tensen CP, Kooiman FP, et al. 1999. An insect homolog of the vertebrate very low density lipoprotein receptor mediates endocytosis of lipophorins. *J. Lipid Res.* 40:973–78

42. Dantuma NP, Van Marrewijk WJA, Wynne HJ, Van der Horst DJ. 1996. Interaction of an insect lipoprotein with its binding site at the fat body. *J. Lipid Res.* 37:1345–55

43. DeFoliart GR. 1999. Insects as food: why the western attitude is important. *Annu. Rev. Entomol.* 44:21–50

44. de Renobles M, Cripps C, Stanley-Samuelson DW, Jurenka RA, Blomquist GJ. 1987. Biosynthesis of linoleic acid in insects. *Trends Biochem. Sci.* 12:346–66

45. Destephano DB, Brady UE, Lovins RE. 1974. Synthesis of prostaglandin by reproductive tissue of the male house cricket, *Acheta domesticus. Prostaglandins* 6:71–79

46. Douglas AE. 1998. Nutritional interactions in insect-microbial symbioses: aphids and their symbiotic bacteria *Buchnera. Annu. Rev. Entomol.* 43:17–37

47. Downer RGH. 1985. Lipid metabolism. See Ref. 70a, 10:77–113

48. Edmunds M. 1974. *Defence in Animals: A Survey of Anti-Predator Defences.* New York: Longman. 357 pp.

49. Evans PD. 1985. Octopamine. See Ref. 70a, 11:499–530

50. Feltwell J. 1978. The distribution of carotenoids in insects. In *Biochemical Aspects of Plant and Animal Coevolution*, ed. JB Harborne, pp. 227–307. London: Academic

51. Fernando-Warnakulasuriya GJP, Tsuchida K, Wells MA. 1988. Effect of dietary lipid content on lipid transport and storage during larval development of *Manduca sexta. Insect Biochem.* 18:211–14

52. Fields PE, Woodring JP. 1991. Octopamine mobilization of lipids and carbohydrates in the house cricket, *Acheta domesticus. J. Insect Physiol.* 37:193–99

53. Ford PS, Van Heusden MC. 1994. Triglyceride-rich lipophorin in *Aedes aegypti* (Diptera: Culicidae). *J. Med. Entomol.* 31:435–41

54. Friend WG, Dadd RH. 1982. Insect nutrition. In *Advances in Nutritional Research,* ed. HH Draper, pp. 205–47. New York: Plenum

55. Goldsworthy GJ, Mordue W. 1989. Adipokinetic hormones, functions and structures. *Biol. Bull.* 177:218–24

56. Gondim KC, Wells MA. 2000. Characterization of lipophorin binding to the midgut of larval *Manduca sexta. Insect Biochem. Mol. Biol.* 30:405–13

57. Gordon HT. 1959. Minimum nutritional requirements of the German roach, *Blattella germanica. Ann. NY Acad. Sci.* 77:290–351

58. Grieneisen ML. 1994. Recent advances in our knowledge of ecdysteroid biosynthesis in insects and crustaceans. *Insect Biochem. Mol. Biol.* 24:115–32

59. Haunerland NH. 1997. Transport and utilization of lipids in insect flight muscles. *Comp. Biochem. Physiol.* 117B:475–82

60. Heed WB, Kircher HW. 1965. Unique sterol in the ecology and nutrition of *Drosophila pachea. Science* 149:758–61

61. Hobson RP. 1935. On a fat soluble growth factor requirement by blowfly larvae. II. Identity of growth factor with cholesterol. *Biochem. J.* 29:2023–36

62. Howard RW, Stanley-Samuelson DW. 1999. The tie that binds: eicosanoids in invertebrate biology. *Ann. Entomol. Soc. Am.* 92:880–90

63. Hui TY, Bernlohr DA. 1997. Fatty acid transporters in animal cells. *Front. Biosci.* 2:222–31

64. Joshi M, Agarwall HC. 1977. Site of cholesterol absorption in some insects. *J. Insect Physiol.* 23:403–4

65. Jouni ZE, Wells MA. 1996. Purification and partial characterization of a lutein-binding protein from the midgut of the silkworm, *Bombyx mori. J. Biol. Chem.* 271:14722–26

66. Kanost MR, Kawooya JK, Law JH, Ryan RO, Van Heusden MC, Ziegler R. 1990. Insect haemolymph proteins. *Adv. Insect Physiol.* 22:299–396

67. Kaplanis NJ, Robbins WE, Monroe RE, Shortino TJ, Thompson MJ. 1965. The utilization and the fate of $\beta$-sitosterol in the larva of the housefly, *Musca domestica L. J. Insect Physiol.* 11:251–58

68. Kawooya JK, Law JH. 1988. Role of lipophorin in lipid transport to the insect egg. *J. Biol. Chem.* 263:8748–53

69. Kawooya JK, Osir EO, Law JH. 1988. Uptake of the major hemolymph lipoprotein and its transformation in the insect egg. *J. Biol. Chem.* 263:8740–47

70. Kayser H. 1985. Pigments. See Ref. 70a, 10:367–415

70a. Kerkurt GA, Gilbert LI, eds. 1985. *Comprehensive Insect Physiology, Biochemistry and Pharmacology.* Oxford, UK: Pergamon

71. Komnick H, Giesa U. 1994. Intestinal absorption of cholesterol, transport in the haemolymph, and incorporation into the fat body and Malpighian tubules of the larval dragonfly *Aeshna cyanea. Comp. Biochem. Physiol.* 107A:553–57

72. Kutty RK, Kutty G, Kambadur R, Duncan T, Koonin EV, et al. 1996. Molecular characterization and developmental expression of a retinoid- and fatty acid-binding glycoprotein from *Drosophila. J. Biol. Chem.* 271:20641–49

73. Law JH, Wells MA. 1989. Insects as biochemical models. *J. Biol. Chem.* 264:16335–38

73a. Lehane MJ, Billingsley PF, eds. 1996. *Biology of Insect Midgut.* London: Chapman & Hall

74. Leroy B, Chararas C, Chipoulet JM. 1984. Etude des activites osidasques du tube digestif des adultes et des larves de la bruchhe du haricot, *Acanthoscelides obtectus* (Coleoptera: Bruucidae). *Entomol. Exp. Appl.* 35:269–73

75. Liu H, Ryan RO. 1991. Role of lipid transfer particle in transformation of lipophorin in *Manduca sexta* oocytes. *Biochim. Biophys. Acta* 1085:112–18

76. Lok CM, Van der Horst DJ. 1980. Chiral 1,2-diacylglycerols in the haemolymph of the locust, *Locusta migratoria. Biochim. Biophys. Acta* 618:80–87

77. McFarlane JE. 1976. Vitamin K: growth factor for the house cricket (Orthoptera: Gryllidae). *Can. Entomol.* 108:391–94

78. McFarlane JE. 1983. Lipid factors in insect growth and reproduction. In *Metabolic Aspects of Lipid Nutrition in Insects*, ed. TE Mittler, RH Dadd, pp. 149–57. Boulder, CO: Westview

79. Merritt RW, Dadd RH, Walker ED. 1992. Feeding behavior, natural food, and nutritional relationships of larval mosquitoes. *Annu. Rev. Entomol.* 37:349–76

80. Mitchell MJ, Smith SL. 1986. Characterization of ecdysone 20-monoonxygenase activity in wandering stage larvae of *Drosophila melanogaster.* Evidence of mitochondrial and microsomal cytochrome P-450 dependent systems. *Insect Biochem.* 16:525–37

81. Morgan MRJ. 1975. A qualitative survey of the carbohydrates of the alimentary tract of the migratory locust, *Locusta migratoria migratorioides. J. Insect Physiol.* 21:1045–53

82. Nair A, Agarwall H. 1977. Sterols and sterol esters in nutrition of the beetle *Trogoderma granarium* Everts. *Indian J. Exp. Biol.* 15:576–78

83. Ness WD, Lopez M, Zhou W, Guo D, Dowd PF, Northon RA. 1997. Sterol

utilization and metabolism in *Heliothis zea. Lipids* 32:1317–23

84. Orchard I. 1987. Adipokinetic hormones—an update. *J. Insect Physiol.* 33:451–63

85. Orchard I, Loughton BG. 1985. Neurosecretion. See Ref. 70a, 7:61–67

86. Passier PC, Vullings HG, Diederen JH, Van der Horst DJ. 1995. Modulatory effects of biogenic amines on adipokinetic hormone secretion from locust corpora cardiaca *in vitro. Gen. Comp. Endocrinol.* 97:231–38

87. Pease RJ, Harrison GB, Scott J. 1991. Co-translocational insertion of apolipoprotein B into the inner leaflet of the endoplasmic reticulum. *Nature* 353:448–50

88. Petzel DH, Stanley-Samuelson DW. 1992. Inhibition of eicosanoids biosynthesis modulates basal fluid secretion in the Malpighian tubules of the yellow fever mosquito (*Aedes aegypti*). *J. Insect Physiol.* 38:1–8

89. Prasad SV, Fernando-Warnakulasuriya GJ, Sumida M, Law JH, Wells MA. 1986. Lipoprotein biosynthesis in the larvae of the tobacco hornworm, *Manduca sexta. J. Biol. Chem.* 261:17174–76

90. Rimoldi OM, Peluffo RO, Gonzalez SM, Brenner RR. 1985. Lipid digestion, absorption and transport in *Triatoma infestans. Comp. Biochem. Physiol.* 82B:187–90

91. Rusinol AE, Jamil H, Vance JE. 1997. *In vitro* reconstitution of assembly of apolipoprotein B48-containing lipoproteins. *J. Biol. Chem.* 272:8019–25

92. Rustaeus S, Lindberg K, Stillemark P, Claesson C, Asp L, et al. 1999. Assembly of very low density lipoprotein: a two-step process of apolipoprotein B core lipidation. *J. Nutr.* 129:463–66S

93. Ryan RO. 1990. Dynamics of insect lipophorin metabolism. *J. Lipid Res.* 31:1725–39

94. Ryan RO, Prasad SV, Henriksen EJ, Wells MA, Law JH. 1986. Lipoprotein interconversions in an insect, *Manduca sexta.* Evidence for a lipid transfer factor in the hemolymph. *J. Biol. Chem.* 261:563–68

95. Ryan RO, Schmidt JO, Law JH. 1984. Chemical and immunological properties of lipophorins from seven insect orders. *Arch. Insect Biochem. Physiol.* 1:373–83

96. Ryan RO, Van der Horst DJ. 2000. Lipid transport biochemistry and its role in energy metabolism. *Annu. Rev. Entomol.* 45:233–60

97. Ryan RO, Wells MA, Law JH. 1986. Lipid transfer protein from *Manduca sexta* hemolymph. *Biochem. Biophys. Res. Commun.* 136:260–65

98. Sakura S, Warren TJ, Gilbert LI. 1989. Mediation of ecdysone synthesis in *Manduca sexta* by a hemolymph enzyme. *Arch. Insect Biochem. Physiol.* 10:179–97

99. Schal C, Sevala VL, Young HP, Bachmann JAS. 1998. Sites of synthesis and transport pathways of insect hydrocarbons: cuticle and ovary as target tissues. *Am. Zool.* 38:382–93

100. Seki T, Fujishita S, Ito M, Matsuoka N, Tsukida K. 1986. A fly, *Drosophila melanogaster*, forms 11-cis 3-hydroxyretinal in the dark. *Vis. Res.* 26:255–58

101. Seki T, Isono K, Ozaki K, Tsukahara K, Shibata-Katsuta Y, et al. 1998. The metabolic pathway of visual pigment chromophore formation in *Drosophila melanogaster.* All-*trans* (3S)-3-hydroxyretinal is formed from all retinal via (3R)-3-hydroxyretinal in the dark. *Eur. J. Biochem.* 257:522–27

102. Shapiro JP, Law JH, Wells MA. 1988. Lipid transport in insects. *Annu. Rev. Entomol.* 33:297–318

103. Shelness GS, Ingram MF, Huang XF, DeLozier JA. 1999. Apolipoprotein B in the rough endoplasmic reticulum: translation, translocation and the initiation of lipoprotein assembly. *J. Nutr.* 129:456–62S

104. Smith AF, Tsuchida K, Hanneman E, Suzuki TC, Wells MA. 1992. Isolation,

characterization, and cDNA sequence of two fatty acid-binding proteins from the midgut of *Manduca sexta. J. Biol. Chem.* 267:380–84

105. Soulages JL, Salamon Z, Wells MA, Tollin G. 1995. Low concentrations of diacylglycerol promote the binding of apolipophorin-III to a phospholipid surface: a surface plasmon resonance spectroscopy study. *Proc. Natl. Acad. Sci. USA* 92:5650–54

106. Soulages JL, Van Antwerpen R, Wells MA. 1996. Role of diacylglycerol and apolipophorin-III in regulating the physiochemical properties of the lipophorin surface: metabolic implications. *Biochemistry* 35:5191–98

107. Soulages JL, Wells MA. 1994. Effect of diacylglycerol content on some physicochemical properties of the insect lipoprotein, lipophorin. Correlation with the binding of apolipophorin-III. *Biochemistry* 33:2356–62

108. Soulages JL, Wells MA. 1994. Lipophorin, the structure of an insect lipoprotein and its role in lipid transport in insects. *Adv. Prot. Chem.* 45:371–415

109. Soulages JL, Wells MA. 1994. Metabolic fate and turnover rate of hemolymph free fatty acids in adult *Manduca sexta. Insect Biochem. Mol. Biol.* 24:79–86

110. Spring DJ, Chen-Liu LW, Chatterton JE, Elovson J, Schumaker VN. 1992. Lipoprotein assembly: apolipoprotein B size determines lipoprotein core circumference. *J. Biol. Chem.* 267:14839–45

111. Stagg LE, Candy DJ. 1996. The effect of adipokinetic hormones on the levels of inositol phosphates and cyclic AMP in the fat body of the desert locust *Schistocerca gregaria. Insect Biochem. Mol. Biol.* 26:537–44

112. Stahl A, Hirsch DJ, Gimeno RE, Punreddy S, Ge P, et al. 1999. Identification of the major intestinal fatty acid transport protein. *Mol. Cell* 4:299–308

113. Stanley-Samuelson DW. 1994. Prosta-

glandins and related eicosanoids in insects. *Adv. Insect Physiol.* 24:115–212

114. Stanley-Samuelson DW, Jensen E, Nickerson KW, Tiebel K, Ogg CL, Howard RW. 1992. Insect immune response to bacterial infections is mediated by eicosanoids. *Proc. Natl. Acad. Sci. USA* 88:1064–68

115. Stanley-Samuelson DW, Pedibholta VK. 1996. What can we learn from prostaglandins and related eicosanoids in insects? *Insect Biochem. Mol. Biol.* 26: 223–34

116. Sundermeyer K, Hendricks JK, Prasad SV, Wells MA. 1996. The precursor protein of the structural apolipoproteins of lipophorin: cDNA and deduced amino acid sequence. *Insect Biochem. Mol. Biol.* 26:735–38

117. Svoboda JA. 1999. Variability of metabolism and function of sterols in insects. *Crit. Rev. Biochem. Mol. Biol.* 34:49–57

118. Svoboda JA, Feldlaufer MF. 1991. Neutral sterol metabolism in insects. *Lipids* 26:614–28

119. Svoboda JA, Herbert EW Jr, Thompson MJ, Shimanuki H. 1981. The fate of radiolabeled $C_{28}$ and $C_{29}$ phytosterols in the honey bee. *J. Insect Physiol.* 27:183–88

120. Svoboda JA, Lusby WR. 1986. Sterols of phytophagous and omnivorous species of Hymenoptera. *Arch. Insect Biochem. Physiol.* 3:13–18

121. Svoboda JA, Robbins WE, Cohen CE, Shortino TJ. 1972. Phytosterol utilization and metabolism in insects: recent studies with *Tribolium confusum.* In *Insect and Mite Nutrition,* ed. JG Rodriguez, pp. 505–16. Amsterdam: North-Holland

122. Svoboda JA, Thompson MJ. 1985. Steroids. See Ref. 70a, 10:137–75

123. Terra WR. 1990. Evolution of digestive systems of insects. *Annu. Rev. Entomol.* 35:181–200

124. Terra WR, Ferreira C, de Bianchi AG. 1979. Distribution of digestive enzymes

among the endo- and ectoperitrophic spaces and midgut cells of *Rhynchosciara* and its physiological significance. *J. Insect Physiol.* 25:487–94

125. Terra WR, Ferreira C, Jordao BP, Dillon RJ. 1996. Digestive enzymes. See Ref. 73a, pp. 153–94

126. Thompson MJ, Weirich GF, Svoboda JA. 1990. Metabolism of insect molting hormone: bioconversion and titer regulation. In *Morphogenetic Hormones of Arthropods: Discovery, Synthesis, Metabolism, Evolution, Modes of Action, and Technique,* ed. AP Gupta, pp. 325–60. New Brunswick, NJ: Rutgers Univ. Press

127. Tran K, Boren J, Macri J, Wang Y, McLeod R, et al. 1988. Functional analysis of disulfide linkages clustered within the amino terminus of human apolipoprotein B. *J. Biol. Chem.* 273:7244–51

128. Tsuchida K, Wells MA. 1988. Digestion, absorption, transport and storage of fat during the last larval stadium of *Manduca sexta.* Changes in the role of lipophorin in the delivery of dietary lipid to the fat body. *Insect Biochem.* 18:263–68

129. Tsuchida K, Wells MA. 1990. Isolation and characterization of a lipoprotein receptor from the fat body of an insect, *Manduca sexta. J. Biol. Chem.* 265:5761–67

130. Turunen S. 1985. Absorption. See Ref. 70a, 4:241–78

131. Turunen S. 1993. Metabolic pathways in the midgut epithelium of *Pieris brassicae* during carbohydrate and assimilation. *Insect Biochem. Mol. Biol.* 23:681–89

132. Turunen S, Chippendale GM. 1977. Lipid absorption and transport: sectional analysis of the larval midgut of the corn borer, *Diatraea grandiosella. Insect Biochem.* 7:203–8

133. Turunen S, Crailsheim K. 1996. Lipid and sugar absorption. See Ref. 73a, pp. 293–320

134. Van Antwerpen R, Law JH. 1992. Lipophorin lipase from the yolk of *Manduca sexta* eggs: identification and partial characterization. *Arch. Insect Biochem. Physiol.* 20:1–12

135. Van Antwerpen R, Linnemans WAM, Van der Horst DJ, Beenakkers AMT. 1988. Immunocytochemical localization of lipoproteins in the flight muscles of the migratory locust (*Locusta migratoria*) at rest and during flight. *Cell Tissue Res.* 252:661–68

136. Van Antwerpen R, Linnemans WAM, Van der Horst DJ, Beenakkers AMT. 1989. Binding of lipophorin to the fat body of the migratory locust. *Insect Biochem.* 19:809–14

137. Van Antwerpen R, Salvador K, Tolman K, Gentry C. 1998. Uptake of lipids by developing oocytes of the hawkmoth *Manduca sexta.* The possible role of lipoprotein lipase. *Insect Biochem. Mol. Biol.* 28:399–408

138. Van der Horst DJ. 1990. Lipid transport function of lipoproteins in flying insects. *Biochim. Biophys. Acta* 1047:195–211

139. Van der Horst DJ, Van Marrewijk WJA, Vullings HGB, Diederen JHB. 1999. Metabolic neurohormones: release, signal transduction and physiological responses of adipokinetic hormones in insects. *Eur. J. Entomol.* 96:299–308

140. Van der Horst DJ, Weers PMM, Van Marrewijk WJA. 1993. Lipoproteins and lipid transport. In *Insect Lipids: Chemistry, Biochemistry, and Biology,* ed. DW Stanley-Samuelson, DR Nelson, pp. 1–24. Lincoln: Univ. Nebr. Press

141. Van Heusden MC. 1993. Characterization and identification of a lipoprotein lipase from *Manduca sexta* flight muscle. *Insect Biochem. Mol. Biol.* 23:785–92

142. Van Heusden MC, Law JH. 1989. An insect lipid transfer particle promotes lipid loading from fat body to lipoprotein. *J. Biol. Chem.* 264:17287–92

143. Van Heusden MC, Thompson F, Dennis J. 1998. Biosynthesis of *Aedes aegypti* lipophorin and gene expression of

its apolipoproteins. *Insect Biochem. Mol. Biol.* 28:733–38

144. Van Heusden MC, Van der Horst DJ, Van Doorn JM, Beenakkers AMT. 1987. Partial purification of locust flight muscle lipoprotein lipase (LpL): apparent differences from mammalian LpL. *Comp. Biochem. Physiol.* 88B:523–27

145. Van Heusden MC, Van der Horst DJ, Voshol J, Beenakkers AMT. 1987. The recycling of protein components of the flight-specific lipophorin in *Locusta migratoria. Insect Biochem.* 17:771–76

146. Van Kerkove E, Pirotte P, Petzel DH, Stanley-Samuelson DW. 1995. Eicosanoid biosynthesis inhibitors modulate basal fluid secretion rates in the Malpighian tubule of the ant, *Formica polyctena. J. Insect Physiol.* 41:435–41

147. Van Marrewijk WJA, Van den Broek ATM, Gielbert ML, Van der Horst DJ. 1996. Insect adipokinetic hormone stimulates inositol phosphate metabolism, roles for both $Ins,1,4,5.P_3$ and $Ins,1,3,4,5.P_4$ in signal transduction? *Mol. Cell Endocrinol.* 122:141–50

148. Venkatesh K, Lenz CJ, Bergman DK, Chippendale GM. 1987. Synthesis and release of lipophorin in larvae of the southwestern corn borer, *Diatraea grandiosella*: an *in vitro* study. *Insect Biochem.* 17:1173–80

149. Vogt K. 1983. Is the fly visual pigment a rhodopsin? *Z. Natureforsch. Sect. C* 38: 329–33

150. Vogt K. 1984. Chromophores of insect visual pigments. *Photobiochem. Phytobiophys. Suppl.* 7:273–96

151. Vogt K. 1988. Naming visual pigments. *J. Photochem. Photobiol. B* 2:133–34

152. Warren JT, Sakurai S, Rountree DB, Gilbert LI. 1988. Synthesis and secretion of ecdysteroids by the prothoracic glands of *Manduca sexta. J. Insect Physiol.* 34:571–76

153. Weer PMM, Van der Horst DJ, Van Marrewijk WJA, Van den Eijnde M, Van Door JM, Beenakker AMT. 1992. Biosynthesis and secretion of insect lipoprotein. *J. Lipid Res.* 33:485–91

154. Weintrab H, Tietz A. 1973. Triglyceride digestion and absorption in the locust, *Locusta migratoria. Biochim. Biophys. Acta* 306:31–41

155. Weer PMM, Van Marrewijk WJA, Beenakker AMT, Van der Horst DJ. 1993. Biosynthesis of locust lipophorin. Apolipophorins I and II originate from a common precursor. *J. Biol. Chem.* 268:4300–3

156. Wheeler CH, Goldsworthy GJ. 1985. Specificity and localization of lipoprotein lipase in the flight muscles of *Locusta migratoria. Biol. Chem. Hoppe-Seyler* 366:1071–77

157. Wu X, Sakata N, Lele KM, Zhou M, Jiang H, Ginsberg HN. 1997. A two-site model for apoB degradation in HepG2 cells. *J. Biol. Chem.* 272:11575–80

Annu. Rev. Nutr. 2001. 21:47–71

# NUTRITIONAL CONSEQUENCES OF THE AFRICAN DIASPORA

Amy Luke,[1] Richard S Cooper,[1] T Elaine Prewitt,[1] Adebowale A Adeyemo,[2] and Terrence E Forrester[3]

[1]*Department of Preventive Medicine and Epidemiology, Loyola University School of Medicine, Maywood, Illinois 60153; e-mail: aluke@luc.edu, rcooper@luc.edu, tprewit@luc.edu*
[2]*Department of Paediatrics/Institute of Child Health, University College Hospital, University of Ibadan, Ibadan, Nigeria; e-mail: andrew@ibadan.skannet.com*
[3]*Tropical Medicine Research Institute, University of the West Indies, Mona, Kingston, Jamaica; e-mail: tmru@infochan.com*

**Key Words** black populations, nutrition transition, undernutrition, obesity, hypertension

■ **Abstract** Along with their foods and dietary customs, Africans were carried into diaspora throughout the Americas as a result of the European slave trade. Their descendants represent populations at varying stages of the nutrition transition. West Africans are in the early stage, where undernutrition and nutrient deficiencies are prevalent. Many Caribbean populations represent the middle stages, with undernutrition and obesity coexisting. African-Americans and black populations in the United Kingdom suffer from the consequences of caloric excess and diets high in fat and animal products. Obesity, non–insulin-dependent diabetes mellitus, hypertension, coronary heart disease, and certain cancers all follow an east-to-west gradient of increasing prevalence. Public health efforts must focus not only on eradicating undernutrition in West Africa and the Caribbean but also on preventing obesity, hypercholesterolemia, and their consequences. Fortunately, a coherent and well-supported set of recommendations exists to promote better nutrition. Implementation of it founders primarily as a result of the influence of commercial and political interests.

## CONTENTS

## INTRODUCTION

In the 400 years following Columbus' landing on the island of Hispanola, 11–
13 million people were transported from sub-Saharan Africa to provide the primary productive force in the New World colonies. The Africans carried into diaspora by the European slave trade have grown into large populations in North
America, the Caribbean, Brazil and northern South America, and, via more recent
secondary migration, the United Kingdom. Smaller populations dot the coast of
Central America or have merged with the European majority in Argentina and
other Andean countries. The contemporary social and economic environments for
Africans vary more than for any other recognized macro-population group, ranging from traditional subsistence agriculture in much of West Africa and parts of
the Caribbean, to urban and peri-urban small-market economies in other parts of
the Caribbean, to post-industrialized societies in the United States and the United
Kingdom. The contrasts in economic conditions between these populations mir-
ror health and nutrition contrasts. In keeping with the historical experience of
other populations, moving across this spectrum of social settings from traditional
agriculture to industrialization, and as national and individual wealth increases,
nutrition-related concerns shift from privation (e.g. childhood stunting) to surfeit
(e.g. obesity). The African diaspora therefore offers a unique opportunity to observe the nutrition transitions among contemporary populations sharing a common
historical and genetic origin.

## HISTORICAL BACKGROUND TO THE
## AFRICAN DIASPORA

The ownership and exploitation of one human being by another has existed as a
societal institution throughout history. Slaves have occupied a surprisingly wide
range of social roles, although in recent history they have most often been consigned
to manual work under brutal conditions, usually with a minimum of food, clothing,
and shelter. Enslaved persons were considered chattel and as such were denied
freedom of activity and movement, had no rights in courts of law, and could be
sold or given away. Until the time of the Atlantic Slave Trade, which had its
beginning in the late fifteenth century, most slaves were war captives or debtors
(men who sold themselves and/or their wives and children to liquidate debt) (9).

Gradually through the Middle Ages, agricultural slavery in Europe evolved into
tenant farm and manorial systems. Tenant farmers were bound to the landowners
by debt, and serfs pledged their labor and loyalty in return for protection and the

use of a piece of land for subsistence. Though infrequently realized, it was legally sanctioned for a serf, through grueling labor and frugality, to buy his plot of land from the lord of the manor and become a freeman.

Slavery was not eradicated from European society, however. The practice of using slaves for domestic work continued, and sometimes people were sold into slavery as punishment. Slavery in Spain and Portugal continued through the Middle Ages, and from the time of first contact, the Hispanic colonists, to satisfy their need for human labor, instituted forced labor systems on the indigenous peoples of South America, the Caribbean, and Mexico. These systems were not sustainable, however, because of the brutality and overwork imposed on the Indian laborers and the susceptibility of the Indians to such diseases as smallpox, diphtheria, and tuberculosis brought by the colonists. Also, being on their home territory, the Indians who survived often escaped or banded together in revolt (9, 107, 118).

Soon, the Hispanic colonists turned to the nascent Portuguese slave trade on the West African coast to satisfy their need for labor. The first Africans enslaved by the Portuguese were settled in Europe in the late 1400s. In 1510, 250 Africans living in Spain were shipped to the island of Hispanola by the king of Spain to work in the gold mines (107). The first direct voyage from the islands of Cape Verde and São Tome off the western coast of sub-Saharan Africa to the Caribbean was made in 1533 and carried more than 500 Africans to labor on the sugar plantations. Hispanic colonists found the use of the Africans advantageous because they were skilled agriculturists, miners, and metalworkers, had a facility for languages, and were amenable to conversion to Christianity, and those who survived the march to the African coast and the passage to the Americas appeared to have immunity to many dangerous diseases. At least these are the historically recorded reasons; undoubtedly the already established European view that Africans were subhuman also played a critical role. By 1619, one million Africans were enslaved in the Americas, mostly on sugar plantations.

In this same year, a Dutch ship needing supplies docked at Jamestown, Virginia, and traded Africans for food. Although the change was gradual, indentured servitude in the United States was ultimately replaced by racial slavery. The demand for labor in the Americas was met by a systematized triangular trade in which English ships transported goods to the west coast of Africa. After exchanging goods for people, they continued on to the Americas, where they exchanged the people for agricultural produce, then sailed back to England. This arrangement grew into one of the most efficient international enterprises of its time, creating huge fortunes in England, France, and Portugal. By the same token, the extensive nature of the slave trade led to endemic warfare, radically changing the indigenous societies of the coast of Africa. Between the first transport of African slaves in 1533 and the last in 1870, approximately 11–13 million Africans were captured and sold at the coast, up to 1.5 million died on the Middle Passage to the Americas, and 10%–20% died within the first year in the Americas (9, 29, 107). Between 75% and 90% of Africans taken to the New World were transported from ports on the west coast of Africa between Senegambia in the north and Angola in the south (21, 29, 107) (Figure 1).

Based on the capture, enslavement, and transport of humans to wholly new cultures, the shipping business, the plantation owners of the South, and the merchants and shipbuilders of the North collectively accumulated much of the capital necessary to fuel the Industrial Revolution. In the broadest sense, therefore, African peoples laid one of the critical foundation pieces of the contemporary capitalist world. Unlike other immigrants, however, this sacrifice has never been rewarded, either in cultural or economic terms.

The former slave-holding colonies and nations in the Americas achieved their large current populations of Africans in separate ways. Brazil, for example, imported the largest number of slaves; Nigeria is the only nation with a larger black population. The United States, destination for only 5% of slaves, experienced rapid natural expansion. The Caribbean islands—Cuba; the former West Indies, including the Dominican Republic, Puerto Rico, Trinidad, and Tobago; the former British West Indies, including Jamaica, Barbados, and the Bahamas; and the former French West Indies, including Haiti—continually imported large numbers of slaves because of high mortality (9, 107). In addition, there are sizeable populations of African origin living in postcolonial Europe, most notably Britain, where people from the West Indies and British West Africa immigrated to meet labor demands after World War II (16, 102).

In addition to the large-scale forced migration of Africans, the triangular trade transferred cultural, agricultural, and dietary practices from Africa to the New World and back again. Crops such as sorghum, pearl millet, African rice, cowpea (black-eyed peas), African yams, okra, watermelon, bottle gourd, and fluted pumpkin were indigenous to Africa (47, 104). Yams were cultivated as early as 17,000–18,000 years ago on the African continent (47).

Although it is uncertain whether deep frying originated in Africa or the middle East, this cooking method traveled to the Americas with Africans. *Akara* from Nigeria, a fritter made by frying cowpea flour in palm oil, is a clear example of the movement of both crops and cooking method. The cowpea, palm oil, and frying method came to the New World with the Africans, probably Yoruba or Hausa slaves. The same fritter is made in Brazil (*acaraje*), Trinidad (*akkra*), and the French islands (*acrats*). Also, the foods in Bahia—the colonial settlement in northeastern Brazil where the Portuguese first brought Africans to work on plantations—are based on tropical oils, palm oil, and coconut. A rice porridge made with coconut milk called *acaca* is made in Colombia and northeastern Brazil. An identical dish with the same name exists in the Republic of Benin and in Nigeria (104).

Crops carried to Africa from the Americas by the Portuguese that became crucial to African agriculture include peanuts, sweet potatoes, and manioc (cassava). Additional foods carried to Africa by Europeans include maize, guavas, lima beans, pumpkins and squash, avocados, tomatoes, pineapples, papayas, and cashew nuts (104).

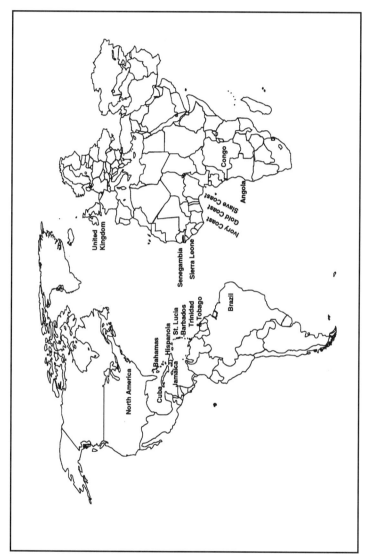

**Figure 1** Map of the Atlantic Ocean showing the primary regions involved in the slave trade between 1533 and 1870. The regions on the West African coast represent primary deportation sites whereas those in the Americas represent primary countries of importation. The United Kingdom is labeled as the site of secondary migration in the twentieth century, primarily from the English-speaking Caribbean.

## DIET IN AFRICA AND THE DIASPORA

Contemporary dietary data are sparse for sub-Saharan Africa in general and for West Africa specifically. Numerous studies list cassavas, yams, maize, or millet and sorghum as the top contributors of energy (8, 11, 80, 94, 108). The most prominent feature of this diet is the high degree of monotony, in terms of both the raw foodstuffs and the methods of preparation. The majority of available data indicate that 20%–25% of kilocalories in both rural and urban diets is supplied by fat (20, 55, 69, 88; E Choboso, unpublished information), most of which is palm, peanut, and corn oil. Recent studies from Cameroon suggest a higher proportion of kilocalories from fat (i.e. more than 40%); however, this estimate seems implausibly high (72, 101). In this study, cassavas, palm wine, and cocoyams were listed as the primary sources of energy in rural areas whereas in urban areas meat and fish were the top energy contributors.

Food-frequency questionnaire data collected in Spanish Town, Jamaica, indicate a higher percentage of kilocalories derived from fat (101; TE Forrester, unpublished information) than was observed in West Africa, 27%–30% versus 20%–25%. The primary energy sources listed in Jamaica were rice and peas (101). Consistent with trends in industrialized nations, it was estimated that the diet of African-Caribbeans living in Manchester, England, had a fat content between 32% and 35% (100). The chief energy contributors for this population were meat, rice, and peas.

Based on the results of the second National Health and Nutrition Examination Survey (NHANES II), the primary sources of kilocalories for all people in the United States were white breads, cookies and donuts, and meat (10, 70). Self-reported dietary data from NHANES III, however, suggest that diets of all ethnic groups have become more healthful, i.e. over the course of 30 years, the percentage of kilocalories from fat dropped from 38% (NHANES I) to 34% (NHANES III) (93). Still, the diet of African-Americans is characterized as high in fat and salt and low in fruits and vegetables (60). A comparison of diets indicated that those of southern-born African-Americans living in Harlem were less healthful than those of African-Americans born in other regions of the United States or in the Caribbean. African-Americans born in the Caribbean reported the lowest intake of fat (43).

In general, dietary data record an increase in the percentage of energy derived from fat as one moves from West Africa, to the Caribbean, to the United States and United Kingdom, as well as a marked increase in the consumption of refined foods and meat products. At the far end of the spectrum, the African influence has been completely submerged by commercial food patterns; a mixed or syncretic pattern remains in some regions of the Americas (e.g. Jamaica and Bahia, Brazil). For the great majority of West Africans, certainly for the 75% of the population living on subsistence farms, every day brings a meal much like the one the day before, and the ones of centuries before.

# NUTRITION TRANSITION AMONG POPULATIONS OF THE DIASPORA

The usual diet of rural, agriculturist West Africa and that of the industrialized United States represent the early and late stages, respectively, of what has been termed the nutrition transition (90). The changes in nutrient intake and dietary patterns effected by populations as social, cultural, and economic changes decisively influence the public health and thereby the course of the epidemiologic transition (90, 111). The epidemiologic transition can be defined as the changes in patterns of health, morbidity, and mortality that result from demographic shifts and associated economic and societal changes (111). Although these processes are most often used to describe the transition one population undergoes in a linear fashion over time, the African diaspora provides an opportunity to examine and compare separate stages of related populations at a single point in time. When viewed as a whole, the populations of the African diaspora represent differing stages of the transition while the individual countries are undergoing the transition at varying rates themselves.

Although the concept of integrated societal transitions is a useful organizing principle, much heterogeneity exists across societies and subpopulations within those societies. The demographic, epidemiologic, and nutrition transitions interact such that in the earliest stage, the high fertility and high mortality rates of traditional societies influence and are influenced by high prevalences of infectious disease and undernutrition. As societies shift to relatively low fertility rates and an increase occurs in the mean age of the population, noncommunicable diseases come to predominate, due in large part to shifts in dietary patterns (30, 90). Historically in countries now fully industrialized, as personal and community resources improved, the nutrition transition involved changes from traditional, agriculturally based low-fat, high-fiber diets to diets rich in animal fats, rich in refined and processed foods, and relatively low in fiber (111). In recent decades, the rapid urbanization of developing countries (44, 98) and the dramatic increase in the availability of inexpensive vegetable fats (30) have altered the historical pattern of the nutrition transition. In much of the developing world, the absolute number of poor and undernourished people living in urban areas has increased, as has the urban share of overall poverty and undernutrition (44). This pattern of urbanization, in combination with increased consumption of dietary fat and refined foods and changes in physical activity levels (30, 34, 91, 98), has created a situation in which the nutrition and epidemiologic transitions are occurring at ever-lower levels of economic development (30), and noncommunicable diseases are coexisting with infectious and nutrient-deficiency diseases (92, 99, 111).

Much of West Africa can be considered as being in the early stage of the transition processes. Sub-Saharan Africans contend with very high rates of morbidity and mortality from infectious disease, a situation that is worsening as the prevalence of HIV/AIDS increases (81), and they continue to struggle with undernutrition, manifested most prominently as stunting in children (5). In many Caribbean and South American countries of the diaspora, the nutrition and epidemiologic transitions are well under way, accompanied by increases in dietary fat intake and the prevalence of obesity and associated chronic diseases (38, 45, 116). At the same time, undernutrition among children continues to exist in many communities (75, 87, 99). The United States and United Kingdom represent the late stage of the epidemiologic and nutrition transitions. Chronic, degenerative diseases of nutrition excess are the leading causes of ill health among both African-Americans and the black populations of the United Kingdom (15, 78).

## UNDERNUTRITION AMONG CHILDREN OF THE DIASPORA

Although in the late twentieth century large-scale famines and frank starvation became relatively rare, except in regions embroiled in war or civil unrest (40, 45), undernutrition is still prevalent in many parts of West Africa and in some regions of the Caribbean and Latin America (33, 87).

Of the regions relevant to this report, West Africa experiences by far the greatest degree of undernutrition. In reporting the proportion of chronically undernourished people, the Food and Agriculture Organization of the United Nations estimates the minimum energy requirements of populations, i.e. 1.54 times the estimated average basal metabolic rate, and compares that with the available food supply (14, 35). Based on these criteria, between 1990 and 1996, 40% of sub-Saharan Africans did not have access to adequate supplies of energy (35). This burden is disproportionately experienced by children and childbearing women and is most extreme in populations undergoing governmental instability and/or armed conflicts (40). In children, depending on the time of deprivation, inadequate energy and/or protein intake manifest as stunting, i.e. height-for-age more than two standard deviations (SD) below the US National Center for Health Statistics reference values, or wasting, i.e. more than two SD below means of weight-for-height (113). Stunting, of course, reflects more than physical insults; more than acute wasting, it has been linked to delayed mental development and measurable deficits in behavior and cognitive performance in school-aged children (3, 42, 112).

A 1993 nutritional survey among Nigerian children between the ages of 6 and 71 months reported a national prevalence of 38% for stunting and 19% for wasting (33). This high degree of stunting has been observed in other West African surveys among preschool children, e.g. 61% stunted and 7% wasted in a smaller group of Nigerian children (2), and 27% stunted and 4% wasted in northern Ghana (106). Stunting is diagnostic of low energy intakes during critical stages of development; however, data collected by our group in rural southwestern Nigeria (Yoruba land) may offer some insight into the potential for catch-up growth in this population. Over 47% of the boys and 17% of the girls between the ages of 12 and 19 years had heights more than two SD below the mean of comparably aged African-American children. By adulthood, however, less than 10% of either gender was of short stature (25). The implications of this apparent adolescent catch-up growth for long-term health and cognitive performance are not clear and need further investigation.

Vitamin A deficiency is highly prevalent in most of the developing world, including West Africa. The overall prevalence of subclinical deficiency was reported as 9%–25% in Ghanian and Nigerian preschoolers (33, 106). The highest rate of clinical vitamin A deficiency, presenting as xerophthalmia, was reported as 1% in the Sahel and the northern arid regions of those countries (1, 5, 33). Although most West African dietary patterns include the intake of red palm oil, which has very high concentrations of carotenoids, and seasonal consumption of vitamin A–containing fruits, there is some evidence that vitamin A–rich foods are introduced into children's diets at a late stage (33). Iron-deficiency anemia among children and women of childbearing age is a significant problem in much of West Africa. Numerous surveys have estimated the prevalence rates of anemia to be from 55% to 92% in children (1, 33, 48, 106), 27% in adults, and 53% in pregnant women (48). There are many contributing factors to the high rates of iron deficiency, including the low intake of meat, fish, and vitamin C–containing fruits, the high intake of plant foods with low concentrations of bioavailable iron, and the endemic malaria parasitemia (33). As noted, most rural diets consist of relatively few foods (101; A Luke, unpublished information), which undoubtedly contributes to documented vitamin A and iron deficiencies and has a negative impact on overall health.

In the Caribbean and Brazil, the prevalence of childhood stunting and wasting have decreased significantly over the past 3–4 decades as economic and social conditions have improved (45, 75, 103). Based on national nutrition survey data, the prevalence of undernutrition in Brazil, defined as weight-for-age more than two SD below the National Center for Health Statistics reference means, fell by more than 60% between 1975 and 1989 (75), with an additional 20% drop between 1989 and 1994 (87). The cities were found to have about half the rate of undernutrition (10%) of the rural areas (19%) (74), and the highest prevalence was in the traditionally poor north and northeast regions of the country (74, 75). Similar decreases over the past three decades have been reported for Jamaica, e.g. between 1970 and 1985, the rate of undernutrition decreased from 10.8% to 8.0% (87, 103). Many of the Caribbean islands currently report similar levels of low weight-for-age (87, 103). The primary exception to this late-twentieth-century improvement in the nutritional status of children has been in economically depressed, politically unstable Haiti, where the prevalence of severe stunting in five-year-old children was greater than 40% in 1996 (87). Much of the regional decrease in rates of undernutrition in the Caribbean and Brazil has been attributed to modest improvement in family incomes associated with a substantial increase in health services and programs (75, 103, 112).

Although undernutrition is present among African-Americans and among the black populations in the United Kingdom and in the wealthier of the Caribbean nations, such as the Bahamas, the far greater concern is that of the dramatically increasing prevalence of overweight, obesity, hypercholesterolemia, and associated health risks among children (41, 103). These findings conform to the expectations for populations in the final stage of the epidemiologic and nutrition transitions. There continues to be a real need among governmental and health organizations to improve the nutritional status among children while avoiding the problems associated with increased buying power.

## ADULT ANTHROPOMETRICS AND OBESITY

The long-term impact of diet and nutrition, as well as overall health status, can be observed from the comparison of adult anthropometric values within and across the populations of the African diaspora. Comparison of heights and weights of adults within a population over time provides an indication of changes in the availability of energy and nutrient sources, balanced against the requirement for physical activity. Anthropometric and dietary data were collected in the late 1950s in seven villages in Nigeria (80) and in urban and rural sites in Jamaica (4). One of the first databases in the United States in which race was identified was the first National Health and Nutrition Examination Survey (NHANES I) (77). Mean height, weight, and body mass index (BMI) from these early studies were compared with data from more recent population-based surveys conducted by the International Collaborative Study on Hypertension in Blacks (ICSHIB) (see Table 1), described in more detail

**TABLE 1**   Change in height, weight, and body mass index (BMI) of Nigerian, Jamaican, and African-American adults[a]

| Determinant | N | Height (cm) M | Height (cm) W | Weight (kg) M | Weight (kg) W | BMI M | BMI W | Reference |
|---|---|---|---|---|---|---|---|---|
| Nigeria | | | | | | | | |
| 1959, rural[b] | 448 | 158.5 | 167.7 | 50.5 | 58.4 | 20.0 | 20.4 | 80 |
| 1995, rural | 1666 | 157.9 | 168.3 | 58.5 | 62.5 | 22.9 | 22.7 | 25 |
| Difference | | −0.6 | +0.6 | +8.0 | +4.1 | +2.9 | +2.3 | |
| Jamaica | | | | | | | | |
| 1963, urban | 736 | 159.0 | 170.2 | 60.3 | 66.1 | 23.9 | 22.8 | 4 |
| 1995, urban | 1031 | 161.9 | 172.9 | 74.0 | 71.7 | 28.2 | 23.9 | 25 |
| Difference | | +2.9 | +2.7 | +13.7 | +5.6 | +4.3 | +1.1 | |
| US | | | | | | | | |
| 1971–1974, national | 1333 | 162.7 | 174.7 | 71.5 | 78.1 | 26.9 | 25.6 | 78 |
| 1995, urban | 1151 | 163.9 | 177.0 | 82.2 | 84.6 | 30.5 | 26.9 | 25 |
| Difference | | +1.2 | +2.3 | +10.7 | +6.5 | +3.6 | +1.3 | |

[a]Mean values; ages 25–55 years. M, Men; W, women.

[b]Includes ages >13 years.

below (25). Although the sampling methods were not the same in the early and recent surveys, there was overlap in the sampling areas. For Nigeria, the 1959 data used in Table 1 were those collected from adults aged 25–55 years in two of the seven total villages in which cassavas and yams were the primary sources of energy; this diet was comparable to that of the ICSHIB sample (80). The 1959 Jamaican data were those collected in urban areas, again comparable to the ICSHIB sample (4). The ICSHIB sample from the United States was not significantly different in terms of height and weight from the African-American NHANES III sample (59).

As can be observed from Table 1, average height increased slightly between the surveys among the Jamaican and US samples but did not change over the 35-year interval in Nigeria. In contrast, weight and BMI increased between the surveys across all sites and for both genders, with the largest increases in BMI occurring among women. These data suggest that the availability of energy for adults has increased in each of these three populations over the 25–35 years between surveys. The lack of change in mean height among Nigerian adults further suggests that there was no increase in the supply of energy and/or protein during the vulnerable growth periods in childhood (113). These comparisons of adult anthropometric values over time provide some evidence of the extent of the nutrition transition within populations; from these data it is clear that women of African origin, particularly in Jamaica and the United States, have been affected by the changes in dietary patterns more than men.

The ICSHIB study was a large-scale project designed to describe the biological evolution of hypertension over the course of the African diaspora (6, 25). The aims of the first phase of the study were to determine the magnitude of associations between blood pressure and known major risk factors in each population, to compare levels of blood pressure and hypertension prevalence, and to determine the extent to which contrasts between populations were due to differences in the level of risk factors (6). The initial phase of the ICSHIB study was a population-based survey of over 10,000 individuals, aged 25–74 years, from West Africa (Nigeria, Cameroon), the Caribbean (Barbados, Jamaica, St. Lucia), the United States (Chicago, Illinois), and the United Kingdom (Manchester). In each site, height, weight, waist and hip circumferences, blood pressure, and urinary sodium and potassium were measured using standardized protocols (6, 25). In Nigeria, Jamaica, and the United States, body composition was estimated using bioelectrical impedance analysis (65, 66).

As illustrated by the reduced data sets presented in Table 1, for each of the measured anthropometric variables there was a distinct gradient in the mean values, with lowest levels observed in Nigeria and rural Cameroon and highest levels found in the United States, for both women and men (95). For example, height increased from a mean of 158.2 cm for Nigerian women to 163.4 cm for African-American women, with values in the middle for Barbados and Jamaica (160.5 cm). The same pattern was observed for height of men, and for weight and waist and hip circumferences of both genders. Mean body weight ranged from 57 kg for Nigerian women to 83 kg for US women, and from 62 kg among Nigerian men to 85 kg for US men. Waist circumferences among women ranged from a low of 74 cm to a high of 91 in Nigeria and the United States, respectively, with the same degree of variation in hip circumference (83, 95). Among men, waist circumferences ranged from 77 cm in Nigeria to 92 cm in the United States. In contrast to the wide variation in waist and hip circumferences, the mean waist-hip ratios did not vary across sites. Men from Nigeria, rural Cameroon, Barbados, and the United States had the same mean waist-hip ratio (0.88–0.89), whereas women from all sites except rural Cameroon did not differ in this measurement (0.79–0.82) (25, 95).

BMI displayed an increasing gradient in mean values from West Africa to the Caribbean to the United States for both men and women (53, 95). Among men, the lowest BMIs were from Nigeria (mean = 21.7) and rural Cameroon (mean = 23.5). BMI values were slightly higher among men in the Caribbean, Jamaica (mean = 23.8), St. Lucia (mean = 24.3), and Barbados (mean = 25.9), and highest in the United States (mean = 27.1). For women, there was a dramatic increase in mean values between West Africa and the Caribbean and the United States. In Nigeria and rural Cameroon, mean BMI of women was 22.6 and 23.5, respectively, whereas in Jamaica it was 27.9, in St. Lucia 27.3, in Barbados 29.4, and in the United States 30.8. There was a marked east-to-west increasing gradient in the prevalence of obesity, defined as a BMI ≥ 30.0 (79, 121) (Figure 2). The prevalence of obesity was lowest for Nigerian men (5%) and highest for African-American women (49%). In the three sites where body composition was estimated, Nigeria, Jamaica, and the United States, the levels of fat-free mass did not differ for

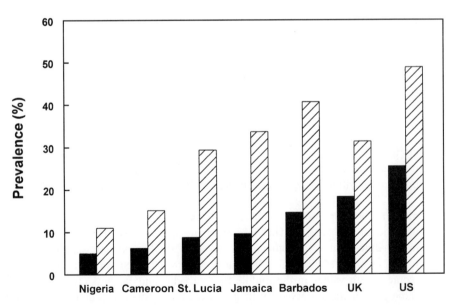

**Figure 2**  Age-adjusted prevalence of obesity, defined as body mass index ≥30, in seven populations of the African diaspora by gender; men are represented by solid bars, women by hatched bars. (Data from References 25 and 95.)

men (mean $=$ 57 kg) or women (mean $=$ 45 kg) (65). The difference in weight between these populations, as described above, was due to significant differences in fat mass within each gender across the three populations. Mean percentages of body fat levels were 11%, 19%, and 25% for men and 25%, 36%, and 40% for women in Nigeria, Jamaica, and the United States, respectively. Not only did adults in Jamaica and the United States have greater mean levels of body fat, the relationships between adiposity and BMI were shifted to the left, such that a BMI of 25 represented a body fat level of 16.4%, 22.2%, and 25.8% for Nigerian, Jamaican, and US men, respectively (65). The same shift was observed in women.

Obesity, of course, is a syndrome with a variety of potential underlying causes. Whatever the specific etiologies for the increases in obesity prevalence across the African diaspora, the consequences are readily observable in the morbidity and mortality patterns resulting from obesity-related chronic diseases, most notably non–insulin-dependent diabetes mellitus (NIDDM), hypertension and cerebrovascular disease, and coronary heart disease (CHD).

## DIABETES IN THE DIASPORA

More than any other chronic disease, NIDDM is most strongly associated with obesity, total body fat, and abdominal fat (82, 89). As a shadow cast by obesity, there is a distinct east-to-west gradient in the prevalence of NIDDM among adults of the diaspora (Figure 3) (26). In 1901, Albert Cook, a medical missionary to Uganda,

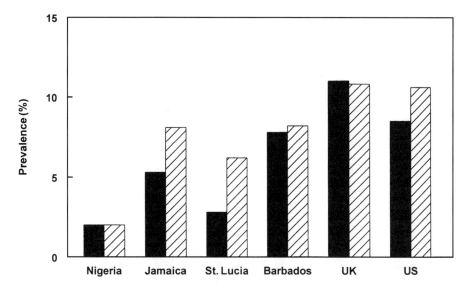

**Figure 3**  Age-adjusted prevalence of non–insulin-dependent diabetes mellitus, by self-report or fasting blood glucose $\geq 6.7$ mmol/liter, in six populations of the African diaspora by gender; men are represented by solid bars, women by hatched bars. (Data from Reference 26.)

recognized that diabetes was relatively rare in sub-Saharan Africa, reporting that "...diabetes is rather uncommon and very fatal..." (see 71). Since the 1960s, several studies have attempted to determine the prevalence of NIDDM in sub-Saharan Africa (57, 71, 86). Based on population samples ranging in age from 30 to 64, prevalences between 0.5% and 4% have been reported (26, 71, 76, 109). The exception appears to be the more urbanized, industrialized South Africa, where rates between 4.8% and 8.0% were recorded, and where obesity is also relatively prevalent (62, 73). The low prevalence rates observed in much of Africa may also be affected by the lack of treatment, and by the consequent high mortality. A recent study in rural and poor urban Nigeria suggests that as many as 20% and 35% of the elderly population were hyperinsulinemic and insulin resistant, respectively (31). It is hard to reconcile these data with estimates from the same communities of the prevalence of frank NIDDM being 2%, however, and this needs to be investigated further (26, 97). Even with the very low prevalence of NIDDM among indigenous Africans [rates are higher among Africans of Asian origin (56, 71)], a consistent positive association has been reported with BMI (26, 62, 109).

The positive association between BMI and NIDDM persists across the African diaspora, at both the individual and the population level. In the Caribbean the prevalence among black adults, especially women, increases sharply compared with those in West Africa (Figure 3). Based on self-report and/or fasting blood glucose concentration $\geq 6.7$ mmol/liter (120), the age-adjusted prevalences were 2.8%, 7.8%, and 5.3% for men and 9.0%, 8.4% and 10.4% for women in St. Lucia, Barbados, and Jamaica, respectively (26). Using a more stringent diagnosis based on an oral glucose-tolerance test in the same Jamaican population, Wilks et al reported a prevalence of 9.8% for men and 15.7% for women for NIDDM (117). In the Jamaican sample, the population's attributable risk for diabetes, i.e. the proportion of NIDDM in the population that is due to the exposure of being overweight (i.e. BMI $\geq 25$) was 66% and of having a waist-to-hip ratio greater than the median (0.80) was 80% (117). A multicenter study on NIDDM conducted in nine Brazilian cities between 1986 and 1988 reported a mean prevalence of 7.6% for the urban population aged 30–69 years, with higher rates in Sao Paulo (9.7%) and Porto Alegre (8.9%) (87). With the rate of obesity increasing in Brazil (74, 99), it is likely that current rates of NIDDM currently exceed these estimates.

In population-based samples from Chicago, Illinois, and Manchester, England, the overall age-adjusted prevalence of NIDDM among blacks was reported to be 10.6% and 10.8%, respectively (26, 97). In the United States, as in the Caribbean populations, the rate was higher for women than men (12.3% vs 8.5%, respectively). Among the African-Caribbean adults living in Manchester, however, no difference between genders was reported in this study (26). Separate studies conducted in London reported the prevalence of NIDDM to be somewhat higher than the Manchester study, about 15% and 18%, respectively, for men and women originating from the West Indies (15, 19).

Not only is NIDDM more prevalent among blacks in the western hemisphere relative to West Africa, it is also more prevalent among blacks than whites in both the United States (17, 56) and the United Kingdom (15). Although obesity is clearly a primary risk factor for the development of NIDDM, it does not completely explain the excess incidence of NIDDM in African-Americans. In a 16-year follow-up to NHANES I, African-American adults had one and a half to two times the incidence of NIDDM at comparable levels of obesity (64). Not only are the prevalence and incidence of NIDDM greater, health outcomes such as end-stage renal disease (28), retinopathy (46), and lower-extremity amputations (61) tend to be more frequent and severe among African-Americans. In contrast, an 18- to 20-year follow-up of diabetics in the United Kingdom reported comparable BMI and blood pressure but lower serum cholesterol levels and much lower risk ratios for all-cause (0.59) and coronary heart disease mortality (0.37) for African-Caribbean relative to European diabetics (19).

The prevalence of NIDDM increases colinearly with obesity among populations of the African diaspora, and blacks in the West currently have higher rates and suffer more comorbidities than do whites. With particular regard to NIDDM, a clear goal of public health nutritionists will be to minimize the increase in obesity that occurs as populations undergo the nutrition transition.

## HYPERTENSION IN THE DIASPORA

Hypertension is the most common cardiovascular condition in the world; the lifetime risk approaches 50% in most populations. Among the known risk factors for hypertension, nutritional aspects of lifestyle figure prominently, including obesity, a low intake of fruits and vegetables, and a high intake of sodium. Persons of African descent in the United States have been recognized since the 1930s to have a higher incidence of this condition than do whites (105). Early on, a tendency developed to think of the black experience with hypertension as an exceptional case and, despite limited evidence, to speculate that the condition was common in Africa (114). Recent large-scale surveys have in fact demonstrated low prevalences in rural Africa, with the expected gradient to urban areas, the Caribbean, and the United States paralleling trends in obesity and sodium intake (25, 53, 54). Among black populations in the West Indies, the hypertension burden is similar to that of US and European whites (i.e. 25%) (25), whereas in the United States, prevalences are significantly higher (i.e. 35%) (see Figure 4). The pattern of vascular disease, especially stroke, follows the gradient one would anticipate given the population levels of hypertension (84). The extent to which these trends are simply the result of multiple environmental exposures or unique predisposition on the part of this population group is much debated (27). In general, however, it is now clear that the pattern observed across populations of the African diaspora is consistent with what might be predicted from the epidemiologic experience.

In effect, the case for "black exceptionalism" rests on the slope of the cross-cultural gradient. That is, it remains possible that the rate of increase, given the exposures, is steeper than would be observed for other groups because the prevalences

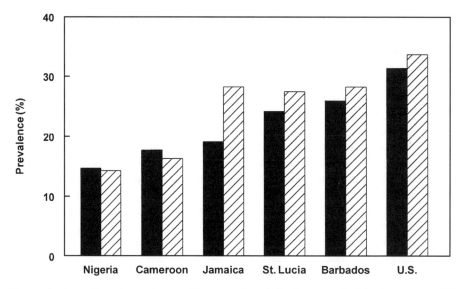

**Figure 4**  Age-adjusted prevalence of hypertension, defined as systolic blood pressure ≥140 mmHg and/or diastolic blood pressure ≥90 mmHg, or having treatment for hypertension, in seven populations of the African diaspora by gender; men are represented by solid bars, women by hatched bars. (Data from Reference 25.)

in the United States and the United Kingdom are higher than for whites. Of course, this exercise ignores the potential contribution of other less well-characterized factors, such as socioeconomic status and psychosocial stressors. Furthermore, it is not often recognized that among Finns, Russians, and Poles, hypertension rates are similar to those of African-Americans (22); whether all these populations achieve this exceptional status by the same route, namely nutritional excesses, or whether different combinations of risk factors are present in each group has not been well studied.

A more quantitative formulation of this question, that is, what proportion of the change in prevalence can be attributed to measured risk factors, quickly reveals the limitations of the epidemiologic method. A multistage analysis is required to answer this question. First, similar relationships need to be observed at the individual level between the exposures and the outcomes, e.g. salt and blood pressure. Second, the trends in exposures need to be collinear across populations, making it possible to ignore interactions, and the absence of unmeasured confounders must be assumed. If these conditions are met, an ecologic analysis could be undertaken, with the population as the unit of analysis and mean risk factor as the exposure. Clearly for diseases like hypertension, where one is trying to model lifetime effect of multiple, poorly characterized exposures, this analysis is approximate. Unfortunately, this imprecision has been interpreted as license to invoke genetic predisposition as the cause of more hypertension among blacks than whites in the United States and the United Kingdom (119).

An examination of the relative impact of specific nutritional factors across the African diaspora is complicated by the imprecision of the survey methods and the interactions that occur between them. Recent data suggest that in such low-risk groups as rural Nigerians, the associations between measurable exposures and blood pressure at the individual level are stronger than among high-risk groups, where multiple exposures coexist (12, 52). Thus, the correlation between 24-h sodium excretion and blood pressure was as high as 0.4 among rural Nigerian men compared with 0.10–0.15 for "westernized" populations (54). Preliminary data also suggest that the blood pressure response to changes in dietary sodium in these communities may be larger than seen elsewhere (A Adeyemo, unpublished information). By the same token, the correlation between BMI was also slightly greater in African groups (53). Parallel research on pathophysiologic measures, such as circulating hormone levels, reinforces the impression that the within-person relationships are better defined among the low-risk groups, implying that the underlying control mechanisms have become less disordered (37). This pattern, which has been confirmed in studies of experimental animals (H Jacobs, unpublished information), suggests that further insights into the evolution of disease patterns could be obtained by comparative studies across these populations (27). The potential also exists to use this "population laboratory" in combination with modern molecular genetic techniques to examine gene-environment interactions, and as a unique epidemiologic resource, the African diaspora could make it possible to address entirely new questions. Excessive concern with prevalence estimates and comparisons between whites and blacks has prevented many investigators from seeing this opportunity (119).

Although the quantitative results are only approximate, it is abundantly clear that nutritional status accounts for the majority of the increase in hypertension risk comparing Africans to African-Americans (53, 83). Not only are black populations in the west more overweight, they also consume much more sodium and have differing dietary patterns than do West Africans, e.g. Nigerians do not add salt to their food once it is prepared (54; A Adeyemo, unpublished information). The opportunities for prevention are therefore substantial. In fact, it is difficult to see how any progress toward prevention of this disease will take place without successful programs to reduce sodium in the food supply, maintain normal body weight, and increase intake of fruits and vegetables.

## OTHER NUTRITION-RELATED OUTCOMES

Data on prevalence and incidence rates for many other nutrition- and obesity-related chronic diseases, e.g. certain cancers, osteoarthritis, and sleep disorders, are sparse or nonexistent for much of sub-Saharan Africa and the Caribbean. The interaction of overall nutritional status and/or specific nutrients and cancer, in particular colon, breast, and prostate cancers, are extremely active areas of research. We hope future cross-cultural studies will shed light on the roles nutrition plays in the development and progression of cancer in black populations. CHD is another such disease; in this case, however, some data are available. Although limited, available data suggest a prevalence pattern among populations of African origin similar to that observed for NIDDM and hypertension, i.e. very low rates in West Africa, increasing rates in the Caribbean, and relatively high rates in the United States and United Kingdom. As with the other two diseases, the pattern for CHD follows the epidemiologic and nutrition transitions of the diaspora.

In Africa and much of the Caribbean, the proportion of mortality attributable to CHD is difficult to estimate with precision because of the overall dearth of vital status information (24). Much of the data for Africa come from the 1960s and 1970s, during which time CHD was documented at autopsy as the cause of death in 0.5% of examined cases in Uganda, 1.5% in Ibadan, Nigeria, and 1.2% in Accra, Ghana (49). In the Caribbean, the available mortality statistics suggest an increased rate of death due to CHD. Approximately 8% of all deaths in Brazil in 1995 and 23% in Cuba in 1996 were attributed to CHD, although it must be remembered that these are not race-specific data and the majority of Brazilians and Cubans are not of African descent (122). In Jamaica, 13.1% of all deaths between 1996 and 1998 were due to CHD (87). In the United States, CHD is the leading cause of death among both blacks and whites, with death rates of 99.4 and 86.4, respectively, per 100,000 resident population in 1996, or about 20% of all deaths for both races (78). Although the overall incidence rates are comparable between the races (23), blacks in the United States suffer a higher rate of fatal events, and for the first time since the CHD data were recorded in vital statistics, the age-adjusted death rates from CHD are higher among black than white men (63). The well-documented decline in CHD mortality since the mid-1960s has been steady among whites whereas the rate of decline has decelerated among blacks such that since 1980, the absolute mortality gap between blacks and whites has steadily increased (63). Among adults in the United Kingdom, black immigrants from the Caribbean and West Africa tend to have a significantly lower incidence of and mortality from CHD than do either their South Asian counterparts or European whites (7, 15, 115).

There are several causal risk factors for CHD, most significantly serum lipid levels, hypertension, smoking, and physical inactivity, which likely impact the differential CHD mortality rates observed in the populations of interest (58, 76). Differences in dietary patterns and obesity prevalence across the diaspora have influenced population-level serum lipid concentrations. Both population-based surveys (51, 85, 96) and those among targeted subgroups, i.e. civil servants (13) and rural and urban elderly (31), reported low total serum cholesterol concentrations among Nigerians relative to contemporary mean values for African-Americans. For example, mean serum cholesterol concentrations for Nigerian and African-American adults from the ICSHIB survey were 3.75 and 5.00 mmol/liter, respectively (96). Jamaican serum cholesterol values from the same survey fell between these two, 4.73 mmol/liter (R Wilks, unpublished information). In each of the NHANES and the Coronary Artery Risk Development in Young Adults studies, total cholesterol concentrations for African-American adults have been comparable to those for whites, whereas high-density lipoprotein cholesterol (HDL) levels tended to be higher among African-Americans, particularly men (23, 39, 110). In contrast, HDL levels for Nigerians and Jamaicans were lower than for African-Americans but comparable to whites (96; R Wilks, unpublished information). The differences in serum lipid levels observed among the populations of the diaspora are likely the result of high intakes of total and saturated fats in the West, which will increase both total and HDL cholesterol levels, and lower intakes of fats in Africa and the Caribbean, resulting in lower serum levels and lower risk for CHD mortality.

## SUMMARY

Millions of Africans were sacrificed through the trans-Atlantic slave trade to lay a critical piece of the foundation for the modern capitalist world. They brought with them many of their foods and dietary customs, which have had an impact on nutritional status throughout the Americas. The descendants of the African slaves in diaspora now represent populations at varying stages of the nutrition transition. West Africans, in the early stages of the transition, consume diets relatively low in fat and containing few highly processed foods. Undernutrition among children exists, and obesity and its adverse health consequences, e.g. NIDDM, hypertension, and CHD, are uncommon in most West African countries. Diets of Caribbean populations tend to have somewhat higher levels of fat, between 25% and 30% of total kilocalories. Undernutrition among children has declined sharply in the past few decades, but the prevalence of obesity and its sequelae are much higher in most Caribbean countries than in West Africa. The United States and the United Kingdom represent the last stages of the transition, in which public health concerns have shifted almost completely from undernutrition and deficiency diseases to those of excess, as illustrated by the very high prevalence of obesity and chronic diseases among black adults in these countries. It is hoped that with the awareness arising from public health research, the last stage of the nutrition transition will eventually be one in which obesity, NIDDM, CHD, and hypertension will be prevented or controlled and the majority of diets will be nutritionally replete. The African diaspora provides the opportunity for the investigation of the nutrition transition and dramatically illustrates the need for public health measures to be implemented in the Caribbean and West Africa to eradicate undernutrition while preventing obesity and its consequences.

**Visit the Annual Reviews home page at www.AnnualReviews.org**

## LITERATURE CITED

1. Adelekan DA, Adeodu OO. 1998. Anaemia in Nigerian mothers and their children: relative importance of infections and iron deficiency. *Afr. J. Med. Sci.* 28:185–87

2. Adelekan DA, Fatusi AO, Fakunle JB, Olotu CT, Olukoga IA, et al. 1997. Prevalence of malnutrition and vitamin A deficiency in Nigerian preschool children subsisting

on high intakes of carotenes. *Nutr. Health* 12:17–24

3. Allen LH. 1993. The nutrition CRSP: What is marginal malnutrition, and does it affect human function? *Nutr. Rev.* 51:255–67

4. Ashcroft MT, Ling J, Lovell HG, Miall WE. 1966. Heights and weights of adults in rural and urban areas of Jamaica. *Br. J. Prev. Soc. Med.* 20:22–26

5. Ashworth A, Dowler E. 1991. Child malnutrition. See Ref. 32, pp. 122–33

6. Ataman SL, Cooper R, Rotimi C, McGee D, Osotimehin B, et al. 1996. Standardization of blood pressure measurement in an international comparative study. *Clin. Epidemiol.* 49:869–77

7. Balarajan R. 1991. Ethnic differences in mortality from ischaemic heart disease and cerebrovascular disease in England and Wales. *Br. Med. J.* 302:560–64

8. Banea-Mayambu J-P, Tylleskar T, Tylleskar K, Gebre-Medhin M, Rosling H. 2000. Dietary cyanide from insufficiently processed cassava and growth retardation in children in the Democratic Republic of Congo (formerly Zaire). *Ann. Trop. Paediatr.* 20:34–40

9. Blackburn R. 1997. *The Making of New World Slavery*. New York: Verso. 602 pp.

10. Block G, Dresser CM, Hartman AM, Carroll MD. 1985. Nutrient sources in the American diet: quantitative data from the NHANES II survey. *Am. J. Epidemiol.* 122:27–40

11. Brieger WR. 1985. Food groups in cultural perspective. *Trop. Dr.* 15:42–43

12. Bunker CH, Okoro FI, Markovic N, Thai N, Pippin B, et al. 1996. Relationship of hypertension to socioeconomic status in a West African population. *Ethn. Health* 1:33–45

13. Bunker CH, Ukoli FA, Okoro FI, Olomu AB, Kriska AM, et al. 1996. Correlates of serum lipids in a lean black population. *Atherosclerosis* 123:215–25

14. Buttel F. 2000. Ending hunger in developing countries. *Contemp. Sociol.* 29:13–27

15. Cappuccio FP, Cook DG, Atkinson RW, Strazzullo P. 1997. Prevalence, detection, and management of cardiovascular risk factors in different ethnic groups in South London. *Heart* 78:555–63

16. Carlson E, Kipps M, Thomson J. 1984. Influences on the food habits of some ethnic minorities in the United Kingdom. *Hum. Nutr. Appl. Nutr.* 38A:85–98

17. Carter JS, Pugh JA, Monterrosa A. 1996. Non-insulin-dependent diabetes mellitus in minorities in the United States. *Ann. Intern. Med.* 125:221–32

18. Chadwick DJ, Cardew G, eds. 1996. *The Origins and Consequences of Obesity*. New York: Wiley. 278 pp.

19. Chaturvedi N, Jarrett J, Morrish N, Keen H, Fuller JH. 1996. Differences in mortality and morbidity in African Caribbeans and European people with non-insulin dependent diabetes mellitus: results of 20-year follow up of a London cohort of a multinational study. *Br. Med. J.* 313:848–52

20. Cole AH, Taiwo OO, Nwagbara NI, Cole CE. 1997. Energy intakes, anthropometry and body composition of Nigerian adolescent girls: a case study of an institutionalized secondary school in Ibadan. *Br. J. Nutr.* 77:497–509

21. Conniff ML, Davis TJ. 1994. *Africans in the Americas*. New York: St. Martin's. 356 pp.

22. Cooper RS. 1998. Geographic patterns of hypertension: a global perspective. In *Hypertension Primer: The Essentials of High Blood Pressure*, ed. LJ Izzo, H Black, pp. 150–53. New York: Lippincott, Williams & Wilkins. 374 pp.

23. Cooper RS, Ford E. 1992. Comparability of risk factors for coronary heart disease among blacks and whites in the NHANES-I Epidemiologic Follow-up Study. *Ann. Epidemiol.* 2:637–45

24. Cooper RS, Osotimehin B, Kaufman JS, Forrester T. 1998. Disease burden in sub-Saharan Africa: What should we conclude

in the absence of data? *Lancet* 351:208–10

25. Cooper RS, Rotimi C, Ataman S, McGee D, Osotimehin B, et al. 1997. The prevalence of hypertension in seven populations of West African origin. *Am. J. Public Health* 87:160–68

26. Cooper RS, Rotimi CN, Kaufman JS, Owoaje EE, Fraser H, et al. 1997. Prevalence of NIDDM among populations of the African diaspora. *Diabetes Care* 20:343–48

27. Cooper RS, Rotimi CN, Ward R. 1999. The puzzle of hypertension in African Americans. *Sci. Am.* 280:56–63

28. Cowie CC, Port PK, Wolfe RA, Savage PJ, Moll PP, Hawthorne VM. 1989. Disparities in incidence of end-stage renal disease according to race and type of diabetes. *N. Engl. J. Med.* 321:1074–79

29. Curtin PD. 1969. *The Atlantic Slave Trade: A Census.* Milwaukee: Univ. Wisconsin Press. 338 pp.

30. Drewnowski A, Popkin BM. 1997. The nutrition transition: new trends in the global diet. *Nutr. Rev.* 55:1905–16

31. Ezenwaka CE, Akanji AO, Akanji BO, Unwin NC, Adejuwon CA. 1997. The prevalence of insulin resistance and other cardiovascular disease risk factors in healthy elderly southwestern Nigerians. *Atherosclerosis* 128:201–11

32. Feachem RG, Jamison DT, eds. 1991. *Disease and Mortality in Sub-Saharan Africa.* London: Oxford Univ. Press. 356 pp.

33. Fed. Ministry Health Soc. Serv./USAID/VITAL/OMNI. 1996. *The Nigeria Micronutrient Survey 1993. Final Report.* Lagos, Nigeria: Fed. Ministry Health Soc. Serv. 105 pp.

34. Ferro-Luzzi A, Martino L. 1996. Obesity and physical activity. See Ref. 32, pp. 207–27

35. Food Agric. Org. 1998. *The State of Food and Agriculture 1998.* Rome: FAO. 396 pp.

36. Ford ES, Giles WH, Croft JB. 2000. Prevalence of nonfatal coronary heart disease among American adults. *Am. Heart J.* 139:371–77

37. Forrester T, Cooper R, Bennet F, McFarlane-Anderson N, Puras A, et al. 1996. Angiotensinogen and blood pressure among blacks: findings from a community survey in Jamaica. *J. Hypertens.* 14:315–21

38. Forrester T, Wilks R, Bennett F, McFarlane-Anderson N, McGee D, et al. 1996. Obesity in the Caribbean. See Ref. 18, pp. 17–36

39. Freedman DS, Strogatz DS, Williamson DF, Aubert RE. 1992. Education, race, and high-density lipoprotein cholesterol among US adults. *Am. J. Public Health* 82:999–1006

40. Goldman R. 1999. Food and food poverty: perspectives on distribution. *Soc. Res.* 66:283–304

41. Gortmaker SL, Dietz WH, Sobol AM, Wehler CA. 1987. Increasing pediatric obesity in the United States. *Am. J. Dis. Child.* 141:535–40

42. Grantham-McGregor SM, Cumper G. 1992. Jamaican studies in nutrition and child development, and their implications for national development. *Proc. Nutr. Soc.* 51:71–79

43. Greenberg MR, Schneider D, Northridge ME, Ganz ML. 1998. Region of birth and black diets: the Harlem Household Study. *Am. J. Public Health* 88:1199–202

44. Haddad L, Ruel MT, Garrett JL. 1999. Are urban poverty and undernutrition growing? Some newly assembled evidence. *World Dev.* 27:1891–904

45. Hagley KE. 1993. Nutrition and health in the developing world: the Caribbean experience. *Proc. Nutr. Soc.* 52:183–87

46. Harris EL, Feldman S, Robinson CR, Sherman S, Georgopoulos A. 1993. Racial differences in the relationship between blood pressure and risk of retinopathy among individuals with NIDDM. *Diabetes Care* 16:748–54

47. Harris JB. 1998. *The Africa Cookbook*. New York: Simon & Schuster. 383 pp.
48. Hercberg S, Galan P, Dupin H. 1987. Iron deficiency in Africa. *World Rev. Nutr. Diet.* 54:201–36
49. Hutt MSR. 1991. Cancer and cardiovascular disease. See Ref. 32, pp. 221–40
50. James WPT, Ferro-Luzzi A, Waterlow JC. 1988. Definition of chronic energy deficiency in adults. Report of a working party of the International Dietary Energy Consultative Group. *Eur. J. Clin. Nutr.* 42:969–81
51. Kadiri S, Salako BL. 1997. Cardiovascular risk factors in middle aged Nigerians. *East Afr. Med. J.* 74:303–6
52. Kaufman J, Rotimi C, Cooper R. 1999. Blood pressure change in Africa. A case study from Nigeria. *Hum. Biol.* 71:641–57
53. Kaufman JS, Durazo-Avizu RA, Rotimi CN, McGee DL, Cooper RS, ICHSHIB Invest. 1996. Obesity and hypertension prevalence in populations of African origin: results from the International Collaborative Study on Hypertension in Blacks. *Epidemiology* 7:398–405
54. Kaufman JS, Owoaje EE, James SA, Rotimi CN, Cooper RS. 1996. Determinants of hypertension in West Africa: contribution of anthropometric and dietary factors to urban-rural and socioeconomic gradients. *Am. J. Epidemiol.* 143:1203–18
55. Kigutha HN. 1997. Assessment of dietary intake in rural communities in Africa: experiences in Kenya. *Am. J. Clin. Nutr.* 65:1168–72S
56. King H, Rewers M, WHO Ad Hoc Diabetes Rep. Group. 1993. Global estimates for prevalence of diabetes mellitus and impaired glucose tolerance in adults. *Diabetes Care* 16:157–77
57. Kinnear TWG. 1963. The pattern of diabetes mellitus in a Nigerian teaching hospital. *East Afr. Med. J.* 40:288–94
58. Knuiman JT, West CE, Katan MB, Hautvast JGAJ. 1987. Total cholesterol and high density lipoprotein cholesterol levels in populations differing in fat and carbohydrate intake. *Arteriosclerosis* 7:612–19
59. Kuczmarski RJ, Flegal KM, Campbell SM, Johnson CL. 1994. Increasing prevalence of overweight among US adults. *JAMA* 272:205–11
60. Kumanyika S. 1993. Diet and nutrition as influences on the morbidity/mortality gap. *Ann. Epidemiol.* 3:154–58
61. Lavery LA, Ashry HR, van Houtum W, Pugh JA, Harkless LB, Basu S. 1996. Variation in the incidence and proportion of diabetes-related amputations in minorities. *Diabetes Care* 19:48–52
62. Levitt NS, Katzenellenbogen JM, Bradshaw D, Hoffman MN, Bonnici F. 1993. The prevalence and identification of risk factors for NIDDM in urban Africans in Cape Town, South Africa. *Diabetes Care* 16:601–7
63. Liao Y, Cooper RS. 1995. Continued adverse trends in coronary heart disease mortality among blacks, 1980–91. *Public Health Rep.* 110:572–79
64. Lipton RB, Liao Y, Cao G, Cooper RS, McGee D. 1993. Determinants of incident non-insulin-dependent diabetes mellitus among blacks and whites in a national sample. *Am. J. Epidemiol.* 138:826–39
65. Luke A, Durazo-Arvizu R, Rotimi C, Prewitt TE, Forrester TE, et al. 1997. Relation between body mass index and body fat in black population samples from Nigeria, Jamaica, and the United States. *Am. J. Epidemiol.* 145:620–28
66. Luke AH, Rotimi CN, Cooper RS, Long AE, Forrester TE, et al. 1998. Leptin and body composition of Nigerians, Jamaicans, and US blacks. *Am. J. Clin. Nutr.* 67:391–96
67. Macfarlane S, Racelis M, Muli-Muslime F. 2000. Public health in developing countries. *Lancet* 356:841–46
68. Martorell R, Kettel Khan L, Hughes ML, Grummer-Strawn LM. 2000. Obesity in women from developing countries. *Eur. J. Clin. Nutr.* 54:247–52

69. Mazengo MC, Simell O, Lukmanji Z, Shirima R, Karvetti R-L. 1997. Food consumption in rural and urban Tanzania. *Acta Trop.* 68:313–26

70. McDowell MA, Briefel RR, Alaimo K, Bischof AM, Caughman CR, et al. 1994. Energy and micronutrient intakes of persons age 2 months and over in the United States: Third National Health and Nutrition Examination Survey, Phase 1, 1988–91. *Adv. Data Natl. Cent. Health Stat.* 255:1–23

71. McLarty DG, Pollitt C, Swai ABM. 1990. Diabetes in Africa. *Diabetes Med.* 7:670–84

72. Mennen LI, Mbanya JC, Cade J, Balkau B, Sharma S, et al. 2000. The habitual diet in rural and urban Cameroon. *Eur. J. Clin. Nutr.* 54:150–54

73. Mollentze WF, Moore AJ, Steyn AF, Joubert G, Steyn K, et al. 1995. Coronary heart disease risk factors in a rural and urban Orange Free State black population. *S. Afr. Med. J.* 85:90–96

74. Mondini L, Monteiro CA. 1997. The stage of nutrition transition in different Brazilian regions. *Arch. Latinoam. Nutr.* 47:17–24

75. Monteiro CA, Benicio MH, Iunes R, Gouveia NC, Taddei JAAC, Cardoso MAA. 1992. Nutritional status of Brazilian children: trends from 1975 to 1989. *Bull. WHO* 70:657–66

76. Muna WFT. 1993. Cardiovascular disorders in Africa. *World Health Stat. Q.* 46:125–32

77. Natl. Cent. Health Stat. 1979. *Weight by Height and Age for Adults 18–74 Years: United States, 1971–1974. Vital and Health Stat., Ser. 11, No. 208.* Washington, DC: US Gov. Print. Off.

78. Natl. Cent. Health Stat. 1998. *Health, United States, 1998 with Socioeconomic Status and Health Chartbook.* Hyattsville, MD: Natl. Cent. Health Stat. 460 pp.

79. Natl. Inst. Health. 1998. Clinical guidelines on the identification, evaluation, and treatment of overweight and obesity in adults—

the evidence report. *Obes. Res.* 6:51–209S

80. Nicol BM. 1959. The protein requirement of Nigerian peasant farmers. *Br. J. Nutr.* 13:307–20

81. Ofosu-Amaah S. 1991. Disease in sub-Saharan Africa: an overview. See Ref. 32, pp. 119–21

82. Okosun IS, Cooper RS, Rotimi CN, Osotimehin B, Forrester T. 1998. Association of waist circumference with risk of hypertension and type 2 diabetes in Nigerians, Jamaicans, and African-Americans. *Diabetes Care* 21:1836–42

83. Okosun IS, Forrester TE, Rotimi CN, Osotimehin BO, Muna W, Cooper RS. 1999. Abdominal obesity in six populations of West African descent: prevalence and population attributable fraction of hypertension. *Obes. Res.* 7:453–62

84. Okosun IS, Muna WFT, Cooper R. 1998. International epidemiology of stroke in African populations outside the United States. In *Stroke in Blacks: A Guide to Management and Prevention*, ed. PB Gorelick, ES Cooper, RF Gillum, pp. 70–83. New York: Karger. 230 pp.

85. Ononogbu IC. 1979. Comparison of high density lipoprotein and serum cholesterol levels in a European and an African community. *Atherosclerosis* 34:49–52

86. Osuntokun BO, Akinkugbe FM, Francis TI, Reddy S, Osuntokun O, Taylor GOL. 1971. Diabetes mellitus in Nigerians: a study of 832 patients. *West Afr. Med. J.* 20:295–312

87. Pan Am. Health Org. 1999. *Basic Country Health Profiles, Summaries.* http://www.paho.org

88. Phillips PG. 1954. The metabolic cost of common West African agricultural activities. *J. Trop. Med.* 57:12–20

89. Pontiroli AE, Galli L. 1998. Duration of obesity is a risk factor for non-insulin-dependent diabetes mellitus, not for arterial hypertension or hyperlipidaemia. *Acta Diabetol.* 35:130–36

90. Popkin BM. 1994. The nutrition transition

in low-income countries: an emerging crisis. *Nutr. Rev.* 52:285–98

91. Popkin BM, Paeratakul S, Zhai F, Ge K. 1995. A review of dietary and environmental correlates of obesity with emphasis on developing countries. *Obes. Res.* 3:145–53S

92. Popkin BM, Richards MK, Monteiro CA. 1996. Stunting is associated with overweight in children of four nations that are undergoing the nutrition transition. *J. Nutr.* 126:3009–16

93. Popkin BM, Siega-Riz AM, Haines PS. 1996. A comparison of dietary trends among racial and socioeconomic groups in the United States. *N. Engl. J. Med.* 335:716–20

94. Ross PJ, Etkin NL, Muazzamu I. 1996. A changing Hausa diet. *Med. Anthropol.* 17:143–63

95. Rotimi CN, Cooper RS, Ataman SL, Osotimehin B, Kadiri S, et al. 1995. Distribution of anthropometric variables and the prevalence of obesity in populations of West African origin: the International Collaborative Study on Hypertension in Blacks. *Obes. Res.* 3:95–105S

96. Rotimi CN, Cooper RS, Marcovina SM, McGee D, Owoaje E, Ladipo M. 1997. Serum distribution of lipoprotein(a) in African Americans and Nigerians: potential evidence for a genotype-environmental effect. *Genet. Epidemiol.* 14:157–68

97. Rotimi CN, Cooper RS, Okosun IS, Olatunbosun ST, Bella AF, et al. 1999. Prevalence of diabetes and impaired glucose tolerance in Nigerians, Jamaicans and US blacks. *Ethn. Dis.* 9:190–200

98. Ruel MT, Haddad L, Garrett JL. 1999. Some urban facts of life: implications for research and policy. *World Dev.* 27:1917–38

99. Sawaya AL, Dallal G, Solymos G, de Sousa MH, Ventura ML, et al. 1995. Obesity and malnutrition in a shantytown population in the city of São Paulo, Brazil. *Obes. Res.* 3:107–15S

100. Sharma S, Cade J, Griffiths S, Cruickshank K. 1998. Nutrient intakes among UK African-Caribbeans: changing risk of coronary heart disease. *Lancet* 352:114–15

101. Sharma S, Cade J, Jackson M, Mbanya JC, Chungong S, et al. 1996. Development of food frequency questionnaires in three population samples of African origin from Cameroon, Jamaica and Caribbean migrants to the UK. *Eur. J. Clin. Nutr.* 50:479–86

102. Shyllon F. 1993. Blacks in Britain: a historical and analytical overview. In *Global Dimensions of the African Diaspora*, ed. JE Harris, pp. 223–48. Washington, DC: Howard Univ. Press. 532 pp.

103. Sinha DP. 1988. Nutrition in the English-speaking Caribbean: a brief review of the changes over the last three decades. *Cajanus* 21:113–32

104. Sokolov R. 1991. *Why We Eat What We Eat.* New York: Summit. 255 pp.

105. Stamler J, Stamler R, Pullman TN, eds. 1967. *The Epidemiology of Hypertension.* New York: Grune & Stratton. 472 pp.

106. Takyi EEK. 1999. Nutritional status and nutrient intake of preschool children in northern Ghana. *East Afr. Med. J.* 76:510–15

107. Thomas H. 1997. *The Slave Trade.* New York: Simon & Schuster. 908 pp.

108. Thomas HM. 1972. Some aspects of food and nutrition in Sierra Leone. *World Rev. Nutr. Diet.* 14:48–58

109. van der Sande MAB, Bailey R, Faal H, Banya WAS, Dolin P, et al. 1997. Nationwide prevalence study of hypertension and related noncommunicable diseases in the Gambia. *Trop. Med. Int. Health* 2:1039–48

110. Van Horn LV, Ballew C, Liu K, Ruth K, McDonald A, et al. 1991. Diet, body size, and plasma lipids-lipoproteins in young adults: differences by race and sex. *Am. J. Epidemiol.* 133:9–23

111. Vorster HH, Bourne LT, Venter CS, Oosthuizen W. 1999. Contribution of nutrition to the health transition in developing countries: a framework for research and intervention. *Nutr. Rev.* 57:341–49

112. Waterlow JC. 1979. Childhood malnutrition—the global problem. *Proc. Nutr. Soc.* 38:1–9

113. Waterlow JC. 1994. Childhood malnutrition in developing nations: looking backward and looking forward. *Annu. Rev. Nutr.* 14:1–19

114. White PD. 1967. Hypertension and atherosclerosis in the Congo and in the Gabon. See Ref. 105, pp. 150–54

115. Wild S, McKeigue P. 1997. Cross sectional analysis of mortality by country of birth in England and Wales, 1970–92. *Br. Med. J.* 314:705–10

116. Wilks R, McFarlane-Anderson N, Bennett F, Fraser H, McGee D, et al. 1996. Obesity in peoples of the African diaspora. See Ref. 18, pp. 37–53

117. Wilks R, Rotimi C, Bennett F, McFarlane-Anderson N, Kaufman JS, et al. 1999. Diabetes in the Caribbean: results of a population survey from Spanish Town, Jamaica. *Diabetic Med.* 16:875–83

118. Williams E. 1970. *From Columbus to Castro. The History of the Caribbean.* New York: Random House. 576 pp.

119. Wilson TW, Grim CE. 1991. Biohistory of slavery and blood pressure differences in blacks today. *Hypertension* 17:I122–28

120. World Health Org. 1980. *WHO Expert Committee on Diabetes Mellitus. Second Rep.* Geneva, Switzerland: WHO. 262 pp.

121. World Health Org. 1998. *Obesity. Preventing and Managing the Global Epidemic. Rep. WHO Consult. Obes.* Geneva, Switzerland: WHO. 276 pp.

122. World Health Org. 2000. *World Health Statistics Annual Mortality Data. WHO Statistical Information System.* http://www.who.org

Annu. Rev. Nutr. 2001. 21:73–95

# THE "FETAL ORIGINS" HYPOTHESIS: Challenges and Opportunities for Maternal and Child Nutrition

## Kathleen Maher Rasmussen
*Division of Nutritional Sciences, Cornell University, Ithaca, New York 14583, and Danish Epidemiology Science Centre, Institute of Preventive Medicine, Copenhagen University Hospital, Copenhagen, Denmark; e-mail: kmr5@cornell.edu*

**Key Words**　birth weight, maternal nutritional status, programming, supplementation, chronic disease

■ **Abstract**　The "fetal origins" hypothesis postulates that conditions, most likely nutritional, "program" the fetus for the development of chronic diseases in adulthood. Associations between the newborn's size at birth and various determinants or consequences of chronic diseases have been identified in many, but not all, of the available studies. It remains to be established whether these associations are causal. Remarkably little information is available on the specific role of maternal nutritional status. The role of birth weight remains difficult to interpret except as a proxy for events in intrauterine life. Unfortunately, birth weight does not make an important contribution to the population attributable risk of cardiovascular disease; lifestyle factors during adulthood make much greater contributions. Data from experimental species suggest possible mechanisms for the origin of chronic disease early in life. It is too soon to use this research as a basis for new interventions directed at pregnant women for the purpose of reducing chronic disease in their offspring.

## CONTENTS

0199-9885/01/0715-0073$14.00

**73**

# INTRODUCTION

In the late 1980s, Barker introduced what has come to be known as the "fetal origins" hypothesis. It states that "... poor nutrition, health, and development among girls and young women is the origin of high death rates from cardiovascular disease in the next generation.... The fetus responds to undernutrition with permanent changes in its physiology and metabolism, and these lead to coronary heart disease and stroke in adult life" (7). Size at birth is thought to be linked to chronic disease in adulthood via "programming." According to Lucas (67), "programming occurs when an early stimulus or insult, operating at a critical or sensitive period, results in a permanent or long-term change in the structure or function of the organism." This "occurs because different systems and organs of the body develop in fetal life and infancy during critical and sometimes brief periods" (5). Over time and with additional data, Barker has expanded this hypothesis to distinguish between effects that might occur if fetal growth were compromised at different periods of gestation. In particular, he has proposed that compromises to fetal growth in the first trimester of pregnancy might result in hemorrhagic stroke via raised blood pressure; in the second trimester, in coronary heart disease (CHD) via insulin resistance or deficiency, and in the third trimester, in both CHD and thrombotic stroke via growth hormone resistance or deficiency (8).

That there are "critical periods of development" has been known since the 1920s (105). That the events that occur during such periods have consequences far beyond infancy also has been known for many decades. What is novel here is the notion that events in early life might be linked to such chronic degenerative diseases as non–insulin dependent diabetes mellitus (NIDDM) and cardiovascular disease (CVD), which do not usually appear until mid-life or later.

This concept is important because, according to Barker, it represents "a new point of departure for cardiovascular disease research" (6). Such a new point of departure was needed because "the search for influences in the adult environment that lead to the disease has met with limited success" and "adult lifestyle is a poor predictor of individual risk for CVD" (6). If supported, Barker's ideas could aid scientists in identifying new ways of preventing chronic disease. Inasmuch as such chronic conditions now cause the majority of deaths in both developed and developing countries (121), and their contribution to total mortality can only be expected to rise in the coming years, careful attention to the fetal origins hypothesis is certainly warranted.

The fetal origins hypothesis has already been the subject of numerous reviews by Barker and his coworkers (e.g. 5, 6, 9, 10, 12, 13, 32–34, 38), several books (e.g. 7, 11), and many reviews, editorials, and critiques by others (e.g. 2, 24, 39 49, 50, 55, 64, 68–70, 78, 80, 83, 100). In addition, there is now a book on this topic for the lay public (85) that in 1999 was the impetus for a cover story in *Newsweek* (14). In the past year alone, several small scientific meetings that were focused on these ideas were held, and in 2001, the First World Congress on Fetal Origins of Adult Disease will take place in India. To avoid redundancy, this review focuses on the implications of the fetal origins hypothesis for maternal and child health because, if supported, these ideas could change current concepts about, for example, optimal weight at birth and recommendations for maternal weight gain during pregnancy. The fetal origins hypothesis is reviewed from this perspective with particular attention to the importance of maternal nutritional status (MNS) and birth weight (BW). The implications of these findings for public health policy are then explored.

## THE MEANING OF BIRTH WEIGHT

The determinants and consequences of the infant's size at birth are well understood (e.g. 22, 53, 55). Most of the morbidity and mortality associated with small size at birth is related to the duration of gestation, not the rate of growth in utero. In other words, it is preterm birth—not low BW (LBW) per se—that is the primary cause of the excess morbidity and mortality in the perinatal period and shortly thereafter. Worldwide, however, small size at birth is much more common than is premature delivery.

### Low Birth Weight

LBW is usually defined as a weight at delivery of $<2500$ g for an infant born at term ($\geq 37$ completed weeks of gestation) (122). In developed countries, most LBW infants are preterm; the opposite is true in developing countries (112). Infants can also be characterized as small or large for their gestational age relative to an appropriate reference population (118). This approach provides a statistical definition of small size at birth and identifies those who are born at a relatively lower weight, but it does not provide information on the trajectory with which they reached this weight. In other words, it does not distinguish those who grew slowly throughout gestation from those whose growth faltered during gestation (3). It is important to recognize that some small babies have achieved their genetic potential, are not "growth retarded" and are properly in the lower tail of the distribution of BW for gestational age. Others, however, may have suffered from some time-limited insult or long-term condition that suppressed their growth, be properly classified as growth-retarded, and still be of appropriate weight for their gestational age. The classic example of this situation is the infant born to the tall, well-nourished cigarette smoker (23). It also has recently been suggested that babies who are small relative to their mothers' BW are at increased risk of mortality (100a). Thus, it is difficult to identify accurately which infant is growth retarded, yet it is important to know why this condition occurred before choosing a treatment for it.

The postnatal growth of small-for-gestational-age infants is strongly influenced by their length and body mass index at birth as well as by their "target height" (74) and may be modified by the way they are fed (71). However, although there is catch-up growth in the early months of life, babies who are born small—even in developed countries—tend to stay small throughout childhood (44). They remain lighter and shorter and have smaller head circumferences (generally about −0.5 standard deviations) than do babies born at weights appropriate for their gestational ages. Nor do they accumulate fat at greater rates. In fact, at 6 years of age, they have a relative deficit of fat (45). According to Martorell et al (76), in the literature on intrauterine growth retardation, there is no support for a relationship between LBW and greater fatness at follow-up.

It has been postulated that, among term infants, absolute weight is less important than body proportionality for the development of chronic diseases in adulthood. Further, it has been postulated that the different fetal phenotypes are associated with different long-term outcomes: proportionally small and reduced BW with hemorrhagic stroke, thin and reduced BW with CHD, and short and normal BW with CHD and thrombotic stroke (7, 13). These different phenotypes are distinguished by their ponderal index (weight/height$^3$). Body proportionality was first advanced as a way to disentangle the heterogenous determinants of intrauterine growth retardation (97), and it was proposed that body proportionality reflected the timing of the intrauterine insult (111). However, critical analysis does not support this concept or the idea that MNS is an important determination of fetal proportionality—at least in well-nourished populations (58). Rather, it appears that body proportionality at birth reflects the severity of the intrauterine insult (57), and once this is accounted for, proportionality is of little additional use in predicting risk of adverse outcomes in the perinatal period (59). It is perhaps not surprising then that studies on the fetal origins hypothesis that have been based on the concepts of body proportionality have produced inconsistent findings (50).

## High Birth Weight

At the other extreme of the distribution of BW, prematurity is infrequent; babies may be postmature instead. High BW (>4000 g, "macrosomia") is associated with a variety of negative outcomes for both the mother and the infant. Determinants of macrosomia include (*a*) high maternal age, parity, and height, (*b*) maternal obesity before conception, (*c*) high maternal weight gain during pregnancy, and (*d*) gestational diabetes mellitus (16, 120). Women who deliver macrosomic infants are more likely to have a cesarean section and complications of delivery (120). Macrosomia increases the risk for shoulder dystocia, birth injury, low Apgar scores, and perinatal death (101, 120). Nationally representative data in the United

States (1988–1994) show that 10% of infants are large for gestational age (for those born at term, 77% weighed more than 4000 g at birth) (44). As a group, these infants experienced catch-down growth in the first 6 months of life but thereafter remained heavier and longer and had larger head circumferences (generally about +0.5 standard deviations) than did babies born at weights appropriate for their gestational ages. In addition, unlike infants born at gestation age–appropriate weights, the large-for-gestational-age group consistently accumulated fat after 2 years of age (45).

## Normal Birth Weight

It is noteworthy that most of the reports by Barker and his coworkers include few (if any) LBW infants. The "BW effect" in these papers refers to associations between BW values primarily within the normal range (i.e. 2500–4000 g) and outcomes in later life. In fact, according to Barker, "[i]t is clear from our data that growth retardation in early life is not limited to a rather small number of extremely underweight babies who are at risk of dying or of complications after birth. That is a hospital obstetric view of growth retardation. Rather, growth retardation occurs in humans across the whole spectrum of growth. There are many babies of average or even above average birth weight who are growth retarded" (5). In another review article, he states that "[i]f the criteria for successful fetal growth include good health in adult life and longevity, these findings reinforce the view that babies with significant intrauterine growth retardation need not necessarily be 'light for gestational age'" (6).

As described above, it is indeed possible for babies to be born with a normal BW and be growth retarded (particularly with BW values <3000 g). In the relatively affluent areas studied by Barker and his coworkers in the early 1900s (8), as well as in developed countries currently, the frequency of this condition is likely to have been low and be low. However, the prevalence of true growth retardation within the normal range of BW is unknown (19). This is because determining the prevalence would require either serial measurements of intrauterine size from which growth retardation can be ascertained or the use of a customized BW reference (79, 117), resources that are, respectively, unavailable or not in wide use.

It can be argued that infants who experience "catch-up" growth (i.e. who cross weight-for-age percentiles upward) are those who experienced some restraint of growth prenatally. Therefore, the proportion of such children provides an estimate of prenatal growth retardation. Such an estimate is available from the Avon longitudinal study of pregnancy and childhood, a geographically defined cohort of children born in Avon, United Kingdom, in 1991–1992 (87). Size at birth was similar to national data, but 30.7% of the children showed catch-up growth in weight (defined as an increase of 0.67 standard deviation score from birth to age 2). Those who experienced catch-up growth had mothers with lower BW values themselves and were more likely to be the first child of a smoker—all known predictors of small size at birth. They also had taller fathers, which suggests a genetic component to the rate of postnatal growth. It is noteworthy that they were significantly less likely to have been breastfed at 3 mo than those who did not change growth percentiles or experienced catch-down growth, leaving open the possibility of mode of infant feeding as an important cause of the difference in growth trajectory. This is because appropriate-for-gestational-age infants who are fed infant formula grow more rapidly than those fed human milk. In addition, 24.5% of the cohort showed catch-down growth in weight (defined as a decrease of 0.67 standard deviation score from birth to age 2). They were larger at birth, but their growth pattern was not explained by characteristics of their parents. In this sample it was the pattern of postnatal growth, not BW per se, that explained differences in body weight and fatness at 5 years of age. Furthermore, although the proportion of children who might be regarded as having experienced prenatal growth restraint was higher than might have been expected, the proportion who experienced growth excess was also high—an additional cause for concern. It is likely that both of these proportions are too high because the authors did not account for the statistical phenomenon of regression to the mean.

## THE EVIDENCE FROM EPIDEMIOLOGIC STUDIES

There is a paucity of information on maternal nutrition in the context of the fetal origins hypothesis. MNS is one of the few determinants of BW that is modifiable immediately before and during pregnancy (53), and observations about the conditions of women have had a central role in the presentation of the fetal origins hypothesis (7). The available evidence is considered as three groups of studies: those of well-nourished women living under good circumstances, those of previously well-nourished women subjected to famine, and women living under poor circumstances.

## Maternal Nutritional Status

*Data From Well-Nourished Women in Developed Countries*    Historical data on the domestic conditions and probable diets of young women at the time of Barker's initial work have been collected from interviews of women aged 80 and over (27). Godfrey and Barker have presented data from three samples of well-nourished women that identify associations between some measure of MNS (e.g. anemia) (37) and the BW of their infants or between dietary intake and BW (31, 35). They also have presented studies that link measures of MNS to blood pressure at age 10–12 in Jamaica (36) and that link diet during pregnancy to blood pressure at age 40 in Aberdeen, Scotland (17). The relationships between MNS and childhood blood pressure were complex and not readily explainable. Maternal triceps skin-fold thickness apparently explained the observed association between maternal anemia and raised blood pressure in the children. Both low triceps skin-fold thickness and weight gain during pregnancy were associated with raised blood pressure in the children (36). The data on dietary intake during pregnancy in the study of adults come from a classic investigation conducted by Thomson in the 1950s (107a). In this study there was also a complex relationship between the dietary characteristics and later blood pressure that is not easily interpreted within the framework of the fetal origins hypothesis. As expected for well-nourished women, others (76a) who have studied them have been unable to find an association between maternal dietary intake and BW.

To explore the relationship between MNS and blood pressure in late adolescence, data on MNS that were obtained as part of the Jerusalem Perinatal Study were linked to data from physical examinations of men being inducted into military service. Mothers' body weight and body mass index before pregnancy—but not weight gain during pregnancy or the BW of the baby—were positively associated with both systolic and diastolic blood pressures at age 17 (62). The finding on BW is opposite that predicted by the fetal origins hypothesis and the findings on MNS are opposite those of Godfrey et al (36). These results cannot easily be explained by confounding by socioeconomic status or length of gestation, as both were included in the analysis. It is noteworthy that, even with these opposite findings, in both cases there was an association between measures of MNS and blood pressure in the offspring without a significant relationship between BW and blood pressure.

The longest-term follow-up of MNS, by Forsén et al (28) using the national registry, linked birth data (1924–1933) from a hospital in Helsinki, Finland, to deaths (1971–1995). The authors identified a positive association between mothers' body mass index (among those below the median height) and mortality of their sons from CHD; they also found a negative association of the infant's ponderal index with this outcome. In this study on mortality, as for the two discussed above on blood pressure in children and draftees, there was no association between BW and the later outcome—even with an association between the measure of MNS and that outcome. These findings do not support a biological pathway between MNS and these outcomes via BW, as suggested by the fetal origins hypothesis.

***Data From Famine-Stricken Women in Developed Countries***    Links between maternal malnutrition during pregnancy and long-term outcomes for the fetus are available from follow-up studies of three famines. Two of these are ecologic studies because they lack data on the specific exposure of individuals. However, each was so severe and prolonged that it is reasonable to assume that everyone was affected. Three sequential crop failures caused a famine and then epidemics in Finland in 1866–1868 that resulted in the death of 8% of the population; infant mortality was 40% in 1868 (52). Survival from birth to age 17 was significantly lower in the cohorts born before and during the famine than in those born afterwards. However, there was no difference in adult survival among cohorts born before, during, or after the famine (52). The 872-day siege of Leningrad during World War II created a famine during which at least 30% of the city's inhabitants died, most of starvation (102); BW dropped by >500 g during the siege (4). Stanner et al (102) found no differences between those exposed and those not exposed to the famine in glucose intolerance, dyslipidemia, hypertension, or CVD in adulthood.

Although both these investigations provide evidence counter to the fetal origins hypothesis, the conditions were so severe that it is possible only the healthier individuals survived. This could account for the lack of difference between the exposed and unexposed groups.

Data from the famine during the "Dutch hunger winter" of 1944–1945 have been used to evaluate the association between MNS during pregnancy and determinants of chronic disease at about age 50: glucose tolerance, blood pressure, and obesity. It has previously been shown that exposure to this famine was associated with reduced BW, increased perinatal and infant mortality, and obesity in men at the time of induction into military service (only with famine exposure in the first trimester; later exposure was associated with a reduction in obesity) (107). In these three investigations, subjects born in one hospital in Amsterdam and exposed to the famine were compared with a random sample of infants from the same hospital born before or after the famine. In women, but not in men, exposure to famine was associated with obesity, but only when the exposure to famine occurred early in gestation (94). Exposure to famine during gestation was associated with some but not all measures of decreased glucose tolerance. The effects were greatest in those who became obese as adults, but the association was not mediated by obesity (93). In contrast, exposure to famine during gestation was not associated with blood pressure, even though those who were small at birth had higher blood pressures (96). Thus, the findings from these three "natural experiments" provide only occasional support for the fetal origins hypothesis.

***Data From Developing Countries***   Studies from developing countries, where maternal malnutrition remains common, are recent additions to epidemiological studies on the fetal origins hypothesis. Data from Mysore, India, show the predicted negative association between BW and CHD for those older than 45 years (103). The mean BW in this population was low (about 2750 g) and mothers' weights also were low, but no data on maternal height were presented so body mass index cannot be calculated and, thus, MNS is unknown. Maternal weight was not related to the prevalence of CHD, but it was only available in a subset of the cases, so adequate statistical power may have been a problem in this analysis. In contrast to data from developed countries, there was no association between BW and NIDDM (26), and there were positive associations between BW and blood pressure (61) and measures of lung function (men only) (104) in this population.

Distinct differences in seasonal food availability and agricultural work load create differences in MNS in Gambia. In the harvest season, MNS is normal, but in the hungry season, women lose weight and BW declines by 200–300 g; this is reversed by maternal supplementation (18). In three rural villages, those born in the rainy (hungry) season had the highest blood pressures at 8–9 years of age; a proxy for MNS (mother's weight at 6 months of pregnancy) was not related to the child's blood pressure. The opposite was true for younger children: Those born in the dry season had the highest blood pressures, and MNS was positively associated with their blood pressure (75). Using demographic data collected since 1949, Moore et al (82) observed that those born in the hungry season had a significantly higher mortality rate after age 15 and, especially, between 35 and 50 years of age. However, mortality in this population was dominated by infections and pregnancy-related deaths, and no deaths were attributed to chronic degenerative diseases. In a further case-control analysis of these data, the authors found no differences between cases and controls in measures of nutritional status at 18 months of age, but they observed a close correlation between temporal pattern of BW and that of death (81). They speculated that their findings might have resulted from nutritional programming of immune function, which could have occurred prenatally, postnatally, or both. Thus, the findings from these two developing countries provide no support for an association between MNS and the predictors or consequences of chronic diseases. The mortality data from Gambia suggest that something about season of birth is related to mortality at 15–48 years, but what this might be is unknown.

In summary, evidence is lacking for a link between MNS and the determinants or consequences of chronic disease in offspring as children or adults. This same conclusion was reached by Leon & Koupilová, who called this "a priority area for future work" (65). The following question then arises: Is any association of BW with later outcomes really driven by MNS? Lucas (69) has labeled this a "key area for debate," noting that "[p]oor intrauterine growth might be associated with other, non-nutritional derangements that could be responsible for long-term programming."

## The Role of Catch-Up Growth

The role of postnatal catch-up growth in modifying the association between BW and CVD has begun to receive some attention. Cianfarani et al (21) have proposed that the metabolic adaptations that permit survival for growth-retarded infants are a liability postnatally and result in a higher-than-expected risk of NIDDM in adulthood. An evaluation of a variation of this proposition is provided by Eriksson et al (25). They used data on growth from school records combined with information on MNS during pregnancy and mortality from CHD that was already available (28). Body mass index at age 11 was associated with CHD; adjustment for ponderal index at birth strengthened this association. As described previously, there was no association between BW and mortality in this population. The authors interpreted these findings as evidence of a detrimental effect of catch-up growth. It is not clear from these data whether the children experienced catch-up growth (that is, crossed percentile lines upward shortly after birth as a reflection of prenatal growth restriction) or became fat at some time later during childhood. Osmond et al (88) had previously reported an association between weight at age 1 and premature death from CVD that was even stronger than that for BW. It is not possible to tell from the analyses they presented whether catch-up growth was responsible for this association. Thus, at this point there is no persuasive data from human subjects to establish a relationship between true catch-up growth and determinants or consequences of chronic disease. This lack of evidence, however, does not rule out the possibility of effect modification by postnatal events, such as method of infant feeding. This is an important area for additional research, as the feeding and growth of infants and children are changing rapidly worldwide (99).

## Assessment of the Associations Between Maternal Nutritional Status or Birth Weight and Outcomes

Barker and his coworkers have published a very large number of papers in which associations between some characteristics of the newborn, particularly BW, and various later outcomes are documented. These later outcomes include hypertension, diabetes mellitus, CHD, stroke, chronic obstructive lung disease, renal failure, ovarian cancer and other disorders. This work is summarized in Barker's most recent book (11). Other groups of investigators also have contributed similar findings from different population groups. However, there also have been important contrary findings. When examined in more detail, the relationships between specific characteristics of the newborn and specific conditions in later life are much less consistent. They appear in some studies but not others, or in some population subgroups (e.g. males or the obese) but not others (47, 50, 89).

The general problems with these epidemiological studies on BW also apply to those described above on MNS. These difficulties have been enumerated and discussed in detail (24, 48, 50, 55, 56). They include (a) substantial losses to follow-up because members of the cohort have died, moved, or refused to participate, (b) absent or inadequate control for obvious potential confounding factors (often because such information was not available in the data set)—an important concern in evaluating an association with such a long latency period, and (c) inconsistencies in findings between one study and another, compounded by the use of multiple combinations of dependent and independent variables. In addition, the hypothesis itself does not explain temporal and international trends in BW and CVD (56). It is especially difficult to control for confounding by behavioral, lifestyle, and socioeconomic factors and, even when this is attempted, to provide assurance that all residual confounding has been eliminated. Joseph (49) has made this point clearly in his examination of the BW/blood pressure relationship.

Arguably the strongest epidemiological study published to date is that of Leon and his coworkers (66), in which birth records from a large cohort of Swedish men and women born between 1915 and 1929 were linked to census data (to provide information on socioeconomic status at multiple times during follow-up) and to death registers. A high proportion of the subjects were traced. These features of the study design addressed two of the major critiques of prior investigations. For men only, they found an inverse association between BW and all-cause mortality after 65 years of age; this resulted from a reduction in ischemic heart disease and circulatory disease in general. The investigators were able to adjust for the duration of gestation and, thereby, to distinguish between BW (attained size) and growth rate (weight for gestational age). They used this information to conclude that it is the rate of fetal growth, not attained size at birth, that is important for long-term mortality from ischemic heart disease.

One of the best possibilities for eliminating confounding in an epidemiological design is to study twins because for those raised together, there is no difference in socioeconomic conditions during infancy and childhood, and for monozygotic twins, there is no difference in genetic characteristics. Twins are also of interest for testing the fetal origins hypothesis because their BW is substantially lower than that of singletons, and there is reason to suppose they experienced a "suboptimal intra-uterine environment" in the third trimester of pregnancy (108). Compared with nontwins in the general Swedish (108) or Danish populations (20), twins had no excess mortality. However, these kinds of studies have been criticized for (*a*) failing to control as well as desired for socioeconomic status because dizygotic twinning does not occur randomly in the population (98) and (*b*) using an inappropriate model because twins, although small, do not have the hypoinsulinemia characteristic of growth-retarded infants (109). In another study, twins had lower blood pressures than singletons at ages 9 and 18 years (119), contrary to expectations from the fetal origins hypothesis. These authors used path analysis to explore the relationships between available variables and concluded that the effect of BW may have been overestimated by previous authors because they did not account for current height or body mass index. Differences within twin pairs have now been examined in several studies. In one study (90), 55–74-year-old subjects were drawn from the Danish twin registry. Oral glucose tolerance tests were used to identify pairs who were discordant for NIDDM. Among both mono- and dizygotic twins, the twin with NIDDM had a lower BW than the twin without NIDDM. A within-pair design has been used in two studies to examine the association between BW and blood pressure at age 8 (23a) in adulthood (90a). In both studies, large decreases in blood pressure were associated with increases in BW, but these associations were not statistically significant. These three studies make the best use of the twin design and support the idea of in utero programming of later effects. However, they do not support the postulate that programming results from variation in MNS as both twins were exposed to the same maternal conditions. In summary, the studies of twins provide some improvement in methodology, but the two strongest of the studies come to conflicting conclusions about the fetal origins hypothesis.

## Future Directions

Particularly problematic in this literature is the lack of well-articulated, testable causal sequences that include both biological and nonbiological factors (89) and also allow for effect modification by factors acting after birth. Barker has provided various biological models for the fetal origins hypothesis (7) and has acknowledged the possible importance of lifestyle factors (10). Including such factors will require richer data sources than those used to date and appropriate modeling (91). Several researchers (47, 60) have recently called for using a "life course" approach. This approach suggests that "throughout the life course exposures or insults gradually accumulate through episodes of illness, adverse environmental conditions and behaviours increasing the risk of chronic disease and mortality. Accumulation of risk is different from programming in that it does not require (nor does it preclude) the notion of a critical period" (60). Such an approach would not only allow for effect modification in the postnatal and other subsequent periods, but would also include consideration of other modifying or confounding factors. Using this approach may be a more appropriate way to proceed, rather than continuing with efforts to eliminate all confounding while ignoring the important contributions of adult circumstances and characteristics (64).

## Summary

The studies described above are all observational and, thus, are unsuitable for establishing a causal relationship. Although their results suggest various causal sequences depending on the outcome of interest, such sequences cannot be taken as causal "until the result repeatedly and consistently survives rigorous tests that might disprove the hypothesis" (89). To date, such a refutation has only been attempted in one study (119), and the fetal origins hypothesis did not turn out to be robust (106). Unfortunately, as a result of the lack of specificity in the independent variable as well as the multiplicity of dependent variables, these many associations remain difficult to interpret except via the more specific biologic information now being accumulated. Furthermore, it is not appropriate to describe these relationships between BW and later outcomes as associations between intrauterine growth retardation and some later outcome, as evidence is lacking that the infants studied were actually growth retarded.

There is no persuasive evidence of a causal pathway that leads from MNS through BW to determinants or consequences of chronic disease among either well-nourished or presumably undernourished women. This may be because the investigations that included individual-level data on MNS were obtained from well-nourished women, and no relationship between MNS and BW would be expected among these women. Unfortunately, there was also no association between BW and later outcome in these studies, so interpreting any association found between MNS and the later outcome is problematic. It is well known that MNS is important for fetal growth (53, 55). However, MNS is not the only determinant of fetal condition in utero, so attention could more profitably be directed to these other determinants in the search for an early origin for CVD.

## THE EVIDENCE FROM INTERVENTION STUDIES

Intervention studies provide stronger evidence with which to evaluate the fetal origins hypothesis, but these are few in number and limited to outcomes observed in childhood or young adulthood. Individuals in Guatemala whose mothers were supplemented during pregnancy and lactation and who themselves were supplemented up to 3 years of age between 1969 and 1977 have been studied as young adults. These results show, for example, that later physical work capacity is improved for the males, with a positive dose response to the amount of supplemental energy consumed (40). In this trial, pre- and postnatal contributions to the observed outcome cannot be distinguished.

Two trials with still stronger designs provide data on blood pressure following supplementation of pregnant women with calcium (15) or preterm infants with various formulas (72). In neither case was there a significant overall effect on blood pressure when children were 5–9 years old or 7.5–8 years old, respectively. However, the subgroup of children whose mothers received the calcium supplement and were currently above the median body mass index had lower systolic blood pressures than those whose mothers did not receive the supplement.

Two other outcomes have been measured at 7.5–8 years in the study of preterm infants: growth and cognitive function. As was the case for blood pressure, there was no difference between the treatments (in this case standard compared with preterm formula among women who did or did not choose to provide their own milk for their infants) in growth at 9 or 18 months or 7.5–8 years of age (84). In contrast, boys (but not girls) fed the standard formula as their sole diet had a significantly lower intelligence quotient measured at 7.5–8 years of age than those fed the preterm formula (73). The authors interpreted these findings as evidence that for preterm babies, the period between birth and hospital discharge is one during which nutritional programming takes place for cognitive function, but not for growth or blood pressure. Losses to follow-up in these trials were minimal, and their designs permit causal inference. As a group, these studies provide mixed support for the fetal origins hypothesis. As is the case in the epidemiologic studies, "programming" seems to occur erratically in these studies as well—for some outcomes, at some times, for some subgroups of the population.

# THE EVIDENCE FROM STUDIES USING EXPERIMENTAL SPECIES

Studies using experimental species have provided strong evidence for the concept of programming across a wide range of organ systems and for both short- and long-term outcomes (69, 100). It is clear that the critical period depends both on the species used and on the outcome studied and that both pre- and postnatal periods are important. Some of these studies have produced results that are concordant in direction and effect with the fetal origins hypothesis, and some have not (69, 114). Recent reviews of the metabolic and endocrine responses to undernutrition that may be relevant to the later development of chronic disease in human subjects are available from a variety of model systems (e.g. 29, 42, 46, 77, 95, 110).

Research to date has generated additional hypotheses, with a change in emphasis from environmental to genetic factors. Hattersley & Tooke (43) propose in the fetal insulin hypothesis that "the association between low birthweight and adult insulin resistance is principally genetically mediated." This could result in poor growth in utero mediated by insufficient insulin as well as by insulin resistance in childhood and adulthood; thus, all these conditions would be manifestations of the same insulin-resistant genotype. This raises the interesting problem of genetic confounding; that is, the same factors that caused the fetus to be small at birth would also cause later chronic disease. They go on to state that "Central to this fetal insulin hypothesis is the concept that insulin-mediated fetal growth will be affected by fetal genetic factors that regulate either fetal insulin secretion or the sensitivity of fetal tissues to the effects of insulin" (43). These possibilities are now being investigated. However, others disagree with their assertion of a genetic basis for the association between BW and later insulin resistance (78).

More recently, Waterland & Garza (114) have taken the concept of programming further and used the term metabolic imprinting to describe "the basic biological phenomena that putatively underlie relations among nutritional experiences of early life and later diseases." The term is intended to encompass adaptive responses to specific nutritional conditions in early life and to assist in the development of a concise list of underlying mechanisms. Metabolic imprinting is characterized by "(a) a susceptibility limited to a critical ontogenic window early in development, (b) a persistent effect lasting through adulthood, (c) a specific and measurable outcome (that may differ quantitatively among individuals), and (d) a dose-response or threshold relation between a specific exposure and outcome" (114). This definition allowed them to identify five specific candidate mechanisms by which metabolic imprinting could occur: "(a) organ structure (morphological development, (b) alterations in cell number, hepatocyte polyploidization or myocyte multinucleation, (c) clonal selection, (d) apoptotic remodeling and (e) metabolic differentiation" (115). In reviewing this list, it is clear that these mechanisms of metabolic imprinting could—and do—occur after the fetal period as well as during it (115). In addition, experimental evidence for an effect of perinatal nutrition on epigenetic gene expression is now available (113).

## POSSIBLE IMPLICATIONS FOR PUBLIC HEALTH ACTION

The many studies that link BW to the development of chronic disease challenge us to rethink our definition not only of growth retardation but also of optimal BW. Currently, the optimal BW is considered to be that with the minimal perinatal mortality. Perinatal mortality is lowest for infants of 3501–4000 g born at a gestational age of 38–42 weeks (122). This target BW is lower than the BW values with the lowest CVD mortality in the studies by Barker (9–9.5 lb, or 4091–4328 g) (7) and also the recent study by Leon et al (3750–4249 g) (66) and is much lower than the maximum reported BW values. From a public health perspective, the question to address is which of these possibilities should be used as the target—our current approach (the lower end of the range for minimal perinatal mortality) or some higher number that could be based on minimizing chronic disease in off-spring? It is important to recognize that setting any higher-target BW will require some intervention(s) to achieve it because it is even farther away from the mean BW than the current target for BW. Possible interventions include actions to reduce the rate of LBW (alleviation of poverty, more adequate provision of pre-natal care, distribution of food supplements to needy women, smoking cessation programs for smokers who want to quit, etc) and/or to shift the entire BW distribution to the right (by using some of the same interventions as above, as well as by using campaigns to encourage women to weigh more when they conceive and eat more while pregnant, etc). Other possibilities also have been discussed (41).

Nutritional interventions designed to increase BW (in populations in which the majority of small babies are born at term) have had only modest success. Such interventions may raise the lower tail of the BW distribution (i.e. lower the proportion of LBW births) and/or raise the mean BW. A meta-analysis of well-designed intervention trials revealed that the increase in mean BW with energy and protein supplementation during pregnancy was only 30 g (54). Larger effects (about 100 g) have been observed in less-well-controlled studies conducted among poorer populations (e.g. 54, 63) as well as in a primary health care setting in Gambia, where BW was increased by 136 g over the whole year and 201 g in the "hungry" season (18). There are still larger effects in the needier women, as high as 400–600 g among Guatemalan women with specific characteristics or combinations of characteristics (86). These findings provide an upper bound for the extent to which BW might be improved by nutritional interventions in poor populations (92). Thus, these studies provide causal evidence that maternal supplementation increases BW in populations with relatively low mean BW values, but even in these populations, the effect is small.

If one assumes that association shown by Barker and his coworkers between BW and mortality CVD is causal, would increasing BW improve cardiovascular outcomes? Joseph & Kramer (51) have done these calculations and the results are sobering. They estimated that a 100-g increase in BW (an achievable goal) would result in a 2.5% and 1.9% decrease in mortality from CHD in women and men, respectively. The change in mortality that has been documented with reductions in risk factors during adulthood is much larger (51). The results of these calculations suggest that although studying factors in early life has offered some new ways of thinking about the origins of CVD, increasing BW is likely to be much less effective in reducing mortality than modifying the traditional risk factors observed during adulthood.

Even if increasing BW within the normal range decreased mortality from CVD, is this an intervention worth doing? Answering this question requires consideration of possible negative consequences of this action (30, 51). The possible risks to the mother include an increase in the rate of cesarean section and the prevalence of obesity (via high maternal weight at conception or failure to lose the extra weight that was gained to increase BW). The possible risks to the infant include those associated with being macrosomic at birth, as well as an increased risk of death from various kinds of cancer that is at least as large as the reduction in CVD mortality that could be achieved with a similar increase in BW.

These calculations all assume that the fetal origins act through BW and, therefore, that one would have to change the BW distribution to have an effect on later chronic disease. To the extent that BW is most likely only a proxy, and perhaps a poor one at that, for a process or processes that have affected the fetus, changing BW may not even be an appropriate target. As our understanding improves about how and when "programming" or "metabolic imprinting" occurs, different interventions may be suggested. Until that time, it seems inappropriate to intervene during pregnancy to reduce the development of chronic disease. However, there remain—in both developed and, especially, developing countries—ample other reasons to continue to intervene now in various ways to promote a good outcome of pregnancy for both mother and infant.

## CONCLUSIONS

Barker's promotion of the idea that events during intrauterine life might have implications for the development of CVD has generated substantial interest as well as controversy. Both the importance of the idea and the controversy that has surrounded it have led to much additional research. Some of this research was similar to the investigations of Barker's group but in different populations; this has helped establish the robustness of the association between BW and various chronic conditions of later life and suggested specific avenues for future research. It still remains to be established, however, whether this association is causal.

Numerous studies in experimental species also have contributed to our understanding of the biological phenomena underlying the "fetal origins" hypothesis. These studies confirm the concept that different organs have different critical periods of development. These different critical periods, as well as the use of different experimental conditions, may help to explain the erratic associations that have been observed in the epidemiologic studies. Additional specific ways of investigating these phenomena have recently been proposed, with greater importance placed on genetic factors.

To date, remarkably little additional information has become available on the specific role of MNS before or during pregnancy, a central feature of the fetal origins hypothesis. What little information is available provides only minimal support for it.

The role of BW remains difficult to interpret except as a proxy for events in intrauterine life that are reflected in size at birth. Not all events that might be relevant for the later development of chronic disease would be expected to influence BW, and not all factors that influence BW would also be expected to affect the later development of chronic disease. In addition, compensatory changes occur after birth, some in response to BW and others in response to various environmental conditions. These compensatory changes are likely to be important and, to date, have not been well studied.

Unfortunately, these investigations have not revealed any significant contribution of BW to the attributable risk of CVD; lifestyle factors during adulthood make a much greater contribution. BW also does not provide any appreciable improvement in the prediction of individual risk of chronic disease, which was Barker's hope when this research began.

Although it is tempting to use the excitement generated by this research to encourage policy makers to develop interventions aimed at pregnant women based on these findings, calculations of the reduction in CVD mortality as well as the increase in deleterious outcomes that might occur as a result suggest this would be inadvisable at this time.

Finally, it is difficult to justify continuing to refer to this body of knowledge as the fetal origins hypothesis because prior knowledge and more recent epidemiologic studies of humans and experimental studies using animals suggest that, in addition to effects that occur during adulthood, chronic disease may have it origins before, during, or after the fetal period.

**Visit the Annual Reviews home page at www.AnnualReviews.org**

## LITERATURE CITED

1. Deleted in proof
2. Adair LS, Kuzawa CW. 2001. Early growth retardation and Syndrome X: conceptual and methodological issues surrounding the programming hypothesis. In *Nutrition and Growth*, ed. R Martorell, F Haschke. New York: Lippincott-Raven. In press
3. Altman DG, Hytten FE. 1989. Intrauterine growth retardation: Let's be clear about it. *Br. J. Obstet. Gynaecol.* 96:1127–32
4. Antonov AN. 1947. Children born during the siege of Leningrad in 1942. *J. Pediatr.* 30:250–59
5. Barker DJP. 1992. The fetal origins of diseases of old age. *Eur. J. Clin. Nutr.* 46(Suppl. 3):S3–9
6. Barker DJP. 1993. The intrauterine origins of cardiovascular disease. *Acta Paediatr. Scand.* 391:93–99
7. Barker DJP. 1994. *Mothers, Babies, and Disease in Later Life*. London: BMJ
8. Barker DJP. 1995. Fetal origins of coronary heart disease. *Br. Med. J.* 311:171–74

9. Barker DJP. 1997. Intrauterine programming of coronary heart disease and stroke. *Acta Paediatr. Scand.* 423(Suppl.):178–82
10. Barker DJP. 1997. Maternal nutrition, fetal nutrition, and disease in later life. *Nutrition* 13:807–13
11. Barker DJP. 1998. *Mothers, Babies and Health in Later Life*. Edinburgh, Scotland: Churchill Livingstone
12. Barker DJP. 1999. In utero programming of cardiovascular disease. *Theriogenology* 53:555–74
12a. Barker DJP, ed. 2000. *Fetal Origins of Cardiovascular and Lung Disease*. New York: Dekker
13. Barker DJP, Gluckman PD, Godfrey KM, Harding JE, Owens JA, Robinson JS. 1993. Fetal nutrition and cardiovascular disease in adult life. *Lancet* 341:938–41
14. Begley S. 1999. Shaped by life in the womb. *Newsweek*. Sept. 27, pp. 50–57
15. Belizán JM, Villar J, Bergel E, del Pino A,

Di Fulvio S, et al. 1997. Long term effect of calcium supplementation during pregnancy on the blood pressure of offspring: follow up of a randomised controlled trial. *Br. Med. J.* 315:281–85

15a. Black R, Michaelsen KF, eds. 2001. *Public Health Issues in Infant and Child Nutrition.* Vevey, Switzerland: Nestlé. In press

16. Bromwich P. 1986. Big babies. *Br. Med. J.* 293:1387–88

17. Campbell DM, Hall MH, Barker DJP, Cross J, Shiell AW, Godfrey KM. 1996. Diet in pregnancy and the offspring's blood pressure 40 years later. *Br. J. Obstet. Gynaecol.* 103:273–80

18. Ceesay S, Prentice AM, Cole TJ, Foord FJ, Weaver LT, et al. 1997. Effects on birth weight and perinatal mortality of maternal dietary supplements in rural Gambia: 5 year randomised controlled trial. *Br. Med. J.* 315:786–90

19. Chard T, Young A, Macintosh M. 1993. The myth of fetal growth retardation at term. *Br. J. Obstet. Gynaecol.* 100:1076–81

20. Christensen K, Vaupel JW, Holm NV, Yashin AI. 1995. Mortality among twins after age 6: fetal origins hypothesis versus twin method. *Br. Med. J.* 310:432–36

21. Cianfarani S, Germani D, Branca F. 1999. Low birthweight and adult insulin resistance: the "catch-up growth" hypothesis. *Arch. Dis. Child. Fetal Neonatal Ed.* 81:F71–73

22. Cnattingius S, Haglund B, Kramer MS. 1998. Differences in late fetal death rates in association with determinants of small for gestational age fetuses: population based cohort study. *Br. Med. J.* 316:1483–87

23. de Onis M, Blössner M, Villar J. 1998. Levels and patterns of intrauterine growth retardation in developing countries. *Eur. J. Clin. Nutr.* 52(S1):S5–15

23a. Dwyer T, Blizzard L, Morley R, Ponsonby A-L. 1999. Within pair association

between birth weight and blood pressure at age 8 in twins from a cohort study. *Br. Med. J.* 321:1325–33

24. Elo IT, Preston SH. 1992. Effects of early-life conditions on adult mortality: a review. *Popul. Index* 58:186–212

25. Eriksson JG, Forsén T, Tuomilehto J, Winter PD, Osmond C, Barker DJP. 1999. Catch-up growth in childhood and death from coronary heart disease: longitudinal study. *Br. Med. J.* 318:427–31

26. Fall CHD, Stein CE, Kumaran K, Cox V, Osmond C, et al. 1998. Size at birth, maternal weight, and type 2 diabetes in South India. *Diabet. Med.* 15:220–27

27. Fellague Ariouat J, Barker DJP. 1993. The diet of girls and young women at the beginning of the century. *Nutr. Health* 9:15–23

28. Forsén T, Eriksson JG, Tuomilehto J, Teramo K, Osmond C, Barker DJP. 1997. Mother's weight in pregnancy and coronary heart disease in a cohort of Finnish men: follow up study. *Br. Med. J.* 315:837–40

29. Fowden AL, Forhead AJ. 2000. The role of hormones in intrauterine development. See Ref. 12a, pp. 199–228

30. Garner P, Kramer MS, Chalmers I. 1992. Might efforts to increase birthweight in undernourished women do more harm than good? *Lancet* 340:1021–23

31. Godfrey K, Robinson S, Barker DJP, Osmond C, Cox V. 1996. Maternal nutrition in early and late pregnancy in relation to placental and fetal growth. *Br. Med. J.* 312:410–14

32. Godfrey KM. 1998. Maternal regulation of fetal development and health in adult life. *Eur. J. Obstet. Gynecol.* 78:141–50

33. Godfrey KM, Barker DJP. 1995. Maternal nutrition in relation to fetal and placental growth. *Eur. J. Obstet. Gynecol.* 61:15–22

34. Godfrey KM, Barker DJP. 2000. Fetal nutrition and adult disease. *Am. J. Clin. Nutr.* 71(Suppl.):1344–52S

35. Godfrey KM, Barker DJP, Robinson S, Osmond C. 1997. Maternal birthweight and

diet in pregnancy in relation to the infant's thinness at birth. *Br. J. Obstet. Gynaecol.* 104:663–67

36. Godfrey KM, Forrester T, Barker DJP, Jackson AA, Landman JP, et al. 1994. Maternal nutritional status in pregnancy and blood pressure in childhood. *Br. J. Obstet. Gynaecol.* 101:398–403

37. Godfrey KM, Redman CWG, Barker DJP, Osmond C. 1991. The effect of maternal anaemia and iron deficiency on the ratio of fetal weight to placental weight. *Br. J. Obstet. Gynaecol.* 98:886–91

38. Godfrey KM, Robinson S. 1998. Maternal nutrition, placental growth and fetal programming. *Proc. Nutr. Soc.* 57:105–11

39. Goldberg GM, Prentice AM. 1994. Maternal and fetal determinants of adult diseases. *Nutr. Rev.* 52:191–200

40. Haas JD, Murdoch S, Rivera J, Martorell R. 1996. Early nutrition and later phyical work capacity. *Nutr. Rev.* 54:S41–48

41. Harding JE, Bauer MK, Kimble RM. 1997. Antenatal therapy for intrauterine growth retardation. *Acta Paediatr. Scand.* 423(Suppl.):196–200

42. Harding JE, Gluckman PD. 2000. Growth, metabolic and endocrine adaptations to fetal undernutrition. See Ref. 12a, pp. 181–97

43. Hattersley AT, Tooke JE. 1999. The fetal insulin hypothesis: an alternative explanation of the association of low birth weigth with diabetes and vascular disease. *Lancet* 353:1789–92

44. Hediger ML, Overpeck MD, Maurer KR, Kuczmarski RJ, McGlynn A, Davis WW. 1998. Growth of infants and young children born small or large for gestational age. *Arch. Pediatr. Adolesc. Med.* 152:1225–31

45. Hediger ML, Overpeck MD, McGlynn A, Kuczmarski RJ, Maurer KR, Davis WW. 1999. Growth and fatness at three to six years of age in children born small- or large-for-gestational age. *Pediatrics* 104:e33

46. Holness MJ. 1999. The impact of dietary protein restriction on insulin secretion. *Proc. Nutr. Soc.* 58:647–53

47. Järvelin M-R. 2000. Fetal and infant markers of adult heart disease. *Heart* 84:219–26

48. Jones ME, Swerdlow AJ. 1996. Bias caused by migration in case-control studies of prenatal risk factors for childhod and adult diseases. *Am. J. Epidemiol.* 143:823–31

49. Joseph KS. 2001. Validating the fetal origins hypothesis: an epidemiologic challenge. See Ref. 15a. In press

50. Joseph KS, Kramer MS. 1996. Review of the evidence on fetal and early childhood antecedents of adult chronic disease. *Epidemiol. Rev.* 18:158–74

51. Joseph KS, Kramer MS. 1997. Should we intervene to improve fetal growth? See Ref. 60a, pp. 277–95

52. Kannisto V, Christensen K, Vaupel JW. 1997. No increased mortality in later life for cohorts born during famine. *Am. J. Epidemiol.* 145:987–94

53. Kramer MS. 1987. Intrauterine growth and gestational duration determinants. *Pediatrics* 80:502–11

54. Kramer MS. 1993. Effects of energy and protein intakes on pregnancy outcome: an overview of the research evidence from controlled clinical trials. *Am. J. Clin. Nutr.* 58:627–35

55. Kramer MS. 1997. Social and environmental determinants of intrauterine growth retardation. *Eur. J. Clin. Nutr.* 52:S29–33

56. Kramer MS, Joseph KS. 1996. Enigma of fetal/infant-origins hypothesis. *Lancet* 348:1254–55

57. Kramer MS, McLean FH, Olivier M, Willis DM, Usher RH. 1989. Body proportionality and head and length "sparing" in growth-retarded neonates: a critical reappraisal. *Pediatrics* 84:717–23

58. Kramer MS, Olivier M, McLean FH, Dougherty GE, Willis DM, Usher RH. 1990. Determinants of fetal growth and body proportionality. *Pediatrics* 86:18–26

59. Kramer MS, Olivier M, McLean FH, Willis

DM, Usher RH. 1990. Impact of intrauterine growth retardation and body proportionality on fetal and neonatal outcome. *Pediatrics* 86:707–13

60. Kuh D, Ben-Schlomo Y. 1997. Introduction: a life course approach to the aetiology of adult chronic disease. See Ref. 60a, pp. 3–14

60a. Kuh D, Ben-Schlomo Y, eds. 1997. *A Life Course Approach to Chronic Disease Epidemiology*. Oxford, UK: Oxford Univ. Press

61. Kumaran K, Fall CHD, Martyn CN, Vijayakumar M, Stein C, Shier R. 2000. Blood pressure, arterial compliance, and left ventricular mass: no relation to small size at birth in south Indian adults. *Heart* 83:272–77

62. Laor A, Stevenson DK, Shemer J, Gale R, Seidman DS. 1997. Size at birth, maternal nutritional status in pregnancy, and blood pressure at age 17: population based analysis. *Br. Med. J.* 315:449–53

63. Lechtig A, Habicht J-P, Delgado H, Klein RE, Yarbrough C, Martorell R. 1975. Effect of food supplementation during pregnancy on birthweight. *Pediatrics* 56:508–20

64. Leon DA. 1998. Fetal growth and adult disease. *Eur. J. Clin. Nutr.* 52(S1):S72–82

65. Leon DA, Koupilová I. 2000. Birth weight, blood pressure, and hypertension. See Ref. 12a, pp. 23–48

66. Leon DA, Lithell HO, Vågerö D, Koupilová I, Mohsen R, et al. 1998. Reduced fetal growth rate and increased risk of death from ischaemic heart disease: cohort study of 15,000 Swedish men and women born 1915–29. *Br. Med. J.* 317:241–45

67. Lucas A. 1991. Programming by early nutrition in man. In *The Childhood Environment and Adult Disease*, ed. GR Bock, J Whelan, pp. 38–55. Chichester, UK: Wiley

68. Lucas A. 1994. Role of nutritional programming in determining adult morbidity. *Arch. Dis. Child.* 71:288–90

69. Lucas A. 1998. Programming by early nutrition: an experimental approach. *J. Nutr.* 128:401–6S

70. Lucas A, Fewtrell MS, Cole TJ. 1999. Fetal origins of adult disease—the hypothesis revisited. *Br. Med. J.* 319:245–49

71. Lucas A, Fewtrell MS, Davies PSW, Bishop NJ, Clough H, Cole TJ. 1997. Breastfeeding and catch-up growth in infants born small for gestational age. *Acta Paediatr.* 86:564–69

72. Lucas A, Morley R. 1994. Does early nutrition in infants born before term programme later blood pressure? *Br. Med. J.* 309:304–8

73. Lucas A, Morley R, Cole TJ. 1998. Randomised trial of early diet in preterm babies and later intelligence quotient. *Br. Med. J.* 317:1481–87

74. Luo Z-C, Albertsson-Wikland K, Karlberg J. 1998. Length and body mass index at birth and target height influences on patterns of postnatal growth in children born small for gestational age. *Pediatrics* 102:e72

75. Margetts BM, Rowland MGM, Foord FJ, Cruddas AM, Cole TJ, Barker DJP. 1991. The relation of maternal weight to the blood pressures of Gambian children. *Int. J. Epidemiol.* 20:938–43

76. Martorell R, Ramakrishnan U, Schroeder D, Melgar P, Neufeld L. 1998. Intrauterine growth retardation, body size, composition and physical performance in adolescence. *Eur. J. Clin. Nutr.* 52:S43–53

76a. Mathews F, Yudkin P, Neil A. 1999. Influence of maternal nutrition on outcome of pregnancy: prospective cohort study. *Br. Med. J.* 319:339–43

77. Matthews SG, Challis JRG, Cox DB, Sloboda DM, McMillen C, et al. 2000. The hypothalamic-pituitary-adrenal and hypothalamic-pituitary-gonadal axes in early life: problems and perspectives. See Ref. 12a, pp. 229–48

78. McKeigue PM. 1999. Fetal effects on insulin resistance and glucose tolerance. In *Insulin Resistance: The Metabolic Syndrome X*, ed. GM Reaven, A Laws, pp. 35–49. Totowa, NJ: Humana

79. Mongelli M, Gardosi J. 1996. Reduction of false-positive diagnosis of fetal growth restriction by application of customized fetal growth standards. *Obstet. Gynecol.* 88:844–48

80. Moore SE. 1998. Nutrition, immunity and the fetal and infant origins of disease hypothesis in developing countries. *Proc. Nutr. Soc.* 57:241–47

81. Moore SE, Cole TJ, Collison AC, Poskitt EME, McGregor IA, Prentice AM. 1999. Prenatal or early postnatal events predict infections deaths in young adulthood in rural Africa. *Int. J. Epidemiol.* 28:1088–95

82. Moore SE, Cole TJ, Poskitt EME, Sonko BJ, Whitehead RG, et al. 1997. Season of birth predicts mortality in rural Gambia. *Nature* 388:434

83. Morley R, Dwyer T. 2001. Early exposures and later health and development. See Ref. 15a. In press

84. Morley R, Lucas A. 2000. Randomized diet in the neonatal period and growth performance until 7.5–8 y of age in preterm infants. *Am. J. Clin. Nutr.* 71:822–28

85. Nathanielsz PW. 1999. *Life in the Womb: The Origin of Health and Disease.* Ithaca, NY: Promethean

86. Olson RK. 1994. *Developing indicators that predict benefit from prenatal energy supplementation.* PhD thesis. Cornell Univ., Ithaca, NY. 326 pp.

87. Ong KKL, Ahmed ML, Emmett PM, Preece MA, Dunger DB, et al. 2000. Association between postnatal catch-up growth and obesity in childhood: prospective cohort study. *Br. Med. J.* 320:967–71

88. Osmond C, Barker DJP, Winter PD, Fall CHD, Simmonds SJ. 1993. Early growth and death from cardiovascular disease in women. *Br. Med. J.* 307:1519–24

89. Paneth N, Susser M. 1995. Early origin of coronary heart disease (the "Barker hypothesis"). *Br. Med. J.* 310:411–12

90. Poulson P, Vaag AA, Kyvik KO, Jensen DM, Beck-Nielsen H. 1997. Low birth weight is associated with NIDDM in discordant monozygotic and dizygotic twin pairs. *Diabetologia* 40:439–46

90a. Poulter NR, Chang CL, MacGregor AJ, Sneider H, Spector TD. 1999. Association between birth weight and adult blood pressure in twins: historical cohort study. *Br. Med. J.* 321:1325–29

91. Rasmussen KM. 1998. Commentary. *Eur. J. Clin. Nutr.* 52(S1):S78–81

92. Rasmussen KM. 1999. Causes of intrauterine growth restriction. In *Prenatal Care: Effectiveness and Implementation*, ed. MC McCormick, JE Siegel, pp. 153–74. Cambridge, UK: Cambridge Univ. Press

93. Ravelli ACJ, van der Muelen JHP, Michels RPJ, Osmond C, Barker DJP, et al. 1998. Glucose tolerance in adults after prenatal exposure to famine. *Lancet* 351:173–77

94. Ravelli ACJ, van der Muelen JHP, Osmond C, Barker DJP, Bleker OP. 1999. Obesity at the age of 50 y in men and women exposed to famine prenatally. *Am. J. Clin. Nutr.* 70:811–16

95. Robinson JS, McMillen C, Edwards L, Kind K, Gatford KL, Owens J. 2000. Maternal and placental influences that program the fetus. See Ref. 12a, pp. 273–95

96. Roseboom TJ, van der Muelen JHP, Ravelli ACJ, van Montfrans GA, Osmond C, et al. 1999. Blood pressure in adults after prenatal exposure to famine. *J. Hypertens.* 17:325–30

97. Rosso P, Winick M. 1974. Intrauterine growth retardation: a new systematic aproach based on the clinical and biochemical characteristics of this condition. *J. Perinat. Med.* 2:147–51

98. Rothwell PM. 1994. Low birth weight and ischaemic heart disease. *Lancet* 343:731

99. Schroeder D, Martorell R, Flores R. 1999.

Infant and child growth and fatness and fat distribution in Guatemalan adults. *Am. J. Epidemiol.* 149:177–85

100. Seckl JR. 1998. Physiologic programming of the fetus. *Clin. Perinatol.* 25:939–62

100a. Skjærven R, Wilcox AJ, Øyen N. Magnus P. 1997. Mothers' birth weight and survival of their offspring: population based study. *Br. Med. J.* 314:1376–80

101. Spellacy WN, Miller S, Winegar A, Peterson PQ. 1985. Macrosomia—maternal characteristics and infant complications. *Obstet. Gynecol.* 66:158–61

102. Stanner SA, Bulmer K, Andrès C, Lantseva OE, Borodina V, et al. 1997. Does malnutrition in utero determine diabetes and coronary heart disease in adulthood? Results from the Leningrad seige study, a cross sectional study. *Br. Med. J.* 315:1342–49

103. Stein CE, Fall CHD, Kumaran K, Osmond C, Cox V, Barker DJP. 1996. Fetal growth and coronary heart disease in South India. *Lancet* 348:1269–73

104. Stein CE, Kumaran K, Fall CHD, Shaheen SO, Osmond C, Barker DJP. 1997. Relation of fetal growth to adult lung function in South India. *Thorax* 52:895–99

105. Stockard CR. 1920. Developmental rate and structural expression: an experimental study of twins, "double monsters" and single deformities, and the interaction among embryonic organs during their origin and development. *Am. J. Anat.* 28:115–277

106. Susser M, Levin B. 1999. Ordeals for the fetal programming hypothesis: the hypothesis largely survives one ordeal but not another. *Br. Med. J.* 318:885–86

107. Susser M, Stein Z. 1994. Timing in prenatal nutrition: a reprise of the Dutch Famine Study. *Nutr. Rev.* 52:84–94

107a. Thomson AM. 1958. Diet in pregancy. 1. Dietary survey technique and the nutritive value of diets taken by primigravidae. *Br. J. Nutr.* 12:446–61

108. Vågerö D, Leon DA. 1994. Ischaemic heart disease and low birth weight: a test of the fetal-origins hypothesis from the Swedish Twin Registry. *Lancet* 343:260–63

109. Van Assche FA, Aerts L, Holemans K. 1994. Low birth weight and ischaemic heart disease. *Lancet* 343:731–32

110. Van Assche FA, Holemans K, Aerts L. 1998. Fetal growth and consequences for later life. *J. Perinat. Med.* 26:337–46

111. Villar J, Belizan J. 1982. The timing factor in the pathophysiology of the intrauterine growth retardation syndrome. *Obstet. Gynecol. Surv.* 37:499–506

112. Villar J, Belizán J. 1982. The relative contribution of prematurity and fetal growth retardation to low birth weight in developing and developed countries. *Am. J. Obstet. Gynecol.* 143:793–98

113. Waterland RA. 2000. *Mechanisms underlying the persistent effects of divergent sucking-period litter size on the rat insulin axis.* PhD thesis. Cornell Univ., Ithaca, NY. 148 pp.

114. Waterland RA, Garza C. 1999. Potential mechanisms of metabolic imprinting that lead to chronic disease. *Am. J. Clin. Nutr.* 69:179–97

115. Waterland RA, Garza C. 2001. Potential for metabolic imprinting by nutritional perturbation of epigenetic gene regulation. See Ref 15a. In press

116. Deleted in proof

117. Wilcox MA, Johnson IR, Maynard PV, Smith SJ, Chilvers CED. 1993. The individualised birthweight ratio: a more logical outcome measure of pregnancy than birthweight alone. *Br. J. Obstet. Gynaecol.* 100:342–47

118. Williams RL, Creasy RK, Cunningham CG, Hawes WE, Norton FD, Tashiro M. 1982. Fetal growth and perinatal viability in California. *Obstet. Gynecol.* 59:624–32

119. Williams S, Poulton R. 1999. Twins and

maternal smoking: ordeals for the fetal origins hypothesis? A cohort study. *Br. Med. J.* 318:897–900

120. Wollschlaeger K, Nieder J, Köppe I, Härtlein K. 1999. A study of fetal macrosomia. *Arch. Gynecol. Obstet.* 263:51–55

121. World Health Org. 1990. *Prevention in Childhood and Youth of Adult Cardio-vascular Disease. WHO Technical Rep. Ser. No. 792.* Geneva, Switzerland: World Health Org.

122. World Health Org. Expert Comm. Phys. Status. 1995. *Physical Status: The Use and Interpretation of Anthropometry. WHO Tech. Rep. Ser. No. 854.* Geneva, Switzerland: World Health Org.

Annu. Rev. Nutr. 2001. 21:97–119

# THE GENETICS OF FATTY ACID METABOLISM IN SACCHAROMYCES CEREVISIAE

## Pamela J Trotter

*The Division of Nutritional Sciences and the Institute for Cellular and Molecular Biology, The University of Texas at Austin, Austin, Texas 78712; e-mail: trotter@mail.utexas.edu*

**Key Words**   $\beta$-oxidation, peroxisome, biosynthesis, regulation, yeast

■ **Abstract**   Long-chain fatty acids are a vital metabolic energy source and are building blocks of membrane lipids. The yeast *Saccharomyces cerevisiae* is a valuable model system for elucidation of gene-function relationships in such eukaryotic processes as fatty acid metabolism. Yeast degrades fatty acids only in the peroxisome, and recently, genes encoding core and auxiliary enzymes of peroxisomal $\beta$-oxidation have been identified. Mechanisms involved in fatty acid induction of gene expression have been described, and novel fatty acid–responsive genes have been discovered via yeast genome analysis. In addition, a number of genes essential for synthesis of the variety of fatty acids in yeast have been cloned. Advances in understanding such processes in *S. cerevisiae* will provide helpful insights to functional genomics approaches in more complex organisms.

## CONTENTS

## INTRODUCTION: Yeast As a Model System
## and Tools of the Trade

The budding yeast *Saccharomyces cerevisiae* has long been the model eukaryote of choice for the investigation of basic, yet complex, cellular processes, including the cell cycle, protein targeting and secretion, transcription, and metabolism. Yeast combines an array of characteristics desirable in a model system, including a well-described biochemistry and ease of genetic experimentation. Additionally, the official disclosure of the genome sequence of *S. cerevisiae* in April 1996 (41) provided the first complete sequence of a eukaryotic genome. As observed by Bussey in 1997 (13), with this achievement came "a complete parts list for a eukaryotic cell" and an opportunity to work toward "a comprehensive understanding of how a yeast cell works."

Many genes encoding enzymes in *S. cerevisiae*, such as those encoding core enzymes of fatty acid oxidation and biosynthesis (see below), were characterized using classical genetic approaches. These advances were made possible because *S. cerevisiae* is easily cultivated in a chemically defined medium. Thus, the investigator can precisely control the experimental conditions, both physically and biochemically. Generation, isolation, and analysis of mutant strains can be performed with comparable ease because yeast can be grown in either the haploid or diploid form. Identification of genes [i.e. your favorite gene 1 (*YFG1*)] by complementation of a strain with a mutation in the *yfg1* gene is facilitated by a large collection of plasmids and genomic libraries available for use in *S. cerevisiae* (88). In addition, yeast is especially adept at gene conversion or recombination, so replacement of the genomic copy of *YFG1* with a null allele ( *yfg1Δ* ) or an allele carrying a specific mutation (*yfg1-1*) is relatively straightforward (90).

The completion of the entire *S. cerevisiae* genome sequence has added several new dimensions to the utility of this organism as a model eukaryote. The yeast genome encodes about one gene every 2 kb, in contrast to the estimated 30 kb or more of DNA required per gene in the human (41). In addition, only 4% of yeast genes contain introns. This relative simplicity of the yeast genome has facilitated the systematic analysis of the sequence data, allowing the identification of probable protein-encoding reading frames. Having this information has led to a new approach to the investigation of gene-function relationships, or functional genomics (13, 53), using "reverse genetics" (86). In the classical genetic approach, one begins with a function, inferred from a mutant phenotype, for which the gene involved is determined. In reverse genetics, one begins with the sequence of a gene and must, based on sequence analysis, devise experiments to determine its biological function. For example, homology information may place a protein into a functional group such as transcription factors, but the challenge lies in determining which genes it might regulate. Databases such as the *Saccharomyces* genome database (15), the Yeast proteome database (23), and the MIPS Yeast Genome

Database (78) provide comprehensive compilations of available functional information on open reading frames in yeast. At the writing of this review, the Yeast Proteome Database listed 6145 proteins: 3717 characterized by biochemical or genetic methods, 587 with predicted function based on homology, and 1841 without a known function (23). It is expected that nearly every gene in *S. cerevisiae* will have a homolog in other eukaryotic organisms (11, 41). Thus, progress toward the elucidation of how the 6000 proteins encoded in the genome work to make a functional yeast cell should prove valuable for functional genomics investigations in more complex organisms (86).

Many areas of eukaryotic cell biology have been positively impacted by the utilization of the *S. cerevisiae* as a model organism. As in other eukaryotes, fatty acids serve important roles as a source of metabolic energy and as building blocks of membrane lipids. An increase in the past decade in the number of investigative tools available has led to a greater understanding of gene-function associations and of the regulation of gene expression in fatty acid metabolism in *S. cerevisiae*. This review discusses recent progress in yeast on the peroxisomal $\beta$-oxidation of fatty acids and its regulation, and the biosynthesis and remodeling of endogenous fatty acids.

## PEROXISOME BIOGENESIS

Yeast can grow in medium containing fatty acids as the sole carbon source, as the glyoxylate cycle allows for gluconeogenesis. When de novo fatty acid synthesis is blocked, cells can be rescued by addition of fatty acids to the growth medium. In contrast to mammalian cells, in which $\beta$-oxidation occurs in both the mitochondria and the peroxisome, yeast lack the enzymes required for mitochondrial $\beta$-oxidation (71). Examination of fatty acid oxidation in yeast is thus limited to one organelle and metabolic pathway.

Transfer of *S. cerevisiae* from a glucose-containing medium to a medium containing oleic acid as the sole carbon source is accompanied by a proliferation of peroxisomes and an increase in the activity of $\beta$-oxidation enzymes (112). Although peroxisome proliferation had been observed in several other fungi, demonstration that this process occurs in *S. cerevisiae* permitted its investigation using this genetically well-characterized model system. Peroxisome assembly mutants were isolated by screening for an inability to grow on oleic acid, cytosolic localization of peroxisomal matrix enzymes, and absence of the organelles by electron microscopy analysis (34). These initial studies led to an ongoing extensive investigation of the biogenesis of peroxisomes and of the targeting and transport of proteins to the organelle as well as to the identification of more than 20 required proteins, termed peroxins. Targeting of proteins to the peroxisome matrix has been particularly well described. Synthesized by cytosolic ribosomes, these proteins usually contain either a C-terminal (PTS1) or N-terminal (PTS2) signal sequence that is recognized by PTS receptors in the peroxisomal membrane. They are then moved across the membrane to the matrix by a mechanism requiring a number of proteins. Insertion of peroxisomal membrane proteins, which are also translated in the cytosol, proceeds via a less-well-characterized mechanism. Several recent reviews provide further discussion of peroxisome biogenesis and protein targeting (50, 70, 116). As is discussed below, similar screens for strains unable to grow on fatty acids have led to significant progress in the metabolism of exogenous fatty acids by *S. cerevisiae.*

## FATTY ACID TRANSPORT

### Uptake and Activation

Before a fatty acid can be catabolized by the yeast cell, it must be transported across the plasma and peroxisomal membranes along with its conversion to a coenzyme A (CoA) derivative. The mechanism of extracellular fatty acid transport across the plasma membranes of cells is a point of debate (1, 47). On one hand, in vitro studies have demonstrated that free fatty acids can very rapidly ($t_{1/2} < 1$ s) traverse synthetic lipid bilayers at physiological pH (47). Others argue that although such a diffusion mechanism may be important at relatively high fatty acid concentrations, at physiological levels saturable, facilitated transport appears to predominate (5). Several membrane proteins have been proposed as possible fatty acid transporters or receptors (1, 27, 55), and acyl-CoA synthetases have been shown to enhance fatty acid uptake into cells (27). In *E. coli,* import of fatty acids requires the coupling of FadL, an outer membrane binding and translocation protein, and acyl-CoA synthetase, located in the inner membrane (27). In addition, a putative eukaryotic transporter, FATP, as well as acyl-CoA synthetase were identified in a screen for cDNAs that, when expressed in cultured murine 3T3-L1 adipocytes, increase fatty acid uptake (92).

Saturable uptake of exogenous fatty acids has also been demonstrated in several yeasts, including *S. cerevisiae* (65, 68, 108). A yeast homolog to the adipocyte FATP was identified by comparison of its predicted amino acid sequence to the open reading frames in the *Saccharomyces* genome database (35). The protein encoded by the yeast *FAT1* gene had 54% overall similarity to FATP and contained an AMP-binding motif common to such proteins as acyl-CoA synthetases. When the fatty acid synthase inhibitor cerulenin is added to the medium, normal yeast can be rescued by supplementation with fatty acids. Cells carrying a disruption of the *FAT1* gene (*fat1Δ*), however, have difficulty growing in the presence of cerulenin even in the presence of fatty acid. Incorporation of fatty acids into lipids was also impaired in the *fat1Δ* cells. Yet, acyl-CoA synthetase activity for 14:0, 16:0, and 18:1 fatty acids in *fat1Δ* cells did not differ from the wild-type *FAT1* cells. Thus, in this initial report, Fat1p was proposed to function as a fatty acid transporter protein, as had been proposed for the murine FATP (35, 92).

Recent observations, however, indicate that the impaired fatty acid uptake observed in *fat1Δ* cells is secondary to a defect in the metabolism of the fatty acid. Subcellular localization experiments suggest that Fat1p is associated with the endoplasmic reticulum and peroxisomal membranes, rather than the plasma membrane (18). Also, the initial *FAT1* sequence in the database contained an error, and the correction significantly improved the homology to rat very-long-chain acyl-CoA synthetase (VLCS) (18, 117). Significant accumulation of fatty acids with greater than 22 carbons and severely reduced VLCS activity was observed in *fat1Δ* cells (18, 117). Furthermore, heterologous expression of the *FAT1* gene indicates that Fat1p is a VLCS enzyme (18). Fat1p appears to be involved in the maintenance of very-long-chain fatty acid homeostasis, only indirectly affecting utilization of exogenous fatty acids. It is interesting that the murine FATP has also recently been reported to be a VLCS (21).

Five additional genes (*FAA1-4* and *FAT2*) encoding proteins with homologies to acyl-CoA synthetases have been described in *S. cerevisiae* (7, 117). The *FAA1* and *FAA4* genes encode acyl-CoA synthetases (see Figure 1) required for activation of imported exogenous fatty acids (30, 58, 65). Faa1p exhibits a preference for fatty acids with between 12 and 16 carbons (64), and genetic evidence indicates that it is functionally exchangeable with Faa4p or rat liver acyl-CoA synthetase (65). Faa1p and Faa4p account for 99% of the total 14:0 and 16:0 activation activity in *S. cerevisiae*, and when endogenous fatty acid synthesis is blocked, at least one is required for rescue on medium containing exogenous fatty acids (65). Cells carrying disruptions in both genes, *faa1Δ faa4Δ*, appear to have normal initial rates of free fatty acid import (65), but bulk accumulation in cell lipids is negligible (18). Thus, it seems that these cells are defective in the activation, but not the transport, of the fatty acids.

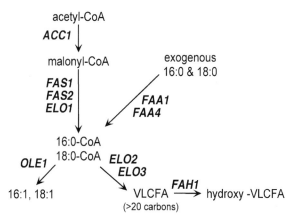

**Figure 1** Schematic of fatty acid biosynthesis in *Saccharomyces cerevisiae*. Processes of de novo synthesis, desaturation, elongation, and hydroxylation are shown. The names of genes encoding enzymes that catalyze each step appear in bold italics. Abbreviations: 16:0, palmitic acid; 16:0-CoA, palmitoyl-coenzyme A; 16:1, palmitoleic acid; 18:0, stearic acid; 18:0-CoA, stearoyl-coenzyme A; 18:1, oleic acid; VLCFA, very-long-chain fatty acid. Further details are in the text.

Disruption of the *FAA2* and *FAA3* genes has no affect on the ability of cells to use exogenously supplied fatty acids, indicating that the acyl-CoA synthetases encoded by these genes can access only fatty acids synthesized within the cell (59). Analysis of the fatty acyl specificity of these enzymes indicates that Faa2p can utilize a wide range of fatty acids but that the greatest activity is toward fatty acids with 9–13 carbons. Faa2p has been localized to the matrix side of peroxisomal membranes (52) and accounts for the residual VLCS activity present in cells lacking Fat1p (18). Faa3p has comparatively lower enzyme activity than Faa2p, favors fatty acids with 16–18 carbons, and displays activity toward very-long-chain fatty acids (64). The *FAT2* gene product (Fat2p, previously named Psc60p) is localized in the peroxisomal matrix but is not necessary for growth on oleic acid (7). The cellular roles of Faa3p and Fat2p remain uncertain.

## Cytoplasmic Pools

*S. cerevisiae* expresses at least one acyl-CoA binding protein encoded by the *ACB1* gene (89). Acyl-CoA binding proteins are polypeptides of 86–103 amino acids that bind acyl-CoAs of 14–22 carbons, but not free fatty acids, and are thought to function in acyl-CoA pool formation as well as in regulation of the metabolic and regulatory functions of long-chain fatty acids (66, 67). Disruption of the *ACB1* gene causes cellular acyl-CoA levels to rise 1.5- to 2.5-fold, primarily because of a sevenfold accumulation of newly synthesized steaoryl-CoA, without affecting the overall fatty acid composition of the cell (93). The yeast Acb1p is thought to play a role in the release of newly synthesized stearoyl-CoA from fatty acid synthase for utilization throughout the cell (93). Because disruption of the gene fails to affect cell survival and membrane fatty acid composition, it is predicted that other mechanisms for acyl-CoA trafficking exist (93).

## Peroxisomal Import

X-linked adrenoleukodystrophy is a human disease characterized by accumulation of very-long-chain fatty acids, and the affected gene has been identified as a member of the ATP binding cassette transporter family (82, 83). Genes encoding two ATP binding cassette half transporters with significant homology to the human adrenoleukodystrophy protein are present in yeast: *PAT1* (or *PXA2*) and *PAT2* (or *PXA1* or *PAL1*) (10, 51, 52, 98, 105). Disruption of either gene results in decreased growth of the cells on medium containing long-chain fatty acid as the sole carbon source, without any affect on the biogenesis of the peroxisomal organelle (52, 97, 105). Long-chain fatty acid oxidation is impaired in whole cells lacking the proteins, but when cells and organelles are disrupted, oxidation is normal. Thus, these proteins appear to be involved in fatty acid import across the peroxisomal membrane. Moreover, immunoprecipitation studies indicate a physical interaction between the encoded proteins, Pat1p and Pat2p (97), which suggests they are two components of the same complex. Finally, the substrate of the transporter is apparently an acyl-CoA derivative because when peroxisomal acyl-CoA synthetase activity is removed by disruption of the *FAA2* gene, oxidation of long-chain fatty acids is completely dependent on Pat1p/Pat2p. The mechanism by which the Pat1p/Pat2p transporter functions remains unclear. It has been suggested that it may act on membrane-associated fatty acyl-CoAs to facilitate the flip of the polar CoA group across the membrane (8, 51).

Cells lacking the Pat1p/Pat2p transporter are capable of growth on such medium-chain fatty acids as laurate, 12:0 (52). In addition, the peroxisomal acyl-CoA synthetase Faa2p (see above) is required for oxidation of medium- but not long-chain fatty acids. Thus, it appears that fatty acids of medium length enter the peroxisome before their activation, which explains their independence of the Pat1p/Pat2p long-chain acyl-CoA transporter. Mislocalization of Faa2p to the cytosol causes medium-chain fatty acids to be activated to their CoA derivatives outside the peroxisome, and their oxidation becomes entirely dependent on the presence of Pat1p/Pat2p (52). In summary, to enter $\beta$-oxidation, long-chain fatty acyl-CoAs are formed in the cytosol and enter the peroxisome via Pat1p/Pat2p, whereas medium-chain fatty acids first reach the peroxisomal lumen, where they are then activated by Faa2p.

# FATTY ACID OXIDATION

## Saturated Fatty Acids

The core reactions of peroxisomal $\beta$-oxidation in *S. cerevisiae* (see Figure 2) are comparable to nonmitochondrial pathways in other organisms (71). The process begins with oxidation of acyl-CoA to *trans*-$\Delta^2$-enoyl-CoA by acyl-CoA oxidase, encoded by the *POX1* (or *FOX1*) gene (29), producing hydrogen peroxide that is detoxified by peroxisomal catalase, encoded by the *CTA1* gene (22, 101). The *trans*-$\Delta^2$-enoyl-CoA hydratase and NAD$^+$-dependent D-3-hydroxyacyl-CoA dehydrogenase steps producing 3-ketoacyl-CoA are catalyzed by a bifunctional protein encoded by the *FOX2* gene (54). The NAD$^+$ required for this reaction is not obtained from the cytosol, as the peroxisomal membrane is impermeable to NAD(H) (110). Rather, NADH is reoxidized by a peroxisomal malate dehydrogenase (Mdh3p) as part of a predicted redox shuttle mechanism across the peroxisomal membrane (51, 110). The final cleavage of the ketoacyl-CoA to yield acetyl-CoA and the shortened acyl-CoA is catalyzed by ketoacyl-CoA thiolase encoded by the *FOX3* (or *POT1*) gene (32, 57). Disruption of *POX1*, *FOX2*, or *FOX3* results in an inability of cells to grow with fatty acids as sole carbon source (29, 54, 57).

The final product of fatty acid oxidation in yeast is acetyl-CoA, which is exported to the mitochondria for utilization in the citric acid cycle. Two pathways for export of acetyl-CoA from peroxisomes have been described (110). In one pathway, acetyl-CoA produced in the peroxisome is transported to the mitochondria as an acetyl-carnitine derivative. One nuclear gene, *CAT2*, encodes the acetyl-carnitine acyltransferases found in both the peroxisome and the mitochondria (33). Alternatively, the acetyl-CoA may be metabolized via the glyoxylate cycle, which serves

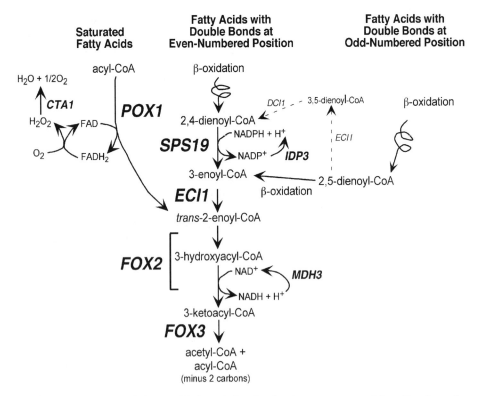

**Figure 2** Schematic of fatty acid degradation in *Saccharomyces cerevisiae*. Reactions for β-oxidation of saturated fatty acids (left), and fatty acids containing double bonds at even (middle) or odd-numbered (right) carbons are shown. The names of genes encoding enzymes that catalyze each step appear in larger bold italics, and genes encoding auxiliary enzymes are in smaller bold italics. The dispensable alternative pathway for 2,5-dienoyl-CoA metabolism is depicted by dotted arrows. Further details are in the text.

to produce four carbon units from the two-carbon acetyl-CoA. Intermediates of this pathway include isocitrate and/or succinate, which can be imported into the mitochondria (110). Genetic experiments indicate that at least one of these pathways must be active to support fatty acid oxidation in yeast peroxisomes (110).

## Unsaturated Fatty Acids

*S. cerevisiae* also catabolizes an array of unsaturated and polyunsaturated fatty acids with *cis* double bonds at odd or even positions (see Figure 2). A recent report indicates yeast can also degrade *trans*-unsaturated fatty acids (43). During β-oxidation of fatty acids that are *cis* unsaturated at an odd position, such as oleic acid (18:1Δ9), a 2,5-dienoyl-CoA intermediate is formed. After an additional round of oxidation, a 3-*cis* double bond is created and isomerized by

$\Delta^3$-*cis*-$\Delta^2$-*trans*-enoyl-CoA isomerase, allowing oxidation to continue. A peroxisomal form of this enzyme is encoded by the *ECI1* gene in *S. cerevisiae* (39, 44). Cells carrying an *eci1*$\Delta$ disruption are unable to utilize oleic acid (18:1$\Delta$9) as their sole carbon source. Heterologous expression of a cDNA for the rat mitochondrial enzyme was effective in rescuing the *eci1*$\Delta$ mutant (44). Eci1p is also required for degradation of fatty acids with odd-numbered *trans*-double bonds, indicating it is actually a $\Delta^3$-*cis/trans*-$\Delta^2$-*trans*-enoyl-CoA isomerase (43). An additional enzyme, $\Delta^{3,5}$, $\Delta^{2,4}$-dienoyl-CoA isomerase, involved in an alternate and dispensable pathway of 2,5-dienoyl-CoA metabolism (Figure 2) is encoded by the *DCI1* gene in *S. cerevisiae* (45).

Oxidation of fatty acids with *cis*-double bonds in an even position gives rise to a 2-*trans*-4-*cis*-dienoyl-CoA intermediate (Figure 2). Further oxidation requires reduction of this intermediate to 3-enoyl-CoA by an NADPH-dependent 2,4-dienoyl-CoA reductase, followed by isomerization to 2-enoyl-CoA by the $\Delta^3$-*cis*-$\Delta^2$-*trans*-enoyl-CoA isomerase (Eci1p). As expected, growth of *eci1*$\Delta$ mutants on fatty acids with a *cis*-double bond in an even or odd position is impaired (44). In contrast, the gene for yeast 2,4-dienoyl-CoA reductase, *SPS19*, is required for growth on petroselinic acid (18:1$\Delta$6), but not oleic acid (18:1$\Delta$9), confirming its essential role in metabolism of fatty acids with a double bond at an even position (46). Degradation of fatty acids with *trans*-double bonds at even positions does not require Eci1p, Sps19p, or Dci1p (43).

It is unlikely that the 2,4-dienoyl-CoA reductase Sps19p obtains NADPH from the cytosol (110). The necessary NADPH (Figure 2) appears to be provided by an oleic acid–inducible, peroxisomal isocitrate dehydrogenase activity encoded by the *IDP3* gene (49, 111). Cells containing an *idp3*$\Delta$ disruption are unable to grow on fatty acids with double bonds at even positions (i.e. 18:1$\Delta$6 or 18:2$\Delta$9,12) but retain growth on stearic acid (18:0) and oleic acid (18:1$\Delta$9) (49, 111). It has been suggested that Idp3p functions in a redox shuttle across the peroxisomal membrane to maintain the levels of NADPH within the organelle (111).

# FATTY ACID INDUCTION OF GENE EXPRESSION

As mentioned above, peroxisome biogenesis and function is induced by exposure to fatty acids. In yeast, expression of such peroxisomal proteins as $\beta$-oxidation enzymes is subject to several types of regulation, primarily at the level of transcription (72). Transcription of most of these genes is repressed by glucose, which requires several proteins, including Abf1p, RP-A, and Car80p. Derepression by removing glucose and growing cells on a nonfermentable carbon source, such as acetate or glycerol, allows a modest increase in expression. Adr1p, Snf1p, and Snf4p are proteins required for general derepression of glucose repressible genes. Expression of many genes encoding peroxisomal proteins is not only derepressed by the removal of glucose, it is also further induced by such fatty acids as oleic acid. For instance, when cells are cultured in medium containing $\geq 2\%$ glucose,

the activities of acyl-CoA oxidase (Pox1p) and thiolase (Fox3p) are nearly undetectable. Growth in a nonfermentable carbon source causes these activities to rise
by 20 times. Exposure to oleic acid increases the activities of these enzymes a
further 20-fold (72). Efficient fatty acid induction of genes encoding peroxisomal
enzymes is contingent on removal of glucose repression. Thus, the derepression
proteins Adr1p and Snf1p are also necessary for complete oleic acid induction
of several genes encoding peroxisomal proteins (72, 84, 99, 100). Mechanisms of
glucose repression and derepression are not considered further here, and the reader
is referred to recent reviews (14, 38, 72).

## Regulation Via Oleate Response Elements

The promoters of many yeast genes encoding peroxisomal proteins contain an
upstream activating sequence responsible for oleic acid regulation of transcription,
dubbed the oleate response element (ORE) (31, 32, 36, 115). The element, which
contains palindromes of CGG with a spacer of 15–18 bp that contains conserved
T and A nucleotides, may be present in one or two copies, depending on the
gene (91, 115). The ORE consensus has been deduced as either $CGG\text{-}N_{15-18}\text{-}$
CCG (91) or $CGGNNNTNA\text{-}N_{9-12}\text{-}CCG$ (63). Initial footprint and gel retardation
analysis demonstrated binding of a protein to the element that coincided with
transcriptional activation. Mutational analysis within the ORE motif interfered with
protein binding as well as gene activation (31, 36, 115). One half of the palindromic
element of *FOX3* was found to bind a small amount of protein and allow some
transcriptional activation. Thus, it was proposed that activation of transcription via
the ORE occurs via binding of an activator dimer complex (31).

Genes encoding two proteins that interact with OREs have been identified. The
*PIP2(OAF2)* gene, identified in screens for peroxisome induction mutants (62, 91),
is induced by oleic acid and encodes a protein that exhibits DNA binding activity
and is capable of oleic acid–specific transcriptional activation of a reporter gene.
Cells containing a *pip2Δ* disruption display no defect in derepression but are unable to grow on oleic acid or induce peroxisome biogenesis because of impaired
oleic acid induction of gene expression. A second protein named Oaf1p was purified using an affinity column to which oligonucleotides encoding an ORE had
been coupled (74). Microsequence analysis of Oaf1p allowed the identification of
the gene by database searching. Cells containing the *oaf1Δ* null allele are unable to
grow on oleic acid, presumably because gene induction by oleic acid and binding
of protein(s) to OREs is impaired in *oaf1Δ* cells. Expression analysis of more than
20 oleic acid–induced genes containing putative OREs found that most are dependent on Oaf1p and Pip2p for complete induction (63, 91). However, not all genes
containing a consensus ORE are regulated in a manner requiring Oaf1p/Pip2p, and
at least one Oaf1p/Pip2p-regulated gene appears to lack an ORE (63).

Immunoprecipitation experiments indicate that Oaf1p interacts physically with
Pip2p, leading to the suggestion that the two transcription factors interact with the
ORE and activate transcription as a heterodimer (62). The domain structure of the

two proteins is similar; each contains an N-terminal $Zn_2Cys_6$ DNA binding domain, two inhibitory domains and an auxiliary domain near the middle of the protein, and a C-terminal 26–27 amino acid activation domain (3). The individual role of each protein in the oleic acid activation of transcription has been addressed using protein fusions and reporter constructs. The data led to a proposed model (3) in which Pip2p activity is inhibited under derepressing conditions via its interaction with inactive Oaf1p. When oleic acid is present, Oaf1p becomes activated and the Oaf1p/Pip2p complex binds the ORE and activates transcription. When glucose is added back, the activity of both Oaf1p and Pip2p is repressed directly. As yet, what the precise molecular nature is by which the Oaf1p/Pip2p complex is activated by oleic acid and repressed by glucose remains unknown.

## Identification of Novel Fatty Acid–Responsive Genes

The availability of the *S. cerevisiae* genomic database has facilitated the identification of novel genes induced by oleic acid using genome sequence analysis. The *Saccharomyces* genome database has been searched for genes containing a possible Oaf1p/Pip2p–binding site using a consensus oleate response element (ORE) sequence (63). Forty genes contained the putative binding site within the first 500 bp upstream of the start codon, and 22 were actually induced by oleic acid. Many of the genes encoded known peroxisomal proteins required for $\beta$-oxidation. Seven novel oleic acid–regulated open reading frames were identified, one of which was later identified as peroxisomal $\Delta^3$-*cis*-$\Delta^2$-*trans*-enoyl-CoA isomerase (*ECI1*) (39, 44).

A similar search utilizing a computer algorithm called CoSMoS (for context-sensitive motif searches), in which motif searches are combined with position or context specifications within the open reading frame, has recently been used to identify novel peroxisomal proteins (40). CoSMoS was used to scan the yeast genome for genes encoding proteins with 100 or more amino acids containing peroxisomal targeting sequence type 1 at the C terminus or a peroxisomal targeting sequence type 2 within the first 25 amino acids. The tool was also used to identify open reading frames with 100 or more codons with an ORE consensus within 500 bp upstream. CoSMoS identified most of the proteins known to contain peroxisomal targeting sequences (7 of 8) or to be induced by oleic acid (13 of 14). Additionally, genes encoding 18 candidate peroxisomal proteins as well as 300 putative oleic acid–regulated genes were identified. Subcellular localization and mutational analysis has confirmed the role of some of these proteins in peroxisomal function. The *DCI1* gene encoding $\Delta^{3,5}$-$\Delta^{2,4}$-dienoyl-CoA isomerase was originally identified in this screen (40, 45).

The *Saccharomyces* genome database has also facilitated the genome-wide analysis of mRNA expression. SAGE (serial analysis of gene expression) can be used to generate a profile of gene expression for cells under different conditions (113, 114). Short, oligonucleotide sequence tags (10–14 bp) containing unique sequences corresponding to certain transcripts are used to assay the abundance of mRNAs in the mixture. The number of times each sequence tag occurs in a SAGE library is generally proportional to the level of expression of the mRNA. This technique has recently been used to compare the profile of mRNA expression (termed the transcriptome) of glucose and oleic acid–grown yeast cells (60). As expected, transcripts of genes encoding $\beta$-oxidation enzymes were more highly expressed on oleic acid than on glucose. The induction of mRNAs for enzymes involved in putative redox shuttles across peroxisomal and mitochondrial membranes was also high. A transcript profile was also determined for cells carrying the $oaf1\Delta$ and $pip2\Delta$ null alleles. Comparison of this profile to that of wild-type cells identified genes dependent on these transcription factors; it also identified genes induced as the cell's response to this defect. Data from this type of analysis provides the basis for detailed knowledge of the metabolic changes underlying utilization of different carbon sources, as well as ascribing possible function to novel genes identified via the genome sequencing project.

## FATTY ACID BIOSYNTHESIS

Fatty acids provided to *S. cerevisiae* in the medium are readily incorporated into complex lipids, especially when fatty acid synthesis is inhibited (19). Thus, altering the membrane lipid composition to study its effects on function is quite feasible. The profile of fatty acids actually synthesized de novo by *S. cerevisiae*, however, is relatively uncomplicated. The vast majority are saturated and monounsaturated fatty acids containing 16 and 18 carbons (24, 118). In addition, 1%–2% of the total fatty acids synthesized are very-long-chain fatty acids from 20–30 carbons, of which 26:0 is reported to be most abundant (118).

### Saturated Fatty Acids

Like other eukaryotes, de novo biosynthesis of saturated fatty acids in *S. cerevisiae* (see Figure 1) requires acetyl-CoA carboxylase and the fatty acid synthase complex. The gene encoding acetyl-CoA carboxylase, called *ACC1* (or *FAS3*), encodes a protein of approximately 250 kDa (2, 48). The deduced amino acid sequence of the encoded protein displays approximately 34% homology to the rat enzyme and contains typical biotin carboxylase, biotin binding, and transcarboxylase domains (2). Haploid yeast containing an *acc1* mutation are incapable of vegetative growth, even in the presence of exogenous fatty acids, which indicates that the gene is necessary for function(s) in addition to fatty acid biosynthesis (48). Fatty acid synthase in yeast is composed of two nonidentical, multifunctional subunits, $\alpha$ and $\beta$, organized as a hexamer ($\alpha_6\beta_6$). The 208-kDa $\alpha$ subunit, encoded by the *FAS2* gene, is trifunctional, containing the $\beta$-ketoacyl synthase, $\beta$-ketoacyl reductase, and acyl carrier protein functions (81, 95). The pentafunctional, 220-kDa $\beta$ subunit is encoded by the *FAS1* gene and possesses acetyl-, malonyl-, and palmitoyl-transferase, as well as dehydratase and enoyl reductase activities (17, 95, 96). Haploid yeast strains containing mutations in the fatty acid synthase complex are not viable unless the medium is supplemented with exogenous myristic (14:0), palmitic (16:0), stearic (18:0), or oleic (18:1) acid (94).

Like other eukaryotes, fatty acid biosynthesis in yeast is repressed by the presence of fatty acids (16, 61). Growth of yeast in the presence of exogenous fatty acids decreases both acetyl-CoA carboxylase and fatty acid synthase activities by 50%–70%. Transcription of the *FAS1*, *FAS2*, and *ACC1* are all decreased by fatty acids. If *FAS2* is overexpressed in cells, the expression of *FAS1* and *ACC1* is increased, indicating coordinate regulation of the three genes. In addition to fatty acid repression, these three genes are coordinately regulated by an inositol/choline response element, along with a number of genes involved in phospholipid biosynthesis (16, 48).

## Desaturation

*S. cerevisiae* is only able to synthesize monounsaturated fatty acids containing a $\Delta 9$ double bond, primarily palmitoleic (16:1) and oleic (18:1) acids. The $\Delta 9$ desaturase that produces these fatty acids in the endoplasmic reticulum is encoded by the *OLE1* gene (79, 104). In order to grow, yeast strains carrying an *ole1* mutation require supplementation with exogenous monounsaturated or polyunsaturated fatty acids containing either a $\Delta 9$ unsaturation or, in certain fatty acids, a $\Delta 10$, $\Delta 11$, or $\Delta 5$ double bond (76, 103). *OLE1* was also independently cloned as a gene involved in mitochondrial movement and transfer into daughter cells during mitosis, indicating a role for unsaturated fatty acids in this process (102). *OLE1* encodes a protein with an internal region that is 60% homologous to rat stearoyl-CoA desaturase. A fusion protein containing the N-terminal 27 amino acids of Ole1p fused to the rat stearoyl-CoA desaturase is able to complement the defect of an *ole1* mutant (104). Despite this functional interchangeability and unlike the mammalian enzyme, the yeast desaturase fails to exhibit a dependence on cytochrome *b5*, which is thought to be the electron donor for fatty acid desaturases. Rather, the yeast protein has an essential C-terminal extension with high homology to cytochrome *b5* that may serve to facilitate electron transfer (79). Ole1p is considered to be the only desaturase required for synthesis of monounsaturated fatty acids in yeast (103).

Regulation of *OLE1* expression has received a significant amount of attention recently. Transcription of *OLE1* is weakly induced by saturated fatty acids (1.6-fold) and severely repressed (up to 60-fold) by unsaturated fatty acids (19, 76), which is also reflected in desaturase enzyme activity (9). In fact, when yeast cells are grown in the presence of exogenous unsaturated fatty acids, such as linoleic acid (18:2 $\Delta 9$, 12), the cells readily incorporate them into membrane lipids, replacing nearly all the monounsaturated fatty acids (9, 103). *OLE1* gene regulation is dependent on acyl-CoA formation by acyl-CoA synthetases Faa1p and Faa4p as well as the acyl-CoA binding protein Acb1p, which indicates that metabolism of the fatty acid is required (19). Regulation of *OLE1* mRNA expression occurs both at the level of transcription (76) and via mRNA stability (42). A number of mutants insensitive to *OLE1* repression by unsaturated fatty acids (37, 77) or unable to derepress *OLE1* in response to saturated fatty acids (37) have been identified. Two redundant transcription factors, encoded by the *SPT23* and *MGA2* genes, were found to be required for *OLE1* transcription. Expression of *OLE1* on a plasmid or supplementation with oleic or palmitoleic acids suppresses the lethality of the *spt23Δ mga2Δ* double mutant (120). A recent report suggests that Spt23p processing from an inactive membrane-bound form to an active soluble form is regulated by the cellular fatty acid pool via a novel ubiquitin/proteosome–dependent process (56). Further studies of Spt23p activation will likely enrich our understanding of the role of the biophysical state of membranes in regulation of gene expression.

## Elongation

*S. cerevisiae* has enzyme systems capable of elongating fatty acyl-CoAs formed from de novo synthesis or acquired from the medium up to 26 carbons (see Figure 1). Elongation activity in homogenates is dependent on malonyl-CoA as the two-carbon donor, NADPH, and a medium- or long-chain fatty acyl-CoA primer with greater than 10 carbons (28). Several different membrane-bound elongation systems localized to the endoplasmic reticulum or mitochondria have been described, including systems capable of elongation of medium-chain fatty acyl-CoAs (12 and 14 carbons to 16 and 18 carbons) and a system that converts 18-carbon fatty acids to fatty acids with 20 or more carbons (6, 28, 107).

Recent genetic approaches in yeast have identified several genes involved in fatty acid elongation. Two groups have recently independently identified a gene essential for elongation of medium- (12 carbons) to long-chain (16–18 carbons) fatty acyl-CoAs (28, 107). Strains unable to elongate 12- to 14-carbon fatty acids were isolated by mutagenizing strains lacking fatty acid synthase (*fas-*) and identifying mutants that could be rescued with fatty acids of 16 or greater carbons but not with fatty acids with ≤15 carbons. The *ELO1* gene was identified as encoding an enzyme involved in lengthening fatty acids from 14 to 16 carbons. Strains carrying an *elo1Δ* disruption in the presence of functional fatty acid synthase (*FAS+*) exhibit no phenotype, indicating that the FAS complex is also capable of producing the required 16-carbon species. Sequence analysis by Toke & Martin (107) shows that the *ELO1* gene encodes a protein containing a putative NADPH binding site, a motif (HXXHH) characteristic of nonheme, iron deoxy cluster enzymes such as desaturases, and a cluster of lysine residues that may represent a sequence for retrieval of the protein from the Golgi to the endoplasmic reticulum.

Comparison of the deduced amino acid sequence of Elo1p to the *Saccharomyces* genome database revealed two additional genes, *ELO2* and *ELO3*, involved in formation of very-long-chain fatty acids (85). The predicted amino acid sequences of *ELO2* (previously cloned as *GNS1* and *FEN1*) and *ELO3* (previously identified as *APA1*, *SUR4*, and *SRE1*) exhibit 76% and 72% homology to Elo1p, respectively.

Both Elo2p and Elo3p contain the deoxy iron cluster motif, but neither has a recognizable NADPH binding site. Disruption of both genes in cells is lethal, but loss of either one alone results in a loss or large decrease in the formation of 26:0 fatty acid from 16- or 18-carbon fatty acids. Analysis of fatty acid profiles in *elo2Δ* and *elo3Δ* mutants indicate that Elo2p is involved in elongation up to 24 carbons, whereas Elo3p has a broader specificity and is required for elongation from 24 carbons to 26 carbons.

Sphingolipids in yeast contain a ceramide composed of a long-chain base such as phytosphingosine or dihydrosphingosine N-acylated with either a 26-carbon (26:0) or hydroxylated 26-carbon (HO-26:0) fatty acid (73). As one might expect, in *elo2Δ* or *elo3Δ* strains unable to synthesize 26:0, there is an accumulation of long-chain bases and an absence of ceramide (85). An additional gene, *TSC13*, has recently been identified as encoding an enoyl-CoA reductase required for very-long-chain fatty acid synthesis (T Dunn, S Kohlwein, personal communication). Strains containing a *tsc13* defect also accumulate long-chain bases and exhibit decreased levels of very-long-chain fatty acids. This phenotype is exacerbated by the introduction of a mutation in either *ELO2* or *ELO3*. Finally, hydroxylation of 26:0 to HO-26:0 requires the *FAH1* gene (80). Thus, the *ELO2*, *ELO3*, and *TSC13* gene products appear to play essential roles in the formation of very-long-chain fatty acids (see Figure 1) vital in sphingolipid biosynthesis.

## FUNCTIONAL GENOMICS AND THE FUTURE

The new era of yeast functional genomics brought on by the availability and analysis of the genome sequence has already facilitated the characterization of many novel genes, including several involved in fatty acid metabolism (i.e. *FAT1*, *ECI1*, *DCI1*, *IDP3*, *OAF1*, *ELO2*, *ELO3*). This, however, only represents a first step toward developing a working model for the eukaryotic cell (13). The genome project and international cooperation has led to the development of an array of new genomics tools and experimental approaches that will aid in the continued effort (12, 87). A collection of yeast strains carrying disruptions in almost all open reading frames encoding 100 or more amino acids (∼6000) became available for purchase in July 2000 (15, 119). Collections of strains carrying transposon-tagged or fusion-tagged alleles, which should prove useful for biochemical studies, have also been created (69, 75). Large-scale screens for novel protein-protein interactions in yeast have also become possible and can provide new clues as to the biological function of previously unclassified proteins (109).

Comprehensive analysis of gene expression via serial analysis of gene expression (SAGE) (60, 113, 114) or microarray technology (26) can provide a profile of the expression of the complete set of yeast genes under specific conditions (the transcriptome). Also, an effort using two-dimensional gel electrophoresis is being used to describe the proteome or the complete set of proteins synthesized in specific situations (87). Finally, quantitative metabolite profiles (the metabolome) of wild-type versus deletion strains may aid in elucidating the cellular roles of proteins with unknown function (106).

Experience and knowledge gained from the large effort in yeast functional genomics should prove valuable for analysis of more-complex genomes by providing a basis for comparative genomics (20, 86). A clue to the function of a novel gene from a more-complex organism may come via "in silico" experiments on the computer, revealing homology to a gene or a domain of a gene more completely studied in *S. cerevisiae*. In addition, indication of function for a new gene might come from the phenotype of yeast carrying a mutation in a similar gene, from the ability of the new gene to complement the corresponding yeast mutant when expressed on a plasmid, or from comparable patterns of gene expression or protein subcellular localization. To cite an example from fatty acid metabolism, advances made toward elucidating the roles of Pat1p and Pat2p in yeast peroxisomal fatty acid import shed light on the function of the homologous protein defective in X-linked adrenoleukodystrophy (52). Finally, yeast can be utilized as a living test tube for heterologous reconstitution of processes specific to higher organisms by introducing the necessary gene(s); recent examples include the biosynthesis of *n*-3 and *n*-6 polyunsaturated fatty acids (4) and editing of the mRNA of apolipoprotein B (25). Through these and other creative approaches, yeast will continue as a valuable tool during future analysis of more-complex genomes. Thus, continued effort toward understanding how the genes of yeast work together to make a functioning cell is critical. With better understanding of yeast biology comes greater potential for insight into the functional analysis of novel genes from higher organisms.

## ACKNOWLEDGMENTS

I thank Teresa Dunn and Sepp Kohlwein for generously sharing data prior to its publication. I am also indebted to Chuck Martin, Dean Appling, and Anne Tibbetts for their critical reading of the manuscript and helpful comments. Research in my laboratory on genes required for yeast growth on fatty acids is supported by the National Institutes of Health.

**Visit the Annual Reviews home page at www.AnnualReviews.org**

## LITERATURE CITED

1. Abumrad N, Coburn C, Ibrahimi A. 1999. Membrane proteins implicated in long-chain fatty acid uptake by mammalian cells: CD36, FATP and FABPm. *Biochim. Biophys. Acta* 1441:4–13

2. Al-Feel W, Chirala SS, Wakil SJ. 1992. Cloning of the yeast *FAS3* gene and the primary structure of yeast acetyl-CoA carboxy-lase. *Proc. Natl. Acad. Sci. USA* 89:4534–38

3. Baumgartner U, Hamilton B, Piskacek M, Ruis H, Rottensteiner H. 1999. Functional analysis of the $Zn_2Cys_6$ transcription factors Oaf1p and Pip2p. *J. Biol. Chem.* 274:22208–16

4. Beaudoin F, Michaelson LV, Hey SJ, Lewis

MJ, Shewry PR, et al. 2000. Heterologous reconstitution in yeast of the polyunsaturated fatty acid biosynthetic pathway. *Proc. Natl. Acad. Sci. USA* 97:6421–26

5. Berk PD, Stump DD. 1999. Mechanisms of cellular uptake of long-chain free fatty acids. *Mol. Cell. Biochem.* 192:17–31

6. Bessoule JJ, Lessire R, Rigoulet M, Guerin B, Cassagne C. 1988. Localization of the synthesis of very-long-chain fatty acid in mitochondria from *Saccharomyces cerevisiae. Eur. J. Biochem.* 177:207–11

7. Blobel F, Erdmann R. 1996. Identification of a yeast peroxisomal member of the family of AMP-binding proteins. *Eur. J. Biochem.* 240:468–76

8. Borst P, Schinkel AH. 1997. Genetic dissection of the function of mammalian P-glycoproteins. *Trends Genet.* 13:217–22

9. Bossie MA, Martin CE. 1989. Nutritional regulation of yeast Δ-9 fatty acid desaturase activity. *J. Bacteriol.* 171:6409–13

10. Bossier P, Fernandes L, Vilela C, Rodrigues-Pousada C. 1994. The yeast YKL741 gene situated on the left arm of chromosome XI codes for a homologue of the human ALD protein. *Yeast* 10:681–86

11. Botstein D, Chervitz SA, Cherry JM. 1997. Yeast as a model organism. *Science* 277:1259–60

12. Brown AJP, Tuite MF. 1998. Yeast gene analysis in the next millennium. *Methods Micro.* 26:451–61

13. Bussey H. 1997. 1997 ushers in an era of yeast functional genomics. *Yeast* 13:1501–3

14. Carlson M. 1999. Glucose repression in yeast. *Curr. Opin. Microbiol.* 2:202–7

15. Cherry JM, Ball C, Dolinski K, Dwight S, Harris M, et al. 2000. *Saccharomyces Genome Database.* http://genome-www.stanford.edu/Saccharomyces/

16. Chirala SS. 1992. Coordinated regulation and inositol-mediated and fatty acid mediated-repression of fatty acid synthase genes in *Saccharomyces cerevisiae. Proc. Natl. Acad. Sci. USA* 89:10232–36

17. Chirala SS, Kuziora MA, Spector DM, Wakil SJ. 1987. Complementation of mutations and nucleotide sequence of *FAS1* gene encoding β subunit of yeast fatty acid synthase. *J. Biol. Chem.* 262:4231–40

18. Choi J-Y, Martin CE. 1999. The *Saccharomyces cerevisiae FAT1* gene encodes an acyl-CoA synthetase that is required for maintenance of very long-chain fatty acid levels. *J. Biol. Chem.* 274:4671–83

19. Choi J-Y, Stukey J, Hwang S-Y, Martin CE. 1996. Regulatory elements that control transcription activation and unsaturated fatty acid-mediated repression of the *Saccharomyces cerevisiae OLE1* gene. *J. Biol. Chem.* 271:3581–89

20. Clark MS. 1999. Comparative genomics: the key to understanding the Human Genome Project. *BioEssays* 21:121–30

21. Coe NR, Smith AJ, Frohnert BI, Watkins PA, Bernlohr DA. 1999. The fatty acid transport protein (FATP1) is a very long-chain acyl-CoA synthetase. *J. Biol. Chem.* 274:36300–4

22. Cohen G, Fessl F, Traczyk A, Rytka J, Ruis H. 1985. Isolation of the catalase A gene of *Saccharomyces cerevisiae* by complementation of the *cta1* mutation. *Mol. Gen. Genet.* 200:74–79

23. Costanzo MC, Hogan JD, Cusick ME, Davis BP, Fancher AM, et al. 2000. The yeast proteome database (YPD) and *Caenorhabditis elegans* proteome database (WormPD): comprehensive resources for the organization and comparison of model organism protein information. *Nucleic Acids Res.* 28:73–76

24. Cottrell M, Viljoen BC, Kock JLF, Lategan PM. 1986. The long-chain fatty acid compositions of species representing the genera *Saccharomyces, Schwanniomyces and Lipomyces. J. Gen. Microbiol.* 132:2401–3

25. Dance GS, Sowden MP, Yang Y, Smith HC. 2000. APOBEC-1 dependent cytidine to uridine editing of apolipoprotein B RNA in yeast. *Nucleic Acids Res.* 28:424–29

26. DeRisi JL, Iyer VR, Brown PO. 1997.

Exploring the metabolic and genetic control of gene expression on a genomic scale. *Science* 278:680–86

27. DiRusso CC, Black PN. 1999. Long-chain fatty acid transport in bacteria and yeast. Paradigms for defining the mechanism underlying this protein-mediated process. *Mol. Cell. Biochem.* 192:41–52

28. Dittrich F, Zajonc D, Hühne K, Hoja U, Ekici A, et al. 1998. Fatty acid elongation in yeast: biochemical characteristics of the enzyme system and isolation of elongation-defective mutants. *Eur. J. Biochem.* 252:477–85

29. Dmochowska A, Dignard D, Maleszka R, Thomas DY. 1990. Structure and control of the *Saccharomyces cerevisiae POX1* gene encoding acyl-coenzyme A oxidase. *Gene* 88:247–52

30. Duronio RJ, Knoll LJ, Gordon JI. 1992. Isolation of a *Saccharomyces cerevisiae* long-chain fatty acyl:CoA synthetase gene (*FAA1*) and assessment of its role in protein N-myristoylation. *J. Cell Biol.* 117:515–29

31. Einerhand AWC, Kos WT, Distel B, Tabak HF. 1993. Characterization of a transcriptional control element involved in proliferation of peroxisomes in yeast in response to oleate. *Eur. J. Biochem.* 214:323–31

32. Einerhand AWC, Voorn-Brouwer TM, Erdmann R, Kunau W-H, Tabak HF. 1991. Regulation of transcription of the gene coding for peroxisomal 3-oxoacyl-CoA thiolase of *Saccharomyces cerevisiae. Eur. J. Biochem.* 200:113–22

33. Elgersma Y, van Roermund CWT, Wanders RJA, Tabak HF. 1995. Peroxisomal and mitochondrial carnitine acetyltransferases of *Saccharomyces cerevisiae* are encoded by a single gene. *EMBO J.* 14:3472–79

34. Erdmann R, Veenhuis M, Mertens D, Kunau W-H. 1989. Isolation of peroxisome-deficient mutants of *Saccharomyces cerevisiae. Proc. Natl. Acad. Sci. USA* 86:5419–23

35. Faergeman NJ, DiRusso CC, Elberger A, Knudsen J, Black PN. 1997. Disruption of the *Saccharomyces cerevisiae* homologue to murine fatty acid transport protein impairs uptake and growth on long-chain fatty acids. *J. Biol. Chem.* 272:8531–38

36. Filipits M, Simon MM, Rapatz W, Hamilton B, Ruis H. 1993. A *Saccharomyces cerevisiae* upstream activating sequence mediates induction of peroxisome proliferation by fatty acids. *Gene* 132:49–55

37. Fujimori K, Anamnart S, Nakagawa Y, Sugioka S, Ohta D, et al. 1997. Isolation and characterization of mutations affecting expression of the Δ9-fatty acid desaturase gene, *OLE1*, in *Saccharomyces cerevisiae. FEBS Lett.* 413:226–30

38. Gancendo JM. 1998. Yeast carbon catabolite repression. *Micro. Mol. Biol. Rev.* 62:334–61

39. Geisbrecht BV, Zhu D, Schulz K, Nau K, Morrell JC, et al. 1998. Molecular characterization of *Saccharomyces cerevisiae* $\Delta^3, \Delta^2$-enoyl-CoA isomerase. *J. Biol. Chem.* 273:33184–91

40. Geraghty MT, Bassett D, Morrell JC, Gatto GJ Jr, Bai J, et al. 1999. Detecting patterns of protein distribution and gene expression *in silico. Proc. Natl. Acad. Sci. USA* 96:2937–42

41. Goffeau A, Barrell BG, Bussey H, Davis RW, Dujon B, et al. 1996. Life with 6000 genes. *Science* 274:546–67

42. Gonzalez CI, Martin CE. 1996. Fatty acid-responsive control of mRNA stability: unsaturated fatty acid-induced degradation of the *Saccharomyces OLE1* transcript. *J. Biol. Chem.* 271:25801–9

43. Gurvitz A, Hamilton B, Ruis H, Hartig A. 2001. Peroxisomal degradation of trans-unsaturated fatty acids in the yeast *Saccharomyces cerevisiae. J. Biol. Chem.* In press

44. Gurvitz A, Mursula AM, Firzinger A, Hamilton B, Kilpeläinen SH, et al. 1998. Peroxisomal $\Delta^3$-*cis*-$\Delta^2$-*trans*-enoyl-CoA isomerase encoded by *ECI1* is required for growth of the yeast *Saccharomyces cerevisiae* on unsaturated fatty acids. *J. Biol. Chem.* 273:31366–74

45. Gurvitz A, Mursula AM, Yagi AI, Hartig A, Ruis H, et al. 1999. Alternatives to the isomerase-dependent pathway for the β-oxidation of oleic acid are dispensable in *Saccharomyces cerevisiae*. *J. Biol. Chem.* 274:24514–21

46. Gurvitz A, Rottensteiner H, Kilpeläinen SH, Hartig A, Hiltûnen JK, et al. 1997. The *Saccharomyces cerevisiae* peroxisomal 2,4-dienoyl-CoA reductase is encoded by the oleate-inducible gene *SPS19*. *J. Biol. Chem.* 272:22140–47

47. Hamilton JA. 1998. Fatty acid transport: difficult or easy? *J. Lipid Res.* 39:467–81

48. Hasslacher M, Ivessa AS, Paltauf F, Kohlwein SD. 1993. Acetyl-CoA carboxylase from yeast is an essential enzyme and is regulated by factors that control phospholipid metabolism. *J. Biol. Chem.* 268:10946–52

49. Henke B, Girzalsky W, Berteaux-Lecellier V, Erdmann R. 1998. *IDP3* encodes a peroxisomal NADP-dependent isocitrate dehydrogenase required for the β-oxidation of unsaturated fatty acids. *J. Biol. Chem.* 273:3702–11

50. Hettema EH, Distel B, Tabak HF. 1999. Import of proteins into peroxisomes. *Biochim. Biophys. Acta* 1451:17–34

51. Hettema EH, Tabak HF. 2000. Transport of fatty acids and metabolites across the peroxisomal membrane. *Biochim. Biophys. Acta* 1486:18–27

52. Hettema EH, van Roermund CWT, Distel B, van den Berg M, Vilela C, et al. 1996. The ABC transporter proteins Pat1 and Pat2 are required for import of long-chain fatty acids into peroxisomes of *Saccharomyces cerevisiae*. *EMBO J.* 15:3813–22

53. Hieter P, Boguski M. 1997. Functional genomics: It's all how you read it. *Science* 278:601–2

54. Hiltûnen JK, Wenzel B, Beyer A, Erdmann R, Fosså A, Kunau W-H. 1992. Peroxisomal multifunctional β-oxidation protein of *Saccharomyces cerevisiae*: molecular analysis of the *FOX2* gene and gene product. *J. Biol. Chem.* 267:6646–53

55. Hirsch D, Stahl A, Lodish HF. 1998. A family of fatty acid transporters conserved from mycobacterium to man. *Proc. Natl. Acad. Sci. USA* 95:8625–29

56. Hoppe T, Matuschewski K, Rape M, Schlenker S, Ulrich HD, Jentsch S. 2000. Activation of a membrane-bound transcription factor by regulated ubiquitin/-proteosome-dependent processing. *Cell* 102:577–86

57. Igual JC, Matallana E, Gonzalez-Bosch C, Franco L, Perez-Ortin JE. 1991. A new glucose-repressible gene identified from the analysis of chromatin structure in deletion mutants of yeast *SUC2* locus. *Yeast* 7:379–89

58. Johnson DR, Knoll LJ, Levin DE, Gordon JI. 1994. *Saccharomyces cerevisiae* contains four fatty acid activation (*FAA*) genes: an assessment of their role in regulating protein N-myristoylation and cellular lipid metabolism. *J. Cell Biol.* 127:751–62

59. Johnson DR, Knoll LJ, Rowley N, Gordon JI. 1994. Genetic analysis of the role of *Saccharomyces cerevisiae* acyl-CoA synthetase genes in regulating protein N-myristoylation. *J. Biol. Chem.* 269:18037–46

60. Kal AJ, van Zonneveld AJ, Benes V, van den Berg M, Koerkamp MG, et al. 1999. Dynamics of gene expression revealed by comparison of serial analysis of gene expression transcript profiles from yeast grown on two different carbon sources. *Mol. Biol. Cell* 10:1859–72

61. Kamiryo T, Parthasarathy S, Numa S. 1976. Evidence that acyl coenzyme A synthetase activity is required for repression of yeast acetyl coenzyme A carboxylase by exogenous fatty acids. *Proc. Natl. Acad. Sci. USA* 73:386–90

62. Karpichev IV, Luo Y, Marians RC, Small GM. 1997. A complex containing two transcription factors regulates peroxisome proliferation and the coordinate induction of

$\beta$-oxidation enzymes in *Saccharomyces cerevisiae. Mol. Cell. Biol.* 17:69–80

63. Karpichev IV, Small GM. 1998. Global regulatory functions of Oaf1p and Pip2p (Oaf2p), transcription factors that regulate genes encoding peroxisomal proteins in *Saccharomyces cerevisiae. Mol. Cell. Biol.* 18:6560–70

64. Knoll LJ, Johnson DR, Gordon JI. 1994. Biochemical studies of three *Saccharomyces cerevisiae* acyl-CoA synthetases, Faa1p, Faa2p, and Faa3p. *J. Biol. Chem.* 269:16348–56

65. Knoll LJ, Johnson DR, Gordon JI. 1995. Complementation of *Saccharomyces cerevisiae* strains containing fatty acid activation gene (*FAA*) deletions with a mammalian acyl-CoA synthetase. *J. Biol. Chem.* 270:10861–67

66. Knudsen J, Jensen MV, Hansen JK, Faergeman NJ, Neergaard TBF, Gaigg B. 1999. Role of acylCoA binding protein in acyl-CoA transport, metabolism and cell signaling. *Mol. Cell. Biochem.* 192:95–103

67. Knudsen J, Neergaard TBF, Gaigg B, Jensen MV, Hansen JK. 2000. Role of acyl-CoA binding protein in acyl-CoA metabolism and acyl-CoA-mediated cell signalling. *J. Nutr.* 130:294S–98S

68. Kohlwein SD, Paltauf F. 1983. Uptake of fatty acids by the yeasts, *Saccharomyces uvarum* and *Saccharomycopsis lipolytica. Biochim. Biophys. Acta* 792:310–17

69. Kumar A, Cheung K-H, Ross-Macdonald P, Coelho PSR, Miller P, Snyder M. 2000. TRIPLES: a database of gene function in *Saccharomyces cerevisiae. Nucleic Acids Res.* 28:81–84

70. Kunau W-H. 1998. Peroxisome biogenesis: from yeast to man. *Curr. Opin. Microbiol.* 1:232–37

71. Kunau W-H, Bühne S, de la Garza M, Kionka C, Mateblowski M, et al. 1988. Comparative enzymology of $\beta$-oxidation. *Biochem. Soc. Transact.* 16:418–20

72. Lazarow PB, Kunau W-H. 1997. Peroxisomes. In *The Molecular and Cellular Biology of the Yeast Saccharomyces*, Vol. III. *Cell Cycle and Cell Biology*, ed. JR Pringle, JR Broach, EW Jones, pp. 547–605. Cold Spring Harbor, NY: Cold Spring Harbor Lab.

73. Lester RL, Wells GB, Oxford G, Dickson RC. 1993. Mutant strains of *Saccharomyces cerevisiae* lacking sphingolipids synthesize novel inositol glycerophospholipids that mimic sphingoid structures. *J. Biol. Chem.* 268:845–56

74. Luo Y, Karpichev IV, Kohanski RA, Small GM. 1996. Purification, identification, and properties of a *Saccharomyces cerevisiae* oleate-activated upstream activating sequence-binding protein that is involved in the activation of POX1. *J. Biol. Chem.* 271:12068–75

75. Martzen MR, McCraith SM, Spinelli SL, Torres FM, Fields S, et al. 1999. A biochemical genomics approach for identifying genes by the activity of their products. *Science* 286:1153–55

76. McDonough VM, Stukey JE, Martin CE. 1992. Specificity of unsaturated fatty acid-regulated expression of the *Saccharomyces cerevisiae OLE1* gene. *J. Biol. Chem.* 267:5931–36

77. McHale MW, Kroening KD, Bernlohr DA. 1996. Identification of a class of *Saccharomyces cerevisiae* mutants defective in fatty acid repression of gene transcription and analysis of the *frm2* gene. *Yeast* 12:319–31

78. Mewes HW, Heumann K, Kaps A, Mayer K, Pfeiffer F, et al. 1999. MIPS: a database for genomes and protein sequences. *Nucleic Acids Res.* 27:44–48

79. Mitchell AG, Martin CE. 1995. A novel cytochrome b5-like domain is linked to the carboxyl terminus of the *Saccharomyces cerevisiae* $\Delta$-9 fatty acid desaturase. *J. Biol. Chem.* 270:29766–72

80. Mitchell AG, Martin CE. 1997. Fah1p, a *Saccharomyces cerevisiae* cytochrome $b_5$ fusion protein, and its *Arabidopsis thaliana* homolog that lacks the cytochrome $b_5$

domain both function in the α-hydroxylation of sphingolipid very long-chain fatty acids. *J. Biol. Chem.* 272:28281–88

81. Mohamed AH, Chirala SS, Mody NH, Huang W-Y, Wakil SJ. 1988. Primary structure of the multifunctional α subunit protein of yeast fatty acid synthase derived from *FAS2* gene sequence. *J. Biol. Chem.* 263:12315–25

82. Mosser J, Douar A-M, Sarde C-O, Kioschis P, Feil R, et al. 1993. Putative X-linked adrenoleukodystrophy gene shares unexpected homology with ABC transporters. *Nature* 361:726–30

83. Mosser J, Lutz Y, Stoeckel ME, Sarde C-O, Kretz C, et al. 1994. The gene responsible for adrenoleukodystrophy encodes a peroxisomal membrane protein. *Hum. Mol. Genet.* 3:265–71

84. Navarro B, Igual JC. 1994. *ADR1* and *SNF1* mediate different mechanisms in transcriptional regulation of yeast *POT1* gene. *Biochem. Biophys. Res. Commun.* 202:960–66

85. Oh C-S, Toke DA, Mandala S, Martin CE. 1997. *ELO2* and *ELO3*, homologues of the *Saccharomyces cerevisiae ELO1* gene, function in fatty acid elongation and are required for sphingolipid formation. *J. Biol. Chem.* 272:17376–84

86. Oliver SG. 1997. Yeast as a navigational aid in genome analysis; 1996 Kathleen Barton-Wright Memorial Lecture. *Microbiology* 143:1483–87

87. Oliver SG, Winson MK, Kell DB, Baganz F. 1998. Systematic functional analysis of the yeast genome. *Trends Biotechnol.* 16:373–78

88. Rose MD, Broach JR. 1991. Cloning genes by complementation in yeast. *Methods Enzymol.* 194:195–238

89. Rose TM, Schultz ER, Todaro GJ. 1992. Molecular cloning of the gene for the yeast homology (*ACB*) of diazepam binding inhibitor/endozepine/acyl-CoA-binding protein. *Proc. Natl. Acad. Sci. USA* 89:11287–91

90. Rothstein R. 1991. Targeting, disruption, replacement, and allele rescue: integrative DNA transformation in yeast. *Methods Enzymol.* 194:281–301

91. Rottensteiner H, Kal AJ, Filipits M, Binder M, Hamilton B, et al. 1996. Pip2p: a transcriptional regulator of peroxisome proliferation in the yeast *Saccharomyces cerevisiae*. *EMBO J.* 15:2924–34

92. Schaffer JE, Lodish HF. 1994. Expression cloning and characterization of a novel adipocyte long-chain fatty acid transport protein. *Cell* 79:427–36

93. Schjerling CK, Hummel R, Hansen JK, Børsting C, Mikkelsen JM, et al. 1996. Disruption of the gene encoding the acyl-CoA-binding protein (*ACB1*) perturbs acyl-CoA metabolism in *Saccharomyces cerevisiae*. *J. Biol. Chem.* 271:22514–21

94. Schweizer E, Bolling H. 1970. A *Saccharomyces cerevisiae* mutant defective in saturated fatty acid biosynthesis. *Proc. Natl. Acad. Sci. USA* 67:660–66

95. Schweizer M, Lebert C, Höltke J, Roberts LM, Schweizer E. 1984. Molecular cloning of the yeast fatty acid synthetase genes, *FAS1* and *FAS2*: illustrating the structure of the *FAS1* cluster gene by transcript mapping and transformation studies. *Mol. Gen. Genet.* 194:457–65

96. Schweizer M, Roberts LM, Höltke H-J, Takabayashi K, Höllerer E, et al. 1986. The pentafunctional *FAS1* gene of yeast: its nucleotide sequence and order of the catalytic domains. *Mol. Gen. Genet.* 203:479–86

97. Shani N, Valle D. 1996. A *Saccharomyces cerevisiae* homolog of the human adrenoleukodystrophy transporter is a heterodimer of two half ATP-binding cassette transporters. *Proc. Natl. Acad. Sci. USA* 93:11901–6

98. Shani N, Watkins PA, Valle D. 1995. *PXA1*, a possible *Saccharomyces cerevisiae* ortholog of the human adrenoleukodystrophy gene. *Proc. Natl. Acad. Sci. USA* 92:6012–16

99. Simon M, Adam G, Rapatz W, Spevak W,

Ruis H. 1991. The *Saccharomyces cerevisiae ADR1* gene is a positive regulator of transcription of genes encoding peroxisomal proteins. *Mol. Cell. Biol.* 11:699–704

100. Simon M, Binder M, Adam G, Hartig A, Ruis H. 1992. Control of peroxisome proliferation in *Saccharomyces cerevisiae* by *ADR1, SNF1 (CAT1, CCR1)* and *SNF4 (CAT3). Yeast* 8:303–9

101. Skoneczny M, Chelstowska A, Rytka J. 1988. Study of the coinduction by fatty acids of catalase A and acyl-CoA oxidase in standard and mutant *Saccharomyces cerevisiae* strains. *Eur. J. Biochem.* 174:297–302

102. Stewart LC, Yaffe MP. 1991. A role for unsaturated fatty acids in mitochondrial movement and inheritance. *J. Cell Biol.* 115:1249–57

103. Stukey JE, McDonough VM, Martin CE. 1989. Isolation and characterization of *OLE1*, a gene affecting fatty acid desaturation from *Saccharomyces cerevisiae*. *J. Biol. Chem.* 264:16537–44

104. Stukey JE, McDonough VM, Martin CE. 1990. The *OLE1* gene of *Saccharomyces cerevisiae* encodes the Δ9 fatty acid desaturase and can be functionally replaced by the rat stearoyl-CoA desaturase gene. *J. Biol. Chem.* 265:20144–49

105. Swartzman EE, Viswanathan MN, Thorner J. 1996. The *PAL1* gene product is a peroxisomal ATP-binding cassette transporter in the yeast *Saccharomyces cerevisiae*. *J. Cell Biol.* 132:549–63

106. Teusink B, Baganz F, Westerhoff HV, Oliver SG. 1998. Metabolic control analysis as a tool in the elucidation of the function of novel genes. *Methods Micro.* 26:297–336

107. Toke DA, Martin CE. 1996. Isolation and characterization of a gene affecting fatty acid elongation in *Saccharomyces cerevisiae*. *J. Biol. Chem.* 271:18413–22

108. Trigatti BL, Baker AD, Rajaratnam K, Rachubinski RA, Gerber GE. 1992. Fatty acid uptake in *Candida tropicalis*: induction of a saturable process. *Biochem. Cell Biol.* 70:76–80

109. Uetz P, Giot L, Cagney G, Mansfield TA, Judson RS, et al. 2000. A comprehensive analysis of protein-protein interactions in *Saccharomyces cerevisiae*. *Nature* 403:623–27

110. van Roermund CWT, Elgersma Y, Singh N, Wanders RJA, Tabak HF. 1995. The membrane of peroxisomes in *Saccharomyces cerevisiae* is impermeable to NAD(H) and acetyl-CoA under *in vivo* conditions. *EMBO J.* 14:3480–86

111. van Roermund CWT, Hettema EH, Kal AJ, van den Berg M, Tabak HF, Wanders RJA. 1998. Peroxisomal β-oxidation of polyunsaturated fatty acids in *Saccharomyces cerevisiae*: isocitrate dehydrogenase provides NADPH for reduction of double bonds at even positions. *EMBO J.* 17:677–87

112. Veenhuis M, Mateblowski M, Kunau W-H, Harder W. 1987. Proliferation of microbodies in *Saccharomyces cerevisiae*. *Yeast* 3:77–84

113. Velculescu VE, Zhang L, Vogelstein B, Kinzler KW. 1995. Serial analysis of gene expression. *Science* 270:484–87

114. Velculescu VE, Zhang L, Zhou W, Vogelstein J, Basrai MA, et al. 1997. Characterization of the yeast transcriptome. *Cell* 88:243–51

115. Wang T, Luo Y, Small GM. 1994. The *POX1* gene encoding peroxisomal acyl-CoA oxidase in *Saccharomyces cerevisiae* is under control of multiple regulatory elements. *J. Biol. Chem.* 269:24480–85

116. Waterham HR, Cregg JM. 1997. Peroxisome biogenesis. *BioEssays* 19:57–66

117. Watkins PA, Lu J-F, Steinberg SJ, Gould SJ, Smith KD, Braiterman LT. 1998. Disruption of the *Saccharomyces cerevisiae FAT1* gene decreases very long-chain fatty acyl-CoA synthetase activity and elevates intracellular very long-chain

fatty acid concentrations. *J. Biol. Chem.* 273:18210–19

118. Welch JW, Burlingame AL. 1973. Very long-chain fatty acids in yeast. *J. Bacteriol.* 115:464–66

119. Winzeler EA, Shoemaker DD, Astromoff A, Liang H, Anderson K, et al. 1999. Functional characterization of the *S. cere-* *visiae* genome by gene deletion and parallel analysis. *Science* 285:901–6

120. Zhang S, Skalsky Y, Garfinkel DJ. 1999. *MGA2* or *SPT23* is required for transcription of the $\Delta 9$ fatty acid desaturase gene, *OLE1*, and nuclear membrane integrity in *Saccharomyces cerevisiae*. *Genetics* 151:473–83

Annu. Rev. Nutr. 2001. 21:121–40

# DIETARY REGULATION OF EXPRESSION OF GLUCOSE-6-PHOSPHATE DEHYDROGENASE

## Lisa M Salati and Batoul Amir-Ahmady

*Department of Biochemistry, West Virginia University School of Medicine, Morgantown, West Virginia 26506; e-mail: lsalati@hsc.wvu.edu*

**Key Words**   polyunsaturated fat, carbohydrate, posttranscriptional regulation, RNA processing, lipogenesis

■ **Abstract**   The family of enzymes involved in lipogenesis is a model system for understanding how a cell adapts to dietary energy in the form of carbohydrate versus energy in the form of triacylglycerol. Glucose-6-phosphate dehydrogenase (G6PD) is unique in this group of enzymes in that it participates in multiple metabolic pathways: reductive biosynthesis, including lipogenesis; protection from oxidative stress; and cellular growth. G6PD activity is enhanced by dietary carbohydrates and is inhibited by dietary polyunsaturated fats. These changes in G6PD activity are a consequence of changes in the expression of the G6PD gene. Nutrients can regulate the expression of genes at both transcriptional and posttranscriptional steps. Most lipogenic enzymes undergo large changes in the rate of gene transcription in response to dietary changes; however, G6PD is regulated at a step subsequent to transcription. This step is involved in the rate of synthesis of the mature mRNA in the nucleus, specifically regulation of the efficiency of splicing of the nascent G6PD transcript. Understanding the mechanisms by which nutrients alter nuclear posttranscriptional events will help uncover new information on the breadth of mechanisms involved in gene regulation.

## CONTENTS

0199-9885/01/0715-0121$14.00    **121**

## INTRODUCTION

Glucose-6-phosphate dehydrogenase (G6PD) activity is needed in all cell types for the production of NADPH and for control of carbon flow through the pentose phosphate pathway. G6PD catalyzes the first reaction of this pathway, oxidizing glucose-6-phosphate to 6-phosphogluconolactone and in the process reducing $NADP^+$ to $NADPH + H^+$ (Figure 1). This reaction is the rate-determining step of the oxidative portion of the pentose phosphate pathway. Together with 6-phosphogluconate dehydrogenase, these enzymes provide NADPH for reductive biosynthetic reactions, such as fatty acid, cholesterol, and amino acid synthesis, and for maintenance of reduced glutathione concentrations. In addition, it regulates the rate of glucose conversion to ribose-5-phosphate, the precursor for nucleotide biosynthesis.

The G6PD gene spans 18 kb on the X chromosome (xq 28) and contains 13 exons. The G6PD promoter is embedded in a CpG island that is conserved from mice to humans (50, 85). The promoter of the G6PD gene contains a TATA-like

**Figure 1**   Role of glucose-6-phosphate dehydrogenase in cellular metabolism.

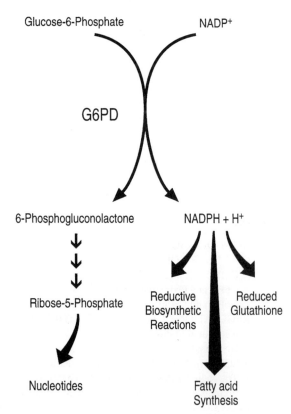

sequence, TTAAAT, and numerous stimulatory protein 1 (Sp1) elements, but no CAAT element (50, 65, 67, 85). S1 nuclease and primer extension analyses of mouse G6PD mRNA indicate that the transcriptional start site used in liver and adipose tissue, in which lipogenesis is regulated, is the same as in kidney, in which G6PD is expressed constituitively (37). These results indicate that the 5'-end of the mRNA is the same in all cell types. Three DNase I hypersensitive sites have been localized in the 5'-end of the G6PD gene. Hss-1 ($-1000$ bp) and Hss-2 ($-400$ bp) are present in all tissues, but Hss-3, which is located in intron 2 ($+1500$ bp), is liver specific (37). The translation start site is located in exon 2 and has been mapped in rats, mice, and humans (19, 36, 50, 79). The number of exons and introns and the size and sequence of the exons are conserved in higher eukaryotes. The sequence similarity between the human G6PD cDNA and that of mice or rats is 87%. The similarity between the mouse and rat cDNA sequences is even greater (93% identity). Most of the dissimilarity is in the 3'-untranslated region (3'-UTR). Exon 13 is at least 800 nucleotides long and contains the translation stop codon. The 3'-UTR is approximately 600 nucleotides long and contains a single poly(A) site (LP Stabile & LM Salati, unpublished data). The structure of the gene is unusual in that the second intron is 11 kb and accounts for almost half of the gene; the large size of this intron is also conserved between humans, rats, and mice.

The amount of G6PD activity and mRNA abundance differs between tissues (27, 37) and most likely reflects tissue-specific differences in growth rate, reductive biosynthetic reactions, and oxidative stress. Moreover, G6PD expression is regulated by hormonal and nutritional factors in only a few tissues. G6PD expression is regulated in liver and adipose tissue, and its activity correlates with the rate of fatty acid biosynthesis. It is also induced in lactating mammary glands by dietary carbohydrate (31). The majority of the research on the nutritional regulation of G6PD expression has been in liver; thus, this review predominantly covers regulation of G6PD in liver tissue.

# CELLULAR ROLES OF G6PD

## G6PD: A Lipogenic Enzyme

The family of lipogenic enzymes includes fatty acid synthase, acetyl-coenzyme A (CoA) carboxylase, ATP-citrate lyase, malic enzyme, and G6PD; these enzymes catalyze reactions for the de novo synthesis of fatty acids. G6PD is considered a lipogenic enzyme because it provides a substrate, NADPH, for production of palmitate by fatty acid synthase. NADPH is also produced by the malic enzyme reaction using malate supplied by the ATP-citrate lyase and malate dehydrogenase reactions and reducing equivalents from cytosolic NADH. The relative contribution of these two pathways, as sources of NADPH for the fatty acid synthase reaction, varies with species. In rodents, and presumable other mammals, the contribution of each pathway is equivalent (18, 42, 68). In contrast, in avians, most of the NADPH is provided by the malic enzyme reaction, and flux through the oxidative reactions of the pentose phosphate pathway is very low (29, 61). The redundancy of the NADPH supply protects the animal from mutations that would influence this supply. In this regard, mice homozygous for a null mutation of malic enzyme are viable and have normal lipid stores (48). In humans, G6PD deficiency, also called favaism, causes disease, with varying levels of severity, but the deleterious symptoms are a consequence of reduced glutathione depletion, not attenuated lipogenesis. Yet the importance of G6PD as a source of NADPH for fatty acid synthesis is highlighted by the decrease in lipogenic rate and in serum lipoprotein concentrations in individuals with G6PD deficiency (17, 57).

The activities of the lipogenic enzymes, including G6PD, change in parallel with lipogenic rates in cells. Their activities increase coordinately to achieve high rates of lipogenesis when substrate is in excess, such as after a high-carbohydrate meal, and their activities are inhibited when substrate is limiting, such as during starvation. The humoral factors signaling these changes effect the expression of all members of this enzyme family, yet the details of the intracellular mechanisms resulting in the changes in enzyme activity differ greatly between enzymes. The lipogenic enzymes are all regulated at a pretranslational step (34). In most cases, these genes undergo large changes in the rate of transcription. In contrast, G6PD is regulated post-transcriptionally. Acetyl-CoA carboxylase is unique in the lipogenic family in that it also undergoes both allosteric and covalent modifications, resulting in short-term changes in its activity in the absence of changes in the amount of enzyme protein.

## G6PD and Oxidative Stress

Physiological conditions resulting in oxidative stress can also result in changes in G6PD activity. NADPH is required for detoxification of free radicals and peroxides. G6PD gene expression is essential for protection of the cell against even mild oxidative stress (6, 62). It provides the only means of generating NADPH to maintain reduced glutathione levels in mature erythrocytes, and in its absence, the erythrocytes are particularly vulnerable to hemolysis. Induction of G6PD expression due to oxidative stress has been observed in many cell types (71, 87). G6PD expression is increased along with other antioxidant enzymes when rat alveolar type II cells are exposed to oxidative stress (44). Incubation of rat hepatocytes with acetaldehyde or ethanol also increases G6PD activity and mRNA abundance (43, 76, 78). Moreover, maintenance of high levels of G6PD activity protects both neuronal cells and fibroblasts from hydrogen peroxide–induced cell death (81). In contrast, a high glucose concentration in the medium of endothelial cells results in a decrease in G6PD activity and cellular death (97). This adverse regulation of G6PD is thought to be involved in the pathogenesis of diabetes mellitus. The complete inactivation of the G6PD gene results in extreme sensitivity to oxidative stress in cells in culture (62). In humans, G6PD deficiency is not extreme; clinical manifestations occur primarily when an exogenous stress, such as an oxidative agent or a viral disease, is present. Of the more than 300 reported mutations in the G6PD gene, most are point mutations; there are no large deletions or insertions (88). Thus, a null mutant for G6PD is most certainly lethal to an animal.

## G6PD and Cellular Growth

Changes in G6PD activity occur in parallel with changes in the rate of cell growth. This may stem in part from the role of the pentose phosphate pathway in providing the ribose-5-phosphate needed for nucleotide biosynthesis, and in part by the role G6PD plays in regulating redox state of the cell. Similar to the regulation of G6PD activity by oxidative stress, the coincident changes in both cell growth and G6PD activity have been observed in multiple cell types. G6PD activity is elevated in proliferating nodules and tumors (27, 47). Growth stimulation by factors such as serum, epidermal growth factor (EGF), and platelet-derived growth factor increase both G6PD activity and DNA synthesis in fibroblast and epithelial cell lines (75, 82). Stimulation of hepatocyte growth by EGF also results in parallel changes in G6PD activity and DNA synthesis (59, 94). Within the same cells, incubation with EGF resulted in a decrease in malic enzyme expression, which suggests that EGF was enhancing G6PD activity to provide ribsose-5-phosphate and NADPH to support cellular growth and not lipogenesis. The mechanisms resulting in this increase in G6PD activity have not been fully examined. Although nutritional regulation of G6PD is not thought to involve allosterism or phosphorylation, G6PD regulation by growth factors may involve the release and thereby activation of G6PD enzyme from intracellular membranes (75). The details of this mechanism will most likely prove to be quite complex. Investigators examining G6PD regulation by hormonal and nutrient factors in cells in culture must bear in mind that some changes in G6PD mRNA or enzyme activity may be a consequence of changing cellular growth rates.

## REGULATION OF G6PD BY NUTRITIONAL AND HORMONAL STATUS

The purpose of regulating G6PD activity by nutritional and hormonal factors is to provide the cell with the capacity to synthesize fatty acids. Thus, this regulation of G6PD is only observed in tissues with high lipogenic capacity, such as liver and adipose tissue. Identification of relevant humoral factors requires model systems using both intact animals and cells in culture. The latter has been particularly challenging because regulation of G6PD expression by nutrients and hormones is lost in most immortalized cell lines. Thus, primary hepatocytes in monolayer cultures have provided the primary tool for these analyses.

## Nutritional Status

***Starvation and Refeeding Paradigm***    Hepatic G6PD expression has been studied frequently as a model of adaptive regulation by diet. Long-term starvation decreases rat liver G6PD activity (40, 51). Refeeding with a fat-free, high-carbohydrate diet increases the activity of G6PD to an amount greater than that of the "normal" fed state (4, 66). This phenomenon has been termed enzyme overshoot (4). The molecular basis for overshoot is not well understood but appears to require insulin, glucocorticoids, and a high-carbohydrate, low-fat diet. The starvation/ refeeding paradigm remains a useful tool for studying metabolic regulation because these dietary changes are unambiguous and result in large changes in enzyme activity.

*Type and Amount of Dietary Carbohydrate*    Consumption of a high-carbohydrate, fat-free diet causes the largest increase in G6PD activity of any diet. The greatest change in G6PD activity is observed when rats are fed diets containing glucose or fructose, compared with starch, and stimulation by fructose is greater than by glucose (20, 40). Glucose and fructose increase hepatic G6PD activity in a manner apparently independent of hormones. In this regard, hepatic G6PD activity can be increased in diabetic rats by feeding them fructose instead of glucose (23). Furthermore, increasing the concentration of glucose in the medium of primary hepatocytes in culture from 0 to 25 mM increases G6PD activity in the absence of hormones (43, 70); however, these effects are not uniformly observed by all researchers (46, 49). Induction by monosaccharides has been described for other enzymes, such as malic enzyme, $S_{14}$ (spot 14, a putative lipogenic protein of unknown identity), and pyruvate kinase (reviewed in 26, 86). The factor causing the carbohydrate stimulation is thought to be an intermediate in the metabolism of glucose or fructose (26, and the references therein). Variations between laboratories with respect to the effect of glucose may reflect differences in the content of gluconeogenic amino acids in the culture medium resulting in sufficient accumulation of this metabolic intermediate even at low glucose concentrations. Alternatively, the effect of glucose on G6PD expression may be indirect and reflect changes in the growth rate or redox state of the cells.

*Type and Amount of Dietary Fat*    In contrast to the stimulatory effect of carbohydrates, polyunsaturated fatty acids inhibit G6PD both in intact animals and in primary hepatocytes in culture (11, 12, 33, 41, 70, 73, 74). The inhibition of G6PD activity by polyunsaturated fat occurs both when rats are switched from a high-carbohydrate, fat-free diet to one containing polyunsaturated fat (11) and when starved rats are refed a high-carbohydrate diet supplemented with polyunsaturated fat (3). Several lines of evidence indicate that the inhibition of G6PD activity is due specifically to the polyunsaturated fat content of the diet. First, in the presence of a similar carbohydrate intake between rats with and without fat added to the diet, the addition of polyunsaturated fatty acids decreases the activity of G6PD (12). Addition to the diet of saturated fatty acids, such as palmitate (16:0) and stearate (18:0), and of monounsaturated fatty acids, such as oleate (18:1), do not inhibit G6PD activity (11, 12). Furthermore, this indicates that the inhibition of G6PD activity is not merely a consequence of a decrease in carbohydrate intake. Second, inhibition of G6PD activity is not a consequence of reversing essential fatty acid deficiency in the animals because adding additional polyunsaturated fat to a diet adequate in essential fatty acids further inhibits G6PD activity (11). Third, the inhibition by polyunsaturated fat is not a consequence of changing the protein-to-calorie ratio of the animals' diet. In rats, 20% additional dietary energy from safflower oil inhibits the activity of G6PD significantly better than does 20% additional energy from beef tallow (10, 33). Finally, the decrease in G6PD enzyme activity is also observed in primary rat hepatocytes incubated with arachidonate (20:4 n-6) and eicosapentaenoate (20:5 n-3) (70, 74). The inhibition of G6PD gene expression in primary rat hepatocytes is likewise caused by polyunsaturated fatty acids and not saturated or monounsaturated fatty acids, which is similar to results observed in intact animals (74). G6PD expression is highly sensitive to the quantity of polyunsaturated fat in the diet. A significant decrease in enzyme activity in rats is observed with the addition (by weight to a glucose-based diet) of as little as 2.5% safflower oil (11); in mice, addition of 5% corn oil (by weight to a glucose-based diet) maximally inhibits G6PD activity (33). Curiously, addition of 10% corn oil (by weight) is needed to maximally inhibit G6PD activity in mice fed a fructose-based diet (33). The inhibitory effect of polyunsaturated fat is unique to G6PD regulation in the liver. Regulation of G6PD in adipose tissue is not affected by the presence of polyunsaturated fat in the diet (12). What remains elusive with respect to G6PD is the signal transduction pathway by which the cell responds to changes in the polyunsaturated fat content of the diet.

## Hormonal Status

***Role of Hormones in the Response to Nutritional Status***    The effects of starvation and refeeding suggest a role for insulin and glucagon in the regulation of G6PD (51). Rats treated with streptozotocin, which destroys the pancreatic $\beta$-cells, thereby stopping insulin production, fail to induce G6PD activity on refeeding (4). G6PD activity in both the liver and adipose tissue of diabetic rats is similar to the activity in starved animals, and treatment with insulin restores G6PD activity to normal levels, implicating insulin as an important signal of the refed state (5, 25, 28). Glucagon or cAMP have an opposing effect on G6PD activity. Injection of rats with glucagon prevents the induction of hepatic G6PD activity during refeeding and does so by decreasing the rate of enzyme synthesis (24). Because glucagon levels rise during starvation, this hormone is implicated as a primary signal of the starved state.

Hormones from the thyroid and adrenal glands also regulate G6PD activity. Thyroidectomy decreases G6PD expression, and treatment with thyroid hormone (T3) increases G6PD expression through a mechanism that does not involve an increase in G6PD mRNA (21). In contrast, the increase in G6PD activity during the transition from normal thyroid status to hyperthyroidism is accompanied by a parallel increase in enzyme synthesis and mRNA abundance (52). A high-sucrose diet further augments the increase in G6PD activity and mRNA abundance due to hyperthyroidism (52). Adrenalectomy attenuates the large increase in G6PD activity caused by refeeding rats, and the refeeding-induced increase is restored by glucocorticoid administration (4). These effects on activity are the result of changes in the rate of enzyme synthesis (80). Thus, the ability of a fat-free, high-carbohydrate diet to increase the activity of G6PD probably requires a minimum thyroid and adrenal status.

G6PD regulation by hormonal factors is observed in primary rat hepatocytes in culture. The induction of G6PD activity and mRNA level in response to carbohydrate and insulin in hepatocyte cultures mimics the response to refeeding in intact animals. Insulin induces G6PD activity in primary rat hepatocytes in culture (46, 70, 74, 95). The insulin-induced increase in G6PD activity is accompanied by parallel changes in the rate of enzyme protein synthesis and G6PD mRNA abundance (49, 74). Furthermore, inhibitors that block signal transduction by insulin also block its stimulatory effect on G6PD expression (89). Because insulin will also increase the metabolism of glucose in hepatocytes, it is difficult at this point to determine whether insulin acts directly on the expression of G6PD or whether its effect is indirect and via enhanced glucose metabolism. Glucocorticoids also have been shown to be positive regulators of G6PD activity in rat hepatocytes. Glucocorticoids and insulin both stimulate G6PD mRNA accumulation and in an additive manner, but the molecular mechanism of this regulation has not been defined (77). Curiously, glucocorticoids block the inhibition of G6PD expression by linoleate (70).

This interaction between glucocorticoid and fatty acid action may reflect an inhibition of fatty acid metabolism by glucocorticoids, thereby blocking the production of the active metabolite required to inhibit G6PD expression. In contrast, T3 and glucagon, both of which change G6PD activity in intact animals, have no effect on G6PD activity in cultured hepatocytes (58, 95). Therefore, in intact animals, the effect of T3 and glucagon may be indirect, possibly by altering circulating free fatty acid concentrations.

## MECHANISMS REGULATING EXPRESSION OF G6PD

### Translational/Posttranslational Mechanisms

The activity of any enzyme can be regulated at many steps. Modifications can occur that alter the catalytic efficiency of the enzyme and/or change the amount of enzyme present in the cell. The generally excepted dogma is that G6PD activity does not undergo allosteric or covalent modifications in response to nutritional modifications. Early reports have argued for an irreversible inactivation of G6PD enzyme. Palmitoyl-CoA, in vitro, has been shown to covalently bind to and inactivate G6PD and to reduce its apparent level when measured with antibodies (14–16). Furthermore, G6PD activity can be stimulated by growth factors and oxidant stress by a mechanism involving release of bound enzyme from intracellular membranes (75, 83). Most recently, Zhang et al (97) have observed phosphorylation of G6PD and a coincident decrease in G6PD activity in endothelial cells incubated in medium with high glucose concentrations. This phosphorylation is mediated via cAMP and protein kinase A. Changes in amount of G6PD by any of these mechanisms have not been observed during dietary manipulations. As is discussed below, regulation of G6PD by nutritional status can largely be accounted for by changes in its synthesis, and thus, these short-term regulatory mechanisms have not been thought relevant to this type of metabolic control. Yet a change in the catalytic efficiency of G6PD has the potential to provide temporal regulation of cellular G6PD activity.

The effect of nutrients on the activity, the amount of enzyme protein, and the relative synthesis and degradation of G6PD have been widely studied. Using antibodies against G6PD protein and liver supernatants from rats fed a high-carbohydrate diet, the increase in G6PD enzyme activity was shown to parallel the increase in the amount of G6PD protein (63, 90). Likewise, starvation or the consumption of dietary lipids decreases the amount of G6PD protein (30, 63, 91). When examined in a variety of nutritional and hormonal conditions in both liver and adipose tissue, changes in G6PD activity can be accounted for by changes in the rate of enzyme synthesis (24, 25, 30, 52, 55, 63, 69, 84, 90, 92). For example, a 13-fold increase was observed in the relative rate of synthesis of G6PD and in G6PD enzyme activity in the livers of rats switched from a chow to a high-sucrose diet (52). Similarly, the rate of G6PD protein synthesis during dietary fat consumption is decreased 96%, coincident with a 91% inhibition of G6PD enzyme activity (91). Changes in the rate of degradation due to hormonal or nutritional modifications are more controversial. Consumption of a high-fat diet has been reported to decrease the half-life of the enzyme from 16 h to 6 h in rat liver (64). However, in other reports, dietary fat had no effect on the rate of enzyme disappearance (30). Multiple procedural differences could explain these conflicting results. Nonetheless, changes in enzyme synthesis can account for the changes in enzyme activity during nutritional manipulations, whereas any changes in the rate of enzyme protein turnover would serve to enhance the rapidity by which the cell can alter the amount of G6PD activity.

## Pretranslational/Posttranscriptional Mechanisms

Changes observed in the rate of G6PD protein synthesis due to nutritional or hormonal factors are accompanied by similar changes in the amount of mature mRNA (38, 45, 52, 66, 73, 77). Such changes have been observed in intact animals in response to (*a*) changes in type of dietary carbohydrate (52, 53), (*b*) fasting and refeeding (45, 66), (*c*) changes in dietary polyunsaturated fat (73, 84), and (*d*) hyperthyroidism (52, 53); in rat hepatocytes in primary culture, such changes have been observed in response to insulin (49, 74, 77), glucocorticoid (49, 77), and polyunsaturated fatty acids (74). The rate of change in G6PD mRNA accumulation varies with diet. Refeeding mice or rats that had been previously starved results in a lag of 12 h or more before an increase in G6PD mRNA is detectable, and the maximal increase is observed 24 h into refeeding (66, 73). This lag is only observed with the starvation/refeeding paradigm. G6PD mRNA increases up to sevenfold during the diurnal cycle (22, 38). The increase occurs during the eating cycle (dark cycle) and is maximal 8 h into it. The increase in mRNA amount is a consequence of diet rather than diurnal cues because presenting the diet at later times in the dark cycle delays the increase in G6PD mRNA accumulation (LP Stabile & LM Salati, unpublished data). Dietary polyunsaturated fat results in an 80% inhibition in G6PD activity accompanied by a parallel decrease in mRNA accumulation (73, 84). In mice, the decrease in G6PD mRNA abundance is observed within 4 h of polyunsaturated fat consumption and maximal inhibition occurs within 9 h (73). These effects are quite rapid considering the relatively slow rate of triacylglycerol absorption from the gastrointestinal tract. A similar time course has been observed in primary rat hepatocytes. In these experiments, incubation with arachidonic acid for 2 h resulted in a 14% decrease in the amount of G6PD mRNA relative to cells incubated with only insulin, and the maximum inhibition of 80% was observed by 8 h (73). The rapid effect of both dietary fat and fatty acids in culture suggests that the action of polyunsaturated fat on gene expression occurs via a protein(s) already present in the liver. In contrast, the lag in accumulation of G6PD mRNA during refeeding is consistent with a requirement for the synthesis of an intermediary protein involved in the induction. Despite these hypothesized differences in the intracellular details, these results are consistent with regulation at a pretranslational step.

Pretranslational regulation can be due to changes in transcriptional activity of the gene or to posttranscriptional regulation, such as mRNA stability, the processing of the pre-mRNA (including splicing and polyadenylation of the pre-mRNA), and nucleocytoplasmic transport. The transcriptional activity of the G6PD gene has been measured using nuclear run-on assays. The rate of G6PD transcription is not regulated by starvation, refeeding with a high-carbohydrate diet, or the inclusion of polyunsaturated fat in the diet (73). Similar results have been obtained for G6PD regulation by insulin, glucose, and arachidonic acid in rat hepatocytes in primary culture (74). Furthermore, the transcriptional activity of the G6PD gene occurs at a very low rate compared with constituitively expressed genes, such as $\beta$-actin and glyceraldehyde-3-phosphate dehydrogenase. The rate of G6PD transcription is as low as the transcriptional rate of the fatty acid synthase or stearoyl-CoA desaturase genes measured during starvation. Although the transcriptional activity of these genes increases 30-fold or more during refeeding, G6PD gene transcription remains at the same low level despite 27- to 30-fold increases in G6PD mRNA (73). In these experiments, multiple controls were used to make sure the measurements of transcriptional activity were valid (73). These included the use of probes to both the 5' and 3' ends of the gene, as well as single-stranded probes that would only hybridize to G6PD RNA, and not transcripts produced off the opposite strand. All probes were free of repetitive elements that could increase the background hybridization. Together, these results indicate that regulation of G6PD gene expression by nutritional and hormonal factors occurs at a posttranscriptional step.

Posttranscriptional regulation can occur at such steps as pre-mRNA processing in the nucleus or mRNA stability in the nucleus or in the cytoplasm. To investigate whether this posttranscriptional regulation of G6PD occurs in the nucleus or in the cytoplasm, Hodge & Salati (38) compared the abundance of G6PD mRNA in these two cellular compartments. Refeeding starved mice resulted in an 18-fold increase in the cytoplasmic mRNA abundance and a 13-fold increase in pre-mRNA abundance in the nucleus. This suggests that regulation of G6PD in this dietary paradigm occurs primarily in the nucleus. Moreover, the changes in G6PD mRNA abundance in the cytoplasm of mice were parallel to those in the nucleus. Thus, nucleocytoplasmic transport of the mature mRNA does not appear to be regulated.

Regulation of G6PD gene expression by polyunsaturated fat is also by a nuclear posttranscriptional mechanism. Accumulation of G6PD pre-mRNA is inhibited 60–70% in the livers of mice fed high-fat diets compared with animals fed low-fat diets (38). Inhibition of G6PD in total RNA, which is more representative of cytoplasmic RNA, parallels the inhibition seen in the nucleus. Despite the major difference in the amount of nuclear mRNA with different diets, no significant differences in the half-life of either G6PD pre- or mature mRNA have been observed (38). Because dietary status causes little or no difference in the half-life of mRNA, all detected mRNA must be stabile, and changes in the amount of mRNA must involve rapid degradation in the nucleus.

Similar results have been obtained in primary rat hepatocytes in culture using arachidonate to inhibit the induction of G6PD by insulin and glucose (74). Incubation of rat hepatocyte monolayers with arachidonate causes a 50% inhibition of cytoplasmic G6PD mRNA abundance and a 60% inhibition of pre-mRNA abundance in the nucleus. Thus, primary rat hepatocytes mimic the regulation of G6PD observed in intact animals both qualitatively and quantitatively.

Because changes in the amount of G6PD mRNA occur in the nucleus and precede the changes in amount of G6PD mRNA in the cytoplasm, steps involved in processing of the nascent G6PD transcript may be sites for regulation. To isolate a pool of RNA that is enriched for mRNA in the processing pathway and to minimize the isolation of mature mRNA in the nucleus that is undergoing transport to the cytoplasm, we isolated RNA from the insoluble fraction of the nucleus. The insoluble fraction of the nucleus contains the proteins involved in transcription and processing of pre-mRNA as well as the pre-mRNA itself (7, 9, 54, 56, 93, 96). Thus, RNA in this fraction represents newly transcribed RNA that is undergoing processing. By using an RNase protection assay and probes that hybridized across an intron/exon boundary, the change in the amount of G6PD mRNA during splicing could be measured.

In starved mice, the amounts of G6PD RNA at all stages of processing were very low (1). When the animals were refed, the amount of nascent G6PD transcripts (those containing at least the intron represented in the probe) increased in the nucleus but remained low. The amount of more processed forms of the RNA (those that had the intron spliced) increased in the nucleus and was consistently greater than the amount of its precursor. These results suggest that the abundance of G6PD RNA is regulated during the processing of the nascent transcript, steps that could involve either splicing or polyadenylation of the pre-mRNA. To differentiate between these two processing reactions, we first measured the amounts of unspliced, partially spliced, and fully spliced RNA using probes that detected two consecutive exons and two intervening sequences. The amount of unspliced RNA (that still contain both introns) was present in very low amounts in RNA samples from both starved and refed mice. Enhanced accumulation of G6PD partially spliced RNA (RNA from which one intron had been spliced) was observed on refeeding and the accumulation was greatest for the fully spliced RNA (1). The accumulation of the partially and fully spliced RNA was greater in refed animals than in starved animals. Thus, refeeding enhanced the accumulation of splicing intermediates for G6PD, which suggests that the efficiency of splicing has been enhanced.

Next, we measured the amount of G6PD RNA that was nonpolyadenylated versus polyadenylated using a probe that hybridized across the cleavage site in the nascent RNA. The amount of nonpolyadenylated RNA was very low in livers of both starved and refed mice but did increase slightly during refeeding. Refeeding resulted in a four-fold increase in the rate of accumulation of G6PD polyadenylated RNA, to a rate similar to that for partially spliced G6PD RNA. The rate of increase in the amount of fully spliced RNA was greater still (eight-fold greater than nonpolyadenylated RNA). The observation that even nonpolyadenylated RNA was increasing in amount, albeit only slightly, suggests that it is the process of splicing that caused G6PD RNA to accumulate in the nucleus. Clearly, polyadenylation is necessary for the production of a stable mRNA but insufficient to cause the enhanced accumulation of fully processed RNA during refeeding. This enhancement is the result of an increase in the efficiency of splicing of the nascent transcript.

Regulation of G6PD expression by polyunsaturated fat appears to use the same nuclear mechanism. Consumption of a diet high in polyunsaturated fat resulted in a decrease in the rate at which more spliced forms of G6PD RNA accumulated in the nucleus (38). Although dietary polyunsaturated fat inhibits G6PD expression, consumption of a diet high in polyunsaturated fat does not prevent the normal diurnal variation in the expression of G6PD; it merely attenuates the magnitude of the increase. Most likely, the carbohydrate component of the diet stimulates the increase in the amount of G6PD mRNA during each eating (dark) cycle. During the first 2 h of the eating cycle, the amount of G6PD mRNA in the cytoplasm is less in mice fed high-fat diets (6% safflower oil) compared with mice fed low-fat diets (1% safflower oil). The diurnal increase in the amount of G6PD mRNA is not detected until 4 h into the eating period (38). Within the insoluble fraction of the nucleus, at 0 and 2 h into the eating cycle, the amount of G6PD unspliced RNA was the same between diets, consistent with the lack of transcriptional regulation of this gene. However, the amount of processed G6PD mRNA was 50% less in mice fed diets high in polyunsaturated fat (1). Thus, regulation of G6PD expression due to dietary polyunsaturated fat also involves changes in the efficiency of pre-mRNA processing.

Is this mechanism unique to G6PD? Posttranscriptional regulation in the nucleus has also been described for regulation of the $S_{14}$ gene by dietary carbohydrate. Consumption of a diet high in carbohydrate increases the transcription of this gene and the amount of the splicing intermediate for its single intron pre-mRNA (8, 32, 39). We extended these findings by examining amounts of unspliced and spliced $S_{14}$ RNA during refeeding. The amount of $S_{14}$ unspliced RNA increased during refeeding. This increase is greater than that seen for G6PD unspliced RNA and is consistent with transcriptional regulation of the $S_{14}$ gene. Refeeding also resulted in a greater amount of the spliced $S_{14}$ RNA compared with the unspliced RNA (1). The enhanced rate of accumulation of spliced RNA for the $S_{14}$ gene suggests that nutritional regulation of splicing is not unique to G6PD. Regulated processing of the RNA for all the lipogenic genes would enhance the rate at which the cell could change the expression of these enzymes. Thus, we hypothesize that this mechanism is common to most members of the lipogenic enzyme family.

## CONCLUSIONS

During the expression of a gene, steps subsequent to transcription are essential for production of the mature mRNA. In this regard, mutations that effect splicing or polyadenylation result in degradation of the RNA in the nucleus (2, 13). A model for regulation of G6PD expression is shown in Figure 2. Clearly, the reactions are listed in this order for illustration purposes only. Because splicing and polyadenylation occur cotranscriptionally (reviewed in 35, 60), splicing ($k_2$ and $k_4$) most likely occurs coincident with polyadenylation ($k_3$).

In the case of G6PD, the rate of gene transcription is constant ($k_1$) across all dietary states. Consumption of a high-carbohydrate diet results in an increase in the accumulation of partially spliced and mature forms of G6PD mRNA. The slowest rates of accumulation of G6PD RNA were observed for the amount of partially spliced, nonpolyadenylated RNA ($k_2$). The increase in the rate of accumulation of polyadenylated but partially spliced RNA ($k_3$) is insufficient to account for the rate of accumulation of mature mRNA in the nucleus. It is during the process of splicing of G6PD pre-mRNA that the greatest increases in rate occur ($k_2$ and $k_4$), and it is the rate of accumulation of the mature RNA that is most enhanced ($k_4$).

In contrast, during starvation or consumption of a diet high in polyunsaturated fat, the rate of splicing ($k_2$ and $k_4$) is decreased and the inefficiently spliced RNA undergoes degradation in the nucleus ($k_5$, $k_6$, and $k_7$). Once fully processed, G6PD mRNA is stable in the nucleus, and no change in its rate of degradation ($k_8$) is detectable across dietary manipulations (38). What remains to be determined is whether starvation or dietary fat directly interacts with the machinery involved in degradation ($k_5$, $k_6$, or $k_7$) or whether their action is to interfere with the mechanisms resulting in the enhanced rate of splicing ($k_2$ and $k_4$) due to a high-carbohydrate diet. Our data to date favor the latter. In this regard, arachidonic acid decreases the induction of G6PD expression caused by incubation of hepatocytes with insulin and glucose, but arachidonic acid does not block the increase in G6PD expression caused by incubation in a high-glucose medium without insulin (74).

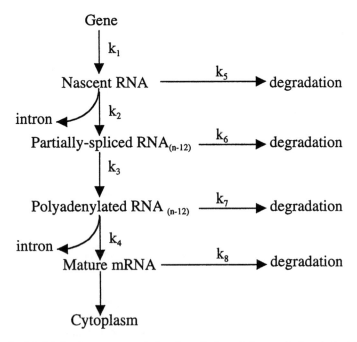

**Figure 2**    Model for the posttranscriptional regulation of glucose-6-phosphate dehydrogenase (G6PD) expression. The rate terms are as follows: $k_1$, the rate of transcription of the gene; $k_2$ and $k_4$, rates of splicing of the 12 introns; $k_3$, rate of polyadenylation; $k_5$ and $k_7$, rate of degradation of RNA that is not correctly or efficiently spliced; $k_6$, rate of degradation of RNA that has not been polyadenylated; and $k_8$, rate of degradation of mature mRNA in the nucleus.

Furthermore, the kinetics of mRNA change during dietary fat consumption are consistent with an interaction between the signal transduction pathway for dietary fat and existing protein(s).

How then can nutrients alter the rate of RNA splicing? Existing examples for regulated splicing have concentrated on alternatively spliced messages. In these cases, splicing enhancers in the RNA molecule appear to mediate this regulation (cf 72). Thus, a potential scenario is the presence of a *cis*-acting element in the G6PD RNA that is a splicing enhancer, and the activity of the protein that binds to this element can be regulated by nutrients. G6PD provides an excellent model to study the regulation of gene expression by dietary factors at a posttranscriptional level. The absence of transcriptional regulation makes interpretation of changes in the pre-RNA pool easier, and its regulation can be studied both in intact animals and in primary rat hepatocytes in culture. Understanding the mechanisms by which nutrients alter nuclear posttranscriptional events will help uncover new information on the breadth of mechanisms involved in gene regulation.

ACKNOWLEDGMENTS

This work was supported by grant DK46897 from the National Institutes of Health. We are grateful to Dr. Huimin Tao and Brian Griffith for critical reading.

**Visit the Annual Reviews home page at www.AnnualReviews.org**

LITERATURE CITED

1. Amir-Ahmady B, Salati LM. 2001. Regulation of the processing of glucose-6-phophate dehydrogenase mRNA by nutritional status. *J. Biol. Chem.* In press

2. Antoniou M, Geraghty F, Hurst J, Grosveld F. 1998. Efficient 3'-end formation of human beta-globin mRNA in vivo requires sequences within the last intron but occurs independently of the splicing reaction. *Nucleic Acids Res.* 26:721–29

3. Baltzell JK, Berdanier CD. 1985. Effect on the interaction of dietary carbohydrate and fat on the responses of rats to starvation-refeeding. *J. Nutr.* 115:104–10

4. Berdanier CD, Shubeck D. 1979. Interaction of glucocorticoid and insulin in the responses of rats to starvation-refeeding. *J. Nutr.* 109:1766–71

5. Berg EA, Wu JY, Campbell L, Kagey M, Stapleton SR. 1995. Insulin-like effects of vanadate and selenate on the expression of glucose-6-phosphate dehydrogenase and fatty acid synthase in diabetic rats. *Biochimie* 77:919–24

6. Beutler E. 1991. Glucose-6-phosphate dehydrogenase deficiency. *N. Engl. J. Med.* 324:169–74

7. Blencowe BJ, Nickerson JA, Issner R, Penman S, Sharp PA. 1994. Association of nuclear matrix antigens with exon-containing splicing complexes. *J. Cell. Biol.* 127:593–607

8. Burmeister LA, Mariash CN. 1991. Dietary sucrose enhances processing of mRNA-S14 nuclear precursor. *J. Biol. Chem.* 266:22905–11

9. Ciejek EM, Nordstrom JL, Tsai MJ, O'Malley BW. 1982. Ribonucleic acid precursors are associated with the chick oviduct nuclear matrix. *Biochemistry* 21:4945–53

10. Clarke SD, Hembree J. 1990. Inhibition of triiodothyronine's induction of rat liver lipogenic enzymes by dietary fat. *J. Nutr.* 120:625–30

11. Clarke SD, Romsos DR, Leveille GA. 1976. Specific inhibition of hepatic fatty acid synthesis exerted by dietary linoleate and linolenate in essential fatty acid adequate rats. *Lipids* 11:85–90

12. Clarke SD, Romsos DR, Leveille GA. 1977. Differential effects of dietary methyl esters of long-chain saturated and polyunsaturated fatty acids on rat liver and adipose tissue lipogenesis. *J. Nutr.* 107:1170–81

13. Custodio N, Carmo-Fonseca M, Geraghty F, Pereira HS, Grosveld F, Antoniou M. 1999. Inefficient processing impairs release of RNA from the site of transcription. *EMBO J.* 18:2855–66

14. Dao ML, Johnson BC, DeLuca C. 1984. Cross-reacting material to monoclonal anti-G6PD in the absence of catalytic activity. *Biochem. Biophys. Res. Commun.* 118:854–58

15. Dao ML, Johnson BC, Hartman PE. 1982. Preparation of a monoclonal antibody to rat liver glucose-6-phosphate dehydrogenase and the study of its immunoreactivity with native and inactivated enzyme. *Proc. Natl. Acad. Sci. USA* 79:2860–64

16. Dao ML, Watson JJ, Delaney R, Johnson BC. 1979. Purification of a new high activity form of glucose-6-phosphate dehydrogenase from rat liver and the effect of

enzyme inactivation on its immunochemical reactivity. *J. Biol. Chem.* 254:9441–47

17. Dessi S, Batetta B, Spano O, Pulisci D, Mulas MF, et al. 1992. Serum lipoprotein pattern as modified in G6PD-deficient children during haemolytic anaemia induced by fava bean ingestion. *Int. J. Exp. Pathol.* 73:157–60

18. Flatt JP, Ball EG. 1966. Studies on the metabolism of adipose tissue. XIX. An evaluation of the major pathways of glucose catabolism as influenced by acetate in the presence of insulin. *J. Biol. Chem.* 241:2862–69

19. Franze A, Ferrante MI, Fusco F, Santoro A, Sanzari E, et al. 1998. Molecular anatomy of the human glucose 6-phosphate dehydrogenase core promoter. *FEBS Lett.* 437:313–18

20. Freedland RA, Murad S, Hurvitz AI. 1968. Relationship of nutritional and hormonal influences on liver enzyme activity. *Fed. Proc.* 27:1217–22

21. Fritz RS, Kletzien RF. 1987. Regulation of glucose-6-phosphate dehydrogenase by diet and thyroid hormone. *Mol. Cell. Endocrinol.* 51:13–17

22. Fukuda H, Iritani N. 1991. Diurnal variations of lipogenic enzyme mRNA quantities in rat liver. *Biochim. Biophys. Acta* 1086:261–64

23. Fukuda H, Iritani N, Tanaka T. 1983. Effects of high-fructose diet on lipogenic enzymes and their substrate and effector levels in diabetic rats. *J. Nutr. Sci. Vitaminol.* 29:691–99

24. Garcia DR, Holten D. 1975. Inhibition of rat liver glucose-6-phosphate dehydrogenase synthesis by glucagon. *J. Biol. Chem.* 250:3960–65

25. Geisler RW, Roggeveen AE, Hansen RJ. 1978. The effects of insulin on the turnover of glucose-6-phosphate dehydrogenase in epididymal adipose tissue of the rat. *Biochim. Biophys. Acta* 544:284–93

26. Girard J, Ferre P, Foufelle F. 1997. Mechanisms by which carbohydrates regulate expression of genes for glycolytic and lipogenic enzymes. *Annu. Rev. Nutr.* 17:325–52

27. Glock GE, McLean P. 1954. Levels of enzymes of the direct oxidative pathway of carbohydrate metabolism in mammalian tissues and tumors. *Biochem. J.* 56:171–75

28. Glock GE, McLean P. 1955. A preliminary investigation of the hormonal control of the hexose monophosphate oxidative pathway. *Biochem. J.* 61:390–97

29. Goodridge AG, Ball EG. 1966. Lipogenesis in the pigeon: in vitro studies. *Am. J. Physiol.* 211:803–8

30. Gozukara EM, Frolich M, Holten D. 1972. The effect of unsaturated fatty acids on the rate of synthesis of rat liver glucose-6-phosphate dehydrogenase. *Biochim. Biophys. Acta* 286:155–63

31. Grigor MR, Gain KR. 1983. The effect of starvation and refeeding on lipogenic enzymes in mammary glands and livers of lactating rats. *Biochem. J.* 216:515–18

32. Hamblin PS, Ozawa Y, Jefferds A, Mariash CN. 1989. Interaction between fructose and glucose on the regulation of the nuclear precursor for mRNA-S14. *J. Biol. Chem.* 264:21646–51

33. Herzberg GR, Janmohamed N. 1980. Regulation of hepatic lipogenesis by dietary maize oil or tripalmitin in the meal-fed mouse. *Br. J. Nutr.* 43:571–79

34. Hillgartner FB, Salati LM, Goodridge AG. 1995. Physiological and molecular mechanisms involved in nutritional regulation of fatty acid synthesis. *Physiol. Rev.* 75:47–76

35. Hirose Y, Manley JL. 2000. RNA polymerase II and the integration of nuclear events. *Genes Dev.* 14:1415–29

36. Ho YS, Howard AJ, Crapo JD. 1988. Cloning and sequence of a cDNA encoding rat glucose-6-phosphate dehydrogenase. *Nucleic Acids Res.* 16:7746; Erratum. 1989. *Nucleic Acids Res.* 17(2):831

37. Hodge DL, Charron T, Stabile LP, Klautky

SA, Salati LM. 1998. Structural characterization and tissue-specific expression of the mouse glucose-6-phosphate dehydrogenase gene. *DNA Cell. Biol.* 17:283–91

38. Hodge DL, Salati LM. 1997. Nutritional regulation of the glucose-6-phosphate dehydrogenase gene is mediated by a nuclear posttranscriptional mechanism. *Arch. Biochem. Biophys.* 348:303–12

39. Jump DB, Bell A, Santiago V. 1990. Thyroid hormone and dietary carbohydrate interact to regulate rat liver S14 gene transcription and chromatin structure. *J. Biol. Chem.* 265:3474–78

40. Kastrouni E, Pegiou T, Gardiki P, Trakatellis A. 1984. Activity changes of glucose-6-phosphate dehydrogenase in response to diet and insulin. *Int. J. Biochem.* 16:1353–58

41. Katsurada A, Iritani N, Fukuda H, Matsumura Y, Noguchi T, Tanaka T. 1989. Effects of nutrients and insulin on transcriptional and post-transcriptional regulation of glucose-6-phosphate dehydrogenase synthesis in rat liver. *Biochim. Biophys. Acta* 1006:104–10

42. Katz J, Rognstad R. 1966. The metabolism of tritiated glucose by rat adipose tissue. *J. Biol. Chem.* 241:3600–10

43. Kelley DS, Kletzien RF. 1984. Ethanol modulation of the hormonal and nutritional regulation of glucose 6-phosphate dehydrogenase activity in primary cultures of rat hepatocytes. *Biochem. J.* 217:543–49

44. Kennedy KA, Crouch LS, Warshaw JB. 1989. Effect of hyperoxia on antioxidants in neonatal rat type II cells in vitro and in vivo. *Pediatr. Res.* 26:400–3

45. Kletzien RF, Prostko CR, Stumpo DJ, McClung JK, Dreher KL. 1985. Molecular cloning of DNA sequences complementary to rat liver glucose-6-phosphate dehydrogenase mRNA. Nutritional regulation of mRNA levels. *J. Biol. Chem.* 260:5621–24

46. Kurtz JW, Wells WW. 1981. Induction of glucose-6-phosphate dehydrogenase in primary cultures of adult rat hepatocytes. Requirement for insulin and dexamethasone. *J. Biol. Chem.* 256:10870–75

47. Ledda-Columbano GM, Columbano A, Dessi S, Coni P, Chiodino C, Pani P. 1985. Enhancement of cholesterol synthesis and pentose phosphate pathway activity in proliferating hepatocyte nodules. *Carcinogenesis* 6:1371–73

48. Lee CY, Lee SM, Lewis S, Johnson FM. 1980. Identification and biochemical analysis of mouse mutants deficient in cytoplasmic malic enzyme. *Biochemistry* 19:5098–103

49. Manos P, Nakayama R, Holten D. 1991. Regulation of glucose-6-phosphate dehydrogenase synthesis and mRNA abundance in cultured rat hepatocytes. *Biochem. J.* 276:245–50

50. Martini G, Toniolo D, Vulliamy T, Luzzatto L, Dono R, et al. 1986. Structural analysis of the X-linked gene encoding human glucose 6-phosphate dehydrogenase. *EMBO J.* 5:1849–55

51. Martins RN, Stokes GB, Masters CL. 1985. Regulation of the multiple molecular forms of rat liver glucose 6-phosphate dehydrogenase by insulin and dietary restriction. *Biochem. Biophys. Res. Commun.* 127:136–42

52. Miksicek RJ, Towle HC. 1982. Changes in the rates of synthesis and messenger RNA levels of hepatic glucose-6-phosphate and 6-phosphogluconate dehydrogenases following induction by diet or thyroid hormone. *J. Biol. Chem.* 257:11829–35

53. Miksicek RJ, Towle HC. 1983. Use of a cloned cDNA sequence to measure changes in 6-phosphogluconate dehydrogenase mRNA levels caused by thyroid hormone and dietary carbohydrate. *J. Biol. Chem.* 258:9575–79

54. Moen PT Jr, Smith KP, Lawrence JB. 1995. Compartmentalization of specific pre-mRNA metabolism: an emerging view. *Hum. Mol. Genet.* 4:1779–89

55. Morikawa N, Nakayama R, Holten D.

1984. Dietary induction of glucose-6-phosphate dehydrogenase synthesis. *Biochem. Biophys. Res. Commun.* 120:1022–29

56. Mortillaro MJ, Blencowe BJ, Wei X, Nakayasu H, Du L, et al. 1996. A hyperphosphorylated form of the large subunit of RNA polymerase II is associated with splicing complexes and the nuclear matrix. *Proc. Natl. Acad. Sci. USA* 93:8253–57

57. Muntoni S, Batetta B, Dessi S, Pani P. 1992. Serum lipoprotein profile in the Mediterranean variant of glucose-6-phosphate dehydrogenase deficiency. *Eur. J. Epidemiol.* 8 (Suppl. 1):48–53

58. Nakamura T, Yoshimoto K, Aoyama K, Ichihara A. 1982. Hormonal regulations of glucose-6-phosphate dehydrogenase and lipogenesis in primary cultures of rat hepatocytes. *J. Biochem.* 91:681–93

59. Nakamura T, Yoshimoto K, Nakayama Y, Tomita Y, Ichihara A. 1983. Reciprocal modulation of growth and differentiated functions of mature rat hepatocytes in primary culture by cell-cell contact and cell membranes. *Proc. Natl. Acad. Sci. USA* 80:7229–33

60. Neugebauer KM, Roth MB. 1997. Transcription units as RNA processing units. *Genes Dev.* 11:3279–85

61. O'Hea EK, Leveille GA. 1968. Lipogenesis in isolated adipose tissue of the domestic chick (*Gallus domesticus*). *Comp. Biochem. Physiol.* 26:111–20

62. Pandolfi PP, Sonati F, Rivi R, Mason P, Grosveld F, Luzzatto L. 1995. Targeted disruption of the housekeeping gene encoding glucose 6-phosphate dehydrogenase (G6PD): G6PD is dispensable for pentose synthesis but essential for defense against oxidative stress. *EMBO J.* 14:5209–15

63. Peavy DE, Hansen RJ. 1975. Immunological titration of rat liver glucose-6-phosphate dehydrogenase from animals fed high and low carbohydrate diets.

*Biochem. Biophys. Res. Commun.* 66:1106–11

64. Peavy DE, Hansen RJ. 1979. Influence of diet on the in vivo turnover of glucose-6-phosphate dehydrogenase in rat liver. *Biochim. Biophys. Acta* 586:22–30

65. Philippe M, Larondelle Y, Lemaigre F, Mariame B, Delhez H, et al. 1994. Promoter function of the human glucose-6-phosphate dehydrogenase gene depends on two GC boxes that are cell specifically controlled. *Eur. J. Biochem.* 226:377–84

66. Prostko CR, Fritz RS, Kletzien RF. 1989. Nutritional regulation of hepatic glucose-6-phosphate dehydrogenase. Transient activation of transcription. *Biochem. J.* 258:295–99

67. Rank KB, Harris PK, Ginsberg LC, Stapleton SR. 1994. Isolation and sequence of a rat glucose-6-phosphate dehydrogenase promoter. *Biochim. Biophys. Acta* 1217:90–92

68. Rognstad R, Katz J. 1979. Effects of 2,4-dihydroxybutyrate on lipogenesis in rat hepatocytes. *J. Biol. Chem.* 254:11969–72

69. Rudack D, Chisholm EM, Holten D. 1971. Rat liver glucose 6-phosphate dehydrogenase. Regulation by carbohydrate diet and insulin. *J. Biol. Chem.* 246:1249–54

70. Salati LM, Adkins-Finke B, Clarke SD. 1988. Free fatty acid inhibition of the insulin induction of glucose-6-phosphate dehydrogenase in rat hepatocyte monolayers. *Lipids* 23:36–41

71. Salvemini F, Franze A, Iervolino A, Filosa S, Salzano S, Ursini MV. 1999. Enhanced glutathione levels and oxidoresistance mediated by increased glucose-6-phosphate dehydrogenase expression. *J. Biol. Chem.* 274:2750–57

72. Smith CW, Valcarcel J. 2000. Alternative pre-mRNA splicing: the logic of combinatorial control. *Trends Biochem. Sci.* 25:381–88

73. Stabile LP, Hodge DL, Klautky SA,

Salati LM. 1996. Posttranscriptional regulation of glucose-6-phosphate dehydrogenase by dietary polyunsaturated fat. *Arch. Biochem. Biophys.* 332:269–79

74. Stabile LP, Klautky SA, Minor SM, Salati LM. 1998. Polyunsaturated fatty acids inhibit the expression of the glucose-6-phosphate dehydrogenase gene in primary rat hepatocytes by a nuclear posttranscriptional mechanism. *J. Lipid Res.* 39:1951–63

75. Stanton RC, Seifter JL, Boxer DC, Zimmerman E, Cantley LC. 1991. Rapid release of bound glucose-6-phosphate dehydrogenase by growth factors. Correlation with increased enzymatic activity. *J. Biol. Chem.* 266:12442–48

76. Stapleton SR, Stevens GJ, Teel JF, Rank KB, Berg EA, et al. 1993. Effects of acetaldehyde on glucose-6-phosphate dehydrogenase activity and mRNA levels in primary rat hepatocytes in culture. *Biochimie* 75:971–76

77. Stumpo DJ, Kletzien RF. 1984. Regulation of glucose-6-phosphate dehydrogenase mRNA by insulin and the glucocorticoids in primary cultures of rat hepatocytes. *Eur. J. Biochem.* 144:497–502

78. Stumpo DJ, Kletzien RF. 1985. The effect of ethanol, alone and in combination with the glucocorticoids and insulin, on glucose-6-phosphate dehydrogenase synthesis and mRNA in primary cultures of hepatocytes. *Biochem. J.* 226:123–30

79. Takizawa T, Huang IY, Ikuta T, Yoshida A. 1986. Human glucose-6-phosphate dehydrogenase: primary structure and cDNA cloning. *Proc. Natl. Acad. Sci. USA* 83:4157–61

80. Tepperman HM, Tepperman J. 1958. Effects of antecedent food intake pattern on hepatic lipogenesis. *Am. J. Physiol.* 193:55–64

81. Tian WN, Braunstein LD, Apse K, Pang J, Rose M, et al. 1999. Importance of glucose-6-phosphate dehydrogenase activity in cell death. *Am. J. Physiol.* 276:C1121–31

82. Tian WN, Braunstein LD, Pang J, Stuhlmeier KM, Xi QC, et al. 1998. Importance of glucose-6-phosphate dehydrogenase activity for cell growth. *J. Biol. Chem.* 273:10609–17

83. Tian WN, Pignatare JN, Stanton RC. 1994. Signal transduction proteins that associate with the platelet-derived growth factor (PDGF) receptor mediate the PDGF-induced release of glucose-6-phosphate dehydrogenase from permeabilized cells. *J. Biol. Chem.* 269:14798–805

84. Tomlinson JE, Nakayama R, Holten D. 1988. Repression of pentose phosphate pathway dehydrogenase synthesis and mRNA by dietary fat in rats. *J. Nutr.* 118:408–15

85. Toniolo D, Filippi M, Dono R, Lettieri T, Martini G. 1991. The CpG island in the 5' region of the G6PD gene of man and mouse. *Gene* 102:197–203

86. Towle HC, Kaytor EN, Shih HM. 1997. Regulation of the expression of lipogenic enzyme genes by carbohydrate. *Annu. Rev. Nutr.* 17:405–33

87. Ursini MV, Parrella A, Rosa G, Salzano S, Martini G. 1997. Enhanced expression of glucose-6-phosphate dehydrogenase in human cells sustaining oxidative stress. *Biochem. J.* 323:801–6

88. Vulliamy T, Mason P, Luzzatto L. 1992. The molecular basis of glucose-6-phosphate dehydrogenase deficiency. *Trends Genet.* 8:138–43

89. Wagle A, Jivraj S, Garlock GL, Stapleton SR. 1998. Insulin regulation of glucose-6-phosphate dehydrogenase gene expression is rapamycin-sensitive and requires phosphatidylinositol 3-kinase. *J. Biol. Chem.* 273:14968–74

90. Winberry L, Holten D. 1977. Rat liver glucose-6-p dehydrogenase. Dietary regulation of the rate of synthesis. *J. Biol. Chem.* 252:7796–801

91. Wolfe RG, Holten D. 1978. The effect of dietary fat or cholesterol and cholic acid on

the rate of synthesis of rat liver glucose-6-P dehydrogenase. *J. Nutr.* 108:1708–17

92. Wolfe RG, Nakayama R, Holten D. 1979. Regulation of glucose-6-p dehydrogenase synthesis in rat epididymal fat pads. *Biochem. Biophys. Res. Commun.* 89:108–15

93. Xing YG, Lawrence JB. 1991. Preservation of specific RNA distribution within the chromatin-depleted nuclear substructure demonstrated by in situ hybridization coupled with biochemical fractionation. *J. Cell. Biol.* 112:1055–63

94. Yoshimoto K, Nakamura T, Ichihara A. 1983. Reciprocal effects of epidermal growth factor on key lipogenic enzymes in primary cultures of adult rat hepatocytes. Induction of glucose-6-phosphate dehydrogenase and suppression of malic enzyme and lipogenesis. *J. Biol. Chem.* 258:12355–60

95. Yoshimoto K, Nakamura T, Niimi S, Ichihara A. 1983. Hormonal regulation of translatable mRNA of glucose-6-phosphate dehydrogenase in primary cultures of adult rat hepatocytes. *Biochim. Biophys. Acta* 741:143–49

96. Zeitlin S, Parent A, Silverstein S, Efstratiadis A. 1987. Pre-mRNA splicing and the nuclear matrix. *Mol. Cell. Biol.* 7:111–20

97. Zhang Z, Apse K, Pang J, Stanton RC. 2000. High glucose inhibits glucose 6-phosphate dehydrogenase via cAMP in aortic endothelial cells. *J. Biol. Chem.* 275:40042–7

Annu. Rev. Nutr. 2001. 21:141–65

# THE ROLE OF C/EBP IN NUTRIENT AND HORMONAL REGULATION OF GENE EXPRESSION

## William J Roesler

*Department of Biochemistry, University of Saskatchewan, 107 Wiggins Road, Saskatoon, Saskatchewan, Canada S7N 5E5; e-mail: bill.roesler@usask.ca*

**Key Words** transcription factor, phosphoenolpyruvate carboxykinase, cAMP, phosphorylation

■ **Abstract** C/EBPs are a family of transcription factors that play important roles in energy metabolism. Although initially thought to be constitutive regulators of transcription, an increasing amount of evidence indicates that their transactivating capacity within the cell can be modulated by nutrients and hormones. There are several mechanisms whereby this occurs. First, hormones/nutrients are known to directly alter the expression of C/EBPs. Second, hormones/nutrients may cause an alteration in the phosphorylation state of C/EBPs, which can affect their DNA-binding activity or transactivating capacity. Third, C/EBPs can function as accessory factors on gene promoters within a hormone response unit, interacting with other transcription factors to enhance the degree of responsiveness to specific hormones. Given their role in regulating genes involved in a wide variety of metabolic events, advancing our understanding of the molecular mechanism of action of C/EBPs will undoubtedly further our appreciation for the role these transcription factors play in both health and disease.

## CONTENTS

# INTRODUCTION

Nutrients exert a wide variety of biochemical and physiological effects in vivo. They stimulate secretion of hormones and neurotransmitters, act as allosteric regulators of metabolic enzymes, and regulate the expression of certain genes. With regard to the latter, nutrients have been shown to regulate gene expression by both direct and/or indirect mechanisms. Molecules such as fatty acids and their metabolites can directly interact with and alter the activity of transcription factors that control expression of specific genes through *cis*-regulatory elements in the promoter region. Alternatively, most nutrients may regulate genes indirectly by regulating the secretion of one or more hormones, such as insulin, glucagon, glucocorticoids, and thyroid hormone, which themselves go on to alter the expression of specific genes. Furthermore, studies performed in isolated cell cultures have indicated that nutrients such as monosaccharides, amino acids, and fatty acids can indirectly affect gene expression by mechanisms that, although not completely understood, are clearly not hormone dependent. It is not surprising that genes whose expression are regulated by nutrients have been found generally to encode proteins that are somehow involved in the metabolism of those same nutrients.

This review article attempts to provide insight into the mechanisms whereby nutrients alter transcription rates of genes, with the focus on a specific transcription factor family called CCAAT/enhancer binding proteins (C/EBPs). Shortly after its discovery by McKnight and associates, the first member of this family, C/EBP$\alpha$, was dubbed "a central regulator of energy metabolism" on rather scant evidence (54). This included the observation that highest levels of expression of this factor were found in such tissues as liver, adipose, and lung, which are organs that control energy metabolism and/or actively metabolize lipids (8). However, subsequent analysis of this transcription factor demonstrated its importance, for example, in regulating adipocyte differentiation (reviewed in 20), and in controlling the expression of a number of genes encoding proteins that are involved in energy homeostasis, such as leptin (28, 29), insulin receptor substrate 1 (52), peroxisome proliferator-activated receptor-$\gamma$ (15), and phosphoenolpyruvate carboxykinase (PEPCK) (71), as well as controlling its own activity through autoregulation (41, 99). These and other observations have validated the bold prediction and underscored the insight McKnight and colleagues had on the potential biological role for this protein. Although this transcription factor was, and perhaps still is, generally thought to be a constitutive regulator, recent studies highlighted in this review emphasize how nutrients and hormones can alter the transactivating capacity of C/EBPs in the cell, thereby using this protein to mediate their effects onto the transcription of specific genes.

A comment about nomenclature is necessary to avoid confusion. As described below, there are several members in the C/EBP family of transcription factors. The nomenclature suggested by Cao et al (12) has been adopted in this review, whereby the original *c/ebp* gene cloned is designated C/EBPα, and the remaining members are assigned Greek letters indicating their chronological order of discovery. Additionally, the *c/ebpβ* gene has been cloned from several different species and is referred to in the literature by different names, including LAP (rat) (21), IL6-DBP (rat) (75), NF-IL6 (human) (2), CRP-2 (mouse) (109), AGP/EBP (mouse) (13), and NF-M (chicken) (36). For the sake of clarity, all of these are referred to as C/EBPβ, although where appropriate, the species origin is identified. This becomes important when the role of specific amino acid residues within C/EBPβ are discussed because equivalent positions of a specific serine residue in the human and rat C/EBP homologue, for example, have different numbering assignments due to variations in the total number of residues in the protein.

## PROPERTIES OF C/EBPs

The C/EBP transcription factor family consists of over eight isoforms that are encoded by six genes (reviewed in 42). The additional isoforms arise through translation initiation at different in-frame AUG codons, generating full-length and truncated versions of the protein, as well as by differential splicing and use of alternative promoters. All C/EBP family members possess a highly conserved DNA-binding domain known as a basic region–leucine zipper motif (bZIP). The region that is rich in basic amino acids makes direct contact with DNA and determines the sequence-specific binding properties (1, 32) whereas the leucine zipper motif mediates dimerization between C/EBP polypeptides, which is required for DNA binding and for transactivation (39). The implications of the conserved bZIP domain are twofold. First, all C/EBP isoforms with DNA-binding domains are at least potentially capable of binding to a given C/EBP binding site in a promoter, although there is some evidence that phosphorylation of certain residues in the basic region of specific C/EBP isoforms may alter their binding affinity (discussed later in this review). As a result, different C/EBP isoforms may compete for binding to a cognate DNA sequence. Second, the conserved nature of the leucine zippers make them compatible, allowing for the formation of heterodimer species (12). Thus, a tissue that expresses, for example, the α and β isoforms will in effect contain three species of C/EBP transcription factors: the α/α homodimer, the β/β homodimer, and the α/β heterodimer. Dimerization between isoforms, therefore, clearly has the potential to increase the variety of transcriptional responses that can be obtained from these transcription factors.

The domains of C/EBPs that possess the transactivation function lie in the amino terminus (22, 64, 74, 104, 108). C/EBPs typically have been observed to produce transactivation; however, there are a few examples of specific genes whose transcription is inhibited by a particular C/EBP isoform (52, 102). The amino acid sequences of the transactivation domains are generally unique for each isoform, although some short, conserved domains have been identified in C/EBP$\alpha$, -$\beta$, and -$\delta$ that are critical for the transcriptional activity of these isoforms (65). These transactivation domains act more or less independently of the bZIP domain, displaying similar activity when fused to heterologous DNA-binding domains (65, 73, 74, 78, 104, 108). This modularity has been exploited extensively in studies of the function of specific domains and amino acid residues in C/EBP proteins.

It should be noted that several members of the C/EBP family act as dominant negative inhibitors. For example, C/EBP$\gamma$ is a small, 16-kDa protein consisting primarily of a bZIP domain and lacks a transactivation domain (16). As a result, dimerization of this molecule with other C/EBP isoforms produces inactive heterodimers. Another isoform, C/EBP$\zeta$, acts as a dominant negative protein through a different mechanism. It contains a functional leucine zipper domain and thus dimerizes with other C/EBP isoforms. However, the basic region contains two proline residues that effectively disrupt the $\alpha$-helical nature of this domain that is necessary for its DNA-binding activity (85). Thus, heterodimers containing C/EBP$\zeta$ are incapable of binding to DNA and as a result are transcriptionally inactive.

The tissue-specific expression profiles of C/EBPs are isoform specific. C/EBP$\alpha$, -$\beta$, and -$\delta$ have some commonality in their patterns, being coexpressed at their highest levels in liver, lung, adipose, and intestine tissue, with lower levels of expression in a number of other tissues and cell types (reviewed in 42). C/EBP$\varepsilon$ is probably the most limited in its expression, attaining significant levels only in cells of myeloid and lymphoid lineages (3, 61). Conversely, the two inhibitor isoforms of C/EBP, $\gamma$ and $\zeta$, are ubiquitously expressed (reviewed in 42), which suggests that all cell types are to some extent capable of restricting or inhibiting the transactivation potential of C/EBPs. Obviously, the extent of inhibition depends on the relative levels of expression of the dominant negative and full-length, active isoforms. It is clear that in order to obtain a complete understanding of the biological role of C/EBPs, we must gain an understanding of the mechanisms whereby the expression of these two dominant negative forms of C/EBP are regulated.

## RELATIVE ROLES OF C/EBP ISOFORMS IN ENERGY METABOLISM

Advances in our understanding of the specific and relative roles of C/EBP isoforms in energy metabolism have been greatly accelerated by the development of a variety of methodologies that allow inhibition of expression of specific genes. These include expression of antisense RNA and deletion of genomic sequences of interest by knockout approaches. Although these methodologies have been performed in both established cell lines and whole animals, observations made in the latter have allowed the most comprehensive evaluation of the roles of C/EBP isoforms in energy metabolism. The studies described in this section are devoted to a description of the general metabolic alterations that result from inhibition of expression of specific C/EBP isoforms. Some of these studies have focused on the $\alpha$ and $\beta$ isoforms because they have been identified as regulators of energy metabolism. The details that relate specifically to nutrient regulation of gene expression are elaborated on in the two subsections below.

It should be mentioned that another novel approach developed for inhibiting the activity of C/EBP proteins that has been developed involves the overexpression of natural or synthetic dominant negative proteins (59, 69, 85). Dominant negative versions of C/EBPs inhibit the activity of all C/EBP proteins via heterodimerization with compatible bZIP proteins, and thus offer no information about the role of any specific C/EBP isoform. This limitation, however, in no way lessens the impact this approach has had on advancing our understanding of the biological roles of C/EBPs. Indeed, this approach has been exploited to create a novel animal model of metabolic disease.

## Metabolic Effects of Inhibiting C/EBPα Activity

Initial characterization of C/EBPα revealed that this transcription factor is not expressed until about the time of parturition, and that two of the tissues in which it is most highly expressed are liver and adipose (8). The developmental and metabolic characteristics displayed by mice that have the C/EBPα gene disrupted (105) are fully compatible with the expression profile of this gene. The knockout mice are phenotypically normal at birth, with no difference in birth weight and no gross anatomical abnormalities. However, within a few hours of birth, these mice die from hypoglycemia. This hypoglycemia appears to result primarily from two metabolic perturbations in liver. First, the level of liver glycogen, which is normally high at birth, is undetectable in these mice and is most likely the consequence of reduced expression of the gene coding for glycogen synthase. Second, the expression of three liver gluconeogenic enzymes, glucose-6-phosphatase, phosphoenolpyruvate carboxykinase, and tyrosine aminotransferase, is undetectable at birth, which would impair the ability of the neonate to synthesize glucose de novo. Both of these processes, glycogen mobilization and gluconeogenesis, normally provide the neonate with the nutritional buffer it requires to sustain itself until it is able to obtain sufficient amounts of milk from its mother (33). These mice also have reduced lipid deposits in both inguinal white adipose and brown adipose tissues. This reduction in lipid content, in response to an inhibition of C/EBPα expression, has also been observed in cell lines that can be induced to differentiate into adipocytes (44, 87).

One limitation of the C/EBPα knockout mouse model is that the effects of the gene deletion cannot be assessed in adults because the animals die shortly after birth. To address this issue, Lee and coworkers (40) developed a model system whereby the physiological effects of inhibiting C/EBPα expression in the liver of adult mice could be assessed. Development of this model included (*a*) genetic manipulation of a mouse such that the endogenous *c/ebpα* gene was modified so as to be recognized by a specific enzyme (*Cre* recombinase), which would splice out the *c/ebpα* gene from the genome, and (*b*) generation of an adenovirus vector that would deliver the *Cre* recombinase to the liver. The mice were infected with the recombinant adenovirus via tail vein infusion, and 10 days later the expression of specific genes was analyzed. The efficiency of the gene knockout was demonstrated by analysis of C/EBPα expression, which was reduced by 90% in mice that received the recombinant adenovirus. The deletion of this gene was specific because expression of C/EBPβ was unaltered in these same mice. More important, deletion of the *c/ebpα* gene in adult liver resulted in a significant reduction in expression of the PEPCK and glycogen synthase genes, mirroring the alterations that occur in the neonatal knockout mice described above. This observation is important because it indicates that C/EBPα is involved not only in the establishment of PEPCK and glycogen synthase expression at birth, but also in the maintenance of their expression in adult liver.

## Metabolic Effects of Inhibiting C/EBPβ Activity

In comparison with C/EBPα, delineating the metabolic roles of C/EBPβ has been somewhat more difficult owing to the fact that at least three distinct phenotypes of C/EBPβ (−/−) mice have been observed. In the first published studies of these knockout mice, it was observed that the mutant mice were generally healthy and had no obvious histological or anatomical abnormalities (89, 97). However, the number of mutant mice obtained from heterozygous parents was significantly lower than expected based on Mendelian genetics, which suggests that some in utero loss of homozygous mutants had occurred. A second study by Croniger et al (17) also noted two different phenotypes, although in this case the affected phenotype (B phenotype) was characterized by defective glucose homeostasis, similar to C/EBPα knockouts, and the mice died shortly after birth from hypoglycemia. The defects in the glucose homeostatic mechanism in C/EBPβ knockouts appear to be similar but not identical to those in C/EBPα knockouts. Both mouse models show an absence of hepatic PEPCK gene expression at birth, which suggests a reduced capability for gluconeogenesis. However, although C/EBPα knockout mice lack liver glycogen stores, the B phenotype of C/EBPβ knockouts are able to synthesize and store glycogen but unable to effectively mobilize it (17). The net result is that although there are differences in the precise molecular alterations that occur, both of these mouse models display similar defects in overall glucose homeostasis. The basis for the different phenotypes of the C/EBPβ (−/−) mice has not been established, but some evidence suggests that expression of noninbred modifier genes, present in the genetic backgrounds of the mice, is involved (17).

It would not be accurate to leave the impression that the so-called normal C/EBPβ (−/−) mice are physiologically unaffected. Adult females are sterile (93), both sexes display increased susceptibility to infection by certain bacterial pathogens (97), and the mice have subtle alterations in several metabolic parameters (46). For example, these mice experience hypoglycemia after an 18-h fast, due to impaired hepatic glycogenolysis (46). This is likely related to the reduction in both basal and glucagon-stimulated cAMP concentrations observed in the livers of these mice. A defect in free fatty acid release from adipose in response to epinephrine has also been noted (46), which undoubtedly contributes to the 40% decrease in plasma levels of this lipid in these knockout mice. Whole body glucose disposal is also higher and is one of several observations that suggest that insulin sensitivity is enhanced in these mice, particularly in their skeletal muscle. Finally, these mice have significantly lower white adipose tissue mass compared with wild-type mice, which is due to a reduction in the number of adipocytes (46). This is consistent with other model systems that indicate an important role for C/EBPβ in adipocyte differentiation (98).

To summarize, the studies described above suggest that both of the major C/EBP isoforms play important metabolic roles. The characteristics of the knockout models allows the general conclusion that C/EBPα plays a broader, more general role in establishing energy metabolism in mammals whereas C/EBPβ mediates more subtle responses by regulating the expression of genes that allow organisms to adapt metabolically to environmental (e.g. nutritional) changes. This conclusion is to some extent biased by the inability to analyze in detail the metabolic characteristics of C/EBPα (−/−) mice due to their early death. Nor should one forget the observation that in certain genetic backgrounds, C/EBPβ (−/−) mice display generalized metabolic abnormalities similar to C/EBPα knockouts (17). Moreover, as is discussed below, it is now well established that C/EBPα mediates the effects of nutrients and/or hormones onto specific genes. Thus, its role clearly extends beyond simply establishing energy metabolism and includes the regulation of energy homeostasis as well.

## MECHANISMS WHEREBY C/EBPs MEDIATE THE EFFECTS OF NUTRIENTS AND HORMONES ON GENE EXPRESSION

There are two general mechanisms whereby nutrients and hormones can alter the amount of C/EBP activity in the cell. One is through the alteration of C/EBP gene expression, which would increase or decrease the steady state levels of the protein in the cell and thus affect the total amount of C/EBP transcriptional activity that is available for regulating the expression of target genes. Included in this mechanism is the possibility of altering the relative levels of active and dominant negative forms of C/EBP, which would determine the amount of C/EBP activity in the cell by regulating the ratio of active versus inactive C/EBP dimers. The second mechanism whereby nutrients might accomplish this is by regulating the intrinsic activity of existing C/EBP, which would include regulation of either the transactivation potency or DNA-binding activity.

## Nutrient and Hormonal Effects on C/EBP Expression

The regulation of C/EBP gene expression has been examined primarily in adipose and liver tissue or cells, and some tissue-specific differences have been observed. In liver-derived cells, glucocorticoids (or synthetic analogues such as dexamethasone) induce expression of both alpha and beta isoforms at both the level of mRNA and protein (18, 53, 76). Conversely, glucocorticoids inhibit C/EBPα expression in adipocytes (49). It is curious that there have been no reports of the effect of glucocorticoids on C/EBPβ expression in adipose, although in intestinal epithelial IEC-6 cells, glucocorticoids induce expression of this isoform as it does in liver (10). This suggests that the induction of C/EBPβ expression by glucocorticoids may be a ubiquitous regulatory feature.

Cyclic AMP (cAMP) has been shown to induce expression of C/EBPβ in a wide variety of experimental models and cell types. Injection of a hydrophobic analogue of cAMP into rats induced hepatic C/EBPβ mRNA levels within 90 min but had no effect on levels of C/EBPα mRNA (18). In rat hepatoma H4IIE cells, a cAMP analogue was shown to modestly increase C/EBPα mRNA and protein concentrations and more robustly induce expression of C/EBPβ (18). An induction of C/EBPβ expression by cAMP has also been demonstrated in 30A5 preadipocytes (96), and incubation of primary cultured hepatocytes with glucagon, which stimulates cAMP production, also leads to up-regulation of C/EBPβ expression (53). It is interesting that exercise also leads to an increase in C/EBPβ, but not C/EBPα, expression in rat liver, an effect that is likely mediated by cAMP (68). The mechanism of induction of C/EBPβ expression by cAMP appears to be transcriptional, which is supported by the identification of a typical cAMP response element (CRE) in the promoter of the C/EBPβ gene (66). One well-characterized mediator of cAMP responsiveness, CREB (CRE binding protein), has been shown to bind to the CRE in this promoter. Because CREB is phosphorylated and, as a result, activated by protein kinase A (PKA), the presence of a CREB binding site in the promoter likely defines the mechanism whereby cAMP induces expression of C/EBPβ (66).

The effects of insulin on C/EBP expression have generally been shown to be inhibitory or without effect. MacDougald et al (50) reported a 90% drop in C/EBPα in 3T3-L1 adipocytes treated with insulin for 24 h. In this same study, insulin transiently induced expression of C/EBPβ. Wang et al (106) also reported an inhibitory effect of insulin on C/EBPα expression in adipocytes, although this was observable only in the presence of high (24 mM) concentrations of glucose. Bosch et al (9) observed that mice either fed a high-carbohydrate diet or injected with insulin had reduced levels of hepatic C/EBPβ mRNA but unaltered levels of C/EBPα mRNA. In rat hepatoma H4IIE cells, insulin treatment was demonstrated to transiently induce levels of C/EBPβ protein but had little effect on C/EBPα protein even though a modest stimulatory effect on mRNA levels was detected (18). Studies examining the impact of streptozotocin-induced diabetes as well as subsequent insulin treatment offer further support for the conclusion that the effect of insulin on C/EBP expression is either neutral or inhibitory. Crosson et al (18) showed that C/EBP$\beta$ mRNA and protein levels were unaffected in diabetic rat liver whereas C/EBP$\alpha$ expression was inhibited, which could be partially reversed by insulin treatment. At odds with this study is a study by Bosch et al (9), who reported that induction of diabetes had no effect on C/EBP$\alpha$ mRNA levels whereas C/EBP$\beta$ mRNA levels decreased, something insulin treatment was able to fully reverse. Whether the changes in mRNA levels were reflected in corresponding changes in protein concentrations was not assessed. The basis for the discrepancies between these two studies is not readily apparent but could presumably be due to differences in the dose of streptozotocin used to induce diabetes, which might generate animals with diabetes of dissimilar severity and different metabolic derangements.

A final aspect of C/EBP expression regulation that should be addressed is the issue of the relative abundance of the C/EBP isoforms that act as dominant negatives. A shift in the relative abundance of these inhibitor isoforms should affect the overall C/EBP activity in the cell and, as a consequence, the expression of target genes. There is some evidence that the expression of inhibiting isoforms can be regulated. GADD153 (also called CHOP) is the C/EBP$\zeta$ isoform that has a truncated transactivation domain, as well as amino acid substitutions in its basic region that abrogate its DNA-binding activity. Overexpression of GADD153 has been shown to inhibit the ability of C/EBPs to transactivate target genes (85). The expression of this C/EBP isoform is induced both during the acute phase response (95) and under conditions of amino acid limitation (11), indicating that different physiological and metabolic states can determine and/or regulate cellular C/EBP activity. This, in fact, was demonstrated by Batchvarova et al (5), who found that incubation of 3T3-L1 cells in low glucose (2 mM), which represents a metabolic stress, led to the induction of GADD153 expression. More important, it also resulted in the inhibition of adipocytic differentiation, a process known to require the presence and activity of C/EBP$\alpha$ and C/EBP$\beta$. In a separate study, Crosson et al (18) observed that in streptozotocin-induced diabetic rat liver, there was a selective decrease in the concentration of the truncated and less-active 29-kDa isoform of C/EBP$\alpha$ whereas the levels of the full-length, fully active 42-kDa form remained unchanged. It was hypothesized that this could result in elevated C/EBP activity in the cell due to a shift in the equilibrium toward the formation of active homodimers of the full-length protein. It is interesting that insulin treatment of the diabetic rats restored the ratio of 42- and 29-kDa isoforms back to that of controls. Together, these observations strongly suggest that there is hormonal and metabolic influence over the ratio of C/EBP isoforms.

# Regulation of the Intrinsic Activity of C/EBPs Via Phosphorylation

The other mechanism whereby the amount of C/EBP activity can be altered in the cell is through regulation of the intrinsic activity of the molecule. A number of studies have demonstrated that the various functional properties of C/EBP are regulatable, and in many, but not all, instances this involves phosphorylation/ dephosphorylation of the protein. As described below, the phosphorylation state of C/EBPs can affect their transactivation capacity and their DNA-binding properties, as well as play a role in controlling translocation of the protein to the nuclear compartment.

*Phosphorylation of C/EBPα*    C/EBPα is a highly phosphorylated molecule (27), and the results of several studies suggest regulatory roles for this phosphorylation, although none of the studies have attributed an unequivocal regulatory function to either a specific protein kinase or a residue in C/EBPα that can be phosphorylated. Mahoney et al (51) were the first to suggest that phosphorylation may play a role in regulating its DNA-binding activity. They observed that C/EBPα was efficiently phosphorylated by protein kinase C (PKC), but not by PKA, on $Ser^{248}$, $Ser^{277}$, and $Ser^{299}$. Although no role for the first two phosphorylation sites could be established, it was observed that phosphorylation of $Ser^{299}$ decreased its sequence-specific DNA-binding affinity by approximately 80%. However, it was not determined whether this phosphorylation event abrogated the ability of C/EBPα to transactivate a target gene, and if so, whether regulation by PKC is lost when $Ser^{299}$ is mutated. It has never been determined whether $Ser^{299}$ is phosphorylated in vivo. Thus, the issue of whether the DNA-binding activity of C/EBPα is regulated through phosphorylation of $Ser^{299}$ needs further assessment.

There is fairly convincing evidence that insulin regulates the phosphorylation state of C/EBPα. Preliminary analysis indicated that insulin had little effect on the overall level of the phosphorylation state of C/EBPα (27). However, a more detailed examination suggested that insulin stimulated the dephosphorylation of at least two sites in C/EBPα (27). The effect of insulin could be blocked by inhibitors of phosphatidylinositol 3-kinase, but not by inhibitors of mitogen-activated protein kinase (MAPK), which identified the signaling pathway through which the insulin effect is exerted. Further evidence supporting these inhibitor data was from Ross et al (86), who determined that C/EBPα was phosphorylated in vivo on $Thr^{222}$, $Thr^{226}$, and $Ser^{230}$. The two threonine residues were present within amino acid sequences that are known substrates for glycogen synthase kinase 3 (GSK3). This kinase is inhibited by insulin through a phosphatidylinositol 3-kinase–dependent pathway and, thus, offered a possible mechanism for the insulin-stimulated dephosphorylation observed. Further analysis indicated that GSK3 could indeed phosphorylate C/EBPα in vitro on $Thr^{222}$ and $Thr^{226}$. Overexpression of a constitutively active GSK3 mutant in 3T3-L1 adipocytes enhanced the level of phosphorylation of C/EBPα, which could be inhibited by incubation of these cells with lithium, a known inhibitor of GSK3. Lithium also inhibited the differentiation of 3T3-L1 preadipocytes into adipocytes, which suggests one possible role for the phosphorylation of these sites in C/EBPα. The phosphorylated and dephosphorylated forms of C/EBPα appear to have different conformations, which may influence one or more of its biological activities. However, the study of Ross et al (86) was unable to assign any specific functional role to the threonine residues. Neither mutation of the threonine residues nor overexpression of GSK3 altered the ability of C/EBP$\alpha$ to transactivate a target gene. It is possible that the role for one or more of these phosphorylations manifests itself not in the constitutive activity of C/EBP$\alpha$ but in one of its hormone-regulated activities (discussed later in this review). Thus, although there is compelling evidence that GSK3 is an insulin-regulated C/EBP$\alpha$ kinase, the biological significance of this phosphorylation is not yet apparent.

***Phosphorylation of C/EBP$\beta$***     C/EBP$\beta$ is phosphorylated on a number of different residues by several protein kinases, some of which appear to play a role in the regulation of its biological functions. The translocation of C/EBP$\beta$ to the nucleus is one of these. Regulation of its translocation has been observed in several cell types, although it is not universally employed (107). For example, treatment of rat pheochromocytoma PC12 cells with forskolin stimulates translocation of C/EBP$\beta$ from the cytosol to the nucleus (56). A similar redistribution of this protein occurs in hepatocytes incubated with tumor necrosis factor $\alpha$ (112) and in human colon cancer DKO-1 cells treated with antioxidants (14). The observation that (*a*) inhibition of PKA blocks translocation of C/EBP$\beta$ (14), (*b*) mutation of Ser$^{299}$ to an alanine prevents human C/EBP$\beta$ (also called NF-IL6) from translocating into the nucleus and activating the c-*fos* gene (56), and (*c*) PKA directly phosphorylates this serine residue in vitro (14) suggests that phosphorylation of Ser$^{299}$ (Ser$^{240}$ is the equivalent position in rat C/EBP$\beta$) by PKA induces translocation of this transcription factor. Because PKC phosphorylates this same site in vitro (103), the possibility exists that extracellular signals that activate this particular kinase may also increase shuttling of C/EBP$\beta$ into the nucleus.

The phosphorylation status of C/EBP$\beta$ can also modulate its ability to bind to DNA. Trautwein et al (103) showed that phosphorylation of Ser$^{240}$ (in rat C/EBP$\beta$) by PKA or PKC in vitro inhibits its DNA-binding activity. Thus, the data obtained to date suggest that phosphorylation of Ser$^{240}$ stimulates translocation of C/EBP$\beta$ into the nucleus but, on its arrival, may not be able to efficiently bind to its cognate DNA sequence. Other studies have reported that C/EBP$\beta$ is not phosphorylated by PKA in vitro to any significant extent (107), and elevating cAMP levels in cells does not increase its degree of phosphorylation (101). Thus, some uncertainty remains regarding the role of PKA in regulating the intrinsic activities of this C/EBP isoform. Finally, a study by Liao et al (43) demonstrated that treatment of 3T3-F442 fibroblasts with growth hormone rapidly induces the binding of C/EBP$\beta$ to a site in the c-*fos* gene promoter. Some evidence was obtained to suggest that this effect was mediated via dephosphorylation of this transcription factor, although the specific residue involved was not identified.

Phosphorylation has also been demonstrated to alter the intrinsic transactivation ability of C/EBP$\beta$. Wegner et al (107) found that murine C/EBP$\beta$ binds to a DNA sequence that had been shown to confer responsiveness to a $Ca^{2+}$-calmodulin–dependent protein kinase II (CaMKII), which suggests that this C/EBP isoform could mediate the effect of this protein kinase. Subsequent analysis showed that treatment of pituitary G/C cells with an inhibitor of CaMKII resulted in a reduced phosphorylation state of C/EBP$\beta$, whereas treatment with a calcium ionophore increased phosphorylation (107). Phosphorylation by CaMKII altered neither the DNA-binding activity of C/EBP$\beta$ nor the translocation step; instead, it stimulated its transactivation capacity. It is interesting that the site of phosphorylation was determined to be Ser[276] (equivalent to Ser[277] in rat C/EBP$\beta$), which lies in the DNA-binding domain, although the stimulatory effect of the phosphorylation required the presence of the amino-terminal transactivation domain of C/EBP$\beta$. The strength of this study was that a causal relationship was observed between the phosphorylation of Ser[276] by CaMKII and the enhanced transcriptional activity. In a separate study, Trautwein et al (101) showed that activation of the PKC pathway by phorbol esters resulted in enhanced phosphorylation of rat C/EBP$\beta$ on residue Ser[105], which lies in the transactivation domain. This phosphorylation enhanced the transactivation potential without altering the DNA-binding activity of this transcription factor. Because PKC does not appear to phosphorylate Ser[105] directly (103), it was hypothesized that PKC activation affects some other signaling pathway that regulates C/EBP$\beta$ transactivation capacity. And finally, MAPK has been shown to phosphorylate human C/EBP$\beta$ on Thr[235] (equivalent to Thr[189] in rat C/EBP$\beta$), which leads to a significant activation of this transcription factor (63). Phosphorylation of the nearby Ser[231] appears to be a requirement for this MAPK-dependent activation of C/EBP$\beta$. The limitation of this study, and others like it, was that no specific gene target, which is activated through a MAPK-catalyzed phosphorylation of C/EBP$\beta$, was identified. However, because MAPK is a component of a signaling pathway that is activated by a number of growth factors, including insulin, it is intriguing to speculate that C/EBP$\beta$ might mediate some of the stimulatory effects that growth factors have on the expression of specific genes.

## C/EBPs AS ACCESSORY FACTORS IN NUTRIENT AND HORMONAL RESPONSIVENESS OF GENE TRANSCRIPTION

Our understanding of how hormones and nutrients regulate transcription of genes has advanced steadily over the past 15 years. One of the initial advances in this area came from the identification of short sequences within promoters of genes that could mediate the effect of hormones or nutrients. These sequences, termed enhancers or response elements, can in most cases function independently to some extent. Thus, for example, a cAMP response element (CRE) from one promoter can be artificially linked to a different, normally unresponsive promoter that converts it to one whose activity is now stimulated in the presence of cAMP. Enhancer elements that mediate the transcriptional responses to a variety of nutrients and hormones have been identified, including those for cAMP (84), insulin (94), thyroid hormone (25), steroid hormones (6), glucose (100), and amino acids (34). All these response elements function through their capacity to bind specific transcription factors that perform the actual job of mediating the hormone/nutrient effect onto the transcriptional apparatus. These concepts have led to the development of simplistic models to describe how hormones alter the transcription of genes.

However, as more and more promoters were characterized, it became increasingly evident that hormone and nutrient responses are often mediated by a set of cis-elements, called a response unit (48), rather than by a single sequence. Typically, these response units consist of a recognizable or consensus-like cis-element that is known to mediate the response being characterized and one or more accessory elements. Accessory elements usually have no intrinsic ability to mediate hormonal or nutrient response; rather, they either boost the fold responsiveness mediated by the consensus hormone/nutrient response element or act permissively. In the latter case, the accessory element is necessary but not sufficient to mediate the response. A detailed discussion of response units and the regulatory advantages they offer can be found in several reviews (48, 77, 81).

The reason for including a brief description of response units in this review is that in the vast majority of genes where C/EBPs have been shown to participate in mediating the effects of hormones and nutrients onto transcription, C/EBPs play the role of accessory factors that bind to accessory elements. That is, although C/EBPs usually have no intrinsic capacity to mediate a response, they are able to cooperate with other transcription factors to mediate a response to a hormonal or nutritional signal. To date, C/EBPs have been implicated in transcriptional responses to cAMP, glucocorticoids, thyroid hormone, and perhaps insulin and, in each case, are known to function within a response unit (discussed below).

A large portion of the body of information regarding the role C/EBPs play in mediating these responses has come from analyses of the PEPCK gene promoter, where C/EBP$\alpha$ and C/EBP$\beta$ play different roles in mediating responses to several hormones. Because of the significant amount of information available on the role of C/EBPs in the regulation of this gene, it is discussed in a separate section below. Ahead of this section, a brief description of other genes that utilize C/EBPs as accessory factors to mediate hormonal responsiveness is provided.

By far the most common type of hormonal response with which C/EBPs are associated is that of glucocorticoids. These steroid hormones interact with a specific receptor in the cytosol, which then causes its translocation to the nucleus, where the receptor-ligand complex binds to specific DNA sequences in select genes, producing either stimulation or repression of their transcription. However, as mentioned above, the full response to glucocorticoids in a number of genes requires the participation of other transcription factors, which frequently include C/EBPs. In their studies examining the acquisition of glucocorticoid responsiveness in chicken embryonic neural retina, Ben-Or & Okret (7) found that induction of glutamine synthetase expression by glucocorticoids was delayed even though the glucocorticoid receptor was expressed early in ontogeny. Detailed analysis of the glutamine synthetase gene promoter demonstrated that a C/EBP-like factor was required for glucocorticoid responsiveness. Although ectopic expression of murine C/EBP$\alpha$ in nonresponsive embryonic day 7 retinal cells enhanced the responsiveness of the glutamine synthetase promoter to glucocorticoids, other experiments suggested that the actual accessory factor is not C/EBP$\alpha$. The ability of other C/EBP isoforms to reconstitute responsiveness was not examined, and it is possible that chickens express a species-specific isoform that functions in this system.

A study by Nishio et al (67) examining the glucocorticoid responsiveness of the $\alpha$1-acid glycoprotein gene promoter not only provided further support for a generalized role for C/EBPs in glucocorticoid responsiveness, it also offered a possible molecular mechanism as to how it participates in this response. In this particular promoter, there are two C/EBP binding sites located just downstream of a glucocorticoid response element that binds the glucocorticoid receptor. Overexpression of C/EBP$\beta$ enhanced the activity of the promoter in the presence of glucocorticoids. It is interesting that this synergism was observed even when a point mutant of C/EBP$\beta$, which interfered with its DNA-binding activity, was expressed. Subsequent analysis indicated that C/EBP$\beta$ and the glucocorticoid receptor could physically interact in vitro, although whether a causal relationship exists between this interaction and the synergistic activation produced by the two transcription factors was not examined. Because the physical interaction occurred through the bZIP domain of C/EBP$\beta$, which is highly conserved among isoforms, it is possible that other members of the C/EBP family could also substitute as an accessory factor for this response.

C/EBP$\alpha$ appears to be involved in the transcriptional regulation of the prolactin gene by insulin. Jacob & Stanley (31) showed that C/EBP$\alpha$ binds to a multihormonal response element in the promoter, and that overexpression of C/EBP$\alpha$ in GH4 cells increased both the basal and insulin-stimulated activity of the prolactin promoter. It has not been determined whether C/EBP$\alpha$ alone mediates the insulin response, and if so how, or whether it functions within a response unit with other factors. Nor is it clear how such a short sequence (10 bp) can mediate the effects of epidermal growth factor, insulin, and cAMP. Several different transcription factors can bind to this sequence, at least in vitro, although it is unlikely that more than one factor could bind at any one time given the length of the sequence.

## HORMONAL REGULATION OF PEPCK GENE TRANSCRIPTION

The PEPCK gene has played a special role in advancing the field of molecular endocrinology and metabolism. This gene codes for a rate-limiting enzyme of gluconeogenesis, and its rate of transcription and mRNA turnover is responsive to a variety of hormones and metabolic conditions (reviewed in 26). Because of these characteristics, this model is frequently used to examine multihormonal regulation of gene expression. Moreover, its expression is both tissue-specific and ontogenetically controlled, making it attractive to investigators working in these areas.

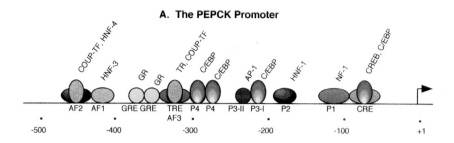

**A. The PEPCK Promoter**

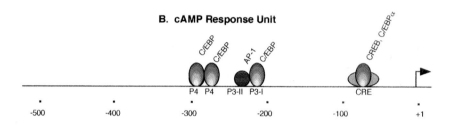

**B. cAMP Response Unit**

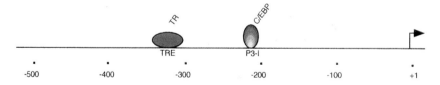

**C. Thyroid Hormone Response Unit**

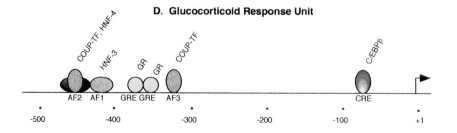

**D. Glucocorticoid Response Unit**

See legend next page

See figure previous page

**Figure 1** The phosphoenolpyruvate carboxykinase (PEPCK) promoter contains a number of hormone response units, some of which share *cis*-elements. (*A*) The various *cis*-elements and their corresponding DNA-binding protein(s). The name of the *cis*-element is shown below the line whereas the name of the transcription factors is placed above the shape depicting the bound protein. It should be noted that for three of the *cis*-elements, more than one potential DNA-binding protein has been identified. The term C/EBP indicates that both alpha and beta isoforms can bind to the site. (*B*) The subset of *cis*-elements and corresponding binding proteins that make up the cyclic AMP (cAMP) response unit. The binding of either cAMP response element binding protein (CREB) or C/EBPa to the cAMP response element (CRE) is permissive for the activity of this response unit. (*C*) The two *cis*-elements and corresponding binding proteins that make up the thyroid hormone response unit. The binding of either C/EBPa or C/EBPb to phosphatidylinositol 3-kinase is permissive for its activity. (*D*) The *cis*-elements and corresponding transcription factors that make up the glucocorticoid response unit. Maximal response to glucocorticoids can be achieved when either chicken ovalbumin upstream promoter transcription factor (COUP-TF) or hepatic nuclear factor 4 (HNF-4) is bound to accessory factor 2 (AF2), whereas there is a specific requirement for the binding of C/EBPb to the CRE. P1–P4, promoter elements 1–4; TR, thyroid hormone receptor; NF-1, nuclear factor 1; GR, glucocorticoid receptor; GRE, glucocorticoid response element.

Transcription of this gene in liver is activated by cAMP, glucocorticoids, retinoic acid, and thyroid hormone and is inhibited by insulin (26). The PEPCK gene promoter was the first in which a CRE was defined (91), which ultimately assisted in the discovery of a specific transcription factor that binds to this sequence (60) and which led to an understanding of one molecular mechanism whereby cAMP induces transcription (90). It was also analysis of this promoter that helped to advance the concept of hormone response units because all the hormonal responses this promoter displays are mediated by more than one *cis*-element. The promoter has several binding sites for C/EBPs (71), one or more of which participate in the hormone response units described below and shown schematically in Figure 1 (see color insert). It was the examination of the involvement of C/EBPs in the regulation of the PEPCK promoter that led to the realization that these transcription factors, more than just constitutive regulators, also assist in mediating the effects of nutrients and hormones onto the transcription rate of specific genes.

## Cyclic AMP Responsiveness

Transcription of the PEPCK gene in liver responds rapidly and robustly to a rise in the level of cAMP (38). This contrasts with a weak response to this second messenger in other tissues, such as kidney (55). Initial analysis of the PEPCK promoter identified a *cis*-element, known as the cAMP response element (CRE), which mediated a cAMP response (91). However, the magnitude of the response mediated by the CRE alone is weak compared with that of a promoter fragment that extends out to nucleotide $-490$ (45, 80). Further analysis of the promoter indicated that there was an upstream region extending from $-355$ to $-200$, which, when coupled with the CRE, conferred a strong response to cAMP although it had little or no activity on its own (80). Detailed analysis of this region ultimately demonstrated that it contained three binding sites for C/EBP and one site for activator protein-1, all of which were required, along with the CRE, for maximal responsiveness to cAMP (83). Thus, five *cis*-elements make up the cAMP response unit (CRU) in this promoter (Figure 1*B*, see color insert). The nature of this response unit (and indeed all response units) likely provides the benefit of allowing for an expanded range of responses the promoter can have to the initial stimulus (77).

Attempts to identify the precise transcription factors that mediate the response to cAMP through the five *cis*-elements was not a straightforward task because some of the *cis*-elements were shown to bind multiple proteins. For example, three different transcription factors can bind, at least in vitro, to the CRE, the CRE-binding protein (CREB) (71), and both $\alpha$- and $\beta$-isoforms of C/EBP (71, 73). And both C/EBP isoforms can bind to the three C/EBP binding sites in the distal portion of the promoter (71, 73). However, using a variety of molecular biological approaches, the roles of specific transcription factors, and the *cis*-elements through which they exert their effects, have been assessed (reviewed in 77, 111).

C/EBP$\alpha$ appears to play a particularly critical role in the ability of the PEPCK promoter to respond to cAMP. Mice with the C/EBP$\alpha$ gene knocked out have an impaired response to cAMP whereas those with a deletion in the C/EBP$\beta$ gene do not (17). Moreover, recent studies by Crosson & Roesler (19) showed that inhibition of C/EBP$\alpha$ gene expression by antisense technology completely abrogated the induction of PEPCK gene expression by cAMP in rat hepatoma cells, whereas antisense directed against C/EBP$\beta$ had no effect. This does not necessarily rule out a role for C/EBP$\beta$ in the CRU; a response to cAMP can be observed when either isoform is bound to the three distal C/EBP binding sites in the promoter (73; PJ McFie, WJ Roesler, unpublished observations).

What remains unclear is the identity of the transcription factor that binds to the CRE, a critical component of the CRU, to confer a robust response to cAMP. The obvious candidate is CREB because it binds in vitro to this site and is a direct substrate of PKA, a cAMP-activated kinase (reviewed in 90). Indeed, tethering of CREB to the CRE reconstitutes a strong cAMP response in hepatoma cells (79). However, both C/EBP isoforms can also bind to this site (71, 73), but with drastically different consequences. When C/EBP$\alpha$ is bound to the CRE, the promoter displays a significant responsivity to cAMP, whereas with C/EBP$\beta$ bound, responsivity is lost (82). These data suggest that the degree to which the PEPCK promoter responds to cAMP is governed by the specific combination of transcription factors that are bound to the components of the CRU at any given time. This in turn might be determined by the relative concentrations of the transcription factors involved. Recently, a model that incorporates the above information has been proposed (77) describing how the PEPCK promoter could exist in various states of cAMP responsivity, depending on the physiological and metabolic signals to which it responds.

The precise role C/EBPs play in the CRU is unknown. C/EBP$\alpha$ is not directly phosphorylated by PKA (51), and although C/EBP$\beta$ may be a substrate for this kinase (103), there is no evidence that it leads to an increase in its activity (101). Structure/function analysis of both C/EBP isoforms have identified the domains that are required for their ability to mediate cAMP responsiveness (73, 82), and some conserved amino acid sequences within these domains exist (65). In the case of C/EBP$\alpha$, mutational analysis has led to the conclusion that the mechanism whereby it mediates constitutive transactivation is distinct from that whereby it mediates cAMP-inducible transactivation (82). This is an important observation because it suggests that unique nuclear targets exist with which C/EBP$\alpha$ makes contact, allowing the manifestation of its cAMP-inducible activity. The identity of these nuclear proteins is unknown, although one potential candidate is the coactivator CBP (CREB-binding protein). This protein mediates the effects of a number of transcription factors by bridging them to the preinitiation complex (35). A functional homologue of CBP, p300, has been shown to physically interact with C/EBP$\beta$ and to enhance its ability to transactivate target promoters (57). In this same study, p300 increased the transcriptional capacity of C/EBP$\alpha$, although no physical interaction between the two was reported. Studies examining a possible role for CBP in the cAMP responsiveness of the PEPCK promoter, as well as experiments attempting to demonstrate a direct interaction between CBP and C/EBP$\alpha$, have been unsuccessful (WJ Roesler, PJ McFie, unpublished observations).

## Thyroid Hormone Responsiveness

A role for thyroid hormone (T$_3$) in the regulation of the PEPCK gene was first suggested when it was detected that the amount of PEPCK activity and its rate of gene transcription were affected by alterations in the thyroid status of animals (47, 62, 92). Analysis of the promoter indicated that there are two *cis*-elements that mediate the T$_3$ response: a typical T$_3$ response element that binds the thyroid hormone receptor, and a binding site for C/EBP (24, 70) (Figure 1C, see color insert). Mutation of either sequence resulted in complete loss of response to the hormone, so the binding of C/EBP to its cognate site is required in order for the promoter to be responsive to T$_3$ (70). Experiments aimed at determining which C/EBP isoform is involved suggested that either C/EBP$\alpha$ or $\beta$ can play the role of accessory factor in this response (72, 73). Here again, the mechanism whereby C/EBPs participate in this hormone response is not known, although it has been speculated that by acting together, thyroid hormone receptor and C/EBP may more efficiently recruit a necessary coactivator to the promoter that mediates the T$_3$ response (73).

## Glucocorticoid Responsiveness

The glucocorticoid responsiveness of the PEPCK promoter is mediated by an extremely complex response unit, which employs two glucocorticoid response elements and four accessory elements (Figure 1D, see color insert) (110). Mutation of any one element results in a significant decrease in fold responsiveness (58, 88). It is interesting that one of the accessory elements in this response unit is the CRE (30), which as mentioned above can bind both CREB and C/EBP family members. Recently, Yamada et al (110) examined which of these CRE-binding proteins acted as an accessory factor for the glucocorticoid response. Their first approach was to change the CRE sequences in the PEPCK promoter to a consensus C/EBP binding site, to which CREB did not bind. This altered promoter was shown to retain full responsiveness to glucocorticoids, which suggests that a C/EBP isoform, and not CREB, was the accessory factor. A second approach was to replace the bZIP (DNA-binding) domain of CREB and C/EBP isoforms with the DNA-binding domain of the yeast transcription GAL4, and to test for their ability to reconstitute glucocorticoid responsiveness on a PEPCK promoter variant that had the CRE replaced by a binding site for GAL4. Using this system, these investigators were able to demonstrate that although CREB and C/EBP$\alpha$ had no accessory factor activity, C/EBP$\beta$ was able to enhance responsiveness to this hormone. Thus, the CRE appears to be a multifunctional *cis*-element, participating in the cAMP response unit when either CREB or C/EBP$\alpha$ is bound to it and acting as an accessory element in the glucocorticoid response unit when C/EBP$\beta$ is bound. Precisely what determines which transcription factor will be bound to the CRE at any point in time, and thus what hormone response unit it will participate in, is a puzzle yet to be solved.

The CRE is not the only *cis*-element that participates in overlapping hormone response units in the PEPCK promoter. The C/EBP binding site at $-230$, for example, which can bind either C/EBP$\alpha$ or -$\beta$, is a component of both the cAMP and $T_3$ response units. This complex of overlapping response units, which collectively has been termed a metabolic control domain (110), likely permits the integration of the various hormonal and nutritional stimuli that regulate the expression of the PEPCK gene. Although the individual components of the various hormone response units have, for the most part, been identified, we do not have any clear vision as to how these bound factors functionally interact in order to mediate their responses. Thus, despite the enormous number of studies that have been performed analyzing the various hormonal responses of the PEPCK promoter, many of the molecular details of its regulation remain a mystery.

## CONCLUDING REMARKS

The studies cited and summarized in this review article have attempted to document the important role that C/EBPs play in the regulation of metabolism, via their ability to mediate the effects of nutrients and hormones onto gene expression. I hope this article has also identified important issues yet unaddressed regarding the functions and mechanisms of action of this family of proteins. For despite their importance in such critical processes as adipocyte differentiation and glucose homeostasis, our understanding of many aspects of their biochemical function remains incomplete. For example, although there are suggestions that individual gene promoters utilize one specific C/EBP isoform in its regulation, we do not have a good grasp as to how selective recruitment of one isoform can occur, given the conserved nature of the bZIP domain. Does differential phosphorylation of isoforms play a role? Perhaps the unique transactivation domains of C/EBP isoforms provide a puzzle-like "fit" with other bound transcription factors on promoters (23, 37). Alternatively, C/EBPs have been shown to distort DNA on binding, with the extent of the distortion dependent on not only the sequence of the binding site but also which isoform(s) it binds (4). Thus, it appears possible that isoforms could be differentially recruited on the basis of their ability to introduce the "correct" distortion into the promoter region that is required for its regulatory effects. Another area that remains entirely unexplored is whether C/EBPs regulate expression of genes that code for proteins that participate in fatty acid oxidation. Given that C/EBPs play a critical role in energy metabolism and alter the expression of genes that code for enzymes involved in carbohydrate metabolism and fatty acid synthesis, it seems probable that genes involved in fatty acid oxidation have been overlooked as a group of C/EBP-regulated genes. Thus, despite the increasing appreciation of the important functions that C/EBPs play in regulating the expression of genes linked to critical metabolic events, there remains much to uncover and understand about this class of transcription factors.

## ACKNOWLEDGMENTS

The work derived from the author's laboratory that is cited in this review was supported by grants from the Canadian Institutes of Health Research and the Canadian Diabetes Association. I would like to thank Ramji Khandelwal and Heather Wilson for critically reviewing the manuscript.

**Visit the Annual Reviews home page at www.AnnualReviews.org**

## LITERATURE CITED

1. Agre P, Johnson PF, McKnight SL. 1989. Cognate DNA binding specificity retained after leucine zipper exchange between GCN4 and C/EBP. *Science* 246:922–26
2. Akira S, Isshiki H, Sugita T, Tanabe O, Kinoshita S, et al. 1990. A nuclear factor for IL-6 expression (NF-IL6) is a member of a C/EBP family. *EMBO J.* 9:1897–906
3. Antonson P, Stellan B, Yamanaka R, Xanthopoulos KG. 1996. A novel human CCAAT/enhancer binding protein gene, C/EBPε, is expressed in cells of lymphoid and myeloid lineages and is localized on chromosome 14q11.2 close to the T-cell receptor alpha/delta locus. *Genomics* 35:30–38
4. Avitahl N, Calame K. 1994. The C/EBP family of proteins distorts DNA upon binding but does not introduce a large directed bend. *J. Biol. Chem.* 269:23553–62
5. Batchvarova N, Wang X-Z, Ron D. 1995. Inhibition of adipogenesis by the stress-induced protein CHOP (Gadd153). *EMBO J.* 14:4654–61
6. Beato M. 1989. Gene regulation by steroid hormones. *Cell* 56:335–44
7. Ben-Or S, Okret S. 1993. Involvement of a C/EBP-like protein in the acquisition of responsiveness to glucocorticoid hormones during chick neural retina development. *Mol. Cell. Biol.* 13:331–40
8. Birkenmeier EH, Gwynn B, Howard S, Jerry J, Gordon JI, et al. 1989. Tissue-specific expression, developmental regulation, and genetic mapping of the gene encoding CCAAT/enhancer binding protein. *Genes Dev.* 3:1146–56
9. Bosch, Sabater J, Valera A. 1995. Insulin inhibits liver expression of the CCAAT/enhancer-binding protein β. *Diabetes* 44:267–71
10. Boudreau F, Blais S, Asselin C. 1996. Regulation of CCAAT/enhancer binding protein isoforms by serum and glucocorticoids in the rat intestinal epithelial crypt cell line IEC-6. *Exp. Cell Res.* 222:1–9
11. Bruhat A, Jousse C, Wang X-Z, Ron D, Ferrara M, Fafournoux P. 1997. Amino acid limitation induces expression of *CHOP*, a CCAAT/enhancer binding protein-related gene, at both transcriptional and post-transcriptional levels. *J. Biol. Chem.* 272:17588–93
12. Cao Z, Umek RM, McKnight SL. 1991. Regulated expression of three C/EBP isoforms during adipose conversion of 3T3-L1 cells. *Genes Dev.* 5:1538–52
13. Chang C-J, Chen T-T, Lei H-Y, Chen D-S, Lee S-C. 1990. Molecular cloning of a transcription factor, AGP/EBP, that belongs to members of the C/EBP family. *Mol. Cell. Biol.* 10:6642–53
14. Chinery R, Brockman JA, Dransfield DT, Coffey RJ. 1997. Antioxidant-induced

nuclear translocation of CCAAT/enhancer-binding protein α. *J. Biol. Chem.* 272: 30356–81

15. Clarke SL, Robinson CE, Gimble JM. 1997. CAAT/enhancer binding proteins directly modulate transcription from the peroxisome proliferator-activated receptor γ2 promoter. *Biochem. Biophys. Res. Commun.* 240:99–103

16. Cooper C, Henderson A, Artandi S, Avitahl N, Calame K. 1995. Ig/EBP (C/EBPγ) is a transdominant negative inhibitor of C/EBP family transcriptional activators. *Nucleic Acids Res.* 23:4371–77

17. Croniger C, Trus M, Lysek-Stupp K, Cohen H, Liu Y, et al. 1997. Role of the isoforms of CCAAT/enhancer-binding protein in the initiation of phosphoenolpyruvate carboxykinase (GTP) gene transcription at birth. *J. Biol. Chem.* 272:26306–12

18. Crosson SM, Davies GF, Roesler WJ. 1997. Hepatic expression of CCAAT/-enhancer binding protein α: hormonal and metabolic regulation in rats. *Diabetologia* 40:1117–24

19. Crosson SM, Roesler WJ. 2000. Hormonal regulation of the phosphoenolpyruvate carboxykinase gene. Role of specific CCAAT/enhancer-binding protein isoforms. *J. Biol. Chem.* 275:5804–9

20. Darlington GJ, Ross SE, MacDougald OA. 1998. The role of C/EBP genes in adipocyte differentiation. *J. Biol. Chem.* 273:30057–60

21. Descombes P, Chojkier M, Lichtsteiner S, Falvey E, Schibler U. 1990. LAP, a novel member of the C/EBP family, encodes a liver-enriched transcriptional activator protein. *Genes Dev.* 4:1541–51

22. Friedman AD, McKnight SL. 1990. Identification of two polypeptide segments of CCAAT/enhancer-binding protein required for transcriptional activation of the serum albumin gene. *Genes Dev.* 4:1416–26

23. Fry CJ, Farnham PJ. 1999. Context-dependent transcriptional regulation. *J. Biol. Chem.* 274:29583–86

24. Giralt M, Park EA, Gurney AL, Liu J, Hakimi P, Hanson RW. 1991. Identification of a thyroid hormone response element in the phosphoenolpyruvate carboxykinase (GTP) gene. *J. Biol. Chem.* 266:21991–96

25. Glass CK, Franco R, Weinberger C, Albert VR, Evans RM, Rosenfeld MG. 1987. A c-erb-A binding site in rat growth hormone gene mediates trans-activation by thyroid hormone. *Nature* 329:738–41

26. Hanson RW, Patel YM. 1994. Phosphoenolpyruvate carboxykinase (GTP): the gene and the enzyme. *Adv. Enzymol.* 69:203–81

27. Hemati N, Ross SE, Erickson RL, Groblewski GE, MacDougald OA. 1997. Signaling pathways through which insulin regulates CCAAT/enhancer binding protein α (C/EBPα) phosphorylation and gene expression in 3T3-L1 adipocytes. *J. Biol. Chem.* 272:25913–19

28. Hollenberg AN, Susulic VS, Madura JP, Zhang B, Moller DE, et al. 1997. Functional antagonism between CCAAT/-enhancer binding protein-α and peroxisome proliferator-activated receptor-γ on the leptin promoter. *J. Biol. Chem.* 272:5283–90

29. Hwang C-S, Mandrup S, MacDougald OA, Geiman DE, Lane MD. 1996. Transcriptional activation of the mouse obese (*ob*) gene by CCAAT/enhancer binding protein α. *Proc. Natl. Acad. Sci. USA* 93:873–77

30. Imai E, Miner JN, Mitchell JA, Yamamoto KR, Granner DK. 1993. Glucocorticoid receptor-cAMP response element binding protein interaction and the response of the phosphoenolpyruvate carboxykinase gene to glucocorticoids. *J. Biol. Chem.* 268:5353–56

31. Jacob KK, Stanley FM. 1999. CCAAT/enhancer-binding protein α is a physiological regulator of prolactin gene expression. *Endocrinology* 140:4542–50

32. Johnson PF. 1993. Identification of C/EBP

basic region residues involved in DNA sequence recognition and half-site spacing preference. *Mol. Cell. Biol.* 13:6919–30

33. Jones CT. 1982. *The Development of the Metabolism in the Fetal Liver.* New York: Elsevier Biomed.

34. Jousse C, Bruhat A, Fafournoux P. 1999. Amino acid regulation of gene expression. *Curr. Opin. Clin. Nutr. Metab. Care* 2:297–301

35. Kamei Y, Xu L, Heinzel T, Torchia J, Kurokawa R, et al. 1996. A CBP integrator complex mediates transcriptional activation and AP-1 inhibition by nuclear receptors. *Cell* 85:403–14

36. Katz S, Kowenz-Leutz E, Müller C, Meese K, Ness SA, Leutz A. 1993. The NF-M transcription factor is related to C/EBPβ and plays a role in signal transduction, differentiation and leukemogenesis of avian myelomonocytic cells. *EMBO J.* 12:1321–32

37. Lamb P, McKnight SL. 1991. Diversity and specificity in transcriptional regulation: the benefits of heterotypic dimerization. *Trends Biochem. Sci.* 16:417–22

38. Lamers WH, Hanson RW, Meisner HM. 1982. cAMP stimulates transcription of the gene for cytosolic phosphoenolpyruvate carboxykinase in rat liver nuclei. *Proc. Natl. Acad. Sci. USA* 79:5137–41

39. Landschultz WH, Johnson PF, McKnight SL. 1989. The leucine zipper: a hypothetical structure common to a new class of DNA binding proteins. *Science* 243:1681–88

40. Lee Y-H, Sauer B, Johnson PF, Gonzalez FJ. 1997. Disruption of the *c/ebpα* gene in adult mouse liver. *Mol. Cell. Biol.* 17:6014–22

41. Legraverend C, Antonson P, Flodby P, Xanthopoulos KG. 1993. High level activity of the mouse CCAAT/enhancer binding protein (C/EBPα) gene promoter involves autoregulation and several ubiquitous transcription factors. *Nucleic Acids Res.* 21:1735–42

42. Lekstrom-Himes J, Xanthopoulos KG. 1998. Biological role of the CCAAT/enhancer-binding protein family of transcription factors. *J. Biol. Chem.* 273:28545–48

43. Liao J, Piwien-Pilipuk G, Ross SE, Hodge CL, Sealy L, et al. 1999. CCAAT/enhancer-binding protein β (C/EBPβ) and C/EBPδ contribute to growth hormone-regulated transcription of *c-fos*. *J. Biol. Chem.* 274:31597–604

44. Lin F-T, Lane MD. 1992. Antisense CCAAT/enhancer-binding protein RNA suppresses coordinate gene expression and triglyceride accumulation during differentiation of 3T3-L1 preadipocytes. *Genes Dev.* 6:533–44

45. Liu JS, Park EA, Gurney AL, Roesler WJ, Hanson RW. 1991. Cyclic AMP induction of phosphoenolpyruvate carboxykinase (GTP) gene transcription is mediated by multiple promoter elements. *J. Biol. Chem.* 266:19095–20102

46. Liu S, Croniger C, Arizmendi C, Harada-Shiba M, Ren J, et al. 1999. Hypoglycemia and impaired hepatic glucose production in mice with a deletion of the C/EBPβ gene. *J. Clin. Invest.* 103:207–13

47. Loose DS, Cameron DK, Short HP, Hanson RW. 1985. Thyroid hormone regulates transcription of the gene for cytosolic phosphoenolpyruvate carboxykinase (GTP) in rat liver. *Biochemistry* 24:4509–12

48. Lucas PC, Granner DK. 1992. Hormone response domains in gene transcription. *Annu. Rev. Biochem.* 61:1131–73

49. MacDougald OA, Cornelius P, Lin F-T, Chen SS, Lane MD. 1994. Glucocorticoids reciprocally regulate expression of the CCAAT/enhancer-binding protein α and δ genes in 3T3-L1 adipocytes and white adipose tissue. *J. Biol. Chem.* 269:19041–47

50. MacDougald OA, Cornelius P, Liu R, Lane MD. 1995. Insulin regulates transcription of the CCAAT/enhancer binding (C/EBP) α, β, and δ genes in

fully-differentiated 3T3-L1 adipocytes. *J. Biol. Chem.* 270:647–54

51. Mahoney CW, Shuman J, McKnight SL, Chen H-C, Huang K-P. 1992. Phosphorylation of CCAAT-enhancer binding protein by protein kinase C attenuates site-selective DNA binding. *J. Biol. Chem.* 267:19396–403

52. Matsuda K, Araki E, Yoshimura R, Tsuruzoe K, Furukawa N, et al. 1997. Cell-specific regulation of IRS-1 gene expression. *Diabetes* 46:354–62

53. Matsuno F, Chowdhury S, Gotoh T, Iwase K, Matsuzaki H, et al. 1996. Induction of the C/EBPβ gene by dexamethasone and glucagon in primary-cultured rat hepatocytes. *J. Biochem.* 119:524–32

54. McKnight SL, Lane MD, Gluecksohn-Waelsch S. 1989. Is CCAAT/enhancer-binding protein α central regulator of energy metabolism? *Genes Dev.* 3:2021–24

55. Meisner HM, Loose DS, Hanson RW. 1984. Effect of hormones on transcription of the gene for cytosolic phosphoenolpyruvate carboxykinase (GTP) in rat kidney. *Biochemistry* 24:421–25

56. Metz R, Ziff R. 1991. cAMP stimulates the C/EBP-related transcription factor rNFIL-6 to *trans*-locate to the nucleus and induce *c-fos* transcription. *Genes Dev.* 5:1754–66

57. Mink S, Haenig B, Klempnauer K-H. 1997. Interaction and functional collaboration of p300 and C/EBPβ. *Mol. Cell. Biol.* 17:6609–17

58. Mitchell J, Noisin E, Hall R, O'Brien R, Imai E, Granner D. 1994. Integration of multiple signals through a complex hormone response unit in the phosphoenolpyruvate carboxykinase gene promoter. *Mol. Endocrinol.* 8:585–94

59. Moitra J, Mason MM, Olive M, Krylov D, Oksana G, et al. 1998. Life without white fat: a transgenic mouse. *Genes Dev.* 12:3168–81

60. Montminy MR, Bilezikjian LM. 1987. Binding of a nuclear protein to the cyclic AMP response element of the somatostatin gene. *Nature* 328:175–78

61. Morosetti R, Park DJ, Chumakov AM, Grillier I, Shiohara M, et al. 1997. A novel, myeloid transcription factor, C/EBPε, is upregulated during granulocytic, but not monocytic, differentiation. *Blood* 90:2591–600

62. Müller MJ, Thomsen A, Sibrowski W, Seitz HJ. 1982. 3,5,3′-Triiodothyronine-induced synthesis of rat liver phosphoenolpyruvate carboxykinase. *Endocrinology* 111:1469–75

63. Nakajima T, Kinoshita S, Sasagawa T, Sasaki K, Naruto M, et al. 1993. Phosphorylation of threonine-235 by a *ras*-dependent mitogen-activated protein kinase cascade is essential for transcription factor NF-IL6. *Proc. Natl. Acad. Sci. USA* 90:2207–11

64. Nerlov C, Ziff EB. 1994. Three levels of functional interaction determine the activity of CCAAT/enhancer binding protein-α on the serum albumin promoter. *Genes Dev.* 8:350–62

65. Nerlov C, Ziff EB. 1995. CCAAT/enhancer binding protein-α amino acid motifs with dual TBP and TFIIB binding ability cooperate to activate transcription in both yeast and mammalian cells. *EMBO J.* 14:4318–28

66. Niehof M, Manns MP, Trautwein C. 1997. CREB controls LAP/C/EBPβ transcription. *Mol. Cell. Biol.* 17:3600–13

67. Nishio Y, Isshiki H, Kishimoto T, Akira S. 1993. A nuclear factor for interleukin-6 expression (NF-IL6) and the glucocorticoid receptor synergistically activate transcription of the rat α1-acid glycoprotein gene via direct protein-protein interaction. *Mol. Cell. Biol.* 13:1854–62

68. Nizielski SE, Arizmendi C, Shteyngarts AR, Farrell CJ, Friedman JE. 1996. Involvement of transcription factor C/EBP-β in stimulation of PEPCK gene expression during exercise. *Am. J. Physiol.* 270:R1005–12

69. Olive M, Williams SC, Deza C, Johnson PF, Vinson C. 1996. Design of a C/EBP-specific, dominant-negative bZIP protein with both inhibitory and gain-of-function properties. *J. Biol. Chem.* 271:2040–47
70. Park EA, Jerden DC, Bahouth SW. 1995. Regulation of phosphoenolpyruvate carboxykinase gene transcription by thyroid hormone involves two distinct binding sites in the promoter. *Biochem. J.* 309:913–19
71. Park EA, Roesler WJ, Liu J, Klemm DJ, Gurney AL, et al. 1990. The role of the CCAAT/enhancer-binding protein in the transcriptional regulation of the gene for phosphoenolpyruvate carboxykinase (GTP). *Mol. Cell. Biol.* 10:6264–72
72. Park EA, Song S, Olive M, Roesler WJ. 1997. CCAAT-enhancer-binding protein $\alpha$ (C/EBP$\alpha$) is required for the thyroid hormone but not the retinoic acid induction of phosphoenolpyruvate carboxykinase (PEPCK) gene transcription. *Biochem. J.* 322:343–49
73. Park EA, Song S, Vinson C, Roesler WJ. 1999. Role of CCAAT enhancer-binding protein $\beta$ in the thyroid hormone and cAMP induction of phosphoenolpyruvate carboxykinase gene transcription. *J. Biol. Chem.* 274:211–17
74. Pei D, Shih C. 1991. An "attenuator domain" is sandwiched by two distinct transactivation domains in the transcription factor C/EBP. *Mol. Cell. Biol.* 11:1480–87
75. Poli V, Mancini FP, Cortese R. 1990. IL-6DBP, a nuclear protein involved in interleukin-6 signal transduction, defines a new family of leucine zipper proteins related to C/EBP. *Cell* 63:643–53
76. Ramos RA, Nishio Y, Maiyar AC, Simon KE, Ridder CC, et al. 1996. Glucocorticoid-stimulated CCAAT/enhancer-binding protein $\alpha$ expression is required for steroid-induced G1 cell cycle arrest of minimal-deviation rat hepatoma cells. *Mol. Cell. Biol.* 16:5288–301
77. Roesler WJ. 2000. What is a cAMP response unit? *Mol. Cell. Endocrinol.* 162:1–7
78. Roesler WJ, Crosson SM, Vinson C, McFie PJ. 1996. The $\alpha$-isoform of the CCAAT/enhancer-binding protein is required for mediating the cAMP responsiveness of the phosphoenolpyruvate carboxykinase promoter in hepatoma cells. *J. Biol. Chem.* 271:8068–74
79. Roesler WJ, Graham JG, Kolen R, Klemm DJ, McFie PJ. 1995. The cAMP response element binding protein synergizes with other transcription factors to mediate cAMP responsiveness. *J. Biol. Chem.* 270:8225–32
80. Roesler WJ, McFie PJ, Puttick DM. 1993. Evidence for the involvement of at least two distinct transcription factors, one of which is liver-enriched, for the activation of the phosphoenolpyruvate carboxykinase gene promoter by cAMP. *J. Biol. Chem.* 268:3791–96
81. Roesler WJ, Park EA. 1998. Hormone response units: One plus one equals more than two. *Mol. Cell. Biochem.* 178:1–8
82. Roesler WJ, Park EA, McFie PJ. 1998. Characterization of CCAAT/enhancer-binding protein $\alpha$ as a cyclic AMP-responsive nuclear regulator. *J. Biol. Chem.* 273:14950–57
83. Roesler WJ, Simard J, Graham JG, McFie PJ. 1994. Characterization of the liver-specific component of the cAMP response unit in the phosphoenolpyruvate carboxykinase (GTP) gene promoter. *J. Biol. Chem.* 269:14276–83
84. Roesler WJ, Vandenbark GR, Hanson RW. 1988. Cyclic AMP and the induction of eukaryotic gene transcription. *J. Biol. Chem.* 263:9063–66
85. Ron D, Habener JH. 1992. CHOP, a novel developmentally regulated nuclear protein that dimerizes with transcription factors C/EBP and LAP and functions as a dominant-negative inhibitor of gene transcription. *Genes Dev.* 6:439–53

86. Ross SE, Erickson RL, Hemati N, Mac-Dougald OA. 1999. Glycogen synthase kinase 3 is an insulin-regulated C/EBPα kinase. *Mol. Cell. Biol.* 19:8433–41

87. Samuelsson L, Strömberg K, Vikman K, Bjursell G, Enerbäck S. 1991. The CCAAT/enhancer binding protein and its role in adipocyte differentiation: evidence for direct involvement in terminal adipocyte development. *EMBO J.* 10: 3787–93

88. Scott DK, Strömstedt P-E, Wang J-C, Granner DK. 1998. Further characterization of the glucocorticoid response unit in the phosphoenolpyruvate carboxykinase gene. The role of the glucocorticoid receptor-binding sites. *Mol. Endocrinol.* 12:482–91

89. Screpanti I, Romani L, Musiani P, Modesti A, Fattori E, et al. 1995. Lymphoproliferative disorder and imbalanced T-helper response in C/EBP beta-deficient mice. *EMBO J.* 14:1932–41

90. Shaywitz AJ, Greenberg ME. 1999. CREB: a stimulus-induced transcription factor activated by a diverse array of extracellular signals. *Annu. Rev. Biochem.* 68:821–61

91. Short JM, Wynshaw-Boris A, Short HP, Hanson RW. 1986. Characterization of the phosphoenolpyruvate carboxykinase (GTP) promoter-regulatory region. II. Identification of cAMP and glucocorticoid regulatory domains. *J. Biol. Chem.* 261:9721–26

92. Sibrowski W, Müller MJ, Seitz HJ. 1982. Rate of synthesis and degradation of rat liver phosphoenolpyruvate carboxykinase in the different thyroid states. *Arch. Biochem. Biophys.* 213:327–33

93. Sterneck E, Tessarollo L, Johnson PF. 1997. An essential role for C/EBPβ in female reproduction. *Genes Dev.* 11:2153–62

94. Streeper RS, Svitek CA, Chapman S, Greenbaum LE, Taub R, O'Brien RM. 1997. A multicomponent insulin response sequence mediates a strong repression of mouse glucose-6-phosphatase gene transcription by insulin. *J. Biol. Chem.* 272:11698–701

95. Sylvester SL, ap Rhys CMJ, Luethy-Martindale JD, Holbrook NJ. 1994. Induction of *GADD153*, a CCAAT/enhancer-binding protein (C/EBP)-related gene, during the acute phase response in rats. *J. Biol. Chem.* 269:20119–25

96. Tae H-J, Zhang S, Kim K-H. 1995. cAMP activation of CAAT enhancer-binding protein-β gene expression and promoter I of acetyl-CoA carboxylase. *J. Biol. Chem.* 270:21487–94

97. Tanaka T, Akira S, Yoshida K, Umemoto M, Yoneda Y, et al. 1995. Targeted disruption of the NF-IL6 gene discloses its essential role in bacteria killing and tumor cytotoxicity by macrophages. *Cell* 80:353–61

98. Tanaka T, Yoshida N, Kishimoto T, Akira S. 1997. Defective adipocyte differentiation in mice lacking the C/EBPβ and/or C/EBPδ gene. *EMBO J.* 16:7432–43

99. Timechenko N, Wilson DR, Taylor LR, Abdelsayed S, Wilde M, et al. 1995. Autoregulation of the human C/EBPα gene by stimulation of upstream stimulatory factor binding. *Mol. Cell. Biol.* 15:1192–202

100. Towle HC. 1995. Metabolic regulation of gene transcription in mammals. *J. Biol. Chem.* 270:23235–38

101. Trautwein C, Caelles C, van der Geer P, Hunter T, Karin M, Chojkier M. 1993. Transactivation by NF-IL6/LAP is enhanced by phosphorylation of its activation domain. *Nature* 364:544–47

102. Trautwein C, Rakemann T, Pietrangelo A, Plümpe J, Montosi G, Manns MP. 1996. C/EBP-β/LAP controls down-regulation of albumin gene transcription during liver regeneration. *J. Biol. Chem.* 271:22262–70

103. Trautwein C, van der Geer P, Karin M, Hunter T, Chojkier M. 1994. Protein kinase A and C site-specific phosphorylation of LAP (NF-IL6) modulate its binding affinity to DNA recognition elements. *J. Clin. Invest.* 93:2554–61

104. Trautwein C, Walker DL, Plümpe J, Manns

MP. 1995. Transactivation of LAP/NF-IL6 is mediated by an acidic domain in the N-terminal part of the protein. *J. Biol. Chem.* 270:15130–36

105. Wang ND, Finegold MJ, Bradley A, Ou CN, Abdelsayed SV, et al. 1995. Impaired energy homeostasis in C/EBP alpha knockout mice. *Science* 269:1108–12

106. Wang Y, Lee-Kwon W, Martindale JL, Adams L, Heller P, et al. 1999. Modulation of CCAAT/enhancer-binding protein-$\alpha$ gene expression by metabolic signals in rodent adipocytes. *Endocrinology* 140:2938–47

107. Wegner M, Cao Z, Rosenfeld MG. 1992. Calcium-regulated phosphorylation within the leucine zipper of C/EBP$\beta$. *Science* 256:370–73

108. Williams SC, Baer M, Dillner AJ, Johnson PF. 1995. CRP2 (C/EBP$\beta$) contains a bipartite regulatory domain that controls transcriptional activation, DNA binding and cell specificity. *EMBO J.* 14:3170–83

109. Williams SC, Cantwell CA, Johnson PF. 1991. A family of C/EBP-related proteins capable of forming covalently linked leucine zipper dimers in vitro. *Genes Dev.* 5:1553–67

110. Yamada K, Duong DT, Scott DK, Wang J-C, Granner DK. 1999. CCAAT/enhancer-binding protein $\beta$ is an accessory factor for the glucocorticoid response from the cAMP response element in the rat phosphoenolpyruvate carboxykinase gene promoter. *J. Biol. Chem.* 274:5880–87

111. Yeagley D, Moll J, Vinson CA, Quinn PG. 2000. Characterization of elements mediating regulation of phosphoenolpyruvate carboxykinase gene transcription by protein kinase A and insulin. *J. Biol. Chem.* 275:17814–20

112. Yin M, Yang SQ, Lin HZ, Lane MD, Chatterjee S, Diehl AM. 1996. Tumor necrosis factor $\alpha$ promotes nuclear localization of cytokine-inducible CCAAT/enhancer binding protein isoforms in hepatocytes. *J. Biol. Chem.* 271:17974–78

Annu. Rev. Nutr. 2001. 21:167–92

# VITAMIN A, INFECTION, AND IMMUNE FUNCTION*

## Charles B Stephensen

*USDA Western Human Nutrition Research Center at UC Davis, and Nutrition Department, University of California, Davis, California 95616; e-mail: cstephensen@ucdavis.edu*

**Key Words** retinoic acid, immunity, T-cells, acute phase response

■ **Abstract** In populations where vitamin A availability from food is low, infectious diseases can precipitate vitamin A deficiency by decreasing intake, decreasing absorption, and increasing excretion. Infectious diseases that induce the acute-phase response also impair the assessment of vitamin A status by transiently depressing serum retinol concentrations. Vitamin A deficiency impairs innate immunity by impeding normal regeneration of mucosal barriers damaged by infection, and by diminishing the function of neutrophils, macrophages, and natural killer cells. Vitamin A is also required for adaptive immunity and plays a role in the development of both T-helper (Th) cells and B-cells. In particular, vitamin A deficiency diminishes antibody-mediated responses directed by Th2 cells, although some aspects of Th1-mediated immunity are also diminished. These changes in mucosal epithelial regeneration and immune function presumably account for the increased mortality seen in vitamin A–deficient infants, young children, and pregnant women in many areas of the world today.

CONTENTS

---

# INTRODUCTION

Physicians and nutritionists have long known that malnutrition increases the severity of infection and that serious or repeated infections increase the risk of malnutrition (91). This is certainly true of vitamin A. In 1928, not long after its identification (62, 74), vitamin A was termed "the anti-infective vitamin" (43). This description was not entirely accurate, however, as more recent work has shown that vitamin A does more to enhance recovery from infection than it does to prevent infection in the first place. Perhaps in recognition of this fact, the therapeutic use of vitamin A became an area of great research interest during the 1930s (for a review, see 94). The advent of antibiotics in the 1940s dampened interest in this area for many years, but interest was rekindled in the 1980s, when the critical role of vitamin A in preventing mortality from infectious diseases was demonstrated anew in clinical and community studies (51, 111). Mechanistic research on the role of vitamin A at the cellular and molecular level also received a substantial boost in the 1980s, when the nuclear receptors for the vitamin A metabolites all-*trans* and 9-*cis* retinoic acid (RA) were discovered (41a, 59, 76). These receptors regulate gene transcription and include the RA receptors (RAR) $-\alpha$, $-\beta$, and $-\gamma$, and the retinoid X receptors (RXR) $-\alpha$, $-\beta$, and $-\gamma$. Thus, the decade of the 1990s was incredibly productive for both public health nutritionists and molecular biologists working on vitamin A.

This review presents an overview of the infection-malnutrition cycle as it applies to vitamin A. As this review is brief, it cannot cover all the relevant research of the past decade. This should not be a shortcoming, however, because many recent review articles (37, 88, 89, 118, 130, 138), as well as the proceedings of a symposium (53) and a comprehensive book covering the health effects of vitamin A deficiency (113), have been published in the past several years.

# INFECTIOUS DISEASE AND VITAMIN A STATUS

## Infectious Diseases Impair Vitamin A Status

Clinicians have long known that preschool age children presenting with xerophthalmia (the ocular disease caused by vitamin A deficiency) often have a concurrent infection or a history of recent infection. Diarrhea, pneumonia, and, in particular, measles are commonly seen preceding or presenting with xerophthalmia (113). This association of xerophthalmia with a history of infection has also been seen in retrospective, case-control studies among pregnant women (24) as well as in prospective, observational studies of children (112). A follow-up of Bangladeshi children who received vitamin A supplements demonstrated that a high incidence of respiratory infection was associated with a failure of the supplements to improve vitamin A status [as assessed by the relative dose-response (RDR) test] just one month after supplementation (80). Similar observations have been made for chickenpox (16). Finally, direct measurement of tissue vitamin A levels in animal studies have shown that acute viral infections can deplete liver vitamin A stores (133). It is thus evident that severe or recurrent infections can lead to the development of vitamin A deficiency, at least in subjects who have a low-to-marginal intake of vitamin A in the first place.

How might infections cause vitamin A deficiency? In general, a micronutrient deficiency may be produced by infectious diseases in five ways: first, by decreasing food intake (anorexia); second, by impairing nutrient absorption; third, by causing direct nutrient losses; fourth, by increasing metabolic requirements or catabolic losses; and fifth, by impairing utilization (e.g. by impairing transport to target tissues) (47, 61, 110). The first three mechanisms certainly affect vitamin A status, although the latter two are not known to be important. These five pathways to deficiency are illustrated in Figure 1 (see color insert).

## Mechanisms

***Decreased Intake***    Acute infections cause anorexia, thus decreasing nutrient intake. In a community study in Guatemala, children with acute respiratory infections or diarrhea consumed 8% and 18% fewer calories per day, respectively, than did asymptomatic children (60). More severe infections have a greater impact on intake. Thus, Kenyan children with severe measles consumed 75% fewer calories when ill than they did after recovery (33). It is important to note that intake of breast milk (a good source of vitamin A) is not diminished by infection. Although total energy intake from non–breast milk sources in a cohort of Peruvian infants decreased by 20%–30% when they had diarrhea or fever, no measurable decrease was seen in breast milk intake (14).

***Malabsorption***    Enteric infections, such as diarrhea and gut helminth infections, directly affect the integrity, morphology, and function of the absorptive mucosa of the intestine and thus may cause malabsorption of vitamin A (61, 110). Impaired digestion and direct competition by parasites may also decrease the availability of some nutrients. It is thus not surprising that infection with the gut helminth *Ascaris lumbricoides* increased the risk of having xerophthalmia in a Nepali case-control study (30). A prospective community study in Indonesia found that diarrhea increases the risk of xerophthalmia (112) whereas a retrospective study in Peru showed that children with longer episodes of diarrhea have lower serum retinol concentrations, which suggests that liver stores may be depleted by infection (3) (although the depressive effect of infection on serum retinol concentration complicates this interpretation, as discussed below). In addition, a recent study found decreased vitamin A absorption in rats with lactose-induced diarrhea, a model of chronic diarrhea in children. The apparent absorption [(intake-fecal loss)/intake] in controls was 90%, compared with 40%–80% in the diarrhea group over the 3-week study period (57). This is a substantial decrease and is similar in magnitude to that seen in isotopic studies, which found that uninfected Indian children absorb 99% of a tracer dose of vitamin A whereas children with diarrhea and *Ascaris* infection absorb 70% and 80%, respectively (106, 107). However, at least one recent study from Bangladesh has shown that intensity of *Ascaris* infection is not associated with impaired vitamin A absorption (using fecal loss as an indicator of absorption) (2), although uninfected controls were not examined. This negative result may also be due to the lower intensity of infection in these study subjects compared with subjects in the earlier study (107). If ascariasis can lead to vitamin A malabsorption, then one would suppose that treating ascariasis should improve vitamin A status. However, a recent study found that treatment of ascariasis did not improve vitamin A status unless supplemental vitamin A was also administered (123). This negative result may not be surprising, as the short time period between deworming and assessment of status (4 weeks) may not have allowed significant increases in vitamin A stores from the unsupplemented diet.

***Direct Loss***    Even after nutrients are absorbed they may still be lost in sweat, vomit, stool, or urine. Vitamin A losses from the first two routes are probably negligible. Loss into the stool can occur during enteric infections that damage the gut mucosa. Such losses may be most pronounced in postmeasles *Shigella* dysentery because of the development of protein-losing enteropathy (90), or during hookworm infection, which causes significant blood loss. However, the amount of vitamin A lost via such routes is probably small. For example, an adult hookworm can cause a loss of up to 0.30 ml of blood/day (49). Even in a heavy hookworm infection (10 adults), this would result in a loss of $<0.003$ $\mu$mol of retinol/day (with serum retinol of 1.0 $\mu$mol/liter), or $<1\%$ of the US recommended dietary allowance for a young child. Urinary retinol losses during severe infection, on the other hand, can be substantial. Adults in intensive care with pneumonia and sepsis lose up to 10 $\mu$mol/day, or nearly three times the recommended dietary allowance, whereas healthy adults lose $<1\%$ of the recommended dietary allowance per day (116). The magnitude of urinary retinol loss is strongly associated with fever and severity of disease. Although children with mild, afebrile infections typically lose little vitamin A in the urine, Bangladeshi children with watery diarrhea, dysentery, pneumonia, or sepsis had maximum observed retinol losses of 0.18, 0.63, 0.38, and 0.60 $\mu$mol/day, respectively, giving maximum estimated losses for each episode (of 10 days estimated duration) of 1.8, 6.3, 3.8, and 6.0 $\mu$mol. In a 2-year-old boy with nearly depleted liver stores (8.6 $\mu$mol), the loss of 6.3 $\mu$mol would represent 73% of reserves (65), indicating that an episode of severe infection could precipitate an episode of xerophthalmia in a child with minimal vitamin A reserves. A principal cause of this urinary retinol loss is impaired tubular reabsorption of low-molecular-weight proteins, including retinol binding protein (RBP) (64), the principal serum transport protein for retinol. Such proteins normally pass from the glomerular capillaries into the collecting tubules and are reabsorbed by the proximal tubular epithelium, as shown in Figure 2 (see color insert). This process is disrupted during febrile episodes when RBP and other low-molecular-weight proteins are lost in the urine. Because most RBP in the blood is normally retained in the serum by its noncovalent association with transthyretin (TTR), a disruption in this association, or decreased TTR production during the acute-phase response (APR), may also contribute to this loss in the most severe cases. Fortunately, children receiving high-dose vitamin A supplements during infection do not have substantially higher urinary retinol losses than do children not receiving vitamin A (C Stephensen, H Hernandez, & LM Franchi, unpublished observations).

***Increased Requirement***    Some nutrient requirements may be increased during infection but this has not been well documented for vitamin A. It is possible, however, that metabolically active tissues that require vitamin A (e.g. lymphoid tissue) may have increased turnover rates during infection, or that retinol may be lost to oxidative cleavage at sites of inflammation. One recent publication suggests that this might occur in children undergoing an APR. Following accidental kerosene ingestion, serum retinol decreased more rapidly after the insult than did serum RBP. The authors suggest that increased tissue uptake rather than decreased liver secretion accounts for this disparity, although this suggestion remains speculative (142).

***Impaired Utilization***    It has been suggested that the APR may impair utilization of vitamin A by decreasing mobilization and transport of retinol from its primary storage site, the liver, to vitamin A–requiring peripheral tissues. The APR is induced when infection or tissue trauma causes the activation of macrophages and neutrophils. The release of tumor necrosis factor (TNF)-$\alpha$, interleukin (IL)-1, and IL-6 by these and other cells at the site of inflammation initiates the systemic APR (8). These cytokines trigger the induction of fever and production of cortisol (to down-regulate inflammation) by the central nervous system and, in the liver, increase the transcription and translation of positive acute-phase proteins [e.g. C-reactive protein (CRP) and $\alpha$-1-acid glycoprotein] while decreasing the production of negative acute-phase proteins, which include transferrin, albumin, TTR (115), and RBP (83). Because RBP is the principal transport protein for delivering vitamin A from liver stores to peripheral tissues (77), this decrease could cause deficiency in peripheral tissue. However, retinol is not a metabolic substrate, like glucose, or precursor for synthesis of macromolecules, as are essential amino acids, and it is not clear that transient decreases have any immediate, detrimental impact on vitamin A–sensitive tissues.

On the other hand, some data do suggest that low serum retinol, even with adequate liver stores of vitamin A, can produce vitamin A deficiency in at least one peripheral tissue, the retina. Very low serum retinol and RBP concentrations are seen in human subjects with specific point mutations in the human RBP gene. These subjects also have night blindness and retinal dystrophy but few other signs of vitamin A deficiency (11). RBP-knockout mice, which have high liver vitamin A stores but low serum retinol concentrations, appear to be largely "normal" but also have impaired retinal function (77). Recent work has also shown that women in Nepal are at significant risk for developing transient night blindness during pregnancy (23). Nepali women with night blindness are more likely to have low serum retinol in association with an active APR than are women without night blindness. Similar observations have been made for children with xerophthalmia (97) and transient retinal whitening during severe episodes of malaria (56). These studies suggest that transient depression in serum retinol causes night blindness. However, as these studies were cross-sectional in design, our ability to make causal inferences is limited. Thus, the impact of the APR on tissue retinol availability remains uncertain.

## THE ACUTE PHASE RESPONSE AND ASSESSMENT OF VITAMIN A STATUS

### Serum Retinol Decreases During the Acute-Phase Response

The decrease in serum retinol which occurs during the APR is seen following trauma as well as infection (for a review, see 37). The greater the severity of infection (as measured by body temperature or serum concentration of a positive acute-phase protein), the greater the decrease in serum retinol. This decrease is transitory and serum retinol typically returns to preinfection levels within a few days (66). Several mechanisms probably contribute to this transient decrease. Increased vascular permeability at sites of inflammation may allow leakage of RBP into extravascular space and thus decrease serum levels. In addition, some retinol will be lost into the urine during infection. In hospitalized children with dysentery, those who lost 0.1 $\mu$mol of retinol per day in the urine (8% of subjects; 15% of the Food and Agriculture Organization/World Health Organization basal requirement) had significantly lower serum retinol concentrations than did subjects who excreted less retinol (66), which suggests that urinary loss contributed to lower serum retinol levels. But this effect may only be significant in severe infections. The lack of significant urinary retinol excretion during mild infections may explain why bacterial lipopolysaccharide (LPS) injection in rats was sufficient to depress serum retinol and liver RBP levels but did not cause a significant urinary retinol excretion (84) (although rats and humans may also have different renal responses to infection). It is likely that the principal reason for decreased serum retinol during relatively mild infections is that synthesis of RBP mRNA by the liver is decreased during the APR, resulting in decreased release of retinol-RBP by the liver (83).

### Impact of Acute Phase Response on Assessing Vitamin A Status

***Serum Retinol Cannot Be Used Uncritically as an Indicator of Vitamin A Status in Subjects with an Active APR***    Serum retinol concentrations are useful in identifying individuals (or, more typically, the percentage of individuals in a population) who have normal liver reserves of vitamin A (serum retinol >1.05 $\mu$mol/liter), marginal reserves ($\leq$1.05 $\mu$mol/liter), depleted reserves ($\leq$0.70 $\mu$mol/liter), or depleted reserves with frank deficiency ($\leq$0.35 $\mu$mol/liter) (128). Transient changes in serum retinol that occur during the APR do not reflect changes in liver reserves. Thus serum retinol concentrations cannot be used to assess vitamin A status during an active APR in the same manner they are used in other subjects. This is obviously true in clinical populations, but community studies of children in Ghana (38) and adults and children in the United States (121) have also found that a significant percentage of asymptomatic subjects with active APRs also have low serum retinol concentrations.

Subjects from the US Third National Health and Nutrition Examination Survey (NHANES III) with active APRs (CRP $\geq$ 10 mg/liter) were significantly more likely to be classified as having marginal liver reserves of vitamin A (odds ratios ranged from 3.1 to 8.6, depending on age and sex) than were subjects without active APRs. [This cross-sectional analysis assumes that serum retinol concentrations were transiently decreased during an active APR, as has been demonstrated in many other studies (66).] Elevated CRP levels were found in from 1% to 14% of the NHANES III population, depending on age and sex, and were associated with infection as well as various chronic diseases, including arthritis, gout, bronchitis, and diabetes. Other tests of vitamin A status that depend on measurements of serum retinol are probably also affected by the APR. For example, a preliminary report indicates that the RDR test does not correctly identify subjects who have recently received high doses of vitamin A as having adequate vitamin A stores when the CRP concentration at the time of the test was $\geq$10 mg/liter (119).

***Can Acute-Phase Proteins Be Used to "Correct" Serum Retinol Levels During the APR?***    Because an active APR may cause misclassification when serum retinol is used to assess vitamin A status, it is reasonable to ask whether serum levels of positive APR proteins might be used to correct this misclassification. Clearly, appropriate cutoff values should be identified for the various positive APR proteins (CRP, $\alpha$-1-acid glycoprotein, $\alpha$-1-antitrypsin, and others) that can be systematically applied in nutrition surveys. But can serum levels of a positive acute-phase protein be used as a correction factor to predict what the "real" concentration of serum retinol would be in the absence of an active APR? Rosales et al have recently suggested that using acute-phase proteins will not adequately correct for transient changes in serum retinol during malaria (86). Furthermore, regression equations to predict serum retinol for NHANES III subjects included age, sex, CRP, and several interaction terms, which suggests that correction for an APR in this manner would be problematic (121).

***Use of the RBP:TTR Ratio to Assess Vitamin A Status***    A better approach to this problem would be to develop an indicator of vitamin A status that is not affected by the APR. Rosales & Ross (85) have recently suggested that the ratio of RBP to TTR may serve this purpose. The basis of the proposed test is as follows:

RBP and TTR form a noncovalent macromolecular complex in serum and have a relatively constant molar ratio, even during the APR. However, serum TTR levels are not affected by vitamin A deficiency whereas serum RBP decreases. This decrease in RBP results in a lower RBP:TTR ratio. This ratio seems not to be affected by the APR and correctly identifies groups of rats on marginal vitamin A diets (as compared with supplemented diets) in both the presence and absence of LPS-induced inflammation (85). Similarly, in a post hoc analysis of samples from children with measles who received vitamin A supplements or placebo, only children in the vitamin A group had a significant increase in the RBP:TTR ratio. A more recent study evaluated the RBP:TTR ratio in children recovering from accidental kerosene ingestion (39). None of these subjects received vitamin A supplements, but their vitamin A status was assessed using the modified RDR (MRDR) test after recovery. The RBP:TTR ratio did not strongly predict categorization of the subjects as adequate or deficient based on the MRDR test. However, some of the subjects had an active APR at the time of the MRDR. Thus, if the MRDR is compromised by an active APR, as occurs with the RDR, the analysis done in this study may underestimate the utility of the RBP:TTR ratio in assessing vitamin A status. Further work on this method is clearly warranted.

## VITAMIN A AND IMMUNE FUNCTION

### Innate Immunity

*Overview*    The innate immune system is, in evolutionary terms, our oldest defense against infection. It consists of epithelial barriers, circulating phagocytes (primarily neutrophils and macrophages), and other cytotoxic cells [e.g. natural killer (NK) cells], as well as constitutive and inflammation-induced serum proteins (e.g. complement proteins and positive acute-phase proteins, respectively). This system is regulated by proinflammatory cytokines produced primarily by macrophages and neutrophils, such as IL-1, TNF-$\alpha$, IL-6, and IL-12, as well as antiinflammatory cytokines, such as IL-10, which down-regulate inflammation once pathogens have been eliminated.

*Barrier Functions*    The skin is an important barrier to infection. Vitamin A deficiency causes a thickening of the outer, keratinized layer of the skin (hyperkeratosis) (25) but does not obviously compromise its barrier function. However, vitamin A deficiency does significantly compromise the mucosal epithelial barriers found in the conjunctiva of the eye as well as in the respiratory, gastrointestinal, and urogenital tracts. One key change caused by vitamin A deficiency is the loss of mucus-producing goblet cells. This loss of the protective mucus blanket diminishes resistance to infection by pathogens that would ordinarily be trapped in the mucus and swept away by the cleansing flow of mucus out of the body (see Figure 3, color insert). In addition, vitamin A deficiency can result in squamous metaplasia (113).

However, vitamin A deficiency that is not complicated by infection causes only minimal epithelial changes. In the respiratory tract, squamous metaplasia is seen only at sites where tissue damage (e.g. caused by viral infection and inflammation) has destroyed the normal epithelium, which is then replaced by metaplastic foci. In the intestine, destruction of epithelial cells in vitamin A–deficient mice results in more severe pathologic changes than is seen in control animals, but squamous metaplasia does not occur (89, 131). It is difficult to directly demonstrate that vitamin A deficiency impairs regeneration of enteric mucosa in humans. However, in a recent preliminary report, Thurnham et al (125) used an indirect test of gut mucosal integrity (lactulose:mannitol differential sugar absorption test) to demonstrate that Gambian children recovering from diarrhea who received vitamin A supplements regained normal mucosal integrity more rapidly than did children receiving a placebo.

The inability of vitamin A–deficient mucosal epithelia to regenerate adequately following damage may allow easier penetration of the gut mucosal barrier by pathogenic bacteria. In support of this argument, increased bacterial translocation from the intestine into regional lymphoid and other tissue has been observed in vitamin A–deficient rats (137). Supplemental vitamin A treatment of rats on normal diets also inhibits bacterial translocation from the gut during lectin-induced diarrhea, a model for chronic diarrhea in humans (102). In the respiratory tract, pathogenic bacteria that would ordinarily be cleared by mucus are able to adhere to damaged epithelium or sites of squamous metaplasia (21) and thus may increase the chance of invasive disease, such as septicemia. Given the importance of the mucosal barriers to infection, it is likely that squamous metaplasia and impaired recovery of normal mucosal integrity—as depicted in Figure 3 (see color insert)— directly contribute to the increased severity of disease and greater risk of mortality that are caused by vitamin A deficiency.

*Neutrophils*    Neutrophils and other granulocytes develop from myeloid stem cells in the bone marrow. RAR-mediated modulation of gene expression controls the development of neutrophils (for a review, see 55). This is illustrated by the fact that a translocation that fuses the RAR-$\alpha$ gene with a gene known as PML (for promyelocytic leukemia) is found in patients with the disease acute promyelocytic leukemia. This fusion disrupts normal neutrophil maturation, triggering the proliferation of promyelocytes. RA therapy for acute promyelocytic leukemia patients can cause reversion of the disease by restoring maturation of promyelocytes to neutrophils.

Vitamin A deficiency also disrupts normal neutrophil development and can result in decreased phagocytosis and killing of bacteria (127). These defects may lead to the decreased clearance of bacteria from the bloodstream that has been seen in vitamin A–deficient rats (73). Recruitment of neutrophils from blood into the site of inflammation may also be affected by vitamin A, as is indicated by the observation that retinoid treatment diminishes neutrophil migration into the skin from capillaries. In addition, treatment with RA and synthetic retinoids can decrease oxidative metabolism that is associated with killing ingested bacteria and promoting inflammation (75).

Although neutrophil function is impaired by vitamin A deficiency, increased numbers of granulocytes have been seen in the peripheral blood of vitamin A–deficient rats (69, 143), and a recent study found that vitamin A deficiency in SENCAR (a strain selectively bred for increased sensitivity to chemical-induced skin carcinogenesis) mice causes an expansion of granulocytes in the bone marrow and peripheral blood, apparently by decreasing neutrophil apoptosis (54). Treatment of these mice with RA returned neutrophil levels to normal, as was also seen in deficient rats (143). Not all mice strains develop neutrophilia during vitamin A deficiency (63), indicating that a genetic predisposition may exist.

Thus, vitamin A deficiency has two disparate effects on neutrophils: It increases numbers but impairs function. On balance, these studies suggest that the protective function of neutrophils is impaired by vitamin A deficiency and will diminish protection against bacterial infections.

*Macrophages*     Macrophages are activated during inflammation and, like neutrophils, are professional phagocytes. Vitamin A deficiency may lead to a significant increase in the total number of macrophages in the secondary lymphoid organs of mice (109), whereas RA treatment can cause a decrease in the number of monocytes found in the bone marrow and spleen (63). In addition to affecting cell numbers, vitamin A deficiency also leads to increased transcription of IL-12 (18), whereas RA inhibits IL-12 production by primary macrophages in vitro (67). IL-12 produced by macrophages, acting as antigen-presenting cells, promotes development of T-helper (Th) 1 cells, which produce interferon (IFN)-$\gamma$ (as discussed below). Increased IFN-$\gamma$ production by Th1 cells can, in turn, lead to increased macrophage activation. Such activation may lead to the higher spontaneous release of nitric oxide (a reactive oxygen metabolite involved in killing ingested bacteria) by peritoneal macrophages that has been observed in vitamin A–deficient mice (136), although this difference disappears after stimulation with LPS. In addition, corneal abrasions in vitamin A–deficient rats result in greater inflammatory damage and production of IL-1 (100). These studies suggest that vitamin A deficiency causes increased inflammation mediated by cytokines from macrophages.

Although data from humans are scarce, a recent clinical study found that patients with common variable immunodeficiency had low serum retinol levels that were increased by supplementation, which suggests a preexisting vitamin A deficiency. The vitamin A supplementation also diminished serum levels and in vitro production of the proinflammatory cytokine TNF-$\alpha$ while increasing serum levels and production of the antiinflammatory cytokine IL-10 (4). Although these data indicate that some macrophage-mediated inflammation is increased by vitamin A deficiency, the phagocytic capacity of macrophages can be impaired by deficiency. For example, vitamin A deficiency decreases the phagocytic activity and bacteria-killing ability of peritoneal macrophages for *Staphylococcus aureus* (141). Peritoneal macrophages from vitamin A–deficient chickens do not have decreased phagocytic ability for yeast but do have reduced oxidative metabolic capacity (104), which is important in bacterial killing. Vitamin A supplementation can also enhance the phagocytic activity of macrophages (for a review, see 88).

These data indicate that vitamin A deficiency enhances macrophage-mediated inflammation by increasing production of IL-12 and IFN-$\gamma$ but impairs the ability of macrophages to ingest and kill bacteria. This latter deficit may lead to increased pathogen replication at sites of infection, thus causing increased pathology, inflammation, and secondary immune responses, as has been observed for bacterial (141) and viral (68) infections in vitamin A deficiency. Thus, macrophage-associated defects in the initial control of infection may lead to more severe infection whereas the enhanced production of proinflammatory cytokines (due both to vitamin A deficiency and increased pathogen load) may also exacerbate inflammation, at least during infections that trigger Th1-mediated responses.

*NK Cells* NK cells are lymphoid cells originally characterized by their anti–tumor cell lytic activity. It is now appreciated that these cells play an important role in innate immunity by killing virus-infected cells as well as tumor cells. Several studies have demonstrated that vitamin A deficiency decreases both NK cell number and lytic activity (for a review, see 89). More recently, these observations have been extended to include aging rats chronically fed diets that produced marginal vitamin A status (31). The protective benefits of NK cells in the early stages of viral infection, or in antitumor responses, clearly is diminished by vitamin A deficiency.

## Pathogen-Specific Immunity

*Overview* Pathogen-specific immunity depends on the recognition of antigen either by antibody produced by plasma cells (which develop from B-cells) or by T-cell receptors on CD4+ Th cells or CD8+ effector T-cells. Antigen-presenting cells (APCs) take up antigen at a site of infection, process it, and display the processed antigen on their surfaces using major histocompatibility class II molecules. When APCs arrive at a regional lymph node, they expose naive T-cells to antigen and initiate proliferation and maturation, as outlined in Figure 4 (see color insert). Memory T-cells develop and persist after primary stimulation to allow a more rapid response on subsequent exposure to the same antigen. Memory Th cells provide help to antibody responses as well as cell-mediated immune responses, such as the development of virus-specific CD8+ cytotoxic T-lymphocytes (CTLs). Some antibody responses to antigens, such as bacterial LPS, do not require help from T-cells. Memory Th cells develop along one of two pathways: Th1 or Th2 (see Figure 4) (92). Put briefly, vitamin A deficiency impairs Th2-mediated antibody responses but does not impair, and may even enhance, Th1-mediated responses.

Th1 cells respond to intracellular pathogens, such as viruses, by producing IFN-$\gamma$ and IL-2. They stimulate CTL responses, macrophage activation, and the delayed-type hypersensitivity (DTH) response and provide limited help to stimulate B-cell development and antibody production [e.g. IFN-$\gamma$ stimulates immunoglobulin (Ig)G2a in mice]. These activities of Th1 cells can be down-regulated by Th2 cytokines. Th2 cells respond to extracellular pathogens and produce IL-4, IL-5, and IL-10, which stimulate B cell help (e.g. for IgG1, IgE, and IgA production), eosinophil and mast cell development, and macrophage deactivation. These activities can be down-regulated by IFN-$\gamma$. The Th1/Th2 patterns are not completely dichotomous. For example, the response to influenza A virus infection elicits a strong IgG2a response, which is driven by IFN-$\gamma$, and a strong secretory IgA response, which is driven by Th2 cytokines.

***Vitamin A Deficiency Diminishes Th2-Mediated Antibody Responses***    Vitamin A deficiency impairs antibody responses to antigens that require Th2-mediated help (for a review, see 88). The serum IgG1 antibody response to purified protein antigens (87, 109) and the serum IgG1 and IgE responses to the intestinal helminth *Trichinella spiralis* are impaired by vitamin A deficiency (20), as is the salivary IgA response to influenza A virus infection (41, 122) and the intestinal IgA response to cholera toxin (139). These changes are caused by a decrease in the number of antigen-specific plasma cells; the amount of antibody produced per cell is not affected (41, 108). Although few human studies have been done, Semba et al (96) have shown that vitamin A supplementation increases the serum antibody response to tetanus toxoid in vitamin A–deficient children, and Rahman et al have made similar observations for the diphtheria vaccine (81).

In contrast, the IgG2a response to influenza A infection is increased in vitamin A–deficient mice (122), and most animal studies find that serum antibody responses to viral infection are not impaired (89). With regard to human studies, vitamin A supplements have been shown to increase the serum IgG response to measles infection (27) and to measles immunization (9), although decreases have also been seen (98; for a review, see 132). The serum antibody response to polio vaccine is not affected by vitamin A supplements given at routine immunization visits (95). The studies using measles and polio vaccine in humans were designed primarily to determine whether administration of high-dose supplements at vaccine visits interfered with the development of protective serum antibody titers (135) and were not designed to examine the role of vitamin A in immune function. In addition, the lack of effect of vitamin A supplements in such studies may also reflect better underlying vitamin A status than in studies that examined the effect of vitamin A deficiency on immune function (96).

In addition to affecting antibody responses, vitamin A deficiency also changes the pattern of Th1/Th2 cytokine production in animal studies. When lymphocytes isolated from the draining lymph nodes of *T. spiralis*–infected mice were restimulated with antigen in vitro, cultures from vitamin A–deficient mice produced more IFN-$\gamma$ and less IL-4, IL-5, and IL-10 than did cultures from control mice (17, 20). Depletion experiments found that CD4+ Th cells were the principal source of the IFN-$\gamma$ (19, 140). Higher IFN-$\gamma$ and IL-2 production have also been seen following mitogen stimulation of lymphocytes from vitamin A–deficient rats (140).

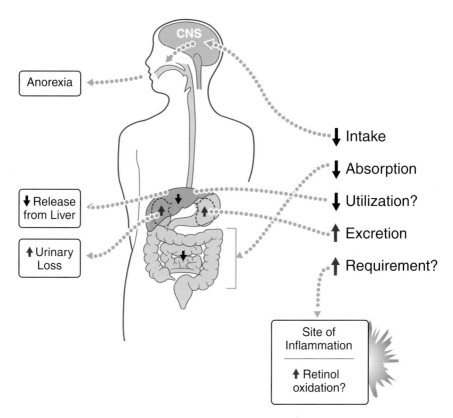

**Figure 1** Infectious diseases impair vitamin A status. This figure illustrates three mechanisms by which infections are known to impair vitamin A status: decreased intake due to anorexia; decreased absorption; and increased urinary excretion. Infection may also affect vitamin A status by impairing utilization of retinol stores in the liver (by diminishing transport from stores to peripheral tissues) or by increasing requirements (e.g. by increasing oxidative degradation of retinol at sites of inflammation), although proof for these two mechanisms is lacking.

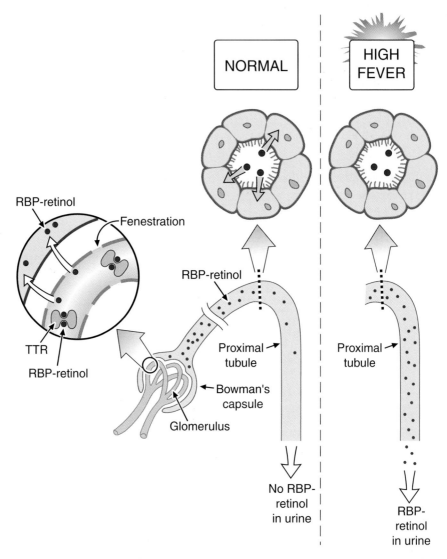

**Figure 2** Mechanism of urinary retinol excretion during infection. Retinol, bound to retinol-binding protein (RBP), is normally retained in the glomerular capillaries by its association with transthyretin (TTR). If not bound to TTR, RBP is small enough to pass through the fenestrations of the glomerular capillaries into the urinary collecting tubules, which begin with Bowman's capsule. Under normal circumstances, RBP passes down the tubules but is reabsorbed by the proximal tubular epithelial cells. During infections, particularly those with high fever, this reabsorption is diminished and RBP, carrying retinol, is lost into the urine.

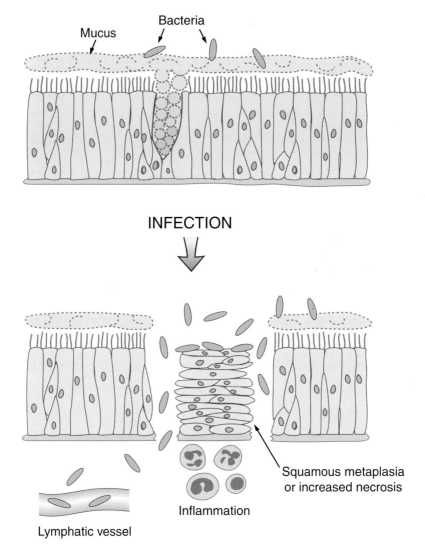

**Figure 3** Vitamin A deficiency impairs regeneration of normal mucosal epithelial barriers during infection. Normal mucosal epithelium (*top*) prevents adherence of many potentially pathogenic bacteria by trapping them in mucus and moving them out of the airways or down the gastrointestinal tract. In vitamin A deficiency, mucosal epithelium that is damaged by infection (and the associated inflammation) does not regenerate normally, and foci of squamous metaplasia (in the respiratory tract) or increased necrosis (in the gut) develop at sites of inflammation. Such foci allow greater adherence of potentially pathogenic bacteria and may allow increased bacterial translocation across the mucosal surface, into lymphatic vessels, and to local lymphoid tissues and beyond, resulting in invasive disease.

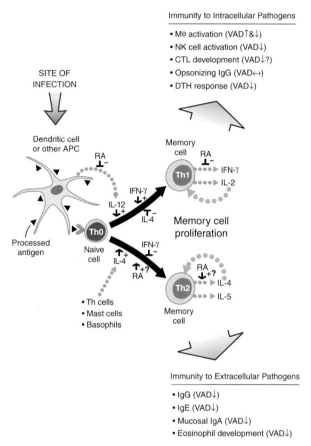

**Figure 4** Effects of retinoic acid (RA) on cytokine production and of vitamin A deficiency (VAD) on mechanisms of immunity. An antigen-presenting cell (APC) arrives in a lymph node carrying processed antigen from an invading pathogen. The antigen-naive T-helper (Th0) cell recognizes the antigen via its T-cell receptor. This recognition, in combination with interleukin (IL)-12 produced by the APC (*green dashed* →), stimulates development of Th1 memory cells or, in the presence of IL-4 (from Th2 cells mast cells or basophils), stimulates development of Th2 memory cells. Th1 cells produce interferon (IFN)-γ to stimulate immunity to intracellular pathogens and IL-2 to promote Th1 cell growth (*blue dashed* →). Th2 cells produce IL-4, which stimulates immunity to extracellular pathogens and Th2 cell growth, as well as other cytokines, such as IL-5. IFN-γ promotes development of Th1 cells (*black* → *with red + sign*) and blocks development of Th2 cells (*black* ⊥ *with red - sign*). IL-4 has the opposite effects. RA blocks IL-12 and IFN-γ production and may enhance development of Th2 cells and IL-4 production (*black* → *with question mark and red + sign*). Immune mechanisms are either enhanced (↑), diminished (↓), or not-changed (↔) by vitamin A deficiency (? indicates equivocal data). Mφ, macrophage; NK, natural killer; CTL, cytotoxic T-lymphocyte; DTH, delayed-type hypersensitivity; Ig, immunoglobulin.

Thus, production of Th2 cytokines is diminished by vitamin A deficiency, whereas production of Th1 cytokines is increased.

***High Dietary Vitamin A May Enhance Th2-Mediated Responses***    Although vitamin A deficiency diminishes the secretory IgA response, we have recently found that high dietary vitamin A significantly enhances the IgA response and IL-10 production, as well as diminishes the serum IgG response and IFN-$\gamma$ production (29). Similarly, RA treatment of mice with experimental allergic encephalomyelitis, a disease mediated by Th1-like T cells following immunization with myelin basic protein (MBP), decreases the severity of disease. In addition, in vitro treatment with all-*trans* RA decreases MBP-specific IFN-$\gamma$ production and increases MBP-specific IL-4 production by lymph node cells (78). Thus, high-dose retinoid treatment can increase the production of Th2 cytokines while decreasing the production of Th1 cytokines.

***How Does Vitamin A Affect the Th1/Th2 Balance?***    The mechanisms underlying the ability of vitamin A deficiency to impair Th2 responses are not fully defined, but work currently in the literature suggests that RA decreases the production of the Th1-enhancing cytokines IL-12 and IFN-$\gamma$ and, thus, indirectly enhances Th2 development because these cytokines down-regulate Th2 responses (as shown in Figure 4). As discussed above, in vitro treatment with RA decreases production of IL-12 p40 by stimulated macrophages (67) and IFN-$\gamma$ production by stimulated Th1-like cells and NK cells (18, 40). In addition, vitamin A–deficient mice have higher levels of IL-12 p40 and IFN-$\gamma$ transcripts in unstimulated lymph node cells than do control mice (18). Higher IFN-$\gamma$ production by CD8+ cells has also been documented by ELISA (18). These data suggest that a lymph node environment conducive to Th1 development is created by vitamin A deficiency. However, because the predominant effect of vitamin A deficiency is to decrease Th2-mediated responses, often without increasing Th1 responses, a direct effect of vitamin A on Th2 development is plausible. A recent preliminary report (117) indicates that RA can directly enhance Th2 development from antigen-naive Th0 cells in vitro. This effect is independent of IL-12 and IFN-$\gamma$ but requires IL-4. Thus, vitamin A may affect Th1/Th2 development by multiple mechanisms.

***Vitamin A Deficiency Can Impair Th1 Responses***    As indicated in Figure 4, data on vitamin A diminishing Th2 and enhancing (or not impairing) Th1-mediated responses are not completely consistent. For example, in three studies, the DTH response to dermal contact sensitization in mice (1, 109) and subcutaneous ovalbumin administration in rats (140) was diminished in vitamin A–deficient rodents. More recently, the DTH response to ovalbumin immunization was enhanced in vitamin A–deficient rats (136). The reasons for these differences are not clear, but taken together, the studies suggest that vitamin A deficiency impairs DTH responses. One human study also found that high-dose vitamin A supplements enhance the DTH response in infants who had improved vitamin A status (as indicated by serum retinol >0.70 $\mu$mol/liter) after supplementation (79).

With regard to another Th1-mediated response, one study has reported that vitamin A deficiency impairs CTL function during Newcastle disease virus infection in chickens (105). In addition, vitamin A deficiency has been shown in some experiments to decrease IL-2 production (20), whereas high-level dietary vitamin A (26) and RA treatment in vitro can enhance IL-2 or IL-2 receptor expression (6), which could enhance proliferation of Th1 cells if this occurs in vivo as well. It is clear that the impact of vitamin A on pathogen-specific immunity is not completely represented by the alterations in Th1/Th2 balance discussed above. Other factors are at work that also impair some aspects of Th1-mediated responses.

*Direct Effects of Vitamin A on B-Cells*    The observation that the antibody response to LPS is not impaired by vitamin A deficiency suggests that B-cell development might be unaffected by vitamin A status. However, the proliferative response of splenocytes to B-cell mitogens is decreased in cells isolated from vitamin A–deficient rats (129). In addition, retinol is a required growth factor for Epstein-Barr virus–transformed B-lymphoblasts, and the retinol metabolite 14-hydroxy-retroretinol has been identified as the required compound (15; for a review, see 88). In contrast, retinol has also been shown to inhibit the proliferation and differentiation of primary human B-cells (12), raising the question of which competing activity is relevant in vivo. In addition, retinoic-acid treatment of B cells can induce greater IgG secretion in vitro (5), can direct class-switching to IgA (126), and affects B-cell apoptosis (58). Clearly, B-cell activity is modulated by vitamin A, but there is not a clear picture of how these different activities come together to regulate B-cell function in vivo.

# VITAMIN A, MORBIDITY, AND MORTALITY

## Community Mortality Studies

It is now well accepted that vitamin A supplements will decrease early childhood mortality in areas of the world where vitamin A deficiency is a public health problem. Very large, placebo-controlled community intervention trials done in Africa and Asia showed an overall decrease in mortality of 30% in children 6 months to 5 years of age. Benefits for infants <6 months of age are less certain. These studies have been reviewed and analyzed together in at least three meta-analyses (34, 42), including one published recently (130). In addition, recent analysis of morbidity and mortality associated with use of immunization visits in infants from Ghana, India, and Peru to deliver vitamin A supplements saw no effects on morbidity or mortality but did show improved vitamin A status (135). Vitamin A supplements have also recently been found to protect against AIDS-associated mortality in this age group (35). The findings of these studies are not recapitulated here other than to highlight a few key points. Not all studies showed a significant benefit and differences between the different study sites (Indonesia, India, Nepal, Sudan, Ghana, Peru) in underlying nutritional status, morbidity patterns, and use of primary and preventive health care no doubt affected the response to vitamin A treatment. When vitamin A was provided in frequent small doses, mortality decreased more dramatically than when infrequent high doses were administered. These studies often had >10,000 subjects and were done in areas where cause of death could not be rigorously assessed. Thus, although most deaths in these studies were from infectious diseases, it was difficult to determine cause of death with certainty. The available data suggest that the deaths averted were from measles, diarrhea, and infections associated with convulsions (perhaps resulting from high fever) but not from pneumonia (130a). More recently, provision of vitamin A supplements to pregnant women has been shown to decrease childbirth-associated mortality (134), although little specific information is available on cause of death. Fetal and infant survival were not improved by this intervention (52). Clearly, vitamin A diminishes risk of death from infectious diseases, with the benefit being seen with some infections but not others. Unfortunately, the mechanistic studies of vitamin A and immune function do not completely explain why this occurs (discussed below).

## Effect of Vitamin A Supplements on Specific Infections

*Measles*    High-dose vitamin A supplements improve recovery from measles, decreasing mortality, duration of disease, and risk of complications (for a review, see 132). Measles is an acute, immunosuppresive viral infection, and children with severe measles often develop opportunistic bacterial pneumonia and diarrhea due to compromised innate and adaptive immunity. The clinical trials of vitamin A supplements during measles primarily studied children brought to hospitals with severe disease. Many of these children also had secondary bacterial infections. It is thus reasonable to ask whether vitamin A improves recovery by affecting measles itself or by affecting the secondary bacterial infections that result from measles (or both). The answer to this question is not clear. Both neutralizing antibody and CTLs are involved in clearing measles infection. Although there are no data on the impact of vitamin A supplements on the CTL response to measles, vitamin A supplements do not appear to enhance, and may impede, the recovery of DTH responses to recall antigens following measles virus infection (82). However, the serum IgG response to measles infection can be increased by vitamin A supplements (27), although effects on vaccine responses are equivocal, as discussed above. Thus, there is not strong evidence for vitamin A supplements enhancing measles-specific immune function. (It should be remembered that the absence of data is not the same as negative data.) However, vitamin A does enhance recovery of mucosal integrity after viral infection, antibody responses to bacterial antigens, and recovery of neutrophil function. These mechanisms can protect against opportunistic bacterial infections. Restoration of these defenses may contribute significantly to the enhanced recovery caused by vitamin A in measles.

*Diarrhea*    In the case of diarrheal diseases, recovery from infection calls on those defense mechanisms that are compromised by vitamin A deficiency: regeneration of intact mucosal epithelium damaged by invasive pathogens, Th2-mediated secretory IgA antibody responses against bacterial toxins, intact phagocytic responses to protect against invasive disease, and Th2-mediated serum IgG responses against bacterial toxins. However, clinical studies of diarrhea offer a mixed picture: Subjects with acute watery diarrhea do not benefit from supplementation whereas, in at least one study, subjects with invasive disease (*Shigella* dysentery) do benefit (for a review, see 130). This benefit in invasive disease may be due to the ability of vitamin A to enhance regeneration of damaged mucosal epithelium and enhance the phagocytic activity of neutrophils and macrophages. It has also been shown that vitamin A supplements can reduce the incidence and duration of diarrhea episodes (7) and is of particular benefit among children who are not breastfed (10). A recent clinical study showed that low-dose vitamin A supplements given daily to hospitalized malnourished children decreased the incidence of severe, nosocomial diarrhea in those with clinically evident protein-energy malnutrition (PEM), but that a single high-dose supplement given on admission increased the risk of such diarrhea in children without underlying PEM (32). The reason for the disparate response to the different doses is not clear, but the improvement in recovery caused by vitamin A supplements in children with PEM is consistent with a recent study showing that in mice, vitamin A restored the decline in the intestinal IgA response and Th2 cytokine production that is produced by PEM (70). Vitamin A enhances the secretory IgA response in animals without PEM as well. This increase in pathogen-specific antibody in the gut could increase resistance to secondary infection and improve recovery from primary infection, thus decreasing incidence, duration, and severity of diarrhea.

***Respiratory Infections***    In community studies, vitamin A supplements have increased the risk of symptomatic respiratory infection, whereas in clinical studies, supplements have typically, although not always, failed to improve recovery (for a review, see 130). In some clinical intervention trials, including those using patients with community-acquired pneumonia in Peru (120) and respiratory syncytial virus infection in the United States (13), use of vitamin A supplements has resulted in more severe disease. Recently, a clinical trial in tuberculosis patients has shown no benefit of vitamin A supplements on recovery (44), although the immune response may have been modified (45). It is interesting that a recent community-based study in Equador found that low-dose supplements given weekly decreased the risk of acute lower respiratory infection (ALRI) in children with weight-for-age $z$-scores two standard deviations below the reference standard while increasing risk of ALRI above this level (99). A similar association of vitamin A enhancing recovery only in children with underlying PEM has also been seen in a clinical study of pneumonia in Vietnam (103). The reason for this association with underlying PEM is not clear but may be due to these children having more severe disease or a greater risk of underlying vitamin A deficiency.

A major puzzle that has yet to be explained is how vitamin A supplements increase the apparent incidence of ALRI in community studies and adversely affect recovery in some clinical studies. In the community studies, it is likely that the incidence of infection is not affected but that the risk of developing disease severe enough to be counted as ALRI (using such indicators as fever, cough, and rapid breathing) is enhanced. How severity is enhanced is not known. However, it is interesting to note that 25%–30% of patients with acute promyelocytic leukemia who receive RA therapy develop what has become known as the RA syndrome (48). This syndrome is characterized by thrombosis, fever, respiratory distress, radiographic evidence of pulmonary infiltrates, and pleural effusions. Although the etiology of the syndrome is unclear, it is known that RA can increase IL-1 production by alveolar macrophages (46), which could, in turn, recruit neutrophils into the lung, thereby increasing inflammation. RA also enhances transcription of the IL-8 gene in respiratory airway epithelium (22). IL-8 is also a chemotactic factor for neutrophils. Could high-dose vitamin A supplements thus produce a low-grade RA syndrome, particularly in children who already have active pulmonary inflammation, including increased vascular permeability and activated macrophages and neutrophils? We do not know the answer to this question, and it is not clear why similar adverse effects are not seen in measles-related pneumonia. However, the possibility that vitamin A enhances some aspect of pulmonary inflammation seems plausible and could explain the adverse effects of vitamin A supplements on respiratory infection in some settings.

*HIV*    HIV, like measles, is a viral infection, and the animal data reviewed above do not predict strong enhancement of antiviral responses by vitamin A supplements. Many studies have examined the association of low serum retinol concentrations with HIV severity or progression of disease in US populations and in the developing world (for a review, see 71, 93). Most data on the association of vitamin A status with severity of HIV infection suffers from the flaw that serum retinol concentrations were used to identify "deficient" subjects. As discussed above, this approach can be unreliable during an ongoing infection. These studies, however, strongly suggested that vitamin A deficiency enhanced the risk of vertical transmission of HIV, at least among women at risk of deficiency in Africa. Placebo-controlled intervention studies in pregnant women at risk of deficiency have now been done, but vitamin A supplementation did not decrease vertical transmission or improve measures of immune function (28, 36). Apart from vertical transmission, short-term interventions in better-nourished adult populations in the United States have also demonstrated no improvement in disease or immune function parameters (50). However, a recent study from Tanzania has shown that vitamin A supplements in HIV-infected children 6 months to 5 years of age reduced diarrhea- and AIDS-related deaths (35). This result is reminiscent of the reduction in deaths seen in HIV-uninfected children and may be attributable to similar mechanisms. Vitamin A supplements may thus diminish the severity of opportunistic infections in populations at risk of vitamin A deficiency, but direct improvement of HIV-specific immunity has not been demonstrated.

*Malaria*    One well-controlled study has shown that vitamin A supplements decrease the severity of malaria infection in children 6 months to 5 years of age

(101). Supplementation reduced the number of febrile episodes, the parasite density, and the proportion of subjects with spleen enlargement. The immune response to malaria, an intracellular parasite, involves innate immunity (NK cells) and IFN-$\gamma$ production, as well as Th2 cytokines (72). Antibody plays a key role in diminishing the severity of disease. This response develops rapidly in young children during their first year or two of exposure to malaria. In the study by Shankar et al (101), subjects 6 months to 3 years of age benefited more from the vitamin A supplements than did older subjects. It is thus tempting to speculate that vitamin A enhanced the acquisition of immunity in these children and thus diminished disease severity, whereas older children already had acquired a more mature antibody response. This interpretation suggests that vitamin A supplements could boost the development of immunity among infants and young children in malaria-endemic areas and thus decrease the burden of malaria morbidity in this age group.

## CONCLUDING REMARKS

In conclusion, we have seen that common infections can increase the risk of vitamin A deficiency by decreasing intake, decreasing absorption, and increasing excretion. Vitamin A deficiency, in turn, impairs both the innate and adaptive immune response to infection. In particular, mucosal integrity and Th2-mediated responses are compromised. These alterations in host defense increase the risk of death from common infections in young children and pregnant women. Correcting vitamin A deficiency decreases mortality from measles, diarrhea, and other infections, although the severity of respiratory infections may be enhanced under some circumstances. Much work remains to be done, as the mechanisms by which vitamin A affects immune function have not been carefully examined at the molecular level. On a clinical and community level, nutrition research would benefit greatly from the development of a method to measure vitamin A status that is simple to apply and not adversely affected by the APR. Pursuing these research priorities will advance our knowledge of how vitamin A affects the infection-malnutrition cycle and will also bolster efforts to develop sustainable programs to eliminate vitamin A deficiency, which, for the reasons described above, should remain a top priority of the international health community.

**Visit the Annual Reviews home page at www.AnnualReviews.org**

## LITERATURE CITED

1. Ahmed F, Jones DB, Jackson AA. 1991. Effect of vitamin A deficiency on the immune response to epizootic diarrhoea of infant mice (EDIM) rotavirus infection in mice. *Br. J. Nutr.* 65:475–85

2. Ahmed F, Mohiduzzaman M, Jackson A. 1993. Vitamin A absorption in children with ascariasis. *Br. J. Nutr.* 69:817–25
3. Alvarez JO, Salazar-Lindo E, Kohatsu J, Miranda P, Stephensen CB. 1995. Urinary

excretion of retinol in children with acute diarrhea. *Am. J. Clin. Nutr.* 61:1273–76

4. Aukrust P, Müller F, Ueland T, Svardal A, Berge R, et al. 2000. Decreased vitamin A levels in common variable immunodeficiency: vitamin A supplementation in vivo enhances immunoglobulin production and downregulates inflammatory responses. *Eur. J. Clin. Invest.* 30:252–59

5. Ballow M, Wang W, Xiang S. 1996. Modulation of B-cell immunoglobulin synthesis by retinoic acid. *Clin. Immunol. Immunopathol.* 80:S73–81

6. Ballow M, Xiang S, Greenberg SJ, Brodsky L, Allen C, et al. 1997. Retinoic acid-induced modulation of IL-2 mRNA production and IL-2 receptor expression on T cells. *Int. Arch. Allergy Immunol.* 113:167–69

7. Barreto ML, Santos LM, Assis AM, Araaujo MP, Farenzena GG, et al. 1994. Effect of vitamin A supplementation on diarrhoea and acute lower-respiratory-tract infections in young children in Brazil. *Lancet* 344:228–31

8. Baumann H, Gauldie J. 1994. The acute phase response. *Immunol. Today* 15:74–80

9. Benn C, Aaby P, Bale C, Olsen J, Michaelsen K, et al. 1997. Randomised trial of effect of vitamin A supplementation on antibody response to measles vaccine in Guinea-Bissau, West Africa. *Lancet* 350:101–5

10. Bhandari N, Bhan MK, Sazawal S. 1994. Impact of massive dose of vitamin A given to preschool children with acute diarrhoea on subsequent respiratory and diarrhoeal morbidity. *Br. Med. J.* 309:1404–7

11. Biesalski H, Frank J, Beck S, Heinrich F, Illek B, et al. 1999. Biochemical but not clinical vitamin A deficiency results from mutations in the gene for retinol binding protein. *Am. J. Clin. Nutr.* 69:931–36

12. Blomhoff H, Smeland E, Erikstein B, Rasmussen A, Skrede B, et al. 1992. Vitamin A is a key regulator for cell growth, cytokine production, and differentiation in normal B cells. *J. Biol. Chem.* 267:23988–92

13. Bresee JS, Fischer M, Dowell SF, Johnston BD, Biggs VM, et al. 1996. Vitamin A therapy for children with respiratory syncytial virus infection: a multicenter trial in the United States. *Pediatr. Infect. Dis. J.* 15:777–82

14. Brown K, Stallings R, de Kanashiro H, Lopez de Romaña G, Black R. 1990. Effects of common illnesses on infants' energy intakes from breast milk and other foods during longitudinal community-based studies in Huascar (Lima), Peru. *Am. J. Clin. Nutr.* 52:1005–13

15. Buck J, Grün F, Derguini F, Chen Y, Kimura S, et al. 1993. Anhydroretinol: a naturally occurring inhibitor of lymphocyte physiology. *J. Exp. Med.* 178:675–80

16. Campos F, Flores H, Underwood B. 1987. Effect of an infection on vitamin A status of children as measured by the relative dose response (RDR). *Am. J. Clin. Nutr.* 46:91–94

17. Cantorna MT, Nashold FE, Hayes CE. 1994. In vitamin A deficiency multiple mechanisms establish a regulatory T helper cell imbalance with excess Th1 and insufficient Th2 function. *J. Immunol.* 152:1515–22

18. Cantorna MT, Nashold FE, Hayes CE. 1995. Vitamin A deficiency results in a priming environment conducive for Th1 cell development. *Eur. J. Immunol.* 25:1673–79

19. Carman JA, Hayes CE. 1991. Abnormal regulation of IFN-gamma secretion in vitamin A deficiency. *J. Immunol.* 147:1247–52

20. Carman JA, Pond L, Nashold F, Wassom DL, Hayes CE. 1992. Immunity to *Trichinella spiralis* infection in vitamin A-deficient mice. *J. Exp. Med.* 175:111–20

21. Chandra R. 1988. Increased bacterial binding to respiratory epithelial cells in vitamin A deficiency. *Br. Med. J.* 297:834–35

22. Chang M, Harper R, Hyde D, Wu R.

2000. A novel mechanism of retinoic acid-enhanced interleukin-8 gene expression in airway epithelium. *Am. J. Respir. Cell. Mol. Biol.* 22:502–10

23. Christian P, Schulze K, Stoltzfus RJ, West KP Jr. 1998. Hyporetinolemia, illness symptoms, and acute phase protein response in pregnant women with and without night blindness. *Am. J. Clin. Nutr.* 67:1237–43

24. Christian P, West KP Jr, Khatry SK, Katz J, Shrestha SR, et al. 1998. Night blindness of pregnancy in rural Nepal—nutritional and health risks. *Int. J. Epidemiol.* 27:231–37

25. Chytil F. 1983. Vitamin A and skin. In *Biochemistry and Physiology of the Skin*, ed. LA Goldsmith, pp. 1187–99. New York: Oxford Univ. Press

26. Colizzi V, Malkovsky M. 1985. Augmentation of interleukin-2 production and delayed hypersensitivity in mice infected with *Mycobacterium bovis* and fed a diet supplemented with vitamin A acetate. *Infect. Immun.* 48:581–83

27. Coutsoudis A, Kiepiela P, Coovadia HM, Broughton M. 1992. Vitamin A supplementation enhances specific IgG antibody levels and total lymphocyte numbers while improving morbidity in measles. *Pediatr. Infect. Dis. J.* 11:203–9

28. Coutsoudis A, Pillay K, Spooner E, Kuhn L, Coovadia H. 1999. Randomized trial testing the effect of vitamin A supplementation on pregnancy outcomes and early mother-to-child HIV-1 transmission in Durban, South Africa. South African Vitamin A Study Group. *AIDS* 13:1517–24

29. Cui D, Moldoveanu Z, Stephensen C. 2000. High-level dietary vitamin A enhances T-helper type 2 cytokine production and secretory immunoglobulin A response to influenza A virus infection in BALB/c mice. *J. Nutr.* 130:1132–39

30. Curtale F, Pokhrel R, Tilden R, Higashi G. 1995. Intestinal helminths and xerophthalmia in Nepal. A case-control study. *J. Trop. Pediatr.* 41:334–37

31. Dawson HD, Li NQ, Decicco KL, Nibert JA, Ross AC. 1999. Chronic marginal vitamin A status reduces natural killer cell number and function in aging Lewis rats. *J. Nutr.* 129:1510–17

32. Donnen P, Dramaix M, Brasseur D, Bitwe R, Vertongen F, et al. 1998. Randomized placebo-controlled clinical trial of the effect of a single high dose or daily low doses of vitamin A on the morbidity of hospitalized, malnourished children. *Am. J. Clin. Nutr.* 68:1254–60

33. Duggan M, Milner R. 1986. Energy cost of measles infection. *Arch. Dis. Child.* 61:436–39

34. Fawzi WW, Chalmers TC, Herrera MG, Mosteller F. 1993. Vitamin A supplementation and child mortality. A meta-analysis. *JAMA* 269:898–903

35. Fawzi WW, Mbise RL, Hertzmark E, Fataki MR, Herrera MG, et al. 1999. A randomized trial of vitamin A supplements in relation to mortality among human immunodeficiency virus-infected and uninfected children in Tanzania. *Pediatr. Infect. Dis. J.* 18:127–33

36. Fawzi WW, Msamanga G, Hunter D, Urassa E, Renjifo B, et al. 2000. Randomized trial of vitamin supplements in relation to vertical transmission of HIV-1 in Tanzania. *J. AIDS* 23:246–54

37. Filteau S. 1999. Vitamin A and the acute-phase response. *Nutrition* 15:326–28

38. Filteau S, Morris SS, Abbott RA, Tomkins AM, Kirkwood BR, et al. 1993. Influence of morbidity on serum retinol of children in a community-based study in northern Ghana. *Am. J. Clin. Nutr.* 58:192–97

39. Filteau S, Willumsen J, Sullivan K, Simmank K, Gamble M. 2000. Use of the retinol-binding protein: transthyretin ratio for assessment of vitamin A status during the acute-phase response. *Br. J. Nutr.* 83:513–20

40. Frankenburg S, Wang X, Milner Y. 1998. Vitamin A inhibits cytokines produced by

type 1 lymphocytes in vitro. *Cell. Immunol.* 185:75–81

41. Gangopadhyay NN, Moldoveanu Z, Stephensen CB. 1996. Vitamin A deficiency has different effects on immunoglobulin A production and transport during influenza A infection in BALB/c mice. *J. Nutr.* 126:2960–67

41a. Giguere V, Ong ES, Segui P, Evans RM. 1987. Identification of a receptor for the morphogen retinoic acid. *Nature* 330:624–9

42. Glasziou PP, Mackerras DE. 1993. Vitamin A supplementation in infectious diseases: a meta-analysis. *Br. Med. J.* 306:366–70

43. Green HN, E Mellanby 1928. Vitamin A as an anti-infective agent. *Br. Med. J.* 2:691–96

44. Hanekom W, Hussey G, Hughes E, Potgieter S, Yogev R, et al. 1999. Plasma-soluble CD30 in childhood tuberculosis: effects of disease severity, nutritional status, and vitamin A therapy. *Clin. Diagn. Lab. Immunol.* 6:204–8

45. Hanekom W, Potgieter S, Hughes E, Malan H, Kessow G, et al. 1997. Vitamin A status and therapy in childhood pulmonary tuberculosis. *J. Pediatr.* 131:925–27

46. Hashimoto S, Hayashi S, Yoshida S, Kujime K, Maruoka S, et al. 1998. Retinoic acid differentially regulates interleukin-1beta and interleukin-1 receptor antagonist production by human alveolar macrophages. *Leuk. Res.* 22:1057–61

47. Herbert V. 1973. The five possible causes of all nutrient deficiency: illustrated by deficiencies of vitamin B 12. *Am. J. Clin. Nutr.* 26:77–86

48. Hong WK, Itri LM. 1994. Retinoids and human cancer. See Ref. 114, pp. 597–630

49. Hotez PJ. 1999. Hookworm infections. In *Tropical Infectious Diseases*, ed. RL Guerrant, DH Walker, PF Weller, 2:966–74. Philadelphia: Churchill Livingstone

50. Humphrey JH, Quinn T, Fine D, Lederman H, Yamini-Roodsari S, et al. 1999. Short-term effects of large-dose vitamin A supplementation on viral load and immune response in HIV-infected women. *J. AIDS Hum. Retrovirol.* 20:44–51

51. Hussey GD, Klein M. 1990. A randomized, controlled trial of vitamin A in children with severe measles. *N. Engl. J. Med.* 323:160–64

52. Katz J, West KJ, Khatry S, Pradhan E, LeClerq S, et al. 2000. Maternal low-dose vitamin A or beta-carotene supplementation has no effect on fetal loss and early infant mortality: a randomized cluster trial in Nepal. *Am. J. Clin. Nutr.* 71:1570–76

53. Kjolhede C, Beisel WR. 1995. *Vitamin A and the Immune Function.* New York: Haworth

54. Kuwata T, Wang I, Tamura T, Ponnamperuma R, Levine R, et al. 2000. Vitamin A deficiency in mice causes a systemic expansion of myeloid cells. *Blood* 95:3349–56

55. Lawson N, Berliner N. 1999. Neutrophil maturation and the role of retinoic acid. *Exp. Hematol.* 27:1355–67

56. Lewallen S, Taylor TE, Molyneux ME, Semba RD, Wills BA, et al. 1998. Association between measures of vitamin A and the ocular fundus findings in cerebral malaria. *Arch. Ophthalmol.* 116:293–96

57. Liuzzi J, Cioccia A, Hevia P. 1998. In well-fed young rats, lactose-induced chronic diarrhea reduces the apparent absorption of vitamins A and E and affects preferentially vitamin E status. *J. Nutr.* 128:2467–72

58. Lomo J, Smeland E, Ulven S, Natarajan V, Blomhoff R, et al. 1998. RAR, not RXR, ligands inhibit cell activation and prevent apoptosis in B-lymphocytes. *J. Cell Physiol.* 175:68–77

59. Mangelsdorf D, Ong E, Dyck J, Evans R. 1990. Nuclear receptor that identifies a novel retinoic acid response pathway. *Nature* 345:224–29

60. Martorell R, Yarbrough C, Yarbrough S, Klein R. 1980. The impact of ordinary

illnesses on the dietary intakes of malnourished children. *Am. J. Clin. Nutr.* 33:345–50

61. Mata L. 1992. Diarrheal disease as a cause of malnutrition. *Am. J. Trop. Med. Hyg.* 47:16–27

62. McCollum EV, Davis M. 1913. The necessity of certain lipins in the diet during growth. *J. Biol. Chem.* 15:167–75

63. Miller S, Kearney S. 1998. Effect of in vivo administration of all *trans*-retinoic acid on the hemopoietic cell populations of the spleen and bone marrow: profound strain differences between A/J and C57BL/6J mice. *Lab. Anim. Sci.* 48:74–80

64. Mitra AK, Alvarez JO, Guay-Woodford L, Fuchs GJ, Wahed MA, et al. 1998. Urinary retinol excretion and kidney function in children with shigellosis. *Am. J. Clin. Nutr.* 68:1095–103

65. Mitra AK, Alvarez JO, Stephensen CB. 1998. Increased urinary retinol loss in children with severe infections. *Lancet* 351:1033–34

66. Mitra AK, Alvarez JO, Wahed MA, Fuchs GJ, Stephensen CB. 1998. Predictors of serum retinol in children with shigellosis. *Am. J. Clin. Nutr.* 68:1088–94

67. Na SY, Kang BY, Chung SW, Han SJ, Ma X, et al. 1999. Retinoids inhibit interleukin-12 production in macrophages through physical associations of retinoid X receptor and NF-kappa-B. *J. Biol. Chem.* 274: 7674–80

68. Nauss K, Anderson C, Conner M, Newberne P. 1985. Ocular infection with herpes simplex virus (HSV-1) in vitamin A-deficient and control rats. *J. Nutr.* 115:1300–15

69. Nauss K, Mark D, Suskind R. 1979. The effect of vitamin A deficiency on the in vitro cellular immune response of rats. *J. Nutr.* 109:1815–23

70. Nikawa T, Odahara K, Koizumi H, Kido Y, Teshima S, et al. 1999. Vitamin A prevents the decline in immunoglobulin A and Th2 cytokine levels in small intestinal mu-

cosa of protein-malnourished mice. *J. Nutr.* 129:934–41

71. Nimmagadda A, O'Brien W, Goetz M. 1998. The significance of vitamin A and carotenoid status in persons infected by the human immunodeficiency virus. *Clin. Infect. Dis.* 26:711–18

72. Omer F, Kurtzhals J, Riley E. 2000. Maintaining the immunological balance in parasitic infections: a role for TGF-beta? *Parasitol. Today* 16:18–23

73. Ongsakul M, Sirisinha S, Lamb A. 1985. Impaired blood clearance of bacteria and phagocytic activity in vitamin A-deficient rats. *Proc. Soc. Exp. Biol. Med.* 178:204–8

74. Osborne TB, Mendel LB. 1913. The influence of butter-fat on growth. *J. Biol. Chem.* 16:423–37

75. Peck GL, DiGiovanna JJ. 1984. Synthetic retinoids in dermatology. See Ref. 114, pp. 631–58

76. Petkovich M, Brand N, Krust A, Chambon P. 1987. A human retinoic acid receptor which belongs to the family of nuclear receptors. *Nature* 330:444–50

77. Quadro L, Blaner W, Salchow D, Vogel S, Piantedosi R, et al. 1999. Impaired retinal function and vitamin A availability in mice lacking retinol-binding protein. *EMBO J.* 18:4633–44

78. Racke MK, Burnett D, Pak SH, Albert PS, Cannella B, et al. 1995. Retinoid treatment of experimental allergic encephalomyelitis. IL-4 production correlates with improved disease course. *J. Immunol.* 154:450–58

79. Rahman M, Mahalanabis D, Alvarez J, Wahed M, Islam M, et al. 1997. Effect of early vitamin A supplementation on cell-mediated immunity in infants younger than 6 mo. *Am. J. Clin. Nutr.* 65:144–48

80. Rahman MM, Mahalanabis D, Alvarez JO, Wahed MA, Islam MA, et al. 1996. Acute respiratory infections prevent improvement of vitamin A status in young infants supplemented with vitamin A. *J. Nutr.* 126:628–33

81. Rahman MM, Mahalanabis D, Hossain S, Wahed M, Alvarez J, et al. 1999. Simultaneous vitamin A administration at routine immunization contact enhances antibody response to diphtheria vaccine in infants younger than six months. *J. Nutr.* 129: 2192–95

82. Rosales F, Kjolhede C. 1994. A single 210-Mumol oral dose of retinol does not enhance the immune response in children with measles. *J. Nutr.* 124:1604–14

83. Rosales FJ, Ritter SJ, Zolfaghari R, Smith JE, Ross AC. 1996. Effects of acute inflammation on plasma retinol, retinol-binding protein, and its mRNA in the liver and kidneys of vitamin A-sufficient rats. *J. Lipid Res.* 37:962–71

84. Rosales FJ, Ross AC. 1998. Acute inflammation induces hyporetinemia and modifies the plasma and tissue response to vitamin A supplementation in marginally vitamin A-deficient rats. *J. Nutr.* 128:960–66

85. Rosales FJ, Ross AC. 1998. A low molar ratio of retinol binding protein to transthyretin indicates vitamin A deficiency during inflammation: studies in rats and a posterior analysis of vitamin A-supplemented children with measles. *J. Nutr.* 128:1681–87

86. Rosales F, Topping J, Smith J, Shankar A, Ross A. 2000. Relation of serum retinol to acute phase proteins and malarial morbidity in Papua New Guinea children. *Am. J. Clin. Nutr.* 71:1582–88

87. Ross AC. 1992. Vitamin A status: relationship to immunity and the antibody response. *Proc. Soc. Exp. Biol. Med.* 200:303–20

88. Ross AC, Hammerling UG. 1994. Retinoids and the immune system. See Ref. 114, pp. 521–43

89. Ross A, Stephensen C. 1996. Vitamin A and retinoids in antiviral responses. *FASEB J.* 10:979–85

90. Sarker S, Wahed M, Rahaman M, Alam A, Islam A, et al. 1986. Persistent protein losing enteropathy in post measles diarrhoea. *Arch. Dis. Child.* 61:739–43

91. Scrimshaw NS, Taylor CE, Gordon JE. 1968. *Interactions of Nutrition and Infection.* Geneva, Switzerland: World Health Org.

92. Seder RA, Mosmann TM. 1998. Differentiation of effector phenotypes of CD4+ and CD8+ T-cells. In *Fundamental Immunology*, ed. WE Paul, pp. 879–908. Philadelphia: Lippincott-Raven. 4th ed.

93. Semba R. 1997. Vitamin A and human immunodeficiency virus infection. *Proc. Nutr. Soc.* 56:459–69

94. Semba R. 1999. Vitamin A as "anti-infective" therapy, 1920–1940. *J. Nutr.* 129:783–91

95. Semba R, Muhilal, Mohgaddam N, Munasir Z, Akib A, et al. 1999. Integration of vitamin A supplementation with the expanded program on immunization does not affect seroconversion to oral poliovirus vaccine in infants. *J. Nutr.* 129:2203–5

96. Semba R, Muhilal, Scott AL, Natadisastra G, Wirasasmita S, et al. 1992. Depressed immune response to tetanus in children with vitamin A deficiency. *J. Nutr.* 122:101–7

97. Semba R, Muhilal, West KJ, Natadisastra G, Eisinger W, et al. 2000. Hyporetinolemia and acute phase proteins in children with and without xerophthalmia. *Am. J. Clin. Nutr.* 72:146–53

98. Semba R, Munasir Z, Beeler J, Akib A, Muhilal et al. 1995. Reduced seroconversion to measles in infants given vitamin A with measles vaccination. *Lancet* 345:1330–32

99. Sempertegui F, Estrella B, Camaniero V, Betancourt V, Izurieta R, et al. 1999. The beneficial effects of weekly low-dose vitamin A supplementation on acute lower respiratory infections and diarrhea in Ecuadorian children. *Pediatrics* 104:E1

100. Shams N, Reddy C, Watanabe K, Elgebaly S, Hanninen L, et al. 1994. Increased

interleukin-1 activity in the injured vitamin A-deficient cornea. *Cornea* 13:156–66

101. Shankar A, Genton B, Semba R, Baisor M, Paino J, et al. 1999. Effect of vitamin A supplementation on morbidity due to *Plasmodium falciparum* in young children in Papua New Guinea: a randomised trial. *Lancet* 354:203–9

102. Shoda R, Mahalanabis D, Wahed M, Albert M. 1995. Bacterial translocation in the rat model of lectin induced diarrhoea. *Gut* 36:379–81

103. Si NV, Grytter C, Vy NN, Hue NB, Pedersen FK. 1997. High dose vitamin A supplementation in the course of pneumonia in Vietnamese children. *Acta Paediatr.* 86:1052–55

104. Sijtsma S, Rombout J, Dohmen M, West C, van der Zijpp A. 1991. Effect of vitamin A deficiency on the activity of macrophages in Newcastle disease virus-infected chickens. *Vet. Immunol. Immunopathol.* 28:17–27

105. Sijtsma S, Rombout J, West C, van der Zijpp A. 1990. Vitamin A deficiency impairs cytotoxic T lymphocyte activity in Newcastle disease virus-infected chickens. *Vet. Immunol. Immunopathol.* 26:191–201

106. Sivakumar B, Reddy V. 1972. Absorption of labelled vitamin A in children during infection. *Br. J. Nutr.* 27:299–304

107. Sivakumar B, Reddy V. 1975. Absorption of vitamin A in children with ascariasis. *J. Trop. Med. Hyg.* 78:114–15

108. Smith SM, Hayes CE. 1987. Contrasting impairments in IgM and IgG responses of vitamin A-deficient mice. *Proc. Natl. Acad. Sci. USA* 84:5878–82

109. Smith SM, Levy NS, Hayes CE. 1987. Impaired immunity in vitamin A-deficient mice. *J. Nutr.* 117:857–65

110. Solomons N. 1993. Pathways to the impairment of human nutritional status by gastrointestinal pathogens. *Parasitology* 107(Suppl.):S19–35

111. Sommer A, Tarwotjo I, Djunaedi E, West KP Jr, Loeden AA, et al. 1986. Impact of vitamin A supplementation on childhood mortality. A randomised controlled community trial. *Lancet* 1:1169–73

112. Sommer A, Tarwotjo I, Katz J. 1987. Increased risk of xerophthalmia following diarrhea and respiratory disease. *Am. J. Clin. Nutr.* 45:977–80

113. Sommer A, West KP Jr. 1996. *Vitamin A Deficiency: Health, Survival and Vision.* New York: Oxford Univ. Press

114. Sporn MB, Roberts AB, Goodman DS, eds. 1994. *The Retinoids: Biology, Chemistry and Medicine.* New York: Raven. 2nd ed.

115. Steel D, Whitehead A. 1994. The major acute phase reactants: C-reactive protein, serum amyloid P component and serum amyloid A protein. *Immunol. Today* 15:81–88

116. Stephensen CB, Alvarez JO, Kohatsu J, Hardmeier R, Kennedy JI Jr, et al. 1994. Vitamin A is excreted in the urine during acute infection. *Am. J. Clin. Nutr.* 60:388–92

117. Stephensen CB, Ceddia MA, Weaver CT, Bucy RP. 2000. Retinoic acid (RA) treatment of T-helper (Th) cell cultures modulates Th1/Th2 phenotype development. *FASEB J.* 14:A557

118. Stephensen CB, Drammeh B, Islam MA. 2001. Vitamin A nutriture in developing countries. In *Childhood Nutrition in Developing Countries*, ed. NW Solomons. Boca Raton, FL: CRC. In press

119. Stephensen CB, Franchi LM, Hernandez H, Campos M, Gilman RH, et al. 1998. Use of the relative dose-response test in children recovering from pneumonia. *FASEB J.* 12:A351

120. Stephensen CB, Franchi L, Hernandez H, Campos M, Gilman R, et al. 1998. Adverse effects of high-dose vitamin A supplements in children hospitalized with pneumonia. *Pediatrics* 101:E3–10

121. Stephensen CB, Gildengorin G. 2000.

Serum retinol, the acute phase response, and the apparent misclassification of vitamin A status in the Third National Health and Nutrition Examination Survey. *Am. J. Clin. Nutr.* 72:1170–78

122. Stephensen CB, Moldoveanu Z, Gangopadhyay NN. 1996. Vitamin A deficiency diminishes the salivary immunoglobulin Aa response and enhances the serum immunoglobulin G response to influenza A virus infection in BALB/c mice. *J. Nutr.* 126:94–102

123. Tanumihardjo S, Permaesih D, Muherdiyantiningsih, Rustan E, Rusmil K, et al. 1996. Vitamin A status of Indonesian children infected with *Ascaris lumbricoides* after dosing with vitamin A supplements and albendazole. *J. Nutr.* 126:451–57

124. Deleted in proof

125. Thurnham D, Northrop-Clewes C, McCullough F, Das B, Lunn P. 2000. Innate immunity, gut integrity, and vitamin A in Gambian and Indian infants. *J. Infect. Dis.* V182:S23–28

126. Tokuyama H, Tokuyama Y. 1999. The regulatory effects of all-*trans*-retinoic acid on isotype switching: retinoic acid induces IgA switch rearrangement in cooperation with IL-5 and inhibits IgG1 switching. *Cell. Immunol.* 192:41–47

127. Twining SS, Schulte DP, Wilson PM, Fish BL, Moulder JE. 1997. Vitamin A deficiency alters rat neutrophil function. *J. Nutr.* 127:558–65

128. Underwood BA. 1994. Vitamin A in human nutrition: public health considerations. See Ref. 114, pp. 211–27

129. van Bennekum A, Wong Yen Kong L, Gijbels M, Tielen F, Roholl P, et al. 1991. Mitogen response of B cells, but not T cells, is impaired in adult vitamin A-deficient rats. *J. Nutr.* 121:1960–68; Erratum. 1992. *J. Nutr.* 122(3):588

130. Villamor E, Fawzi W. 2000. Vitamin A supplementation: implications for morbidity and mortality in children. *J. Infect. Dis.* V182:S122–33

130a. Vitamin A Pneumonia Work. Group. 1995. Potential interventions for the prevention of childhood pneumonia in developing countries: a meta-analysis of data from field trials to assess the impact of vitamin A supplementation on pneumonia morbidity and mortality. *Bull. WHO* 73:609–19

131. Warden R, Strazzari M, Dunkley P, O'Loughlin E. 1996. Vitamin A-deficient rats have only mild changes in jejunal structure and function. *J. Nutr.* 126:1817–26

132. West C. 2000. Vitamin A and measles. *Nutr. Rev.* 58:S46–54

133. West C, Sijtsma S, Kouwenhoven B, Rombout J, van der Zijpp A. 1992. Epithelia-damaging virus infections affect vitamin A status in chickens. *J. Nutr.* 122:333–39

134. West KP, Katz J, Khatry S, LeClerq S, Pradhan E, et al. 1999. Double blind, cluster randomised trial of low dose supplementation with vitamin A or beta carotene on mortality related to pregnancy in nepal. The NNIPS-2 Study Group. *Br. Med. J.* 318:570–75

135. WHO/CHD Immunisation-Linked Vitamin A Suppl. Study Group. 1998. Randomised trial to assess benefits and safety of vitamin A supplementation linked to immunisation in early infancy. *Lancet* 352:1257–63

136. Wiedermann U, Chen XJ, Enerbeack L, Hanson LA, Kahu H, et al. 1996. Vitamin A deficiency increases inflammatory responses. *Scand. J. Immunol.* 44:578–84

137. Wiedermann U, Hanson L, Bremell T, Kahu H, Dahlgren U. 1995. Increased translocation of *Escherichia coli* and development of arthritis in vitamin A-deficient rats. *Infect. Immun.* 63:3062–68

138. Wiedermann U, Hanson LA, Dahlgren

UI. 1996. Vitamin A deficiency and the immune system. *Immunologist* 4:70–75

139. Wiedermann U, Hanson LA, Holmgren J, Kahu H, Dahlgren UI. 1993. Impaired mucosal antibody response to cholera toxin in vitamin A-deficient rats immunized with oral cholera vaccine. *Infect. Immun.* 61:3952–57; Erratum. 1993. *Infect. Immun.* 61(12):5431

140. Wiedermann U, Hanson LA, Kahu H, Dahlgren UI. 1993. Aberrant T-cell function *in vitro* and impaired T-cell dependent antibody response *in vivo* in vitamin A-deficient rats. *Immunology* 80:581–86

141. Wiedermann U, Tarkowski A, Bremell T, Hanson LA, Kahu H, et al. 1996. Vitamin A deficiency predisposes to *Staphylococcus aureus* infection. *Infect. Immun.* 64:209–14

142. Willumsen JF, Simmank K, Filteau SM, Wagstaff LA, Tomkins AM. 1997. Toxic damage to the respiratory epithelium induces acute phase changes in vitamin A metabolism without depleting retinol stores of South African children. *J. Nutr.* 127:1339–43

143. Zhao Z, Ross AC. 1995. Retinoic acid repletion restores the number of leukocytes and their subsets and stimulates natural cytotoxicity in vitamin A-deficient rats. *J. Nutr.* 125:2064–73

Annu. Rev. Nutr. 2001. 21:193–230

# PEROXISOMAL β-OXIDATION AND PEROXISOME PROLIFERATOR–ACTIVATED RECEPTOR α: An Adaptive Metabolic System

## Janardan K Reddy and Takashi Hashimoto

*Department of Pathology, Northwestern University Medical School, Chicago, Illinois 60611; e-mail: jkreddy@northwestern.edu*

**Key Words**    fatty acid oxidation, PPARα, gene knockout models

■ **Abstract**    β-Oxidation occurs in both mitochondria and peroxisomes. Mitochondria catalyze the β-oxidation of the bulk of short-, medium-, and long-chain fatty acids derived from diet, and this pathway constitutes the major process by which fatty acids are oxidized to generate energy. Peroxisomes are involved in the β-oxidation chain shortening of long-chain and very-long-chain fatty acyl-coenzyme (CoAs), long-chain dicarboxylyl-CoAs, the CoA esters of eicosanoids, 2-methyl-branched fatty acyl-CoAs, and the CoA esters of the bile acid intermediates di- and trihydroxycoprostanoic acids, and in the process they generate $H_2O_2$. Long-chain and very-long-chain fatty acids (VLCFAs) are also metabolized by the cytochrome P450 CYP4A ω-oxidation system to dicarboxylic acids that serve as substrates for peroxisomal β-oxidation. The peroxisomal β-oxidation system consists of (*a*) a classical peroxisome proliferator–inducible pathway capable of catalyzing straight-chain acyl-CoAs by fatty acyl-CoA oxidase, L-bifunctional protein, and thiolase, and (*b*) a second noninducible pathway catalyzing the oxidation of 2-methyl-branched fatty acyl-CoAs by branched-chain acyl-CoA oxidase (pristanoyl-CoA oxidase/trihydroxycoprostanoyl-CoA oxidase), D-bifunctional protein, and sterol carrier protein (SCP)x. The genes encoding the classical β-oxidation pathway in liver are transcriptionally regulated by peroxisome proliferator–activated receptor α (PPARα). Evidence derived from mice deficient in PPARα, peroxisomal fatty acyl-CoA oxidase, and some of the other enzymes of the two peroxisomal β-oxidation pathways points to the critical importance of PPARα and of the classical peroxisomal fatty acyl-CoA oxidase in energy metabolism, and in the development of hepatic steatosis, steatohepatitis, and liver cancer.

## CONTENTS

0199-9885/01/0715-0193$14.00

# INTRODUCTION

Peroxisomes are cell organelles present in virtually all eukaryotic cells. Currently, more than 60 proteins have been found to be associated with mammalian peroxisomes, with more than half of these participating in lipid metabolism (16, 92). The regulation of lipid and carbohydrate metabolism is central to energy homeostasis and other vital biological functions of cells in higher organisms (21, 24, 25, 71). Peroxisomes, by virtue of their richness in lipid metabolizing enzymes (44, 48, 92), play a critical role in metabolic systems and physiological processes influencing alternate use of carbohydrate and fatty acids to generate ATP. This regulatory energy consumption, referred to as the glucose fatty acid cycle (71), requires the maintenance of efficient hepatic fatty acid oxidation. It is estimated that in adults, free fatty acids and their ketone body derivatives provide $\sim$80% of caloric requirements after 24 h of fasting, as fasting leads to a dramatic depletion of carbohydrate energy source, especially in infants and children (11). As a consequence, both children and adults exhibit greater dependence on efficient free fatty acid oxidation–dependent ketogenesis during starvation, underscoring the importance of fatty acid oxidation in energy metabolism. Fatty acid oxidation occurs in mitochondria, peroxisomes, and smooth endoplasmic reticulum, and some of the critical enzymes of these oxidation systems are transcriptionally controlled by peroxisome proliferator–activated receptor $\alpha$ (PPAR$\alpha$), a member of the nuclear hormone receptor superfamily (17, 21, 32, 39, 40, 43, 61, 74, 76). PPARs, which derive their designation from structurally diverse compounds called peroxisome proliferators, and their ability to induce predictable pleiotropic responses in rodent livers, including the development of liver tumors (72–73, 75, 76), consist of three isotypes, PPAR$\alpha$, PPAR$\delta$ (also called $\beta$), and PPAR$\gamma$, which are products of different genes (4, 17, 39, 81, 98, 102). $\beta$-Oxidation is a major process by which fatty acids are oxidized, and this oxidation occurs both in mitochondria and in peroxisomes (21, 24, 25, 47). Fatty acids are also oxidized by $\omega$-oxidation by a cytochrome P450 CYP4A subfamily; this oxidation occurs almost exclusively in smooth endoplasmic reticulum (14, 22, 31, 61). This review focuses on recent developments in the enzymology and functional organization of peroxisomal $\beta$-oxidation pathways, and on our perspectives on the critical importance of PPAR$\alpha$ in the inducibility of fatty acid oxidation systems that metabolize long-chain and VLCFAs in the pathogenesis of hepatic steatosis, steatohepatitis, and carcinogenesis. Since the previous review on peroxisomal lipid metabolism published in this series (77), several genetically altered mouse models representing some of the enzymatic deficiencies in peroxisomal $\beta$-oxidation have become available. New information on genetically determined metabolic defects at the individual enzyme level in mitochondrial and peroxisomal fatty acid $\beta$-oxidation pathways in humans has also emerged, and these developments have added new dimensions to our understanding of the interdependencies of the intricate metabolic systems.

# FATTY ACID OXIDATION

Fatty acids are energy-rich molecules that are pivotal (*a*) for a variety of cellular processes, such as synthesis of membrane lipids and generation of lipid-containing messengers in signal transduction, and (*b*) for energy storage in the form of triacylglycerol in adipose tissue (21, 24, 28). Adipocytes provide the virtually limitless capacity to store energy in the form of triacylglycerol, which constitutes the most concentrated form of energy storage in higher animals (28). It is rationalized that by its ability to store energy, the adipocyte radically changed the evolutionary hierarchy of life on earth (4, 82, 91). Although most nonadipocytes contain traces of triacylglycerol for homeostatic functions, they are protected from massive accumulation of triacylglycerol during conditions of excess energy consumption. It is hypothesized that leptin functions to confine the storage of energy to the adipocyte, while limiting triacylglycerol storage in nonadipocytes (91). Of all the nonadipocyte cells, the mammalian liver cell is normally capable of storing considerable quantities of triacylglycerol, especially to accommodate plasma nonesterified fatty acids present in excess of the requirement for immediate oxidation and/or secretion as very-low-density lipoproteins (25, 28, 41). The ability of liver to store lipids is viewed as a protective mechanism, neutralizing the potential toxicity of (*a*) long-chain fatty acids and VLCFAs synthesized de novo in individuals consuming excess energy and fat-rich diets and (*b*) those released into the plasma from adipose tissues stores (28, 91). Abnormal quantities of lipids stored in liver manifest as fatty liver (steatosis), a condition most often attributed to the effects of excess alcohol consumption, obesity, diabetes, drugs, and/or metabolic perturbations resulting from alterations in fatty acid oxidation, fatty acid synthesis, and transport from liver (25, 41).

Fatty acid metabolism is one of the major sources of energy for skeletal muscle and heart, but liver plays a critical role in the energy metabolism of these and other extrahepatic tissues in most animals. Fatty acids are oxidized in three organelles, with $\beta$-oxidation confined to mitochondria and peroxisomes, and the CYP4A-catalyzed $\omega$-oxidation occurring in the endoplasmic reticulum. Fatty acid synthesis is enhanced and $\beta$-oxidation is lowered when glucose supply is plenty so that excess energy can be stored in the form of triacylglycerol (21, 24, 28). When glucose availability is diminished, however, the synthesis of fatty acids is depressed and $\beta$-oxidation is enhanced in liver so as to generate ketone bodies for export to serve as fuels for other tissues, such as the skeletal and cardiac muscle (28, 71). This alternate use of energy sources occurs during short-term fluctuations in energy supply. The fatty acid oxidation in an intact organism is roughly proportional to the plasma concentration of free fatty acids released from adipose tissue, and this mobilization of free fatty acids is stimulated by glucagon and other hormones and inhibited by insulin (28, 71). A brief overview of the three fatty acid oxidation systems is given below as a prelude to a comprehensive review of the peroxisomal $\beta$-oxidation system.

## Mitochondrial $\beta$-Oxidation

Mitochondrial $\beta$-oxidation is responsible for the oxidation of the major portion of the of short- ($<C_8$), medium- ($C_8$–$C_{12}$), and long- ($C_{14}$–$C_{20}$) chain fatty acids and, in the process, contributes to energy production via ATP generating oxidative phosphorylation. Because long-chain fatty acids constitute the bulk of dietary fat, their abundance makes them the predominant source of energy under normal conditions, and during fasting-induced lipolysis they become crucial metabolic substrates (21, 32, 33, 55, 77). The dominant role of mitochondria in the oxidation of long-chain fatty acids appears a logical consequence of the fact that mitochondrial $\beta$-oxidation, by means of oxidative phosphorylation, conserves almost double the energy compared with peroxisomes because the energy produced by the first step of the peroxisomal $\beta$-oxidation dissipates as heat (33, 48, 49, 77). One important short-term regulatory mechanism of the mitochondrial $\beta$-oxidation system involves the carnitine palmitoyltransferase I (CPT I), which, for transport of fatty acids across the inner mitochondrial membrane, catalyzes the formation of fatty acylcarnitine at the outer mitochondrial membrane. Because carnitine concentration is near the $K_m$ value of CPT I, changes in carnitine concentration generally affect the mitochondrial $\beta$-oxidation (21, 33). CPT I is inhibited by malonyl-CoA, and therefore, alterations in malonyl-CoA levels affect fatty acid transport (33, 47). Furthermore, two isoforms of CPT I, the liver isoform and the skeletal muscle isoform, exhibit markedly different kinetic characteristics with respect to carnitine and to malonyl-CoA inhibition (33, 47). CPT I is markedly induced by peroxisome proliferators, and by fatty

acids/fatty acyl-CoAs, which activate PPARα, and in this regard this transcription factor plays a critical role in the regulation of mitochondrial β-oxidation (17, 33).

Fatty acids are completely oxidized to acetyl-CoA by mitochondrial β-oxidation, and the acetyl-CoA then either enters the Krebs cycle for further oxidation or condenses to ketone bodies (acetoacetate, acetone, and β-hydroxybutyrate) in liver to serve as oxidizable fuels for extrahepatic tissues (21, 28, 55, 71). The mitochondrial β-oxidation has two distinct components. The first, which is mitochondrial inner-membrane bound, is active with long-chain fatty acyl-CoAs ($C_{12}$–$C_{20}$) and generates chain-shortened fatty acyl-CoAs (Figure 1). This inner-membrane–bound mitochondrial β-oxidation system consists of four reactions and generally oxidizes long-chain fatty acyl-CoAs by two membrane-associated proteins (33, 87). The first protein, a very-long-chain acyl-CoA dehydrogenase (VLCAD), performs the first step of β-oxidation, and the second protein, a long-chain enoyl-CoA hydratase/long-chain 3-hydroxyacyl-CoA dehydrogenase/long-chain 3-ketoacyl-CoA thiolase trifunctional β-oxidation protein complex

# FATTY ACID β-OXIDATION

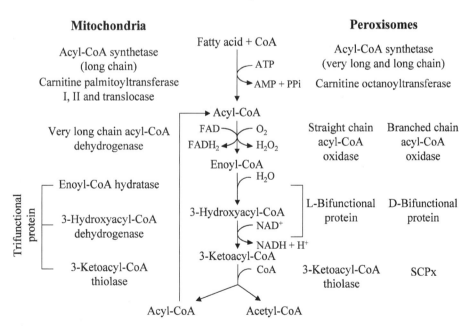

**Figure 1** Enzymology of mitochondrial inner-membrane–bound long-chain fatty acid β-oxidation system involving trifunctional protein, and the peroxisomal-inducible classical striaght-chain and the noninducible branched-chain fatty acid β oxidation systems in humans. SCPx, sterol carrier protein x.

(mitochondrial trifunctional protein), carries out the second, third, and fourth $\beta$-oxidation steps (Figure 1). The resulting optimally chain-shortened fatty acyl-CoAs are then completely $\beta$-oxidized by the second mitochondrial $\beta$-oxidation system located in the matrix. This system is active with long-chain ($C_{14}$–$C_{20}$), medium-chain ($C_8$–$C_{12}$), and short-chain ($C_4$–$C_6$) acyl-CoAs (21, 33, 55, 77). In this matrix-bound $\beta$-oxidation system, the well-known classical chain-length–specific long-chain (LCAD), medium-chain (MCAD), and short-chain acyl-CoA dehydrogenases (SCAD) catalyze the first step (21, 33, 87). The second, third, and fourth steps, respectively, of this $\beta$-oxidation spiral are carried out by the 2-enoyl-CoA hydratase (or crotonse), 3-hydroxyacyl-CoA dehydrogenase, and 3-ketoacyl-CoA thiolase, all of which are present in the mitochondrial matrix as individual enzymes encoded by separate genes.

The mitochondrial inner-membrane–bound trifunctional protein complex, responsible for the oxidation of very-long-chain acyl-CoAs, is a hetero-oct-omer made up of four $\alpha$-subunits with long-chain enoyl-CoA hydratase and 3-hydroxyacyl-CoA dehydrogenase activities and four $\beta$-subunits with long-chain 3-oxo-/or keto-thiolase activity (60). The two subunits ($\alpha$ and $\beta$) are encoded by two adjacent genes linked in a head-to-head fashion, and they are distinctly different from the three genes that encode mitochondrial matrix-bound classical enzymes (60). Comparison of the amino acid sequences of SCAD, MCAD, and LCAD reveal a distinct homology, indicating that these enzymes belong to a gene family, the acyl-CoA dehydrogenase family (21). Primary structures of rat mitochondrial SCAD, MCAD, and LCAD have revealed that their precursors have 414–430 amino acid residues containing a 25- to 30-amino acid signal sequence at the N termini. The subunit of VLCAD is synthesized as a polypeptide with 655 amino acid residues, with a typical cleavable extrapeptide at the N terminus, and the N-terminal region of 98–433 has a high homology with other acyl-CoA dehydrogenases (33). As noted above, long-chain fatty acyl-CoA are actively transported to the mitochondrial matrix, whereas the no-active-transport process involves the transport of short- and medium-chain fatty acids to mitochondrial matrix (21). Enzymes involved in the processing of conjugated double bonds during oxidation of polyunsaturated fatty acids are 2,4-dienoyl-CoA reductase, $\Delta^{3,5}$,$\Delta^{2,4}$-enoyl-CoA isomerase, $\Delta^{3,5}$,$\Delta^{2,4}$-dienoyl-CoA isomerase, and $\Delta^{3,5,7}$,$\Delta^{2,4,6}$-trienoyl-CoA isomerase (21).

## Peroxisomal $\beta$-Oxidation

The presence of a fatty acid $\beta$-oxidation system outside the mitochondrial com-partment was first described in 1969 in glyoxysomes (peroxisomes) present in germinating castor bean seedlings (15), and a similar system was found in 1976 in rat liver peroxisomes (48). It is now clear (*a*) that in animals both the mi-tochondrial and the peroxisomal fatty acid $\beta$-oxidation systems are present in the same cell, (*b*) that they are catalyzed by different enzymes encoded by dif-ferent genes, and (*c*) that they play functionally complementary but different

**TABLE 1**    Enzymes in the peroxisomal fatty acid $\beta$-oxidation system

| |
| --- |
| Very-long-chain acyl-CoA synthetase |
| Long-chain acyl-CoA synthetase |
| Carnitine octanoyltransferase |
| Carnitine acetyltransferase |
| Straight-chain acyl-CoA oxidase |
| Branched-chain acyl-CoA oxidase |
| L-Bifunctional protein |
| D-Bifunctional protein |
| 3-Ketoacyl-CoA thiolase |
| Sterol carrier protein 2/3-ketoacyl-CoA thiolase |
| 2,4-Dienoyl-CoA reductase |
| $\Delta^3,\Delta^2$-Enoyl-CoA isomerase |
| $\Delta^{3,5},\Delta^{2,4}$-Dienoyl-CoA isomerase |

roles (32, 33, 55, 77). The enzymes involved in peroxisomal fatty acid oxidation are listed in Table 1. Although long-chain fatty acids are predominantly $\beta$-oxidized in mitochondria, the peroxisomal $\beta$-oxidation system does indeed participate in the oxidation of these substrates. On the other hand, VLCFAs ($>C_{20}$), are almost exclusively $\beta$-oxidized in peroxisomes because mitochondria are devoid of very-long-chain acyl-CoA synthetase (77, 90, 92). Peroxisomal membranes contain at least two acyl-CoA synthetases: a long-chain acyl-CoA synthetase (89), which activates long-chain fatty acids, and a very-long-chain fatty acyl-CoA synthetase, which activates VLCFAs (89). The peroxisomal $\beta$-oxidation system also metabolizes long-chain dicarboxylic acids, eicosanoids, bile acid precursors, and side chains of some xenobiotics (55, 77). The three enzymes of the peroxisomal $\beta$-oxidation cycle, namely fatty acyl-CoA oxidase (AOX), enoyl-CoA hydratase/L-3-hydroxyacyl-CoA dehydrogenase bifunctional protein (L-PBE), and 3-ketoacyl-CoA thiolase, were purified nearly 20 years ago, but in recent years it has become evident that other enzymes are also involved in the peroxisomal fatty acid oxidation (32, 33, 55, 98). As is discussed later, based on substrate specificity and stereoselectivity of the newly discovered enzymes, two different peroxisomal $\beta$-oxidation pathways have been formulated (Figure 1). The classical pathway catalyzed by AOX, L-PBE, and thiolase is generally accepted to be responsible for the oxidation of straight-chain fatty acids (33, 55), and all three enzymes of this classical system are transcriptionally activated by PPAR$\alpha$ ligands (23, 39, 74). The oxidation of 2-methyl-branched fatty acids and of the bile acid intermediates, di- and trihydroxycoprostanoic acids, occurs via a second pathway (Figure 1) (see below).

The peroxisomal acyl-CoA oxidases, which are the first and rate-limiting enzyme of each of the two $\beta$-oxidation pathways in peroxisomes, reflect distinctive differences between peroxisomal and mitochondrial oxidation pathways (33, 55, 77, 79). The first step in peroxisomal fatty acid $\beta$-oxidation is directly coupled to the molecular oxygen, resulting in the cyanide insensitivity of the system, in contrast to the cyanide sensitivity of the mitochondrial system in which the first step is directly coupled to an electron transfer chain (48). Unlike the mitochondrial system, peroxisomal $\beta$-oxidation system is carnitine independent, and it does not go to completion, as the chain-shortened acyl-CoAs are exported to the mitochondria for the completion of $\beta$-oxidation (21, 32, 33, 77). The peroxisomal acyl-CoA oxidase acts on very-long-chain and long-chain acyl-CoAs but not on medium-chain acyl-CoAs, which are $\beta$-oxidized exclusively in mitochondria (33, 55). Therefore, the carbon-chain of palmitate, for example, is stopped at $C_8$ or so in peroxisomes, and then exported to the mitochondria.

## Microsomal $\omega$-Oxidation

The initial step in $\omega$-oxidation is $\omega$-hydroxylation of fatty acid in the smooth endoplasmic reticulum catalyzed by lauric acid $\omega$-hydroxylase, a member of the CYP4A subfamily (14, 31, 43, 61). The CYP4A family of cytochrome P450 enzymes, which are constitutively expressed in liver and kidney, catalyze the $\omega$- and ($\omega$-1)- hydroxylation of long-chain fatty acids (14). All known CYP4A enzymes in rats, namely CYP4A1, CYP4A2, CYP4A3, and CYP4A8, are constitutively expressed in kidney, but only the first three are expressed in liver (14, 43). The major $\omega$-hydroxylase expressed in human liver and kidney is CYP4A11, which is functionally similar to that of rat CYP4A1 (14, 22, 43). The $\omega$-hydroxy fatty acid produced by the initial hydroxylation reaction is then dehydrogenated to a dicarboxylic acid in the cytosol and converted to its CoA derivative by an acyl-CoA synthetase present in the endoplasmic reticulum (14, 77). In humans, long-chain dicarboxylyl-CoAs derived from $\omega$-oxidation of fatty acids are oxidized almost exclusively by peroxisomal AOX of the classical $\beta$-oxidation pathway (44, 55, 77). In rats, a significant portion of dicarboxylyl-CoAs also appears to be metabolized via pristanoyl-CoA oxidase (55).

The substrate and regiospecificity studies with rat and human CYP4A enzymes showed highest activity of these enzymes for lauric acid ($C_{12:0}$), and no particular preference for longer-chain fatty acids, such as oleic ($C_{18:1}$) and arachidonic acid ($C_{20:4}$) (18). Human and rat CYP4A enzymes, in general, poorly oxidize long-chain fatty acids (37), and in contrast, rabbit CYP4A4, CYP4A6, and CYP4A7 enzymes appear to be highly active toward arachidonic acid (43). Little information exists as to how effectively the VLCFAs are metabolized by the CYP4A subfamily of enzymes in various species. Aminobenzotriazole, a suicide inhibitor of the CYP4A $\omega$-hydroxylases, significantly inhibited the $\omega$-hydroxylation of VLCFAs in cultured human keratinocytes (10). This compound also altered the permeability barrier in the skin of hairless mice as the inhibitor decreased the generation of very-long-chain $\omega$-hydroxyceramide ($C_{\geq 30}$), which is required for corneocyte lipid envelope formation, presumably by inhibiting the $\omega$-hydroxylation of the free fatty acid prior to N-acylation of the sphingolipid base (10). These observations, albeit indirect, strongly implicate a role for the CYP4A subfamily in the $\omega$-oxidation of VLCFAs. However, until the $\omega$-hydroxylation of VLCFAs can be demonstrated in vitro by using highly purified CYP4A isoforms, the possibility that an enzyme other than a CYP4A isoform that is also inactivated by aminobenzotriazole inhibits VLCFA oxidation cannot be excluded. For all four known rat isoforms (CYP4A1, -4A2, -4A3, and -4A8), as well as for the single established human isoform (CYP4A11), the rate of NADPH consumption is always higher than the rate of fatty acid hydroxylation, which implies that the enzymes undergo some degree of uncoupled turnover (U Hoch & P Oritz de Montellano, personal communication). Uncoupled turnover implies that NADPH is being used to reduce oxygen to superoxide and/or $H_2O_2$, and possibly also to $H_2O$ (18, 37). Thus, it is important to note that reactive oxygen species are generated not only during the $\omega$-oxidation of fatty acids to dicarboxylic acids, but also when these dicarboxylic acids undergo $\omega$-oxidation within peroxisomes.

# ENZYMES OF THE PEROXISOMAL $\beta$-OXIDATION SYSTEM

## Fatty Acid Activation and Entry into the Peroxisome

Before a fatty acid can be $\beta$-oxidized by peroxisomes or mitochondria, it must be activated to its CoA derivative. As mentioned above, the peroxisomal membrane contains long-chain and very-long-chain acyl-CoA synthetases (84). Long-chain acyl-CoA synthetase, which activates long-chain fatty acids, is also localized in the mitochondrial outer membrane and in the endoplasmic reticulum (84). The enzymes in these three organelles are indistinguishable from each other at the protein level, which has led to the speculation that they are encoded by the same gene (83). The catalytic site of long-chain acyl-CoA synthetase is exposed to the cytosol (83). Medium straight-chain fatty acids can also be activated by the long-chain acyl-CoA synthetases present in the mitochondrial outer membranes and in the peroxisomal and endoplasmic reticulum membranes (21). Very-long-chain acyl-CoA synthetase, which activates VLCFAs, is present in peroxisomes and in the endoplasmic reticulum but is absent from mitochondria (55, 77, 90). The absence of very-long-chain fatty acyl-CoA synthetase in mitochondria may explain why VLCFAs are $\beta$-oxidized exclusively in peroxisomes (see below). Very-long-chain acyl-CoA synthetase differs from long-chain acyl-CoA synthetase with respect to molecular, catalytic, and immunochemical properties (89, 90). The deduced primary structures of very-long-chain and long-chain acyl-CoA synthetases are quite different, but it is intriguing that the amino acid sequence of very-long-chain fatty acyl-CoA synthetase has 40% amino acid identity with that of fatty acid transport protein isolated from adipocytes (78).

Peroxisomes play a prominent role in the $\beta$-oxidation of pristanic acid and other branched-chain fatty acids (33, 47, 55, 77, 79). Isoprenoid-derived branched-chain fatty acids can be activated by peroxisomes, mitochondria, and the endoplasmic reticulum, possibly via the long-chain acyl-CoA synthetases present in these organelles (83). Whether peroxisomes contain a branched-chain acyl-CoA synthetase remains unclear. Dicarboxylic acids, prostaglandins, and the $C_{27}$ bile acid intermediates, di- and trihydroxycholestanoic acids, are activated solely in the endoplasmic reticulum (55, 98). The bile acid intermediates, synthesized from cholesterol, are activated by a separate enzyme, trihydroxycoprostanoyl-CoA synthetase, which is present only in liver. The observation that dicarboxylic acids and prostaglandins are not activated by mitochondria or peroxisomes implies that these molecules are substrates not for long-chain acyl-CoA synthetase but for a specific enzyme(s). As indicated before, the dicarboxylyl-CoAs are oxidized almost exclusively in peroxisomes by AOX of the classical $\beta$-oxidation pathway (55).

In the mitochondria, the long-chain acyl-CoA esters are transported by a carnitine-dependent mechanism through the inner membrane into the matrix, the place where the $\beta$-oxidation reactions occur (21). Short- and medium-chain fatty acid esters do not require specific transport mechanisms to reach the mitochondrial matrix. The peroxisomal membrane does not contain CPT I and carnitine translocase, and as a consequence, the long-chain acyl-CoAs do not require carnitine for their entry into the peroxisome matrix (21, 33). In essence, the nonspecific permeability of the peroxisomal membrane may facilitate the diffusion of amphiphilic fatty acyl-CoAs. In peroxisomes, both carnitine octanoyltransferase and carnitine acetyltransferase are present in the matrix, but their exact functional role in peroxisomal $\beta$-oxidation remains unclear (33). Peroxisomal membranes also contain adrenoleukodystrophy protein (ALDP), a member of the ATP-binding cassette (ABC) transporter family, and peroxisomal membrane protein (PMP) 70, but their role, if any, in fatty acid or fatty acyl-CoA transport remains unclear (53, 59, 78).

## Presence of Two Sets of Peroxisomal $\beta$-Oxidation Enzymes: Inducible and Noninducible Systems

Although mitochondrial $\beta$-oxidation is primarily involved in the catabolism of short-, medium-, and long-chain fatty acids, the peroxisomal $\beta$-oxidation is largely responsible for the degradation of a number of less-abundant carboxylates of different molecular structure (21, 33, 77). The substrates for peroxisomal $\beta$-oxidation include VLCFAs ($>C_{20}$), 2-methyl-branched fatty acids, dicarboxylic acids, prostanoids, and the $C_{27}$ bile acid intermediates, which are converted to the mature $C_{24}$ bile acid intermediates via $\beta$-oxidation. Similar to mitochondrial $\beta$-oxidation, peroxisomal fatty acid $\beta$-oxidation has four steps: (*a*) an oxidation reaction, in which the acyl-CoA is desaturated to a 2-*trans*-enoyl-CoA; (*b*) a hydration reaction, which converts the enoyl-CoA to a 3-hydroxyacyl-CoA; (*c*) a second oxidation step, which dehydrogenates the hydroxy intermediate to a 3-ketocyl-CoA; and (*d*) thiolytic cleavage, which releases acetyl-CoA and an acyl-CoA that is two carbon atoms shorter than the original molecule and that can reenter the spiral for the next round of $\beta$-oxidation (32, 33, 48). The first step is catalyzed by a $H_2O_2$-generating acyl-CoA oxidase, the second and third steps by a bifunctional protein (hydration plus dehydrogenation), and the fourth (last) step by a thiolase (thiolytic cleavage). During the past 5 years, it has become evident that two or more acyl-CoA oxidases, two different bifunctional proteins, and two different thiolases exist in most mammals (6, 8, 9, 13, 19, 20, 33, 42). Based mostly on substrate specificity of the oxidase that initiates the first and rate-limiting step, two different $\beta$-oxidation pathways have been proposed to operate within the peroxisome (Figure 1). The classical pathway generally utilizes straight-chain saturated fatty acyl-CoAs as substrates, whereas the recently discovered second $\beta$-oxidation pathway acts on 2-methyl-branched fatty acids and on the bile acid intermediates (33, 55, 98). In the L-hydroxy–specific classical $\beta$-oxidation spiral, dehydrogenation of acyl-CoA esters to their corresponding *trans-2-enoyl*-CoAs is catalyzed by AOX, whereas the second and third reactions, hydration and dehydrogenation, of enoyl-CoA esters, to 3-ketoacyl-CoA, are carried out by a single enzyme, enoyl-CoA hydratase/L-3-hydroxyacyl-CoA dehydrogenase [L-bifunctional enzyme (L-PBE); also known as multifunctional protein-1] (33, 55, 77). The third enzyme of this classical system, 3-ketoacyl-CoA thiolase, cleaves 3-ketoacyl-CoAs to acetyl-CoA and an acyl-CoA that is two carbon atoms shorter than the original molecule and that can reenter the $\beta$-oxidation spiral (49, 77). All enzymes of this classical pathway are found in various species and can be strongly induced by peroxisome proliferators and other biological ligands of PPAR$\alpha$ in the liver of rats and mice (23, 74). In the second, D-3-hydroxy–specific $\beta$-oxidation pathway, dehydrogenation of acyl-CoA esters to their corresponding *trans*-2-enoyl-CoAs is catalyzed in humans by the branched-chain acyl-CoA oxidase (8, 9, 33, 79, 96). The recently identified D-3-hydroxyacyl-CoA dehydratase/D-3-hydroxyacyl-CoA dehydrogenase [D-bifunctional enzyme (D-PBE); also known as multifunctional protein-2], then converts enoyl-CoAs to 3-ketoacyl-CoAs via D-3-hydroxyacyl-CoAs (19, 20, 33, 42, 56, 70, 98). The third enzyme of this second system is designated sterol carrier protein (SCP)x, the N-terminal part of which exerts thiolytic activity (33, 44, 55, 57, 99). The first desaturation step in this D-3-hydroxy–specific $\beta$-oxidation spiral is executed by either trihydroxycoprostanoyl-CoA oxidase (which acts on bile acid intermediates) or pristanoyl-CoA oxidase (which facilitates pristanic acid breakdown) in rats, but in humans this first and rate-limiting step of this second $\beta$-oxidation pathway is executed by one enzyme only, the branched-chain acyl-CoA oxidase, which is the counterpart of rat trihydroxycoprostanoyl-CoA oxidase (8). Emerging evidence strongly indicates that separation between two peroxisomal $\beta$-oxidation pathways may not be that rigid after the initial first desaturation step catalyzed by specific oxidase (6, 67). It appears that the L- and D-hydroxy intermediates generated in the two $\beta$-oxidations systems can be metabolized to a variable extent by either L-PBE or D-PBE (see below).

## Individual Peroxisomal $\beta$-Oxidation System Enzymes

***First Step of the $\beta$-Oxidation Cycle Catalyzed by Acyl-CoA Oxidases***    The first reaction of peroxisomal $\beta$-oxidation is catalyzed by FAD-containing oxidases that donate electrons directly to molecular oxygen, thereby generating $H_2O_2$ (33, 48, 77). In the classical $\beta$-oxidation spiral, which deals with straight-chain acyl-CoAs, this step is catalyzed by acyl-CoA oxidase, a single enzyme, in all species examined. In the branched-chain $\beta$-oxidation spiral, the first reaction is also catalyzed by only one oxidase (branched-chain acyl-CoA oxidase) in humans, which appears to be active for both 2-methyl-branched fatty acids and bile acid intermediates (8). However, in rats, two different oxidases are present, namely pristanoyl-CoA oxidase and trihydroxycoprostanoyl-CoA oxidase, which catalyze, respectively, the branched-chain fatty acids and the bile acid intermediates (9, 55, 79).

The acyl-CoA oxidase of the classical $\beta$-oxidation system is 140 kDa and consists of two subunits of 72 kDa (component A), which can be proteolytically cleaved into 52-kDa (component B) and 21-kDa (component C) products within the peroxisome matrix (32, 62, 97). This enzyme oxidizes the CoA-esters of medium-chain, long-chain, and VLCFAs, medium-chain and long-chain dicarboxylic acids, and prostaglandins (33, 55). The enzyme is highly active toward substrates with longer carbon chain length but inactive toward substrates having acyl moieties of eight or fewer carbon atoms (77). The human acyl-CoA oxidase gene, localized to chromosome band 17q25, is present as a single copy per haploid genome, with 13 introns in the protein coding region, and it is structurally similar to the rat gene (97). There are two different sequences for exon 3 (3-I and 3-II), resulting from alternate use of exon 3 in splicing. Human acyl-CoA oxidase gene encodes a 660–amino acid residue, whereas the rat gene encodes a 661–amino acid protein. Both rat and human acyl-CoA oxidase cDNAs contain a Ser-Lys-Leu peroxisomal targeting signal (PTS1) in the COOH-terminal end. The enzyme probably exists in three forms: $A_2$, ABC, and $B_2C_2$ (32). By immuofluorescence and immunocytochemical methods, this enzyme is localizable to peroxisome matrix and is present in liver cells as well as in extrahepatic tissues. This enzyme is inducible by peroxisome proliferators by activating PPAR$\alpha$ (see below).

In humans, the branched-chain acyl-CoA oxidase functions as the first and rate-limiting step (*a*) of the second $\beta$-oxidation pathway acting on 2-methyl-branched fatty acids, such as pristanic acid, which is derived from phytol contained in food, and (*b*) of the bile acid intermediates, di- and trihydroxycoprostanoic acids, which also contain a 2-methyl substitution in their side chain (8, 96). Unlike in humans, the branched-chain $\beta$-oxidation pathway in rats can be initiated by two different noninducible oxidases, namely pristanoyl-CoA oxidase and trihydroxycoprostanoyl-CoA oxidase (33, 55, 79). Pristanoyl-CoA oxidase acts on the CoA esters of

2-methyl-branched fatty acids, whereas the trihydroxycoprostanoyl-CoA oxidase uses bile acid intermediates as substrates. The human branched-chain AOX cDNA encodes a protein of 681 amino acids, calculated to be 76,739 Da (8). The enzyme is encoded by a single-copy gene, present on chromosome 3p14.3, and is expressed in liver and several other extrahepatic tissues (8). Sequence comparison with the other acyl-CoA oxidases shows that despite its broader substrate specificity, the human branched-chain acyl-CoA oxidase is the homologue of rat trihydroxycoprostanoyl-CoA oxidase and separate gene-duplication events led to the occurrence in mammals of peroxisomal acyl-CoA oxidases with different substrate specificities (8, 55). Rat trihydroxycoprostanoyl-CoA oxidase is 139 kDa and consists of two identical subunits of 69 kDa (9). Rat pristanoyl-CoA oxidase, which mostly uses CoA esters of 2-methyl-branched fatty acids as substrates, also exhibits some activity with the CoA esters of straight-chain fatty acids, but this enzyme does not appear to be sufficient to carry out the straight-chain fatty acid β-oxidation in mice deficient in classical inducible AOX (95). It is 420 kDa and consists of identical subunits of 70 kDa (95). All three AOXs possess a C-terminal PTS 1 signal (9, 70, 83, 95).

***Second and Third Steps Catalyzed by Two Different Bifunctional Proteins***    The second step of the peroxisomal β-oxidation is the hydration of the enoyl-CoAs to 3-hydroxyacyl-CoAs, which are then dehydrogenated to generate 3-ketoacyl-CoAs in the third step (32, 33, 48, 55, 77). A single protein, with both enoyl-CoA hydratase/3-hydroxyacyl-CoA dehydrogenase activities, hence called peroxisomal bifunctional enzyme (PBE), catalyzes these two steps. Because this protein also exhibits enoyl-CoA isomerase activity, it is also referred to as trifunctional or multifunctional protein (33, 47, 64). Peroxisomes contain two bifunctional proteins: The first is the L-hydroxy–specific enoyl-CoA hydratase/L-3-hydroxyacyl-CoA dehydrogenase [called L-bifunctional protein (L-PBE) because the hydrated species it generates has the L-configuration] of the classical peroxisome proliferator-inducible β-oxidation spiral, and the second is the D-3-hydroxyacyl-CoA dehydratase/D-3-hydroxyacyl-CoA dehydrogenase [called D-bifunctional protein (D-PBE)] of the branched-chain noninducible β-oxidation system.

The L-PBE, which has been purified from rat and human liver, is a monomeric protein of 79 kDa (32, 33). The enoyl-CoA hydratase activity lies in the N-terminal portion and the L-3-hydroxyacyl-CoA dehydrogenase activity lies in the C-terminal part of the protein. The structure of the N-terminal and C-terminal sides of L-PBE are similar to that of enoyl-CoA hydratase (crotonase) and 3-hydroxyacyl-CoA dehydrogenase, respectively, of the mitochondrial matrix-bound β-oxidation enzymes (33). D-PBE, on the other hand, is a homodimer of two 77-kDa subunits, and it has been shown that D-PBE cleaves in vivo within the peroxisome matrix into the enoyl-CoA hydratase component (45 kDa) and the D-3-hydroxyacyl-CoA dehydrogenase component (35 kDa) (19, 20). The D-PBE also has a C-terminal PTS 1 signal (50). Unlike that of L-PBE, the N-terminal portion of D-PBE contains the D-3-hydroxyacyl-CoA dehydrogenase activity (note that in L-PBE, the N-terminal part contains enoyl-CoA hydratase activity), and the central part contains the enoyl-CoA hydratase activity (33). In this regard the structure of D-PBE is similar to that of yeast multifunctional proteins catalyzing the two reactions with the D-isomer of 3-hydroxyacyl-CoA (33). The C-terminal part of D-PBE exhibits homology to SCP2 (56, 57). Comparison of the L-PBE and D-PBE cDNAs reveals that they have very little sequence homology and differ markedly in their structure. First, in rats, the L-PBE gene spans about 31 kb and consists of seven exons and six introns. The human L-PBE gene is localized to chromosome 3q26.3-3q28 (38), and its structure is similar to that of the rat L-PBE (M Malki & JK Reddy, unpublished data). On the other hand, the D-PBE gene spans >100 kb and consists of 24 exons and 23 introns (50). The substrate specificities of both enzymes differ in that both enzymes can metabolize straight-chain enoyl-CoAs as substrates, but they differ markedly with respect to branched-chain fatty enoyl-CoAs, with respect to $3\alpha$-, $7\alpha$-, and $12\alpha$-hydroxy-$5\beta$-cholest-24-enoyl-CoA, and with respect to $3\alpha$- and $7\alpha$-dihyroxy-$5\beta$-cholest-24-enoyl-CoA, which seem to be more desirable as substrates for D-PBE (33, 55). Finally, the L-PBE, but not the D-PBE, is markedly induced by peroxisome proliferators (33, 77).

***Last Reaction is Also Catalyzed by Two Different Enzymes***    Peroxisomes contain two distinct enzymes capable of thiolytically cleaving 3-ketoacyl-CoA into a chain-shortened acyl-CoA and acetyl-CoA or propionyl-CoA (in case of two methyl branched fatty acids) (13, 33, 55, 57, 62, 77). These two enzymes are the well-known 3-ketoacyl-CoA thiolase of the inducible classic straight-chain $\beta$-oxidation system, and the recently discovered SCPx of the noninducible branched-chain $\beta$-oxidation system (13, 17, 33, 77). 3-Ketoacyl-CoA thiolase is a homodimer of 89 kDa. It is synthesized as a precursor protein of 44 kDa and is proteolytically cleaved to its mature size of 41 kDa (32). In rats, there are two genes (A and B) for peroxisomal 3-ketoacyl-CoA thiolase (32, 62). Gene A is constitutively expressed at a low level, whereas gene B transcript is barely detectable in normal liver but is dramatically inducible by peroxisome proliferators (33, 62). Thiolase A and B proteins show similar biochemical properties and the same substrate specificities except for some difference in N-terminal amino acid sequences (13). Human liver peroxisomes contain only one 3-ketoacyl-CoA thiolase, and the gene encoding this protein, mapped to chromosome 3p23-p22, shows high homology to both rat genes (77). Rat and human 3-ketoacyl-CoA thiolases contain an N-terminal cleavable PTS2 sequence (77, 83).

The thiolytic function of the second $\beta$-oxidation system in peroxisomes is performed by SCPx, a 58-kDa protein with the 3-ketoacyl-CoA thiolase activity in the N-terminal domain and with SCP2 (a lipid carrier or transfer protein) function in the C-terminal domain (33, 57). SCP2 and SCPx are expressed by the same gene, which is mapped to human chromosome 1p32.

The 3-ketoacyl-CoA thiolase and SCPx exhibit distinct substrate specificities: The former enzyme plays a principal but restricted role in the $\beta$-oxidation of straight-chain 3-ketoacyl-CoAs, and the latter plays a broader role in the cleavage not only of branched-chain fatty acids, and the bile acid intermediates, but also of 3-ketoacyl-CoAs of straight-chain fatty acids (33, 55).

## $\beta$-OXIDATION OF POLYUNSATURATED FATTY ACIDS

Polyunsaturated fatty acids (n-3 and n-6) are $\beta$-oxidized in both peroxisomes and mitochondria; however, for this to occur, the double bonds of unsaturated fatty acids must be processed to generate *trans*-2-enoyl-CoA intermediate (36). The removal of preexisting double bonds requires accessory proteins. Two enzymes—a 2,4-dienoyl-CoA reductase and a $\Delta^3$-*cis*,$\Delta^2$-*trans*-enoyl-CoA isomerase—process a double bond in a fatty acid at an even-numbered position (52). Three enzymes—a $\Delta^3$-*cis*,$\Delta^2$-*trans*-enoyl-CoA isomerase, a $\Delta^{3,5}$-$\Delta^{2,4}$-di-enoyl-CoA isomerase, and a 2,4-dienoyl-CoA reductase—process fatty acids with double bonds at odd-numbered positions. The peroxisomal 2,4-dienoyl-CoA reductase has a PTS1 signal, and $\Delta^3$-*cis*,$\Delta^2$-*trans*-enoyl-CoA isomerase is a function of the L-PBE, as indicated before (52). Human and rat peroxisomal $\Delta^{3,5}$-$\Delta^{2,4}$-di-enoyl-CoA isomerase proteins are 36 kDa and contain PTS1 signal (52). Dietary $\gamma$-linolenic acid– and fish oil–containing diets rich in omega-3 polyunsaturated fatty acids, such as docosahexanoic acid (DHA) and eicosapentaenoic acid (EPA), are known to increase peroxisomal $\beta$-oxidation in liver and lower serum triglycerides (3, 47). DHA is essential for normal growth and functional development of brain, and it preferentially binds brain fatty acid binding protein (B-FABP), a member of the fatty acid binding protein family.

The role of peroxisomal $\beta$-oxidation in the synthesis and metabolism of DHA (3, 5, 9, 12, 14, 17–20:6) and retroconversion of DHA to EPA is depicted in Figure 2. Synthesis of DHA requires (*a*) the enzymes in both peroxisomes and smooth endoplasmic reticulum and (*b*) regulated movement of fatty acids between these two compartments (3, 55, 77). Chain elongation of 7, 10, 13, 16, 19–22:5 fatty acid to 9, 12, 15, 18, 21–24:5 and its desaturation to 6, 9, 12, 15, 18, 21–24:6 occurs in microsomes. This fatty acid is then moved to peroxisomes without esterification. In peroxisomes, it is either partially $\beta$-oxidized (3, 5, 9, 12, 14, 17–20:6) or transported to microsomes to form 1-acyl-sn-glycerol-3-phosphocholine, or fully $\beta$-oxidized to yield EPA (4, 7, 10, 15–18:5).

## LIGAND BINDING PROTEINS

Very-long-chain and long-chain fatty acids and their CoA esters are not only the molecules involved in lipid metabolism, as substrates, they also function as PPAR ligands (12, 22, 86). The intracellular concentrations of fatty acids and their derivatives are strictly regulated, which implies the existence of integrated circuits to sense changes in serum and cellular fatty acid levels. Because of extremely low aqueous solubility, the intracellular distribution and trafficking of these PPAR

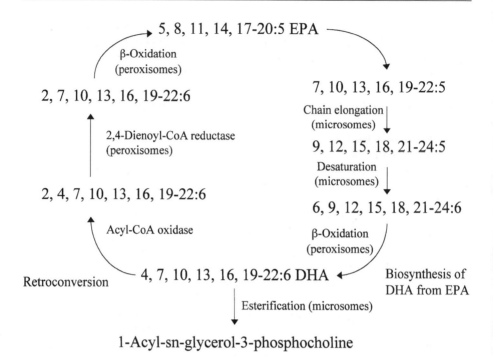

**Figure 2**  Peroxisomal $\beta$-oxidation of polyunsaturated fatty acids and retroconversion of docosa-hexaenoic acid (DHA) to eicosapentaenoic acid (EPA). DHA [22:6(n-3)] and EPA [20:5(n-3)] are interconverted and the process involves the participation of smooth endoplasmic reticulum (microsomes) and peroxisomes.

ligands is modulated by lipid binding proteins (FABP), fatty acyl-CoA binding protein (ACBP), and SCP2 (also called nonspecific lipid carrier protein). These proteins modulate free ligand concentrations in several ways: (*a*) concentrations of binding proteins, (*b*) association constants, (*c*) specificities, (*d*) intracellular localization, and (*e*) cell-tissue–specific expression. FABP and ACBP are cytosolic in distribution, and SCP2 is present exclusively within the peroxisome matrix. Despite the identification of proteins that bind these lipid ligands of PPAR, little is known about the mechanisms by which ligand-binding proteins control receptor-mediated gene expression.

## Fatty Acid Binding Proteins

FABPs form a conserved family of intracellular monomeric lipid binding proteins with low molecular mass ($\sim$15 kDa). The following FABPs are of particular relevance: liver (L-FABP), heart (H-FABP), intestine (I-FABP), and brain (B-FABP). They form 1:1 complexes with fatty acids or other hydrophobic ligands, except that L-FABP is capable of binding two molecules of fatty acids (12). Many of the cell types express more than one type of FABP: L-FABP in liver, L-FABP and H-FABP in kidney, H-FABP and B-FABP in brain, L-FABP and I-FABP in intestine, and H-FABP and I-FABP in stomach. FABPs are thought to bind and target fatty acids to various sites within the cell. L-FABP is induced in response to fatty acids and peroxisome proliferators (12).

## Acyl-CoA Binding Protein

Various cells contain a cytosolic high-affinity acyl-CoA binding protein (ACBP). It is a low-molecular-mass protein (10 kDa) and is identical to a protein known as diazepam-binding inhibitor (86), a modulator of the GABA receptor in brain membranes. The main function of ACBP in lipid metabolism appears to be the modulation of acyl-CoA concentrations within the cell. Acyl-CoA affects the activities of various enzymes. For example, by its ability to bind acyl-CoAs, ACBP effectively opposes the product feedback inhibition of the long-chain acyl-CoA synthetase and shows a string-attenuating effect on the long-chain acyl-CoA inhibition of acetyl-CoA carboxylase. Acyl-CoAs function as ligands for transcription factors and regulate intracellular signaling. ACBP promoter has a sterol regulatory element-like sequence motif (86), which has led to the speculation that ACBP may play a role in steroidogenesis.

## Sterol Carrier Protein-2

SCP2 binds sterols, phospholipids, long-chain isoprenoids, long-chain fatty acids, and long-chain fatty acyl-CoAs. SCP2 also binds branched-chain fatty acids and may be specifically involved in their peroxisomal $\beta$-oxidation (44). SCP2, a 15-kDa protein, contains a PTS1 and is one of the most abundant proteins present in peroxisomes. SCP2 and SCPx are derived from the same gene by alternate use of promoters (57). SCP2 and SCPx share the C-terminal 123–amino acid sequence and a PTS1 (57). SCP2 interacts with long-chain acyl-CoAs and forms specific complexes with acyl-CoA oxidase and other $\beta$-oxidation enzymes. In this capacity, SCP2 appears to facilitate peroxisomal $\beta$-oxidation by supplying fatty acyl-CoA esters and by removing the oxidized or chain-shortened products of $\beta$-oxidation (33). It is conceivable that SCP2 stabilizes $\beta$-oxidation enzymes by protein-protein interaction, a function that may be altered in diabetes because of a change in the SCP2 content in liver (33).

## REGULATORY ROLE OF PPAR$\alpha$

## Peroxisome Proliferators (Ligands for PPAR$\alpha$)

Several structurally diverse chemicals with hypolipidemic properties have been shown to induce peroxisome proliferation in the livers of rats and mice, and a receptor-mediated mechanism for the induction of these pleiotropic responses was proposed (75, 76). These agents, designated as peroxisome proliferators (75), currently encompass a broad spectrum of synthetic and naturally/biologically occurring compounds that function as PPARα ligands (39). Synthetic peroxisome proliferators include certain hypolipidemic drugs, phthalate ester plasticizers, herbicides, food flavors, and leukotriene $D_4$ receptor antagonists (30, 76). In general, peroxisome proliferators exhibit little obvious structural similarity; the only shared chemical feature is that each of these either is or has the potential to be transformed into a carboxylic acid derivative, and these acid properties may be of critical importance to their ability to induce the peroxisome proliferative response. Natural/biological factors that are capable of increasing fatty acid β-oxidation activity and inducing variable degrees of peroxisome proliferation in hepatocytes include high-fat diets [especially diets rich in VLCFAs ($>C_{20}$) and polyunsaturated fatty acids, such as DHA and EPA], phytanic acid, the adrenal steroid dehydroepiandrosterone, and eicosanoids derived from arachidonic acid either via the lipoxygenase pathway, leading to the formation of leukotrienes and dehydroxyeicosatetraenoic acids, or via a cyclooxygenase pathway generating prostaglandins (30). Despite their structural diversity, the synthetic peroxisome proliferators, as a group, induce in rats and mice qualitatively predictable pleiotropic responses consisting of hepatomegaly, proliferation of peroxisomes in liver parenchymal cells, and the induction of several hepatic enzymes, particularly those responsible for lipid metabolism (30, 48, 75, 76). Long-term exposure to synthetic peroxisome proliferators and the sustained induction of peroxisome proliferation in livers leads to the development of hepatocellular carcinoma in rats and mice (30, 72, 72a). Peroxisome proliferators, in general, have been consistently found to be nonmutagenic (nongenotoxic), in that they do not interact with or damage DNA either directly or after metabolic activation, thereby leading to the proposal that the development of liver tumors is attributable to sustained induction of peroxisome proliferation (30, 72a, 76). In this regard, it is pertinent to note that in mice with disrupted AOX gene, sustained peroxisome proliferation occurring spontaneously also causes liver tumors, indicating that substrates for the classical peroxisomal β-oxidation system function as ligands for PPARα and that unmetabolized ligands cause sustained hyperstimulation of PPARα transcriptional activity (23) (see also below). Proliferation of peroxisomes in liver is associated with >15-fold increases in the activities of the enzymes required for peroxisomal β-oxidation of fatty acids, and these now fall under the category of the inducible classical L-hydroxy–specific peroxisomal β-oxidation pathway (72a, 74). Peroxisome proliferation is also associated with profound induction of microsomal CYP4A family of fatty acid ω-oxidation system enzymes (31, 43). The increases in the activities of these enzymes also parallel the increases in the peroxisomal β-oxidation enzyme system and reflect transcriptional activation of the respective genes (31, 74). Several other genes are also induced in livers with peroxisome proliferation, and the recent application of cDNA microarray technology is providing new insights into the hepatic gene expression profiles during peroxisome proliferation.

## PPAR Isotypes

Significant progress has been made during the past decade in understanding the mechanisms responsible for the induction of genes involved in peroxisomal, microsomal, and mitochondrial fatty acid oxidation systems in liver by peroxisome proliferators. The existence of a specific receptor(s) responsible for the action of peroxisome proliferators was first postulated in 1983, based the cell/tissue specificity of pleiotropic responses, rapid transcriptional activation of fatty acid oxidation system genes, response of extrahepatic hepatocytes to the inductive effects of peroxisome proliferators, and the presence of specific binding protein(s) in liver cytosol for amphipathic carboxylates (73, 74, 76). These tenets, in essence, formed the impetus for the identification and molecular cloning of a receptor, now known as PPAR$\alpha$, from mouse liver that is activated by structurally diverse peroxisome proliferators (39). The induction of some of the critical enzymes of the peroxisomal, mitochondrial, and microsomal fatty acid oxidation systems by peroxisome proliferators is transcriptionally controlled by PPAR$\alpha$, as these effects are abrogated in PPAR$\alpha$ null mice (49). Two other PPAR isotypes, PPAR$\gamma$ and PPAR$\delta$, also appear to be important in lipid homeostasis, but they do not participate in the mediation of peroxisome proliferator–induced pleiotropic responses (4, 17, 35, 81). These isotypes are encoded by distinct genes, which are located on different chromosomes in humans and mice (for a review, see 17). The PPAR$\gamma$ gene generates two transcripts, designated PPAR$\gamma$1 and PPAR$\gamma$2, resulting from differential mRNA splicing and promoter usage (103). It plays an important role in adipocyte differentiation and, therefore, storage of fatty acids (4, 82). In conditions associated with excess energy consumption, acetyl-CoA generated from glucose is utilized for fatty acid synthesis, and their subsequent conversion to triglycerides leads to PPAR$\gamma$ promotion of adipogenesis and lipid storage (28, 82, 91). PPAR$\gamma$ null mutation is lethal around embryonic day (E)10, and it appears that this receptor is required for epithelial differentiation of trophoblast tissue, and for proper placental vascularization (7). Lipodystrophy, abnormalities of cardiac development, and multiple hemorrhages occur in tetraploid-rescued mutants surviving to term, indicating that PPAR$\gamma$ orchestrates a spectrum of physiological processes (7). The specific functional role of PPAR$\beta(\delta)$ remains elusive, as little is known about the target genes of this receptor. Disruption of PPAR$\beta$ gene results in myelination and epidermal cell proliferation defects (65).

PPARs, like other members of the nuclear receptor superfamily, display six regions or domains (4, 17, 39, 69, 100). The N-terminal portion of the receptor contains a variable A/B region, which exhibits a ligand-independent transactivation function (AF-1 domain). The central part of the receptor depicts a highly conserved C region composed of two type II zinc fingers that are responsible for sequence-specific DNA recognition and dimerization (DNA-binding domain). The C-terminal half of the PPAR is subdivided into D, E, and F regions, with the E region functioning as the ligand-binding domain. The crystal structures of ligand-binding domain of the human PPARγ and human PPARβ/δ reveal that the ligand-binding pocket is unusually large (~1300 Å$^3$), which may account for the accommodation of a diverse spectrum of synthetic and natural ligands and their variable ability to bind and to transactivate all three PPAR isoforms (100). This E region is relatively large, and highly conserved, and because of its ligand-binding property, it also functions as a ligand-dependent transactivation domain (AF-2 domain). The C-terminal F region is relatively small compared with other regions and is considered important in the interaction of nuclear receptors with nuclear receptor coactivators and corepressors (29, 69, 105).

The tissue distribution of PPARs to some extent reflects their function. PPARα is highly expressed in hepatocytes, enterocytes, proximal tubular epithelium of kidney, and cardiac muscle, and the expression pattern parallels, to a certain extent, the sensitivity of various tissues to the β-oxidation induction by synthetic peroxisome proliferators (4, 17). PPARγ is expressed predominantly in adipose tissue, liver, mammary gland, urinary bladder, and colonic mucosa (4, 17). PPARγ is involved in adipogenesis, and maintenance of differentiation may be an important function of this receptor in breast, colon, and urinary bladder. PPARβ is expressed widely in most tissues, but its function remains largely elusive (17).

## PPAR Response Elements

The PPARs form heterodimers with another nuclear receptor, the 9-*cis*-retinoic acid receptor (RXR), and the PPAR/RXR heterodimers bind to DNA sequences, termed PPAR response elements (PPREs), containing direct repeats (DR) of the hexanucleotide sequence AGGTCA separated by one nucleotide, known as a DR-1 response element, present in the 5'-flanking region of target genes. PPREs transcriptionally activated by peroxisome proliferators and that are present in the promoter sequences of some of the genes, such as AOX, involved in fatty acid oxidation have been characterized (17, 73). Contrary to some of the claims, the PPRE of the human AOX gene is functionally active (97).

## PPAR Cofactors

The biochemical and molecular mechanisms by which nuclear receptors achieve transcriptional activation, in a gene-, tissue-, and species-specific fashion, are the subjects of intense research activity (29). The current models call for participation of a series of cofactors (accessory proteins) that bind to nuclear receptors in a ligand-dependent fashion (29). During the past 5 years, several "coactivator" proteins for nuclear receptors have been identified (29). Of these, steroid receptor coactivator (SRC)-1 (103), PPAR-binding protein (PBP) (106), PPARγ-coactivator-1 (PGC-1) (66), PPAR interaction protein (PRIP) (104), and others have been identified as PPAR coactivators (for a review, see 29, 69). A model depicting the interaction of PPARα-coactivator complexes with the basal transcription machinery is depicted in Figure 3. Mice lacking SRC-1 are viable and

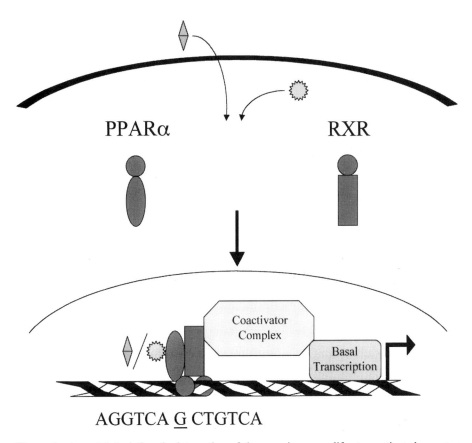

AGGTCA <u>G</u> CTGTCA

**Figure 3**  A model depicting the interaction of the peroxisome proliferator–activated receptor $\alpha$ (PPAR$\alpha$)-coactivator complexes with basal transcription machinery, leading to the enhanced transcription of target genes. Liganded PPAR$\alpha$ interacts with 9-*cis*-retinoic acid receptor (RXR) to form PPAR$\alpha$/RXR heterodimers and recruit nuclear receptor coactivator protein complexes for linking with the basal transcription apparatus. The sequence AGGTCA G CTGTCA represents the PPAR response (DR1) element of the human AOX gene of the classical peroxisomal $\beta$-oxidation spiral. The synthetic ligands (diamonds) and the natural/biological ligands (asterisks) interact with PPAR$\alpha$.

fertile (68, 101) and responded to peroxisome proliferators in a fashion analogous to wild-type mice exposed to peroxisome proliferators, indicating functional redundancy of SRC-1 with regard to PPAR$\alpha$ function (68). In contrast, mice homozygous for PBP null mutation exhibited lethality around E11.5, indicating the critical importance of this coactivator in development (40, 107). Elucidation of the tissue- and cell-specific mechanisms of transcriptional activation of genes involved in peroxisomal $\beta$-oxidation is essential for a greater appreciation of the importance of lipid homeostasis in health and disease.

## DISORDERS OF PEROXISOMAL LIPID METABOLISM

### Peroxisomal Diseases

Since the first description of peroxisomal absence in liver and kidney in patients with Zellweger syndrome, several peroxisomal disorders, a majority manifesting as disturbances in lipid metabolism, have been documented (92, 98). Peroxisomal disorders, classified on the basis of biochemical defects, generally fall into three categories, depending on whether there is a generalized (group A), multiple (group B), or a single (group C) loss of peroxisomal functions (98). Groups A and B are mostly related to defects in posttranslational import of peroxisomal matrix proteins due to mutations in peroxins (83). Peroxins PEX5 and PEX7 function as receptors for PTS1 and PTS2, respectively, and mutations in these receptors lead to defects in the import of PTS1, or PTS1 and PTS2, proteins (83). Because peroxisomal $\beta$-oxidation is not a functional duplication of the mitochondrial system, abnormalities in the peroxisomal $\beta$-oxidation pathway involve specifically the metabolism of VLCFAs, long-chain dicarboxylic acids (DCAs), pristanic acid, certain prostaglandins and leukotrienes, and 15-hydroxyeicosatetraenoic acid, among others (55, 77, 98).

The Zellweger syndrome, neonatal adrenoleukodystrophy, and infantile Refsum's disease are examples of group A with generalized defects in peroxisome assembly, manifesting in the functional loss of many peroxisomal enzymes (98). In these group A diseases, the molecular basis appears to be a dysfunction of *PEX5*, which encodes the PTS1 receptor, necessary for peroxisomal import of such proteins as AOX, L-PBE, D-PBE, and many others with the C-terminal PTS1 (83). Dysfunction of PEX7, which encodes the PTS2 receptor, is also found in group A diseases. These patients reveal abnormalities in the $\beta$-oxidation of VLCFAs and multiple dysmorphogenetic features, including craniofacial, neurological, ocular, hepatological, and skeletal anomalies. Peroxisomes are generally absent, but mitochondrial abnormalities become prominent, in liver cells of Zellweger syndrome patients. Hepatic steatosis is variable, but detailed information on the evolution of hepatic changes in these genetic disorders and the status of PPAR$\alpha$ expression in liver is lacking.

Rhizomelic chondrodysplasia punctata is an example of a group B peroxisomal disorder with defects in ether-phospholipid metabolism due to abnormalities in dihydroxyacetonephosphate acyltransferase and alkyldihydroxyacetonephosphate synthase and to an abnormality in phytanic acid $\alpha$-oxidation (98). The molecular basis is attributed to dysfunction of *PEX7*, which encodes the PTS2 receptor, necessary for peroxisomal import of enzymes such as thiolase, which contain N-terminal PTS2 (83). The hepatic phenotype in this rare genetic disease is not well delineated.

Peroxisomal disorders, characterized by the loss of a single peroxisomal function due to loss/mutation in a single gene, belong to group C (single enzyme deficiency). The several disorders relevant to the discussion of peroxisomal

$\beta$-oxidation include X-linked adrenoleukodystrophy (X-ALD), straight-chain AOX deficiency, D-PBE deficiency, and thiolase deficiency (98). X-ALD, a most frequent peroxisomal genetic disorder, presents either as a lethal childhood form or as a mild "Addison's only" form (98). In this disorder, VLCFAs accumulate because of impaired peroxisomal $\beta$-oxidation. The defect in this condition was initially thought to be a deficiency of very-long-chain acyl-CoA synthetase, which activates VLCFAs to their corresponding CoA esters at the site of peroxisomal membrane, but it is now attributed to a defect in a 80-kDa peroxisomal membrane protein, called adrenoleukodystrophy protein (ALDP), which belongs to the ATP-binding cassette (ABC) transporter superfamily (53, 54, 98). ALDP functions as a homo- or heterodimer and participates in the transport of $C_{26:0}$ CoA esters across the peroxisome membrane into the peroxisome matrix. In X-ALD patients, a variety of mutations, including deletions, point mutations, and insertions, in the ALDP gene have been observed (98). The other diseases belonging to group C include deficiency of one of the enzymes of the straight-chain or branched-chain $\beta$-oxidation systems. Only a few patients with classical AOX deficiency have been reported, and some of these have a large deletion of the oxidase gene (26). The absence of straight-chain AOX leads to deficient oxidation of C26:0 fatty acids only, without affecting the oxidation of branched-chain fatty acids (26). Peroxisomes are present in liver cells in this condition, but detailed descriptions of liver morphology are lacking. Few patients with D-PBE deficiency or 3-ketoacyl-CoA thiolase deficiency have been identified (93, 94, 98). VLCFA and pristanic acid oxidation is affected in D-PBE deficiency, resulting in increased plasma levels. Evidence indicates that D-PBE deficiency is more severe than AOX deficiency but less severe than thiolase deficiency (98). The magnitude of functional anomalies in thiolase deficiency is similar to that encountered in Zellweger syndrome (98). D-PBE deficiency is less severe in part because of the functional redundancy between L-PBE and D-PBE.

The major unresolved issue is how individuals with genetic defects in peroxisomal $\beta$-oxidation or PPAR$\alpha$-inducible genes react to nutritional stress. Data from genetically altered animal models points to the intricacies of basal metabolism and to such rapid, egregious amplification of response to stress as short-term energy deprivation. It is important to note that children with an inherited deficiency of mitochondrial medium-chain acyl-CoA dehydrogenase, a PPAR$\alpha$-inducible mitochondrial $\beta$-oxidation enzyme, develop normally and are mostly asymptomatic, but during fasting-related stress they decompensate and die suddenly (11, 87).

## Fatty Acid Oxidation in Genetically Altered Mice

Of the three PPARs, the PPAR$\alpha$ isotype plays a prominent role in the catabolism of fatty acids and is solely responsible for the peroxisome proliferator–induced pleiotropic responses, including the transcriptional activation of genes involved in fatty acid oxidation in livers of rats and mice (49). Sustained activation of PPAR$\alpha$ and the induction of PPAR$\alpha$-responsive genes that participate in lipid catabolism in the liver leads to the development of liver tumors (23, 30, 72, 76, 72a).

The purported relative nonresponsiveness of human liver cells to the peroxisome proliferator–induced pleiotropic effects may be attributed, in part, to differences in the levels of PPARα expression in rodents and humans (63). The identity of PPARα target genes involved in hepatic lipid catabolism is well delineated, and the use of gene targeting to disrupt PPARα and some of the genes involved in the peroxisomal β-oxidation system has led to major advances in our knowledge about the role of peroxisomal β-oxidation in regulating PPARα activity and in the pathogenesis of macrovesicular and microvesicular hepatic steatosis (5, 6, 23, 35, 44, 49, 67, 80). The studies with genetically altered mice underscore the importance of PPARα and of the peroxisomal β-oxidation systems, in particular the critical role of classical AOX, in hepatic lipid metabolism.

***Classical AOX Deficiency Leads to PPARα Activation***    The fatty acyl-CoA oxidase (AOX) deficiency disease (pseudoneonatal adrenoleukodystrophy) manifests in the neonatal period with hypotonia, varying extent of dysmorphic features, and pyschomotor retardation, with death occurring by 4–5 years of age (26). Mice with a disrupted classical AOX gene (AOX−/−) exhibit, during the first 2–4 months of age, high levels of VLCFAs in the serum, growth retardation, hepatomegaly with severe microvesicular steatohepatitis, and lipogranulomatous reaction (23). Lipogranulomas in liver contain macrophages, lymphocytes, eosinophils, and polymorphonuclear leukocytes, and in many of these lipogranulomas a central fat globule is discernable (23). AOX knockout mice reveal age-progressive hepatocellular regeneration commencing in the periportal region and extending toward the centrizonal region of the liver lobule (23). Between 6 and 8 months of age, almost all steatotic hepatocytes in AOX−/− mice are replaced by regenerated hepatocytes devoid of steatosis, but these cells display an abundance of peroxisomes (23). This spontaneous peroxisome proliferation is associated in liver with increased expression of genes that are transcriptionally regulated by PPARα. Among others that contain PPRE in their 5-flanking regions, these include L-PBE, thiolase, CYP4A1, and CYP4A3 (23). Increased $H_2O_2$ levels are evident in AOX−/− livers compared with age-matched controls. Hepatocellular adenomas and hepatocellular carcinomas develop in AOX−/− mice between 10 and 15 months of age (23). In essence, the phenotypic alterations in AOX−/− mice are similar to wild-type mice exposed chronically to potent synthetic peroxisome proliferators (23, 72a).

The AOX null mouse model serves as a paradigm for several important pathophysiological processes (23). First, disruption of the first and rate-limiting step of the classical peroxisomal β-oxidation system affects the metabolism of VLCFAs and other substrates of AOX, such as the proinflammatory arachidonic acid metabolites, leukotriene $B_4$, and 8(S)-hydroxyeicosatetraenoic acid. Second, it is evident that the unmetabolized acyl-CoAs derived from VLCFAs and DCAs— proinflammatory molecules such as leukotriene $B_4$ and 8(S)-hydroxyeicosatetraenoic acid and possibly other substrates of AOX—function as ligands for PPARα, leading to sustained hyperactivation of this receptor and up-regulation of downstream genes that contain PPRE (23). Sustained induction of CYP4A family genes, which metabolize LCFAs and VLCFAs, results in the excess generation of dicarboxylic acids (14). Rate of NADPH consumption is higher for human (CYP4A11) and rat (CYP4A1, CYP4A2, CYP4A3, and CYP4A8) isoforms than the rate of fatty acid hydroxylation, which implies that the enzymes undergo some degree of uncoupled turnover, indicating reduction of oxygen to superoxide and/or $H_2O_2$ (18, 37; U Hoch & P Oritz de Monetllano, personal communication). The toxic dicarboxylic acids cannot be further metabolized in the absence of AOX in these animals. Third, microvesicular hepatic steatosis and steatohepatitis observed in AOX$-/-$ mice appear to be the result of toxic effects of unmetabolized AOX substrates, which include VLCFAs and DCAs. In addition, the excess production of $H_2O_2$ due to inflammatory changes, to CYP4A-mediated $\omega$-hydroxylation, and to other $H_2O_2$-generating oxidases, such as urate oxidase in the liver of AOX$-/-$ mice (103), can further contribute to the "second hit" capable of inducing necroinflammatory steatohepatitis, leading to the formation of lipogranulomas (41). Fourth, sustained enhanced transcriptional activity of PPAR$\alpha$ on PPAR$\alpha$-regulated genes in liver in this AOX knockout model leads to the development of liver tumors. In AOX$-/-$ mouse liver, increased mRNA levels of genes regulated by PPAR$\alpha$, such as L-PBE, CYP4A1, and CYP4A3, are found, implying sustained activation of this receptor in AOX deficiency. Evidence points to the oncogenic potential of PPAR$\alpha$ (23, 30, 49), and to the fact that AOX gene function is indispensable for the physiological regulation of this receptor (23). It is evident that ligands for PPAR$\alpha$ function as substrates for the AOX, and because the gene encoding this enzyme is transcriptionally regulated by PPAR$\alpha$, this constitutes a critical cross talk because sustained up-regulation of PPAR$\alpha$-controlled genes leads to liver tumor development (23, 103). The principal function of AOX is to keep the PPAR$\alpha$ in check by $\beta$-oxidizing VLCFAs and other biological ligands of this receptor, including DCAs, the products of CYP4A-mediated $\omega$-oxidation. Evidence indicates that the mechanism of liver tumorigenesis in AOX knockout mice is most likely the result of sustained activation of PPAR$\alpha$ and oxidative stress emanating from proinflammatory responses and the induction of $H_2O_2$-generating enzymes.

***Disruption of Peroxisomal $\beta$-Oxidation Pathway Proximal to AOX***   For the $\beta$-oxidation process to begin, very-long-chain fatty acyl-CoAs have to enter peroxisome matrix. In X-ALD, a peroxisomal disorder with impaired VLCFA metabolism, the VLCFAs and/or their acyl-CoAs are not effectively transported into peroxisome because of defective ALDP, which is a transporter (53, 58, 59, 78). In this disease, there is progressive VLCFA accumulation, resulting in mental and motor function deterioration, with demyelination of the central and peripheral nervous system (98). A mouse model for x-linked adrenoleukodystrophy developed by gene targeting (54, 102) reveals no hepatic steatosis and no spontaneous peroxisome proliferation in liver cells, which suggests that disruption of classical peroxisomal $\beta$-oxidation proximal to AOX does not affect the generation and metabolism of PPAR$\alpha$ ligands. Also, because PPAR$\alpha$ is not hyperactivated in this x-linked adrenoleukodystrophy mouse model, the production of toxic dicarboxylic acids by CYP4A is also curtailed, unlike in AOX null mouse (23). These observations imply that VLCFAs are not the direct ligands of PPARα and that intact functional AOX is highly efficient in inactivating these ligands to keep PPARα in check (23).

***Disruption of Peroxisomal β-Oxidation Pathway Distal to AOX***    Mice homozygous for a disruption of the L-PBE gene, which encodes the second enzyme of the β-oxidation spiral, demonstrate that disruption of this classical β-oxidation pathway distal to AOX does not affect the metabolism of natural ligands of PPARα (67). Mice deficient in L-PBE displayed no hepatic steatosis, a feature that is striking in young AOX-deficient mice (23, 67). Disruption of the L-PBE gene also fails to induce spontaneous peroxisome proliferation such as that encountered in the regenerated liver cells of mice lacking AOX. These observations suggest that the hepatic steatogenic stimuli prominent in AOX null background are not present in L-PBE knockout mice, implying that AOX is necessary for their detoxification. The absence of spontaneous peroxisome proliferation in L-PBE null mice also indicates that classical AOX of the L-hydroxy–specific β-oxidation system is responsible for the metabolism of all putative ligands of PPARα (67), and that L-PBE enzyme, which is immediately downstream of AOX, is not essential for the successful completion of the L-hydroxy–specific β-oxidation (67). It would appear that once long and very long straight-chain acyl-CoAs, long-chain dicarboxylyl-CoAs, and the CoA esters of eicosanoids are converted into their respective enoyl-CoAs by the classical AOX, they can be metabolized by D-PBE of the D-hydroxy–specific branched-chain peroxisomal β-oxidation system (67), or even by the mitochondrial β-oxidation system. The AOX and L-PBE null mouse models convincingly prove that classical AOX is pivotal for the metabolic degradation of a bulk of PPARα ligands, and this class of ligands (substrates of classical AOX) is not metabolized by the branched-chain AOX of the second system (23, 67). Thus, it is reasonable to surmise that the functions of AOX (especially the metabolism of critical substrates of AOX, which serve as PPARα ligands) cannot be handled by the branched-chain AOX. Mice with a disrupted D-PBE (6) or SCPx gene (80) of the second system are generally devoid of hepatic steatosis, implying that L-PBE and thiolase of the classical system are capable of completing the β-oxidation reaction of either straight- or branched-chain enoyl-CoAs generated after the initial oxidase step. Further studies are needed to rule out the possibility that if left unmetabolized, straight-chain and branched-chain enoyl-CoAs serve as PPARα ligands (67). Generating mice deficient in both L-PBE and D-PBE and characterizing their liver phenotype should resolve this issue. The observations from these gene knockout mouse models indicate that the two peroxisomal β-oxidation pathways are not strictly separable after the oxidation (desaturation) step.

***Mice Nullizygous for Both PPARα and AOX***    PPARα knockout mice (PPARα −/−) established that this receptor is essential for hepatic peroxisome proliferation and coordinate transcriptional activation of AOX, L-PBE, peroxisomal thiolase, CYP4A1, CYP4A3, and other genes by structurally diverse synthetic peroxisome proliferators (49). PPAR$\alpha$ $-/-$ mice display a normal complement of peroxisomes in hepatocytes, but these mice remain nonresponsive to the inductive influence of synthetic peroxisome proliferators (49). They also fail to develop liver tumors when exposed to peroxisome proliferators, indicating the potential oncogenic nature of PPAR$\alpha$ and the contribution of PPAR$\alpha$-regulated genes to the neoplastic process (30). A mild degree of centrilobular macrovesicular fatty change develops in the liver of these mice. This is attributed to reduction in the constitutive levels of mitochondrial fatty acid $\beta$-oxidation, because the constitutive or basal oxidation of VLCFAs by the peroxisomal $\beta$-oxidation system appears unaffected by PPAR$\alpha$ deficiency, although this system in these mutant mice fails to respond to the inductive effects of peroxisome proliferators (49). The PPAR$\alpha$ null mice have normal levels of the classical peroxisomal AOX, L-PBE, and peroxisomal thiolase but lower constitutive expression of D-PBE. This indicates that this basal activity is sufficient to metabolize the VLCFAs and other AOX substrates and therefore shows no adverse microvesicular steatotic response in liver (49). It is of particular interest, therefore, that disruption of this basal classical $\beta$-oxidation system at the AOX level causes profound microvesicular steatosis in AOX knockout mice, affirming the criticality of AOX in preventing steatohepatitis (23). Mice nullizygous for both PPAR$\alpha$ and AOX (PPAR$\alpha$$-/-$AOX$-/-$) fail to exhibit extensive microvesicular steatohepatitis, spontaneous peroxisome proliferation, and induction of PPAR$\alpha$-regulated genes by biological ligands that remain largely unmetabolized in the absence of AOX (35). In AOX null mice, the hyperactivity of PPAR$\alpha$ enhances the severity of steatohepatitis by inducing CYP4A family proteins that generate DCAs and $H_2O_2$ (18; U Hoch & P Ortiz, personal communication), and because DCAs are not metabolized in the absence of AOX, they damage mitochondria and affect $\beta$-oxidation (Figure 4). Blunting of microvesicular steatosis in PPAR$\alpha$$-/-$AOX$-/-$ mice suggests a role for PPAR$\alpha$-induced genes, especially members of CYP4A family, in determining the severity of steatohepatitis with defective classical peroxisomal $\beta$-oxidation (35). In these PPAR$\alpha$$-/-$AOX$-/-$ mice, under a fed state, only a few scattered hepatocytes in the periportal region show microvesicular fatty change (35).

***Defect in PPAR$\alpha$-Inducible Fatty Acid Oxidation and Severity of Hepatic Steatosis in Response to Fasting***    PPAR$\alpha$ null mice under fed conditions do not manifest hepatic steatosis except for an occasional hepatocyte in the centrizonal area showing large-droplet fatty change as the animals age (35, 49). During starvation, fatty acids entering into the liver constitute the major source of energy, and they require efficient hepatic oxidation to generate ketone bodies to serve as fuels for other tissues (71). It is now well recognized that fasting causes a rapid transcriptional activation of genes encoding peroxisomal, microsomal, and certain mitochondrial fatty acid oxidation enzymes in liver in healthy subjects (45, 46, 51). These observations point to the importance also of regulatory step(s) controlling the levels of inducible fatty acid oxidation enzymes. In response to fasting, any abnormality in the inducibility of such enzymes can, in a manner similar to that encountered

ENERGY METABOLISM

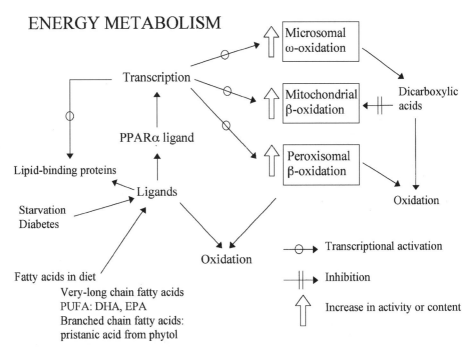

**Figure 4**  Cross talk among fatty acid oxidation systems and the regulatory role of peroxisome proliferator–activated receptor α (PPARα) in the oxidation of fatty acids and energy metabolism. Microsomal ω-oxidation generates dicarboxylic fatty acids, which are further degraded by peroxisomal β-oxidation by the classical fatty acyl-CoA oxidase (AOX). The chain-shortened fatty acyl-CoAs produced by the peroxisomal β-oxidation are shunted to the mitochondrial β-oxidation pathway for completion of oxidation. Substrates for peroxisomal classical β-oxidation system (for AOX) act as ligands for PPARα and increase the transcription of PPARα target genes of the microsomal, mitochondrial, and peroxisomal fatty acid oxidation systems. In the absence of classical peroxisomal β-oxidation (AOX deficiency), the unmetabolized substrates cause hyperstimulation of PPARα-regulated genes. PUFA, polyunsaturated fatty acids; DHA, docosahexaenoic acid; EPA, eicosapentaenoic acid.

with metabolic defects at the enzymatic level, impact energy metabolism and degree of hepatic steatosis. The availability of mice (*a*) deficient in peroxisomal AOX, (*b*) deficient in PPARα (49), and (*c*) nullizygous for both PPARα and AOX (35) enabled studies on the effect of genotype on energy utilization during fasting and on hepatic phenotype (34, 45, 46, 51). In wild-type mice, fasting for 24–72 h caused a modest induction of the hepatic expression of PPARα target genes encoding AOX, L-PBE, PTL, CYP4A1, CYP4A3, mitochondrial medium-chain acyl-CoA dehydrogenase, carnitine palmitoyltransferase I, and very-long-chain acyl-CoA synthetase (34, 45, 46, 51). In the wild-type mice, hepatic steatosis was minimal during 24–72 h of starvation and essentially disappeared when animals were starved for 96 h (34). In contrast, hepatic expression of PPARα-regulated fatty acid oxidation system genes is not induced by fasting in PPAR$\alpha-/-$ mice, and when these mice are stressed by short-term fasting, there is an exaggeration of fatty liver phenotype (45, 46, 51). As these double nulls lack AOX in addition to PPAR$\alpha$, because of added deficiency of peroxisomal $\beta$-oxidation, fasting caused a more pronounced steatotic phenotype in the liver of mice nullizygous for both PPAR$\alpha$ and AOX compared with PPAR$\alpha$ knockout mice (34). Following fasting, the hepatic triglyceride/protein ratio was substantially higher in mice nullizygous for both PPAR$\alpha$ and AOX than that noted in PPAR$\alpha-/-$ mice (34). Fasting for 24–72 h did not lead to significant increases in triglyceride levels in kidney and heart of wild-type, PPAR$\alpha-/-$, AOX$-/-$, and PPAR$\alpha-/-$AOX$-/-$ mice (34). Differences in lipid metabolism between liver and these extrahepatic organs under starvation are attributed to rapid activation of PPAR$\alpha$-responsive genes in liver and to the fact that PPAR$\alpha$-inducible fatty acid oxidation systems in liver play a vital role in energy metabolism and in the prevention of hepatic steatosis. When fasted for 48 and 72 h, both PPAR$\alpha-/-$ and PPAR$\alpha-/-$AOX$-/-$ mice exhibit severe hypoglycemia, hypoketonemia, and elevated serum free fatty acids, indicating a dramatic inhibition of fatty acid oxidation in liver, as the defect in PPAR$\alpha$ essentially negates the induction of fatty acid oxidation systems in response to fasting (34). These observations point to the critical importance of PPAR$\alpha$ in the transcriptional regulatory responses to fasting and in determining the severity of hepatic steatosis. In mice deficient in AOX alone, fasting-related amplification of hepatic steatosis is not prominent (34). Although the basal content of hepatic triglycerides in fed AOX null mice, reflecting the presence of preexisting microvesicular steatosis in some centrizonal hepatocytes, is somewhat higher than that of other groups, fasting only induced a minimal increase in triglyceride/protein ratios. This is attributed to sustained hyperactivation of PPAR$\alpha$ and up-regulation of mitochondrial $\beta$-oxidation and microsomal $\omega$-oxidation systems in liver. As a consequence these animals are highly effective in generating ketone bodies. Increases in plasma 3-hydroxybutyrate levels occurred in AOX$-/-$ mice similar to those observed in fasted wild-type mice (34). In contrast, the 3-hydroxybutyrate levels decreased in fasted PPAR$\alpha-/-$ and PPAR$\alpha-/-$AOX$-/-$ mice. It is also worth noting that the regenerative nature of a majority of hepatocytes containing numerous spontaneously proliferated peroxisomes in the livers of older AOX$-/-$ mice are resistant to fatty change.

***Relevance to Humans***    In humans, the hepatic PPAR$\alpha$ level is reported to be lower than that found in rats and mice (63). This raises issues related to ($a$) species differences in responses to peroxisome proliferators, ($b$) the critical levels of this transcription factor required to maintain lipid homeostasis, and ($c$) the effectiveness of PPAR$\alpha$-inducible fatty acid oxidation systems in different species in dealing with conditions of stress that lead to reduced energy intake and in dealing with dietary energy overload occurring in obesity and other metabolic conditions, such as type 2 diabetes. If the functions of PPAR$\alpha$, vis-à-vis the inducible levels of PPAR$\alpha$-enzymes in liver, are indeed less efficient in humans, the hepatic consequences of starvation, increased energy consumption, and other metabolic conditions involving lipid catabolism may appear more dire in humans than in rats and mice. A PPARα splice variant that may negatively interfere with wild type of PPARα has been described in human liver, which raises the question of countering the induction of PPARα-regulated genes leading to abnormal energy utilization. The relevance of the purported low levels of PPARα and the presence of a splice variant in humans, leading to reduced lipid metabolism and energy storage in hepatic and extrahepatic tissues in obesity, need to be explored (27, 63). If humans have low levels of PPARα, the unmetabolized energy can stimulate PPARγ-mediated adipogenesis for storage functions, which suggests cross talk between PPARα and PPARγ. In PPARα−/− mice as well as in PPARα−/−AOX−/− mice, fasting caused a slight increase in hepatic PPARγ level (34). Detailed quantitative studies are needed to ascertain whether humans have more PPARγ and reduced PPARα levels in general to account for the increased incidence of obesity and associated hepatic steatohepatitis.

## PERSPECTIVE

The demonstration that the phenomenon of peroxisome proliferation can be induced by many structurally diverse synthetic chemicals, now known as peroxisome proliferators, led to the proposal that peroxisome proliferation is linked to lipid metabolism and subsequently to the identification of the peroxisomal β-oxidation system. The tissue/cell specificity of pleiotropic responses and the coordinated rapid transcriptional activation of β-oxidation system genes led to the hypothesis that peroxisome proliferators exert their pleiotropic effects, including the development of liver tumors, by a receptor-mediated mechanism. Ten years ago, the first PPAR, now known as PPARα, was cloned and characterized and the identification of two other isoforms, PPARγ, and PPARβ/δ, soon followed. During the past 5 years, the functional roles of PPARα in peroxisome proliferation and in lipid catabolism, and that of PPARγ in adipogenesis and in lipid storage, have been fully recognized. Fatty acid β-oxidation occurs in both mitochondria and peroxisomes, with peroxisomes playing a specialized role in the metabolism of VLCFAs, long-chain dicarboxylic acids, branched-chain fatty acids, eicosanoids, and bile acid precursors. The genes encoding some of the enzymes responsible for fatty acid oxidation are transcriptionally regulated by PPARα. Recent evidence has demonstrated that in both mitochondria and peroxisomes, two distinct β-oxidation systems operate, and each system has different enzymes with different but some overlapping substrate specificities (Table 2). In peroxisomes, the inducible classical β-oxidation system oxidizes straight-chain fatty acids, dicarboxylic acids, and eicosanoids, whereas the noninducible system oxidizes branched-chain fatty acids and bile acid precursors. Long-chain fatty acids and VLCFAs are also metabolized by the cytochrome P450 CYP4A ω-oxidation system to dicarboxylic acids, which serve as substrates for

**TABLE 2**    Functions of the two fatty acid $\beta$-oxidation systems

| Determinant | Mitochondria | Peroxisomes |
|---|---|---|
| Substrates | Long-chain fatty acids<br>Medium-chain fatty acids | Very-long-chain fatty acids<br>Long-chain fatty acids<br>Long-chain dicarboxylic acids<br>Branched-chain fatty acids<br>Bile acid precursors<br>Some xenobiotics |
| Component | Inner membrane and<br>matrix associated | Enzymes having different<br>fatty acid specificities<br>and enzymes haivng overlapping<br>carbon chain-length specificities |
| Regulation | | |
| Short term | Carnitine, malonyl-CoA | None known |
| Long term | Some enzymes inducible | Enzymes of classical set<br>inducible |
| Clinical mani-<br>festation | Hypoketotic hypoglycemia | Progressive degeneration of<br>central nervous system |
| Main roles | ATP production | Detoxification |

the inducible peroxisomal $\beta$-oxidation system but which inhibit mitochondrial $\beta$-oxidation (Figure 4). The AOX of the classical inducible peroxisomal $\beta$-oxidation system appears critical in metabolizing PPAR$\alpha$ ligands, and in the absence of this enzyme, the unmetabolized natural/biological ligands of PPAR$\alpha$ cause sustained hyperstimulation of PPAR$\alpha$, leading to hepatic steatosis, hepatocellular regeneration, spontaneous peroxisome proliferation, and liver tumors. Thus, the substrates of AOX function as ligands for PPAR$\alpha$, the receptor, which controls the transcription of the enzyme. Because the substrate for the enzyme constitutes the biological/natural ligands of the receptor, this cross talk between the receptor and the enzyme it regulates is an important consideration in extrapolating the species response to peroxisome proliferators and in the blanket dismissal that humans are not susceptible to hepatomegaly, hepatic peroxisome proliferation, induction of peroxisomal $\beta$-oxidation, and liver tumors. The interdependencies between PPAR$\alpha$ and the fatty acid oxidation that occur in three different subcellular organelles, namely peroxisomes, mitochondria, and microsomes, point to delicate, but vital, metabolic circuits (Figure 4). Evidence derived from genetically altered mice with a deficiency of PPAR$\alpha$, peroxisomal AOX, and some of the other enzymes of the two peroxisomal $\beta$-oxidation pathways highlights the critical importance of PPAR$\alpha$ and the classical peroxisomal AOX in energy metabolism, and in the development of hepatic steatosis, steatohepatitis, and liver cancer.

Fatty liver is a common histological finding in human liver biopsies and presents as macrovesicular, with a large fat droplet in hepatocyte cytoplasm displacing the nucleus, or as microvesicular, with numerous small fat droplets surrounding a centrally located nucleus. Macrovesicular steatosis, a reflection of long-standing disturbance of hepatic lipid metabolism, is generally encountered in alcoholic liver injury, obesity, and type 2 diabetes mellitus. Microvesicular steatosis is regarded as a severe condition involving impairment of fatty acid $\beta$-oxidation, and emerging evidence points to the role of abnormalities in the metabolism of VLCFAs, DCAs, and other substrates of peroxisomal AOX that activate PPAR$\alpha$. This nuclear receptor is a key regulator of energy homeostasis and of peroxisomal, mitochondrial, and microsomal fatty acid oxidation systems, and perturbations in the levels of PPAR$\alpha$, and the inducibility of PPAR$\alpha$-regulated enzyme systems that catabolize fatty acids in liver, can play a significant role in the pathogenesis of steatohepatitis and liver tumorigenesis.

## ACKNOWLEDGMENTS

The work from our laboratories mentioned in this article was supported by NIH grant GM23750 and CA84472 and by VA Merit Award. The authors thank Drs. Frank J Gonzalez, Paul R Ortiz de Montellano, and Jorge H Capdevila for valuable discussions, William Cook and Wen-Qing Cao for help in preparing illustrations, and Lola Rivero for typing the manuscript.

**Visit the Annual Reviews home page at www.AnnualReviews.org**

## LITERATURE CITED

1. Antonenkov VD, Van Veldhoven PP, Waelkens E, Mannaerts GP. 1999. Comparison of the stability and substrate specificity of purified peroxisomal 3-oxoacyl-CoA thiolases A and B from rat liver. *Biochim. Biophys. Acta* 1437:136–41
2. Aoyama T, Peters JM, Iritani N, Nasu-Nakajima T, Furihara K, et al. 1998. Altered constitutive expression of fatty acid-metabolizing enzymes in mice lacking the peroxisome proliferator-activated receptor $\alpha$ (PPAR$\alpha$). *J. Biol. Chem.* 273:5678–84
3. Asayama K, Sandhir R, Sheikh FG, Hayashibe H, Nakane T, Singh I. 1999. Increased peroxisomal fatty acid $\beta$-oxidation and enhanced expression of peroxisome proliferator-activated receptor $\alpha$ in diabetic rat liver. *Mol. Cell. Biochem.* 194:227–34
4. Auwerx J. 1999. PPAR$\gamma$, the ultimate thrifty gene. *Diabetologia* 42:1033–49
5. Baes M. 2000. Mouse models for peroxisome biogenesis disorders. *Cell Biochem. Biophys.* 229–37
6. Baes M, Huyghe S, Carmeliet P, Declercq PE, Collen D, et al. 2000. Inactivation of the peroxisomal multifunctional protein-2 in mice impedes the degradation of not only 2-methyl-branched fatty acids and bile acid intermediates but also of very-long-chain fatty acids. *J. Biol. Chem.* 275:16329–36
7. Barak Y, Nelson MC, Ong ES, Jones YZ, Ruiz-Lozano P, et al. 1999. PPAR$\gamma$ is required for placental, cardiac, and adipose tissue development. *Mol. Cell. Biol.* 4:585–95
8. Baumgart E, Vanhooren JC, Fransen M, Marynen P, Puype M, et al. 1996. Molecular characterization of the human peroxisomal

branched-chain acyl-CoA oxidase: cDNA cloning, chromosomal assignment, tissue distribution, and evidence for the absence of the protein in Zellweger syndrome. *Proc. Natl. Acad. Sci. USA* 93:13748–53

9. Baumgart E, Vanhooren JC, Fransen M, Van Leuven F, Fahimi HD, et al. 1996. Molecular cloning and further characterization of rat peroxisomal trihydroxycoprostanoyl-CoA oxidase. *Biochem. J.* 320: 115–21

10. Behne M, Uchida Y, Seki T, Ortiz de Montellano P, Elias PM, Holleran WM. 2000. Omega-hydroxyceramides are required for corneocyte lipid envelope (CLE) formation and normal epidermal permeability barrier function. *J. Invest. Dermatol.* 114:185–92

11. Berk PD. 1999. Acute hepatic failure and defective fatty acid transport: clinical proof of a physiologic hypothesis. *Hepatology* 29:1607–9

12. Bernlohr DA, Simpson MA, Hertzel AV, Banaszack LJ. 1997. Intracellular lipid-binding proteins and their genes. *Annu. Rev. Nutr.* 17:277–303

13. Bun-ya M, Maebuchi M, Kamiryo T, Kurosawa T, Sato M, et al. 1998. Thiolase involved in bile acid formation. *J. Biochem.* 123:347–52

14. Capdevila JH, Falck JR, Harris RC. 2000. Cytochrome P450 and arachidonic acid bioactivation: molecular and functional properties of the arachidonic acid monoxygenase. *J. Lipid Res.* 41:163–81

15. Cooper TG, Beevers H. 1969. $\beta$-Oxidation in glyoxysomes from castor bean endosperm. *J. Biol. Chem.* 244:3514–20

16. deDuve C, Baudhuin P. 1966. Peroxisomes (microbody and related particles). *Physiol. Rev.* 46:323–57

17. Desvergne B, Wahli W. 1999. Peroxisome proliferator-activated receptors: nuclear control of metabolism. *Endocr. Rev.* 20:649–88

18. Dierks EA, Davis SC, Ortiz de Montellano PR. 1998. Glu-320 and Asp-323 are determinants of the CYP4A1 hydroxyla-

tion regiospecificity and resistance to inactivation by 1-aminobenzotriazole. *Biochemistry* 37:1839–47

19. Dieuaide-Noubhani M, Asselberghs S, Mannaerts JP, Veldhoven PP. 1997. Evidence that multifunctional protein 2, and not multifunctional protein 1, is involved in the peroxisomal $\beta$-oxidation of pristanic acid. *Biochem. J.* 325:367–73

20. Dieuaide-Noubhani M, Novikov D, Baumgart E, Vanhooren JCT, Fransen M, et al. 1996. Further characterization of the peroxisomal 3-hydroxyacyl-CoA dehydrogenases from rat liver. Relationship between the different dehydrogenases and evidence that fatty acids and the C27-bile acids di- and trihydroxycoprostanoic acids are metabolized by separate multifunctional proteins. *Eur. J. Biochem.* 240:660–66

21. Eaton S, Bartlett K, Pourfarzam M. 1996. Mammalian mitochondrial $\beta$-oxidation. *Biochem. J.* 320:345–57

22. Engels W, van Bilsen M, Wolffenbuttel BH, van der Vusse GJ, Glatz JF. 1999. Cytochrome P450, peroxisome proliferation, and cytoplasmic fatty acid-binding protein content in liver, heart and kidney of the diabetic rat. *Mol. Cell. Biochem.* 192:53–61

23. Fan C-Y, Pan J, Usuda N, Yeldandi AV, Rao MS, Reddy JK. 1998. Steatohepatitis, spontaneous peroxisome proliferation and liver tumors in mice lacking peroxisomal fatty acyl-CoA oxidase. *J. Biol. Chem.* 273:15639–45

24. Felber J-P, Golay A. 1995. Regulation of nutrient metabolism and energy expenditure. *Metabolism* 44:4–9

25. Fong DG, Nehra V, Lindor KD, Buchman AL. 2000. Metabolic and nutritional considerations in nonalcoholic fatty liver. *Hepatology* 32:3–9

26. Fournier B, Saudubray JM, Benichou B, Lyonnet S, Munnich A, et al. 1994. Large deletion of the peroxisomal acyl-CoA oxidase gene in pseudoneonatal adrenoleukodystrophy. *J. Clin. Invest.* 94:526–31

27. Gervois PP, Grotzinger T, Dubois G, 1999. A truncated human peroxisome proliferator-activated receptor $\alpha$ splice variant with dominant negative activity. *Mol. Endocrinol.* 13:1535–49

28. Gibbons GF, Islam K, Pease RJ. 2000. Mobilisation of triacylglycerol stores. *Biochim. Biophys. Acta* 1483:37–57

29. Glass CK, Rosenfeld MG. 2000. The coregulator exchange in transcriptional functions of nuclear receptors. *Genes Dev.* 14:121–41

30. Gonzalez FJ, Peters JM, Cattley RC. 1998. Mechanism of action of the nongenotoxic peroxisome proliferator-activator receptor $\alpha$. *J. Natl. Cancer Inst.* 90:1702–9

31. Hardwick JP, Song BJ, Huberman E, Gonzalez FJ. 1987. Isolation, complementary DNA sequence, and regulation of rat hepatic lauric acid $\omega$-hydroxylase (cytochrome P450LA$\omega$): identification of new cytochrome P-450 gene family. *J. Biol. Chem.* 262:801–10

32. Hashimoto T. 1996. Peroxisomal $\beta$-oxidation: enzymology and molecular biology. *Ann. NY Acad. Sci.* 804:86–98

33. Hashimoto T. 1999. Peroxisomal $\beta$-oxidation enzymes. *Neurochem. Res.* 24:551–63

34. Hashimoto T, Cook WS, Qi C, Yeldandi AV, Reddy JK, Rao MS. 2000. Defect in peroxisome proliferator-activated receptor $\alpha$-inducible fatty acid oxidation determines the severity of hepatic steatosis in response to fasting. *J. Biol. Chem.* 275:28918–28

35. Hashimoto T, Fujita T, Usuda N, Cook W, Qi C, et al. 1999. Peroxisomal and mitochondrial fatty acid $\beta$-oxidation in mice nullizygous for both peroxisome proliferator-activated receptor $\alpha$ and peroxisomal fatty acyl-CoA oxidase. Genotype correlation with fatty liver phenotype. *J. Biol. Chem.* 274:19228–36

36. Hiltunen JK, Filppula SA, Koivuranta KT, Siivari K, Qin YM, Hayrinen HM. 1996. Peroxisomal $\beta$-oxidation and polyunsaturated fatty acids. *Ann. NY Acad. Sci.* 804:116–28

37. Hoch U, Zhang Z, Kroetz DL, Orritz de Montellano P. 2000. Structural determination of the substrate specificities and regioselectivities of the rat and human fatty acid $\omega$-hydroxylases. *Arch. Biochem. Biophys.* 373:63–71

38. Hoefler G, Forstner M, McGuinness MC, Huulla W, Hiden M, et al. 1994. cDNA cloning of the human peroxisomal enoyl-CoA hydratase:3-hydroxyacyl-CoA dehydrogenase bifunctional enzyme and localization to chromosome 3q26.3–3q28: a free left Alu arm is inserted in the 3′ noncoding region. *Genomics* 19:60–67

39. Issemann I, Green S. 1990. Activation of a member of the steroid hormone receptor superfamily by peroxisome proliferators. *Nature* 347:645–50

40. Ito M, Yuan C-Y, Okano HJ, Darnell RB, Roeder RG. 2000. Involvement of the TRAP220 component of the TRAP/SMCC coactivator complex in embryonic development and thyroid hormone action. *Mol. Cell. Biol.* 5:683–93

41. James O, Day C. 1999. Non-alcoholic steatohepatitis: another disease of affluence. *Lancet* 353:1634–36

42. Jiang LL, Miyazawa S, Hashimoto T. 1996. Purification and properties of rat D-3-hydroxyacyl-CoA dehydratase: D-3-hydroxyacyl-CoA dehydratase/D-3-hydroxyacylCoA dehydrogenase bifunctional protein. *J. Biochem.* 120:633–41

43. Johnson EF, Palmer CAN, Griffin KJ, Hsu M-H. 1996. Role of the peroxisome proliferator-activated receptor in cytochrome P450 4A gene regulation. *FASEB J.* 10:1241–48

44. Kannenberg F, Ellinghaus P, Assmann G, Seedorf U. 1999. Aberrant oxidation of the cholesterol side chain in bile acid synthesis of sterol carrier protein-2/sterol carrier protein-x knockout mice. *J. Biol. Chem.* 274:35455–60

45. Kersten S, Seydoux J, Peters JM, Gonzalez

FJ, Desvergne B, Wahli W. 1999. Peroxisome proliferator-activated receptor $\alpha$ mediates the adaptive response to fasting. *J. Clin. Invest.* 103:1489–98

46. Kroetz DL, Yook P, Costet P, Bianchi P, Pineau T. 1998. Peroxisome proliferator-activated receptor $\alpha$ controls the hepatic CYP4A induction adaptive response to starvation and diabetes. *J. Biol. Chem.* 273:31581–89

47. Kunau WH, Dommes V, Schulz H. 1995. $\beta$-Oxidation of fatty acids in mitochondria, peroxisomes, and bacteria: a century of continued progress. *Prog. Lipid. Res.* 34:267–342

48. Lazarow PB, de Duve C. 1976. A fatty acyl-CoA oxidizing system in rat liver peroxisomes; enhancement by clofibrate, a hypolipidemic drug. *Proc. Natl. Acad. Sci. USA* 73:2043–46

49. Lee SS, Pineau T, Drago J, Lee EJ, Owens JW, et al. 1995. Targeted disruption of the $\alpha$ isoform of the peroxisome proliferator-activated receptor gene in mice results in abolishment of the pleiotropic effects of peroxisome proliferators. *Mol. Cell. Biol.* 15:3012–22

50. Leenders F, Dolez V, Beque A, Moller G, Gloeckner JC, et al. 1998. Structure of the gene for the human 17-$\beta$-hydroxysteroid dehydrogenase type IV. *Mamm. Genome* 9:1036–41

51. Leone TC, Weinheimer CJ, Kelly DP. 1999. A critical role for the peroxisome proliferator-activated receptor $\alpha$ (PPAR$\alpha$) in the cellular fasting response: the PPAR$\alpha$-null mouse as a model of fatty acid oxidation disorders. *Proc. Natl. Acad. Sci. USA* 96:7473–78

52. Liang X, Zhu D, Schulz H. 1999. $\Delta^{3,5,7},\Delta^{2,4,6}$-trienoyl-CoA isomerase, a novel enzyme that functions in the $\beta$-oxidation of polyunsaturated fatty acids with conjugated double bonds. *J. Biol. Chem.* 274:13830–35

53. Lombard-Platet G, Savary S, Sarde CO, Mandel JL, Chimini G. 1996. A close relative of the adrenoleukodystrophy (ALD) gene codes for a peroxisomal protein with a specific expression pattern. *Proc. Natl. Acad. Sci. USA* 91:1265–69

54. Lu J-F, Lawler AM, Watkins PA. 1997. A mouse model for 56-linked adrenoleukodystrophy. *Proc. Natl. Acad. Sci. USA* 94:9366–71

55. Mannaerts GP, Van Veldhoven PP, Casteels M. 2000. Peroxisomal lipid degradation via $\beta$- and $\alpha$-oxidation in mammals. *Cell Biochem. Biophys.* 32:73–87

56. Moller G, Leenders F, van Grunsven EG, Dolez V, Qualmann B, et al. 1999. Characterization of the HSD17B4 gene: D-specific multifunctional protein 2/17$\beta$-hydroxysteroid dehydrogenase IV. *J. Steroid Biochem. Mol. Biol.* 69:441–46

57. Mori T, Tsukamoto T, Mori H, Tashiro Y, Fujiki Y. 1991. Molecular cloning and deduced amino acid sequence of nonspecific lipid transfer protein (sterol carrier protein 2) of rat liver: a higher molecular mass (60 kDa) protein contains the primary sequence of nonspecific lipid transfer protein as its C-terminal part. *Proc. Natl. Acad. Sci. USA* 88:4338–42

58. Mosser J, Douar AM, Sarde CO, Kioschip P, Feil R, et al. 1993. Putative 10X-linked adrenoleukodystrophy gene shares unexpected homology with ABC transporters. *Nature* 361:726–30

59. Netik A, Forss-Petter S, Holzinger A, Molzer B, Unterrainer G, Berger J. 1999. Adrenoleukodystrophy-related protein can compensate functionally for adrenoleukodystrophy protein deficiency (10X-ALD): implication for therapy. *Hum. Mol. Genet.* 8:907–13

60. Orii KE, Orii KO, Souri M, Orii T, Kondo N, et al. 1999. Genes for the human mitochondrial trifunctional protein $\alpha$- and $\beta$-subunits are divergently transcribed from a common promoter region. *J. Biol. Chem.* 274:8077–84

61. Oritz de Montellano P. 1995. *Cytochrome*

*P450. Structure, Mechanism and Biochemistry.* New York: Plenum. 2nd ed.

62. Osumi T. 1993. Structure and expression of the genes encoding peroxisomal $\beta$-oxidation enzymes. *Biochimie* 75:243–50

63. Palmer CNA, Hsu M-H, Griffin KJ, Raucy JL, Johnson EF. 1998. Peroxisome proliferator activated receptor-$\alpha$ expression in human liver. *Mol. Pharmacol.* 53:14–22

64. Palosaari PM, Vihinen M, Mäntsälä PI, Alexson SEH, Pihlajaniemi T, Hiltunen JK. 1991. Amino acid sequence similarities of the mitochondrial short-chain $\Delta^3,\Delta^2$-enoyl-CoA isomerase and peroxisomal multifunctional $\Delta^3,\Delta^2$-enoyl-CoA isomerase, 2-enoyl-CoA hydratase, 3-hydroxyacyl-CoA dehydrogenase enzyme in rat liver. The proposed occurrence of isomerization and hydration in the same catalytic domain of the multifunctional enzyme. *J. Biol. Chem.* 266:10750–53

65. Peters JM, Lee SST, Li W, Wrad JM, Gavrilova O, et al. 2000. Growth, adipose, brain, and skin alterations resulting from targeted disruption of the mouse peroxisome proliferator-activated receptor $\beta(\delta)$. *Mol. Cell. Biol.* 20:5119–28

66. Puigserver P, Wu Z, Park CW, Graves R, Wright M, Spiegleman BM. 1998. A cold-inducible coactivator of nuclear receptors linked to adaptive thermogenesis. *Cell* 92:829–39

67. Qi C, Zhu Y, Pan J, Usuda N, Maeda N, et al. 1999. Absence of spontaneous peroxisome proliferation in enoyl-CoA hydratase/L-3-hydroxyacyl-CoA dehydrogenase-deficient mouse liver. Further support for the role of fatty acyl CoA oxidase in PPAR$\alpha$ ligand metabolism. *J. Biol. Chem.* 274:15775–80

68. Qi C, Zhu Y, Pan J, Yeldandi AV, Rao MS, et al. 1999. Mouse steroid receptor coactivator-1 is not essential for peroxisome proliferator-activated receptor $\alpha$-regulated gene expression. *Proc. Natl. Acad. Sci. USA* 96:1585–90

69. Qi C, Zhu Y, Reddy JK. 2000. Peroxisome proliferator-activated receptors, coactivators, and downstream targets. *Cell Biochem. Biophys.* 32:187–204

70. Qin YM, Poutanen MH, Helander HM, Kvist AP, Siivari KM, et al. 1997. Peroxisomal multifunctional enzyme of $\beta$-oxidation metabolizing D-3-hydroxyacyl-CoA esters in rat liver: molecular cloning, expression and characterization. *Biochem. J.* 321:21–28

71. Randle PJ, Garland PB, Hales CN, Newsholme EA. 1963. The glucose fatty-acid cycle. Its role in insulin sensitivity and the metabolic disturbances of diabetes mellitus. *Lancet* 1:785–89

72. Rao MS, Reddy JK. 1996. Hepatocarcinogenesis of peroxisome proliferators. *Ann. NY Acad. Sci.* 804:573–87

72a. Reddy JK, Azarnoff DL, Hignite C. 1980. Hypolipidemic hepatic peroxisome proliferators form a novel class of chemical carcinogens. *Nature* 283:397–98

73. Reddy JK, Chu R. 1996. Peroxisome proliferator-induced pleiotropic responses: pursuit of a phenomenon. *Ann. NY Acad. Sci.* 804:176–201

74. Reddy JK, Goel SK, Nemali MR, Carrino JJ, Laffler TG, et al. 1986. Transcriptional regulation of peroxisomal fatty acyl-CoA oxidase and enoyl-CoA:hydratase-3-hydroxyacyl-CoA dehydrogenase in rat liver by peroxisome proliferators. *Proc. Natl. Acad. Sci. USA* 83:1747–51

75. Reddy JK, Krishnakantha TP. 1975. Hepatic peroxisome proliferation: induction by two novel compounds structurally unrelated to clofibrate. *Science* 190:787–89

76. Reddy JK, Lalwani ND. 1983. Carcinogenesis by hepatic peroxisome proliferators: evaluation of the risk of hypolipidemic drugs and industrial plasticizers to humans. *CRC Crit. Rev. Toxicol.* 12:1–58

77. Reddy JK, Mannaerts GP. 1994. Peroxisomal lipid metabolism. *Annu. Rev. Nutr.* 14:343–70

78. Schaffer JE, Lodish HF. 1994. Expression

cloning and characterization of a novel adipocyte long-chain fatty acid transport protein. *Cell* 79:427–36

79. Schepers L, van Veldhoven PP, Casteels M, Eyssen HJ, Mannaerts GP. 1990. Presence of three acyl-CoA oxidases in rat liver peroxisomes. An inducible fatty acyl-CoA oxidase, a noninducible fatty acyl-CoA oxidase, and a noninducible trihydroxycoprostanoyl-CoA oxidase. *J. Biol. Chem.* 265:5242–46

80. Seedorf U, Raabe M, Ellinghaus P, Kannenberg F, Fobker M, et al. 1998. Defective peroxisomal catabolism of branched fatty acyl coenzyme A in mice lacking the sterol carrier protein-2/sterol carrier protein-x gene function. *Genes Dev.* 12:1189–201

81. Sher T, Yi HF, McBride OW, Gonzalez FJ. 1993. CDNA cloning, chromosomal mapping, and functional characterization of the human peroxisome proliferator activated receptor. *Biochemistry* 32:5598–604

82. Spiegelman BM, Flier JS. 1996. Adipogenesis and obesity: rounding out the big picture. *Cell* 87:377–89

83. Subramani S. 1998. Components involved in peroxisome import, biogenesis, proliferation, turnover, and movement. *Physiol. Rev.* 78:171–88

84. Suzuki H, Kawarabayashi Y, Kondo J, Abe T, Nishikawa K, et al. 1990. Structure and regulation of rat long-chain acyl-CoA synthetase. *J. Biol. Chem.* 265:8681–85

85. Suzuki Y, Jiang LL, Souri M, Miyazawa S, Fukuda S, et al. 1997. D-3-hydroxyacyl-CoA dehydratase/D-3-hydroxyacyl-CoA dehydrogenase bifunctional protein deficiency: a newly identified peroxisomal disorder. *Am. J. Hum. Genet.* 61:1153–62

86. Swinnen JV, Alen PP, Heynes W, Verhoeven G. 1998. Identification of diazepam-binding inhibitor/acyl-CoA binding protein as a sterol regulatory element binding protein-responsive gene. *J. Biol. Chem.* 273:19938–44

87. Treem WR, Sokol RJ. 1998. Disorders of the mitochondria. *Semin. Liver Dis.* 18:237–53

88. Uchida Y, Izai K, Orii T, Hashimoto T. 1992. Novel fatty acid $\beta$-oxidation enzymes in rat liver. II. Purification and properties of enoyl-coenzyme (CoA) hydratase/3-hydroxyacyl-CoA dehydrogenase/3-ketoacyl-CoA thiolase trifunctional protein. *J. Biol. Chem.* 267:1034–41

89. Uchida Y, Kondo N, Orii T, Hashimoto T. 1996. Purification and properties of rat liver very-long-chain acyl-CoA synthetase. *J. Biochem.* 199:565–71

90. Uchiyama A, Aoyama T, Kamijo K, Uchida Y, Kondo N, et al. 1996. Molecular cloning of cDNA encoding rat very-long-chain acyl-CoA synthetase. *J. Biol. Chem.* 271:30360–65

91. Unger RH, Zhou Y-T, Orci L. 1999. Regulation of fatty acid homeostasis in cells: novel role of leptin. *Proc. Natl. Acad. Sci. USA* 96:2327–32

92. van den Bosch H, Schutgens RB, Wanders RJ, Tager JM. 1992. Biochemistry of peroxisomes. *Annu. Rev. Biochem.* 61:157–97

93. van Grunsven EG, Van Berkel E, Ijlst L, Vreken P, deKlerk JB, et al. 1998. Peroxisomal D-hydroxyacyl-CoA dehydrogenase deficiency: resoluion of the enzyme defect and its molecular basis in bifunctional protein deficiency. *Proc. Natl. Acad. Sci. USA* 95:128–33

94. van Grunsven EG, Van Berkel E, Mooijer PAW, Watkins PA, Moser HW, et al. 1999. Peroxisomal bifunctional protein deficiency revisited: resolution of its true enzymatic and molecular basis. *Am. J. Hum. Genet.* 64:99–107

95. Vanhooren JCT, Fransen M, de Bethune B, Baumgart E, Baes M, et al. 1996. Rat pristanoyl-CoA oxidase. cDNA cloning and recognition of its C-terminal (SQL) by the peroxisomal-targeting signal 1 receptor. *Eur. J. Biochem.* 239:302–9

96. Vanhove GF, van Veldhoven PP, Fransen M, Denis S, Eyssen HJ, et al. 1993. The CoA esters of 2-methyl-branched-chain

fatty acids and of the bile acid inter-mediates di- and trihydroxycoprostanoic acids are oxidized by one single peroxisomal branched-chain acyl-CoA oxidase in human liver and kidney. *J. Biol. Chem.* 268:10335–44

97. Varanasi U, Chu R, Huang Q, Castellon R, Yeldandi AV, Reddy JK. 1996. Identification of peroxisome proliferator-responsive element upstream of the human peroxisomal fatty acylcoenzyme A oxidase gene. *J. Biol. Chem.* 271:2147–55; Erratum. 1998. *J. Biol. Chem.* 273:30842

98. Wanders RJA. 2000. Peroxisomes, lipid metabolism, and human disease. *Cell Biochem. Biophys.* 32:89–106

99. Wanders RJA, Denis S, Wouters F, Wirtz KWA, Seedorf U. 1997. Sterol carrier protein x (SCPx) is a peroxisomal branched-chain β-ketothiolase specifically reacting with 3-oxo-pristanoyl-CoA: a new, unique role for SCPx in branched-chain fatty acid metabolism in peroxisomes. *Biochem. Biophys. Res. Commun.* 236:565–69

100. Willson TM, Brown PJ, Sternbach DD, Henke BR. 2000. The PPARs: from orphan receptors to drug discovery. *J. Med. Chem.* 4 3527–50

101. Xu J, Qiu Y, DeMayo FJ, Ysai MJ, O'Malley BW. 1998. Partial hormone resistance in mice with disruption of the steroid receptor coactivator-1 (SRC-1) gene. *Science* 279:1922–25

102. Yamada T, Shinnoh N, Kondo A, Uchiyama A, Shimozawa N, et al. 2000. Very-long-chain fatty acid metabolism in adrenoleukodystrophy protein-deficient mice. *Cell Biochem. Biophys.* 239–46

103. Yeldandi AV, Rao MS, Reddy JK. 2000. Hydrogen peroxide generation in peroxisome proliferator-induced oncogenesis. *Mutat. Res.* 448:159–77

104. Zhu Y, Kan L, Qi C, Kanwar YS, Yeldandi AV, et al. 2000. Isolation and characterization of peroxisome proliferator-activated receptors (PPAR) interaction protein (PRIP) as a coactivator for PPAR. *J. Biol. Chem.* 275:13510–16

105. Zhu Y, Qi C, Calandra C, Rao MS, Reddy JK. 1996. Cloning and identification of mouse steroid receptor coactivator-1 (mSRC-1), as a coactivator of peroxisome proliferator-activated receptor γ. *Gene Expr.* 6:185–95

106. Zhu Y, Qi C, Jain S, Rao MS, Reddy JK. 1997. Isolation and characterization of PBP, a protein that interacts with peroxisome proliferator-activated receptor. *J. Biol. Chem.* 272:25500–6

107. Zhu Y, Qi C, Jia Y, Nye JS, Rao MS, Reddy JK. 2000. Deletion of PBP/PPARBP, the gene for nuclear receptor coactivator peroxisome proliferator-activated receptor-binding protein, results in embryonic lethality. *J. Biol. Chem.* 275:14779–82

108. Zhu Y, Qi C, Korenberg JR, Chen X-N, Noya D, et al. 1995. Structural organization of mouse peroxisome proliferator-activated receptor γ (mPPAR γ) gene: alternative promoter use and different splicing yield two mPPAR γ isoforms. *Proc. Natl. Acad. Sci. USA* 92:7921–50

Annu. Rev. Nutr. 2001. 21:231–54

# THE ROLE OF APOLIPOPROTEIN A-IV IN THE REGULATION OF FOOD INTAKE

Patrick Tso,[1] Min Liu,[1] Theodore John Kalogeris[2] and Alan BR Thomson[3]

[1]Department of Pathology, University of Cincinnati, Cincinnati, Ohio 45267;
e-mail: tsopp@email.uc.edu; lium@email.uc.edu
[2]Department of Surgery, Louisiana State University Medical Center, Shreveport,
Louisiana 71130; e-mail: tkalog@lsumc.edu
[3]Department of Medicine, University of Alberta, Alberta T6G 2C2 Canada;
e-mail: thomson@ualberta.ca

**Key Words**   obesity, chylomicron, intestine, satiety, Sprague Dawley rats

■ **Abstract**   Apolipoprotein A-IV (apo A-IV) is a glycoprotein synthesized by the human intestine. In rodents, both the small intestine and liver secrete apo A-IV, but the small intestine is the major organ responsible for the circulating apo A-IV. Intestinal apo A-IV synthesis is markedly stimulated by fat absorption and appears not to be mediated by the uptake or reesterification of fatty acids to form triglycerides. Rather, the formation of chylomicrons acts as a signal for the induction of intestinal apo A-IV synthesis. Intestinal apo A-IV synthesis is also enhanced by a factor from the ileum, probably peptide tyrosine-tyrosine. The inhibition of food intake by apo A-IV is mediated centrally. The stimulation of intestinal synthesis and the secretion of apo A-IV by lipid absorption are rapid; thus, apo A-IV likely plays a role in the short-term regulation of food intake. Other evidence suggests that apo A-IV may also be involved in the long-term regulation of food intake and body weight. Chronic ingestion of a high-fat diet blunts the intestinal apo A-IV response to lipid feeding and may explain why the chronic ingestion of a high-fat diet predisposes both animals and humans to obesity.

## CONTENTS

# INTRODUCTION

Apolipoprotein A-IV (Apo A-IV) was discovered over 22 years ago (88), but its physiological role was not firmly established until recently. Apo A-IV is a protein secreted only by the small intestine in humans (5, 35). In rodents, both the small intestine and the liver secrete apo A-IV; however, the small intestine is the major organ responsible for the circulating apo A-IV (30). It has been demonstrated that apo A-IV production by the small intestine is stimulated by active lipid absorption (5, 10, 40, 47). Hayashi et al (39) demonstrated that the stimulation of apo A-IV production by lipid feeding is associated with the formation of chylomicrons. They further demonstrated that the stimulation of apo A-IV production by fat absorption can be abolished by a Pluronic surfactant called Pluronic L-81 (L-81), a potent inhibitor of the formation of chylomicrons (92).

In vitro studies have demonstrated roles for apo A-IV in lipoprotein metabolism (10a, 22, 26, 32, 85). There has been no direct evidence, however, to demonstrate that apo A-IV plays such roles in vivo. Apo A-IV has been shown in vivo to protect apo E–deficient mice from developing atherosclerosis despite the fact that they have a plasma lipid profile that is atherogenic, i.e. increased total plasma cholesterol with no significant change in high-density-lipoprotein cholesterol (21a). This protective effect is further demonstrated by the ability of apo A-IV to protect against diet-induced atherosclerotic lesions (18). These studies demonstrate that both human and mouse apo A-IV protect against atherosclerosis. This might be due to the protective effect of apo A-IV has against lipid oxidation (75). Although there are many exciting proposed functions of apo A-IV, this review focuses on its unique role in regulating short- and long-term food intake, possibly as the satiety factor that is released by the gastrointestinal tract following the ingestion of fat.

# MECHANISMS OF FAT ABSORPTION

Before a discussion of the role of apo A-IV in mechanisms of fat-induced satiety can take place, it is necessary to briefly discuss the process of fat absorption by the small intestine and the intestinal synthesis and secretion of lipoproteins and apolipoproteins.

## Dietary Lipids

Dietary lipids provide as much as 30%–40% of the daily caloric intake in the Western diet. The daily intake of lipids by humans in the Western world ranges between 60–100 g. Triacylglycerol (TG) is the major dietary fat in humans. The major long-chain fatty acids (FAs) present in the diet are palmitate (16:0), stearate (18:0), oleate (18:1), linoleate (18:2), and linolenate (18:3). In most infant diets, fat becomes an even more important source of calories. In human milk and in human formulas, as much as 50% of the total calories are present as fat (36). In human milk, there is also an abundance of medium-chain FAs. The human small intestine is presented daily with other lipids, such as phospholipids (PLs), cholesterol, and plant sterols. Both PL and cholesterol are major constituents of bile. In humans, the biliary PL is a major contributor of luminal PL, and as much as 11–20 g of biliary PL enters the small intestinal lumen daily, whereas the dietary contribution is only between 1 and 2 g (12, 66). The small intestinal epithelium undergoes rapid turnover, thus contributing to the luminal PL and cholesterol. The predominant sterol in the Western diet is cholesterol. Plant sterols account for 20%–25% of total dietary sterol (34, 90), but they are poorly absorbed.

## Luminal Digestion and Uptake of Dietary Lipids

Lipid digestion begins in the stomach. Lipase activity has been reported to be present in human gastric juice (17). In humans, the gastric lipase activity is mainly contributed by the stomach, with the highest activity detected in the fundus of the stomach. Human gastric lipase has a pH optimum ranging from 3.0 to 6.0 and is therefore called acid lipase. It hydrolyzes medium-chain TG (predominantly 8- to 10-carbon chain length) better than long-chain TG (53). The main hydrolytic products of gastric lipase are diacylglycerols and free FAs (70, 76). Gastric lipase does not hydrolyze PL or cholesteryl esters. Gastric lipases play an important role in the absorption of lipids in newborns. It is interesting that in rodents, the main gastric lipase activity is derived from the lipase secreted by the salivary glands and is therefore termed lingual lipase. Though derived from different areas in humans and rodents, and therefore termed differently, gastric and lingual lipase is the same enzyme.

In the stomach, lipid is emulsified (broken into small oil droplets) and enters the small intestinal lumen as fine droplets less than 0.5 $\mu$m in diameter (16, 80). The combined action of bile and pancreatic juice brings about a marked change in the physical and chemical form of the luminal lipid emulsion. Pancreatic lipase is secreted into the duodenum and hydrolyses TG to form 2-monoacylglycerol and FAs (15, 58, 81). The most potent gastrointestinal hormone that stimulates the release of enzymes by the pancreas is cholecystokinin (82), and cholecystokinin-A receptor has been demonstrated to be present in the pancreas (78). In vitro studies using purified pancreatic lipase have demonstrated a potent inhibitory effect of bile salts on the lipolysis of TG at a concentration that is above the critical micellar concentration (9, 62). The inhibitory effect of bile salt, then, is physiological because its concentration in the duodenum is normally higher than what is typically needed to observe an inhibitory effect. Why, then, is pancreatic lipase so efficient in digesting TG? The pancreas secretes another protein that counteracts this inhibition, and this factor is colipase.

Colipase was first isolated by Morgan et al (62) from the pancreatic juice of rats. The structure and mechanism of action of colipase have been elucidated by Maylie et al (59) and Börgstrom et al (13). Colipase acts by attaching to the ester bond region of the TG molecule. In turn, the lipase binds strongly to the colipase by electrostatic interactions, thereby allowing the hydrolysis of the TG by the lipase molecule (24).

Most dietary cholesterol is free sterol, with only 10%–15% being esters. Cholesteryl esters entering the small intestine are hydrolyzed before free cholesterol can be absorbed. The enzyme involved in hydrolyzation is called cholesterol esterase (EC 3.1.1.13—also called carboxylic ester hydrolase, monoglycerol hydrolase, bile salt–dependent lipase, or sterol ester hydrolase), and it is secreted by the pancreatic acinar cells. The digestion of PL occurs in the small intestine. In bile, PL [predominantly phosphatidylcholine (PC)] is found in mixed micelles along with cholesterol and bile salts. Once in the intestinal lumen, the luminal PC distributes between the mixed micelles and the TG droplets; however, PC tends to favor the micellar phase over the oil phase. PC is hydrolyzed by pancreatic phospholipase $A_2$ (EC 3.1.1.4) to yield FA and lysoPC.

Much of our current understanding of the uptake of dietary lipids has been derived from the pivotal work of Hofmann & Borgstrom (43, 44), who identified and emphasized the importance of micellar solubilization of lipid in the uptake of lipid digestion products by enterocytes. Although for a long time uptake of lipids was believed to be passive, a number of more recent studies have raised questions about the validity of this concept. Work by Stremmel et al (86, 87) has raised the possibility that some lipids, especially FAs, may be taken up by enterocytes by carrier-mediated processes. A number of other proteins, including GP330 (also called megalin) (55, 101), CD36 (1, 2), caveolin (64), and FA transporter (1, 37), also bind lipids. Recently, Stahl et al (84) reported having identified a FA transport protein, FATP4 (a member of the family of the FA transport proteins), being abundantly expressed in the intestinal enterocytes, with most of the protein associated with the apical brush border membrane. Considerable excitement has been raised over the ability of these transporters to reduce fat absorption, a potential magic bullet to combat obesity. However, further studies are critical to support such a view.

## Formation and Secretion of Chylomicrons

2-Monoacylglycerol and FA reconstitute to form TG, mainly via the monoacylglycerol pathway (46, 57). The enzymes involved present in a complex called "triglyceride synthetase" (46). Some of the absorbed lysoPC is reacylated to form

PC (65). Cholesterol is transported almost exclusively by the lymphatic system, mainly as esterified cholesterol. The rate of esterification of cholesterol regulates the rate of its lymphatic transport (25). The TG, PL, cholesterol, and cholesteryl esters, together with apolipoproteins, are packaged to form chylomicrons. Chylomicrons are secreted by enterocytes, via a process called exocytosis, and carried by the lymphatic system before being emptied into the circulatory system.

## INTESTINAL APOLIPOPROTEIN SECRETION

Chylomicrons are secreted by the small intestine and have the following proteins associated with them: apolipoprotein apo A-I, apo A-IV, apo B-48, and the apo Cs (Figure 1). Of the various apolipoproteins, only apo A-IV synthesis and secretion is markedly stimulated by fat absorption (two- to threefold) (39, 40).

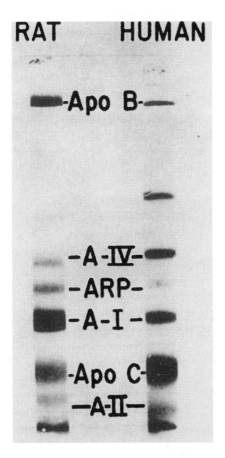

**Figure 1**  Sodium dodecyl sulfate polyacrylamide gels (5.6%) of apolipoproteins of rat lymph chylomicrons and human chylous rine chylomicrons. ARP = apo E. A dye front is apparent at the bottom of each gel. [Reproduced with permission from Bisgaier & Glickman (10)].

## REGULATION OF INTESTINAL APO A-IV SYNTHESIS
## AND SECRETION

Lymphatic apo A-IV secretion by the gastrointestinal tract displays a circadian rhythm with peak output occurring before feeding and just before the first half of the dark period (Figure 2) (30). This pattern is closely correlated with lymphatic, triglyceride, PL, and cholesterol outputs. Bile diversion reduces lymphatic outputs of apo A-IV by 67%, cholesterol by 81%, and both triglyceride and PL by 90%. Moreover, bile diversion completely abolishes the circadian rhythm in outputs of apo A-IV (Figure 2) (30). Davidson et al (19) has demonstrated that bile diversion significantly reduces apo A-IV synthesis by the intestinal mucosa. Thus, an intact enterohepatic circulation is necessary for both normal basal lymphatic output of apo A-IV and its circadian rhythm.

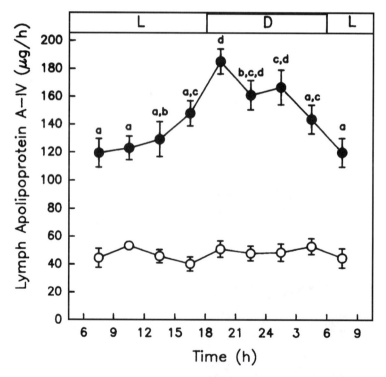

**Figure 2**    Lymph apo A-IV output in 24-h fasted rats with bile diversion (open circles) or without bile diversion (closed circles). Seven rats were used for this study. Values are expressed as the mean plus or minus the standard error. Different letters show that the difference is significant, with $P < 0.05$. L, light period; D, dark period. [Reproduced with permission from Fukagawa et al (30)].

In vivo studies have demonstrated that synthesis and secretion of apo A-IV by the gastrointestinal tract is regulated by the absorption of fat, as well as by a peptide secreted by the lower small intestine, probably peptide YY (49).

## Lipid Absorption

A number of us have demonstrated that intestinal lipid absorption stimulates the synthesis and secretion of apo A-IV (5, 20, 40, 51). Of the major apolipoproteins produced by the gastrointestinal tract (A-I, A-IV, B-48), only apo A-IV is stimulated by lipid absorption (39, 40). Kalogeris et al (47) have demonstrated that intestinal lymphatic transport of apo A-IV increases in a graded fashion with increasing steady state levels of intestinal triglyceride transport. This increase in apo A-IV secretion might be due to graded increases in intestinal mucosal apo A-IV synthesis along a proximal-distal gradient. Evidence thus far suggests that increased synthesis of apo A-IV by fat absorption in adult rats is by a pretranslational mechanism (5).

As previously discussed, intestinal fat absorption involves multiple steps, and knowing which steps of fat absorption are involved in stimulating intestinal apo A-IV synthesis and secretion is crucial. Several lines of evidence support the notion that assembly and transport of chylomicrons is necessary for stimulating intestinal apo A-IV synthesis. Evidence of this first came from studies using L-81. Animals infused with lipid plus L-81 showed no change in intestinal lipid digestion or uptake. The absorbed lipid accumulated in the intestinal mucosa but was not transported (no change in uptake) into lymph (92, 93). It has been further demonstrated that L-81 preferentially blocks chylomicron formation and, thus, intestinal apo A-IV secretion and synthesis, but not the secretion of very-low-density lipoproteins (94). Hayashi et al (40) observed that the increase in apo A-IV synthesis and secretion by the small intestinal mucosa was blocked when L-81 was infused. However, when L-81 was removed, lymphatic lipid transport immediately increased as the accumulated mucosal lipid was cleared from the mucosa as chylomicrons. Removal of L-81 similarly reverses the blockade of apo A-IV transport. A lag period of about 120 min between the maximal output of lipid and that of A-IV (lipid occurring first) with reversal of L-81 blockage suggests that lipid transport stimulates apo A-IV synthesis and secretion (40).

Further evidence that lymphatic apo A-IV output is dependent on chylomicron transport is derived from rat studies that examined the intestinal synthesis and lymphatic secretion of apo A-IV in response to intestinal infusion of FAs that differed in chain length. Infusion of long-chain FAs (myristic, C-14; oleic, C-18; and arachidonic, C-20), which are transported via the lymph in chylomicrons, stimulated synthesis and output of apo A-IV, whereas medium- and short-chain FAs (caprylic, C-8 and butyric, C-4), primarily transported as free FAs in the portal vein, elicited a negligible A-IV response (50). These findings in rats differ from those in neonatal swine where similar increases in jejunal apo A-IV mRNA expression and synthesis in response to infusions of both medium (C8:0 and C10:0) and long-chain triglyceride mixtures were observed (33). Results of the rat studies strongly support the hypothesis that some aspect of chylomicron formation and secretion is required to stimulate apo A-IV synthesis, and thus secretion (39), but contradict the recent findings of the neonatal swine studies. Therefore, it is currently unclear whether the relationship between chylomicron and apo A-IV synthesis and secretion is common to all species or developmental stages. An extremely interesting question worth investigating is how the formation of chylomicrons is signal transduced to stimulate intestinal apo A-IV synthesis.

## Peptide YY

It has recently been determined that the formation and secretion of chylomicrons is not the only mechanism by which apo A-IV synthesis and secretion is stimulated. We administered duodenal infusions of graded doses of TG to rats and quantified both regional lipid distribution and mucosal synthesis of apo A-IV at various sites along the intestine (47). It was determined that despite significant amounts of lipid found only in the proximal half of the small intestine, apo A-IV synthesis was stimulated in the proximal three quarters of the gut, even in segments where there was a negligible amount of lipid. This raised an interesting question of whether factors other than lipid transport are independent of the presence of lipid, which is itself capable of stimulating apo A-IV production by the gut. To address this, a series of experiments were performed comparing the effects of proximal versus distal intestinal infusion of lipid on apo A-IV synthesis. Kalogeris et al (50) found that duodenal lipid infusion elevated both apo A-IV synthesis and mRNA levels two- to threefold compared with control infusions of glucose-saline in the jejunum, and that ileal apo A-IV synthesis and mRNA levels were unaffected. Previous work from our laboratory demonstrated that duodenal lipid infusion only negligibly affected the amount of lipid reaching the ileum, which suggests that insufficient exposure of lipid to the distal gut thereby inhibited a change in apo A-IV secretion.

In contrast to this finding, infusion of lipid to the ileum stimulated both ileal and jejunal apo A-IV synthesis. Subsequent experiments in rats equipped with jejunal or ileal Thiry-Vella fistulas (a segment of intestine isolated luminally from the rest of the gastrointestinal tract) demonstrated the following interesting findings: (a) Ileally infused lipid elicits an increase in proximal jejunal apo A-IV synthesis independent of the presence of jejunal lipid, and (b) both the ileum and more distal sites may be involved in the stimulation. These results strongly suggest that there is a signal in the distal gut that is capable of stimulating apo A-IV synthesis in the proximal gut. These findings have important physiological implications. The distal intestine is known to play an important role in the control of gastrointestinal function. Nutrient (especially lipid) delivered to the ileum results in the inhibition of gastric emptying (54, 56), decreased intestinal motility and transit (56, 83), and decreased pancreatic secretion (38). Ileal nutrient also inhibits food intake (61, 99). The mechanism for these effects has been collectively termed the ileal brake (83) and appears to be related to the release of one or more peptide hormones from the distal intestine (6, 7, 45, 71–73, 79). These effects have traditionally been considered operative only in the abnormal delivery of undigested nutrients to the distal gut, such as the malabsorptive state (83). However, growing evidence supports the notion that nutrient reaches the distal gut, even under normal conditions, because of rapid gastric emptying during the early phases of food ingestion (54, 61, 77). We recently studied the intraluminal and mucosal distribution of a bolus of [$^3$H]triolein-labeled Intralipid (0.5 ml of a 20% emulsion) fed by gavage. By 15–30 min, radiolabeled lipid was spread evenly throughout the gut, with 10%–15% of the load recovered in the ileum and cecum combined. The presence of substantial amounts of lipids in these distal sites persisted for at least 4 h after food ingestion. When we examined apo A-IV synthesis in the small intestine, we discovered that stimulation had occurred rapidly (between 15–30 min), and that it had occurred throughout the entire intestine, including the ileum. Significant stimulation of lymphatic output and plasma levels of apo A-IV occurred as well by 30 min after feeding with a gastric lipid load (77). Consequently, it appears that a much greater length of intestine is involved in the absorption of lipid and in the control of gastric and upper gut functions, even under normal conditions, than has been previously recognized. Thus, the ileal brake may play an important role in the normal control of gut function and control of lipid absorption.

The most likely peptide to mediate the phenomenon of ileal brake is peptide tyrosine-tyrosine (PYY), which is a member of the peptide family that includes pancreatic polypeptide, neuropeptide Y, and fish pancreatic peptide Y (52). PYY is synthesized by the endocrine cells in the ileum and large intestine (3, 6, 41, 89, 91) and is released in response to intestinal nutrients, especially long-chain FAs (41). However, PYY may not be the only mediator of the ileal brake. For example, perfusion of fat in the intestine produces a greater suppression of pentagastrin-stimulated acid secretion than does PYY (79), indicating that the enterogastrone effect of fat is mediated by more than one factor.

We now have evidence that PYY stimulates jejunal apo A-IV synthesis and secretion. Continuous intravenous infusion of physiological doses of PYY elicits significant increases in both synthesis and lymphatic transport of apo A-IV in rats (48). Kalogeris et al (48) further demonstrated that the stimulation of jejunal apo A-IV synthesis by PYY is probably translationally rather than transcriptionally controlled because the apo mRNA level is not altered but synthesis is markedly stimulated. Furthermore, Kalogeris et al (48) showed that vagotomy failed to block the stimulation of jejunal apo A-IV synthesis by fat absorption (Figure 3). However, when lipid was infused directly into the ileum, vagotomy totally abolished an increase in jejunal apo A-IV synthesis (Figure 4). Thus, the stimulation of jejunal apo A-IV synthesis and secretion by fat absorption is mediated by a factor (probably PYY), which, in turn, acts centrally to send a signal via the vagus

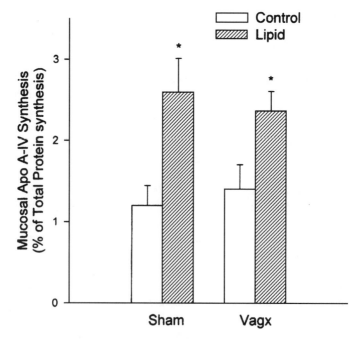

**Figure 3**  Vagotomy has no effect on the stimulation of apo A-IV synthesis in proximal jejunum by duodenal infusion of triacylglycerol emulsion. Vagotomized (Vagx) or sham-vagotomized rats equipped with duodenal infusion cannulas received continuous 8-h duodenal infusions of glucose saline control) or lipid (triolein emulsion, 40 $\mu$mol per h). Values are means plus or minus standard errors for four rats (sham, control), six rats (vagx, control), five rats (sham, lipid), and seven rats (vagx, lipid). (Asterisk) Significant effect of lipid infusion on apo A-IV synthesis ($P < 0.01$). [Reproduced with permission from Kalogeris et al (48)].

nerve to the gut. We believe this to be the first demonstration of a gastrointestinal hormone involved in the control of expression and secretion of an intestinal apolipoprotein, thus bringing together two areas of research in gastrointestinal physiology.

## INTRAVENOUS INFUSION OF APO A-IV INHIBITS FOOD INTAKE

That apo A-IV may play a role in the regulation of food intake is supported by a series of physiological studies that examined (*a*) the effect that intravenous administration of intestinal lymph derived from fasted rats had on food intake, and (*b*) the effect that intestinal lymph derived from rats actively absorbing fat had on food intake. Experimental rats were implanted with indwelling intravenous

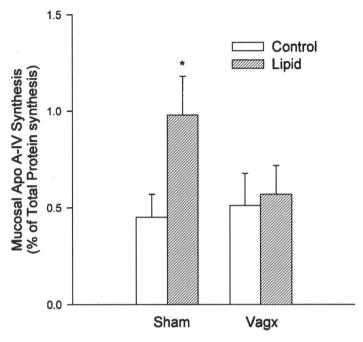

**Figure 4**  Vagotomy prevents increase in jejunal apo A-IV synthesis in a jejunal Thiry-Vella fistula elicited by ileal lipid infusion. Vagotomized (Vagx) or sham-vagotomized rats equipped with jejunal Thiry-Vella fistula and ileal infusion cannulas received continuous 8-h ileal infusions of either glucose-saline (control) or lipid emulsion (lipid). Mucosal apo A-IV synthesis in the Thiry-Vella segment was then measured. Values are mean plus or minus the standard error for six rats (sham, control), five rats (sham, lipid), six rats (vagx, control), and eight rats (vagx, lipid). (Asterisk) Significant effect of lipid ($P = 0.001$). [Reproduced with permission from Kalogeris et al (48)].

infusion cannula and allowed to recover for 1 week before feeding studies began. After a 24-h fasting period, various intestinal lymph samples were taken from donor rats and solutions of apo A-IV and apo A-I infused intravenously to determine whether food intake was affected by a nonpurified diet. Fujimoto et al (27) demonstrated that rats intravenously infused with a physiological dose of saline through the indwelling right atrial catheter ate $3.90 \pm 0.40$ g during the first 30 min of refeeding. Infusion of food-deprived intestinal lymph collected from donor lymph-fistula rats had little effect on food intake compared with the saline-infused rats deprived of food for 24 h. In contrast, the intestinal lymph collected from rats that were actively absorbing lipid markedly suppressed food intake during the first 30 min of refeeding ($P < 0.01$). Suppression of food intake was not observed in the subsequent 30 min of refeeding.

The fact that food intake was inhibited in rats that received intestinal lymph from donor rats actively absorbing fat indicates that one or more factors may be involved in the inhibition of food intake. Because the lipid content of lymph increased as much as 10–15 times during fat absorption, it was hypothesized that the additional lipid in the chylous lymph (in the form of chylomicrons) caused the inhibition of food intake. To test this hypothesis in rats deprived of food for 24 h, a separate group of rats was infused intravenously with a diluted Intralipid solution that mimicked the lipid content of the chylous lymph. When 2 ml of Intralipid (20 g/liter) in saline containing 42 $\mu$mol of triglyceride and 3.1 $\mu$mol of PL (a composition comparable to the lymph collected during active lipid absorption) was infused intravenously, food intake was not suppressed. This result indicated that the effect of chylous lymph on food intake was not caused by its lipid content.

Fujimoto et al (27) reasoned that if it was not the lipid component of the chylous lymph that inhibited food intake, then it must be apo A-IV because it is the only apolipoprotein secreted by the small intestine that is markedly stimulated by lipid feeding (40). L-81 blocks the stimulation of apo A-IV production by the small intestine during lipid absorption. Fujimoto et al (27) therefore tested whether lymph from rats that were fed lipid and L-81 had any effect on food intake. Lymph from L-81–treated rats did not inhibit food intake. However, lymph collected from rats that did not receive L-81 did. This suggests that apo A-IV is probably the factor in chylous lymph that is responsible for the inhibition of food intake.

Fujimoto et al (27) further studied the effect of apo A-IV–deficient chylous lymph on feeding. The chylous lymph treated with normal goat serum suppressed food intake significantly in the first 30 min of feeding. In contrast, chylous lymph that was treated with apo A-IV antiserum had no effect on food intake—the rats consumed an amount of food similar to that consumed by the saline controls. Fujimoto et al demonstrated that the composition of the chylous lymph treated with apo A-IV antiserum was not altered by the treatment, except that the apo A-IV had been removed. In contrast, lymph treated with apo A-I antiserum was just as effective as the untreated lymph in inhibiting food intake.

Apo A-IV or apo A-I (200 $\mu$g) dissolved in 2 ml of physiological saline was infused intravenously in 24-h food-deprived rats. An amount of apo A-IV (200 $\mu$g) comparable to that present in 2 ml of lymph collected from rats actively absorbing lipid suppressed food intake significantly and to the same extent as the chylous lymph collected during 6–8 h of lipid infusion. The inhibition of food intake by apo A-IV was shown to be dose dependent (Table 1). Conversely, 200 $\mu$g of apo A-I did not effect food intake. No nonphysiological reactions, such as sedation, ataxia, or hyperthermia, were observed after apo A-IV and chylous lymph infusion. These studies led Fujimoto et al (27) to first propose that apo A-IV is a circulating signal released by the small intestine in response to fat feeding and is likely the mediator for the anorectic effect of a lipid meal. This function is unique to apo A-IV and is not shared by apo A-I, although all of the functions that are ascribed to apo A-IV in the in vitro studies can also be performed by apo A-I.

**TABLE 1**    Food intake in 24-h fasted rats after infusion of 2 ml of test solution through indwelling atrial catheter[a]

| Test Solutions | Food Consumption After Refeeding (g) | |
| --- | --- | --- |
| | 0–30 Min | 30–60 Min |
| Control (physiological saline) | 3.90 ± 0.40 | 1.31 ± 0.33 |
| Apolipoprotein A-IV | | |
| 60 $\mu$g | 3.35 ± 0.46 | 1.13 ± 0.31 |
| 135 $\mu$g | 2.14 ± 0.16[b] | 1.16 ± 0.26 |
| 200 $\mu$g | 0.90 ± 0.18[b,c] | 1.10 ± 0.19 |
| Apolipoprotein A-I | | |
| 200 $\mu$g | 3.90 ± 0.48 | 1.20 ± 0.25 |

[a]Values are means plus or minus the standard error. Five rats were treated in each group.
[b]$P < 0.01$ compared with values for saline control.
[c]$P < 0.01$ compared with value for 135 $\mu$g of apolipoprotein A-IV.

# CENTRAL ADMINISTRATION OF APO A-IV ALSO INHIBITS FOOD INTAKE

The hypothalamus is a potential site where apo A-IV can elicit an inhibition of food intake because it is intimately involved in regulating food intake and energy metabolism (102). Fujimoto et al (28) reported that administration of apo A-IV into the third cerebroventricular of rats decreased food intake in a dose-dependent manner and with a potency that was ~50-fold higher than intravenous administration (Figure 5). In contrast, apo A-I had no effect on food intake when infused into the third ventricle. When goat anti-rat apo A-IV serum was administered into the third ventricle at 11:00 h (during the light phase when rats usually do not eat), all tested rats began to eat. Thus, Fujimoto et al (28) proposed that apo A-IV antiserum removes any endogenous apo A-IV present.

Evidence suggests that de novo synthesis of apo A-IV in the brain is unlikely (23). Fujimoto et al (28, 29) proposed that apo A-IV (or perhaps a fragment thereof) released by the small intestine may traverse the blood-brain barrier and act in the central nervous system. Using electroimmunosassay, they supported this argument by demonstrating that intact apo A-IV, or a fragment thereof, was present in the third ventricular cerebrospinal fluid. Furthermore, they demonstrated that the concentration of apo A-IV immunoreactivity in the third ventricular cerebrospinal fluid increased as a result of lipid feeding. Later, using immunohistochemical technique, Fukagawa et al (31) demonstrated that specific staining for apo A-IV in astrocytes and tanycytes appears throughout both white and gray matter. The granular nature and perinuclear distribution of apo A-IV immunoreactivity suggests that apo A-IV may be contained in perinuclear organelles or vesicles. The demonstration of immunoreactive apo A-IV in tanycytes does not necessarily

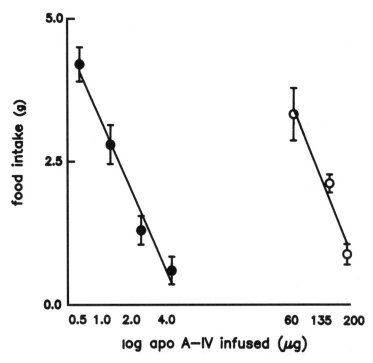

**Figure 5**    The relationship between the suppression of food intake during the first 30 min of refeeding in 24-h fasted rats and the logarithm of the dose in micrograms of apo A-IV infused into the third ventricle (closed circles) or intravenously (open circles). Five animals were studied at each dose, and the values are expressed as mean plus or minus the standard error. [Reproduced with permission from Fujimoto et al (28)].

indicate that there is a selective uptake mechanism because tanycytes take up a variety of neurotransmitters and nonmetabolizable amino acids. The presence of apo A-IV immunostaining in astrocytes does indicate selective uptake of this apolipoprotein by astrocytes. Whether astrocytes are involved in satiety mechanisms associated with lipid feeding is unknown. Extremely preliminary data from our laboratory implies that the brain, particularly the hypothalamus, has apo A-IV mRNA and is therefore capable of synthesizing apo A-IV protein. This interesting finding is being investigated actively in our laboratory.

## IS APO A-IV A SHORT-TERM SATIETY FACTOR?

Although there is compelling evidence that apo A-IV can acutely inhibit food intake during the ingestion of a lipid meal, the temporal relationship between intestinal synthesis and secretion of apo A-IV and satiety has to be considered. The question is whether the increase in plasma levels of apo A-IV in response to lipid feeding is rapid enough and of sufficiently large magnitude to elicit satiety. Rodriguez et al (77) demonstrated that when a gastric bolus of 0.5 ml of an Intralipid solution (200 g/liter) containing 100 mg of triglyceride was fed to rats, there was a significant increase in plasma apo A-IV within 15 min, and the increment remained significant until 30 min following the ingestion of a meal. These changes in plasma apo A-IV concentration were similar to those observed by Fujimoto et al (27), in which the intravenous administration of apo A-IV produced a significant, dose-dependent inhibition of food intake. Rodriguez et al (77) therefore concluded that the increase in plasma levels of apo A-IV produced in response to lipid meals was sufficiently quick and large enough to produce satiety, thereby supporting a role for apo A-IV in the short-term control of food intake in rats.

## POTENTIAL ROLE OF APO A-IV IN THE LONG-TERM CONTROL OF FOOD INTAKE

Evidence from a number of experiments suggests that apo A-IV may be involved in the long-term regulation of food intake and body weight gain. First, it has been demonstrated that intravenous administration of apo A-IV decreases food intake in rats given free access to food (29). This suggests that exogenously administered apo A-IV controls food intake under ad libitum feeding conditions. In rats with free access to food, central administration of apo A-IV antiserum stimulated feeding during the light cycle (28). Similar studies conducted during the dark phase, when rats actively eat, may help clarify the role of apo A-IV in the control of individual meals. Second, evidence shows that there is a link between the regulation of food intake and the circadian rhythm of lymph and serum apo A-IV. Fukagawa et al (30) reported that in rats given free access to food, both serum and intestinal lymph apo A-IV exhibited a circadian rhythm that was significantly higher during the dark hours than during the light hours. When Fukagawa et al (30) examined the serum apo A-IV level in food-deprived rats, they found it to exhibit the same circadian rhythm as in fed rats. However, for all time points, the serum apo A-IV level was significantly higher in rats given free access to food compared with food-deprived rats. This indicated that although ad libitum feeding greatly increased the levels of serum apo A-IV, it did not change the pattern of its inherent circadian rhythm. That serum apo A-IV increased during the dark phase, which corresponds to the most active feeding period of rats, suggests a physiological role for apo A-IV in the regulation of food intake.

Third, Morton et al (63) reported down-regulation of intestinal apo A-IV mRNA levels by leptin. Leptin is a protein made by the adipose tissue and is believed to signal the hypothalamus in the brain (a center for the regulation of food intake and energy metabolism) of how much fat is in the body. Leptin decreases food intake and increases energy metabolism (102). The discovery of leptin by Zhang et al (103) has energized the field of obesity. Preliminary data suggest that leptin decreases apo A-IV synthesis and secretion by the small intestinal epithelial cells. It has also been demonstrated that intestinal apo A-IV synthesis and secretion is up-regulated by insulin in both rodents and humans (8, 11). Energy homeostasis in the body is accomplished by a high integrated and redundant neurohumoral system that prevents the effect of short-term fluctuations in energy balance on fat mass (102). Insulin and leptin are hormones that are secreted in proportion to body adiposity, and they play a critical role in this energy homeostasis. Because leptin and insulin seem to regulate intestinal apo A-IV synthesis, apo A-IV may be involved in the long-term regulation of food intake and body weight. This interesting hypothesis is currently just speculation and must be proven experimentally.

Another point worthy of consideration is that PYY, released by the L cells located in the ileum and the colon, stimulates the production of apo A-IV by the jejunum and the ileum. Several laboratories have demonstrated that PYY is released in response to fat bile salts, glucose, short-chain FAs such as butyrate, and amino acids (4, 74, 95). Thus, the inhibition of food intake by apo A-IV is not just limited to the absorption of long-chain FAs; it could also be initiated by other nutrients and macromolecules in the lumen of the ileum and the colon. This exciting area of apo A-IV research requires further exploration.

## THE ROLE OF APO A-IV ON UPPER GASTROINTESTINAL FUNCTION

Another possible mechanism of action by which apo A-IV inhibits food intake is by affecting gastric motility as well as gastric acid secretion. Okumura et al demonstrated that intracisternal injections of purified apo A-IV inhibited gastric acid secretion (67, 68) and gastric motility (69) in rats in a dose-dependent manner. The doses of apo A-IV chosen for these studies were thought to reproduce the levels of apo A-IV measured in cerebrospinal fluid after lipid feeding (28). Intravenous infusion of similar doses of apo A-I did not elicit gastric responses. This is important because Fujimoto et al (27) demonstrated that intravenous infusion of purified apo A-IV inhibited food intake in a dose-dependent manner, but administration of similar doses of apo A-I had no effect on food intake. Additionally, Fujimoto et al (29) demonstrated that apo A-IV administered into the third ventricle inhibited food intake in a dose-dependent manner but that apo A-I did not. Thus, the studies of Okumura et al (67–69) corroborate the observations made by Fujimoto et al (27, 29). As proposed by Okumura et al (67), apo A-IV acts as an enterogastrone, i.e. a humoral mediator released by the intestine that mediates the humoral inhibition of gastric acid secretion as well as motility by the ingestion of fat. Currently, it is not clear if the effects of apo A-IV on food intake is directly linked to its effects on gastric function. Apo A-IV could directly influence central feeding mechanisms; alternatively, feeding could be affected by the effect of apo A-IV on gastric function, particularly via the inhibition of gastric emptying (60).

Preliminary data seem to indicate that intravenous infusion of apo A-IV also affects intestinal motility as well as the activity of the vagal afferents (H Raybould, personal communication).

# EFFECT OF CHRONIC HIGH-FAT FEEDING ON INTESTINAL APO A-IV SYNTHESIS

The effect that chronic ingestion of a high-fat diet has on intestinal apo A-IV synthesis is interesting, but the mechanisms involved are unclear. Previous studies have determined that acute administration of a lipid meal results in a marked increase in apo A-IV levels and stimulation of apo A-IV synthesis in both the jejunum and the ileum (5). In this same study, Apfelbaum et al (5) determined that chronic consumption of a high-fat diet (30 g/100 g by weight of diet as fat) resulted in the stimulation of apo A-IV synthesis and increased mRNA levels in the jejunum but not the ileum. Does the ileum, then, become less responsive to lipid after chronic ingestion of a high-fat diet, or does the adaptation of the digestive and absorptive process result in fat no longer reaching the ileum? This question warrants further investigation.

In humans, the chronic consumption of a high-fat diet significantly elevates plasma apo A-IV levels. This elevation is observed during the first week of high-fat consumption (97) but disappears during the second week, thus leading investigators to conclude that there is autoregulation of intestinal apo A-IV production in response to diets high in fat. Consequently, both rodent and human data suggest that intestinal apo A-IV synthesis and secretion become less responsive to fat after chronic high-fat diet consumption. Our preliminary data shows that plasma leptin increases dramatically in rats chronically consuming a diet high in fat and while becoming obese. It is interesting that their intestinal apo A-IV responses to lipid feeding were also attenuated. Morton et al (63) demonstrated that intravenous administration of leptin reduces apo A-IV mRNA levels of the small intestine after a lipid load. Our laboratory has also confirmed that leptin greatly suppressed the stimulation of apo A-IV synthesis and secretion by the small intestine in conscious rats (21). It is tempting to speculate that this apparent autoregulation of apo A-IV in response to chronic ingestion of high fat is related to elevated circulating leptin.

Reduction of apo A-IV in response to lipid feeding in both animals and humans that chronically consume a high-fat diet may be physiologically and clinically important because it may explain in part why increasing dietary fat content accelerates the development of obesity. The conclusion that increased consumption of a high-fat diet leads to an increase in body fat is evidenced by numerous experiments with varying diets and species. Excellent reviews on this subject have come from the laboratories of Bray & Popkin (14), Hill et al (42), Warwick et al (96), and West & York (100). Further investigation of why chronic ingestion of a high-fat diet attenuates an apo A-IV response to lipid feeding is extremely important to our understanding of why a high-fat diet predisposes both animals and humans to obesity.

## CONCLUSIONS AND FUTURE DIRECTIONS

Intestinal apo A-IV is a protein stimulated by dietary lipid that has a potentially important physiological role in the integrated control of digestive function and ingestive behavior. It also has a presumed role in cholesterol and lipoprotein metabolism. The role of apo A-IV in the regulation of upper gut function and satiety needs further investigation. For instance, what molecular form of apo A-IV is involved—free monomer, homodimeric (98), high-density-lipoprotein bound, or apo A-IV–derived bioactive peptides? Additional information is urgently needed to help us understand how apo A-IV works in the central nervous system to modify food intake and gastric motility and secretion. Is apo A-IV being made by the central nervous system? If so, where and by what cells? If the brain makes apo A-IV, is it physiologically regulated? Is it regulated in the same way as intestinal apo A-IV? What is the relationship between circulating apo A-IV and brain apo A-IV? Is there a receptor for apo A-IV? If so, where is it located? Is it physiologically regulated? These questions and others need addressing before a comprehensive understanding of the physiology of apo A-IV can be achieved.

Understanding the mechanism of stimulation of apo A-IV synthesis by the formation and secretion of chylomicrons and peptide YY is another area that warrants further investigation. There is evidence that apo A-IV synthesis is stimulated in both the jejunum and ileum when exposed to fat. Lipid exposed to the ileum also results in PYY secretion, which further stimulates the synthesis and release of apo A-IV by the jejunum. Several studies have demonstrated that apo A-IV biosynthesis stimulated by lipid absorption is mediated by a different molecular mechanism than stimulation by PYY because the mRNA levels increase markedly during lipid stimulation but remain the same during PYY stimulation. Future investigation of the mechanisms of regulation of apo A-IV synthesis by lipid absorption, PYY, leptin, chronic consumption of a high-fat diet, and other currently unknown factors will pose both a challenge and a reward in enhancing our understanding of diet-induced obesity.

### ACKNOWLEDGMENT

This work was supported by grants from the National Institutes of Health DK 53444, DK 54504, DK 56863, and DK 56910.

## LITERATURE CITED

1. Abumrad NA, Coburn C, Ibrahimi A. 1999. Membrane proteins implicated in long-chain fatty acid uptake by mammalian cells: CD36, FATP and FABPm. *Biochim. Biophys. Acta* 18:4–13

2. Abumrad NA, Sfeir Z, Connelly MA, Coburn C. 2000. Lipid transporters: membrane transport systems for cholesterol and fatty acids. *Curr. Opin. Clin. Nutr. Metab. Care* 3:255–62

3. Adrian TE, Bacarese HA, Smith HA, Chohan P, Manolas KJ, Bloom SR. 1987. Distribution and postprandial release of porcine peptide YY. *J. Endocrinol.* 113:11–14

4. Anini Y, Fu-Cheng X, Cuber JC, Kervran A, Chariot J, Roz C. 1999. Comparison of the postprandial release of peptide YY and proglucagon-derived peptides in the rat. *Pfugers Arch.* 438:299–306

5. Apfelbaum TF, Davidson NO, Glickman RM. 1987. Apolipoprotein A-IV synthesis in the rat intestine: regulation by dietary triglyceride. *Am. J. Physiol. Gastrointest. Liver Physiol.* 252:G662–66

6. Aponte GW, Fink AS, Meyer JH, Tatemoto K, Taylor IL. 1985. Regional distribution and release of peptide YY with fatty acids of different chain length. *Am. J. Physiol. Gastrointest. Liver Physiol.* 249:G745–50

7. Aponte GW, Park K, Hess R, Garcia R, Taylor IL. 1989. Meal-induced peptide tyrosine-tyrosine inhibition of pancreatic secretion in the rat. *FASEB J.* 3:1949–55

8. Attia N, Touzani A, Lahrichi M, Balafrej A, Kabbaj O, Girard-Globa A. 1997. Response of apolipoprotein A-IV and lipoproteins to glycaemic control in young people with insulin-dependent diabetes mellitus. *Diabet. Med.* 14(3):242–47

9. Benzonana G, Desnuelle P. 1968. Action of some effectors on the hydrolysis of long-chain triglycerides by pancreatic lipase. *Biochim. Biophys. Acta* 164:47–58

10. Bisgaier CL, Glickman RM. 1983. Intestinal synthesis, secretion, and transport of lipoproteins. *Annu. Rev. Physiol.* 45:625–36

10a. Bisgaier CL, Sachdev OP, Lee ES, Williams KJ, Blum CB, Glickman RM. 1987. Effect of lecithin:cholesterol acyl transferase on distribution of apolipoprotein A-IV among lipoproteins of human plasma. *J. Lipid Res.* 28:693–703

11. Black DD, Ellinas H. 1992. Apolipoprotein synthesis in newborn piglet intestinal explants. *Pediatr. Res.* 32:553–58

12. Borgström B. 1974. Fat digestion and absorption. *Biomembranes* 4B:555–620

13. Borgström B, Erlanson-Albertson C, Wieloch T. 1979. Pancreatic colipase-chemistry and physiology. *J. Lipid Res.* 20:805–16

14. Bray GA, Popkin BM. 1998. Dietary fat does affect obesity. *Am. J. Clin. Nutr.* 68:1157–73

15. Brockerhoff H. 1968. Substrate specificity of pancreatic lipase. *Biochim. Biophys. Acta* 159:296–303

16. Carey MC, Small DM, Bliss CM. 1983. Lipid digestion and absorption. *Annu. Rev. Physiol.* 45:651–77

17. Carriere F, Barrowman JA, Verger R, Laugier R. 1993. Secretion and contribution of lipolysis of gastric and pancreatic lipases during a test meal in humans. *Gastroenterology* 105:876–78

18. Cohen RD, Castellani LW, Qiao JH, Van Lenten BJ, Lusis AJ, Reue K. 1997. Reduced aortic lesions and elevated high density lipoprotein level in transgenic mice overexpressing mouse apolipoprotein A-IV. *J. Clin. Invest.* 99:1906–16

19. Davidson NO, Kollmer ME, Glickman RM. 1991. Apolipoprotein B synthesis in rat small intestine: regulation by dietary

triglyceride and biliary lipid. *J. Lipid Res.* 27:30–39

20. Delamatre JG, Roheim PS. 1983. The response of apolipoprotein A-IV to cholesterol feeding in rats. *Biochim. Biophys. Acta* 751:210–17

21. Doi T, Liu M, Seeley RJ, Woods SC, Kalogeris TJ, Tso P. 2000. The effect of leptin on intestinal apolipoprotein AIV synthesis and secretion. *Gastroenterology* 118:A71 (Abstr.)

21a. Duverger N, Tremp G, Caillaud JM, Emmanuel F, Castro G, et al. 1996. Protection against atherogenesis in mice mediated by human apolipoprotein A-IV. *Science* 273:966–68

22. Dvorin E, Gorder NL, Benson DM, Gotto AM. 1988. Apolipoprotein A-IV. A determinant for binding and uptake of high density lipoproteins by rat hepatocytes. *J. Biol. Chem.* 261:15714–18

23. Elsbourhagy NA, Walker DW, Paik YK, Boguski MS, Freeman M, et al. 1987. Structure and expression of the human apolipoprotein A-IV gene. *J. Biol. Chem.* 262:7973–81

24. Erlanson-Albertsson C. 1992. Pancreatic colipase. Structural and physiological aspects. *Biochim. Biophys. Acta* 1125:1–7

25. Field FJ, Cooper AD, Erickson SK. 1982. Regulation of rabbit intestinal acyl coenzyme A-cholesterol acyltransferase in vivo and in vitro. *Gastroenterology* 83:873–80

26. Fielding CJ, Shore VG, Fielding PE. 1972. A protein cofactor of lecithin: cholesterol acyltransferase. *Biochem. Biophys. Res. Commun.* 46:1493–98

27. Fujimoto K, Cardelli JA, Tso P. 1992. Increased apolipoprotein A-IV in rat mesenteric lymph after lipid meal acts as a physiological signal for satiation. *Am. J. Physiol. Gastrointest. Liver Physiol.* 262:G1002–6

28. Fujimoto K, Fukagawa K, Sakata T, Tso P. 1993. Suppression of food intake by apolipoprotein A-IV is mediated through

the central nervous system in rats. *J. Clin. Invest.* 91:1830–33

29. Fujimoto K, Machidori H, Iwakiri R, Yamamoto K, Fujisaki J, et al. 1993. Effect of intravenous administration of apolipoprotein A-IV on patterns of feeding, drinking and ambulatory activity of rats. *Brain Res.* 608:233–37

30. Fukagawa K, Gou HM, Wolf R, Tso P. 1994. Circadian rhythm of serum and lymph apolipoprotein A-IV in ad libitum-fed and fasted rats. *Am. J. Physiol. Regulatory Integrative Comp. Physiol.* 267:R1385–90

31. Fukagawa K, Knight DS, Hamilton HA, Tso P. 1995. Immunoreactivity for apolipoprotein A-IV in tanycytes and astrocytes of rat brain. *Neurosci. Lett.* 199:17–20

32. Goldberg IJ, Scheraldi CA, Yacoub LK, Saxena U, Bisgaier CL. 1990. Lipoprotein C-II activation of lipoprotein lipase. Modulation by apolipoprotein A-IV. *J. Biol. Chem.* 265:4266–72

33. Gonzalez-Vallina R, Wang H, Zhan R, Berschneider HM, Lee RM, et al. 1996. Lipoprotein and apolipoprotein secretion by a newborn piglet intestinal cell line (IPEC-1). *Am. J. Physiol. Gastrointest. Liver Physiol.* 271:G249–59

34. Gould RG, Jones RJ, LeRoy GV, Wissler RW, Taylor CB. 1969. Absorbability of β-sitosterol in humans. *Metabolism* 18:652–62

35. Green PHR, Glickman RM, Riley JW, Quinet E. 1980. Human apolipoprotein A-IV. Intestinal origin and distribution. *J. Clin. Invest.* 65:911–19

36. Hamosh M. 1979. The role of lingual lipase in neonatal fat digestion. In *Development of Mammalian Absorptive Process*, Ciba Found. Symp. 70, ed. K Elliot, J Whelan, pp. 69–98. Amsterdam: Excerpta Med.

37. Harmon CM, Luce P, Beth AH, Abumrad NA. 1991. Labeling of adipocyte membranes by sulfo-N-succinimidyl derivatives of long-chain fatty acids: inhibition

of fatty acid transport. *J. Membr. Biol.* 121:261–68

38. Harper AA, Hood JCA, Mushens J. 1979. Inhibition of external pancreatic secretion by intracolonic and intraileal infusions in the cat. *J. Physiol.* 292:445–54

39. Hayashi H, Nutting DF, Fujimoto K, Cardelli JA, Black D, Tso P. 1990. Fat feeding increases size, but not number, of chylomicrons produced by small intestine. *Am. J. Physiol. Gastrointest. Liver Physiol.* 259:G709–19

40. Hayashi H, Nutting DF, Fujimoto K, Cardelli JA, Black D, Tso P. 1990. Transport of lipid and apolipoproteins A-I and A-IV in intestinal lymph of the rat. *J. Lipid. Res.* 31:1613–25

41. Hill FLC, Zhang T, Gomez G, Greeley GH Jr. 1991. Peptide YY, a new gut hormone. *Steroids* 56:77–82

42. Hill JO, Lin D, Yakubu F, Peters JC. 1992. Development of dietary obesity in rats: influence of amount and composition of dietary fat. *Int. J. Obes.* 16:321–33

43. Hofmann AF, Borgstrom B. 1962. Physico-chemical state of lipids in intestinal content during their digestion and absorption. *Fed. Proc.* 21:43–50

44. Hofmann AF, Borgstrom B. 1964. The intraluminal phase of fat digestion in man: the lipid content of the micellar and oil phases of intestinal content obtained during fat digestion and absorption. *J. Clin. Invest.* 43:247–57

45. Jin H, Gai L, Lee K, Chang TM, Li P, et al. 1993. A physiological role of peptide YY on exocrine pancreatic secretion in rats. *Gastroenterology* 105:208–15

46. Johnston JM, Rao GA, Lowe PA. 1967. The separation of the $\alpha$-glycerophosphate and monoglyceride pathways in the intestinal biosynthesis of triglycerides. *Biochim. Biophys. Acta* 137:578–80

47. Kalogeris TJ, Fukagawa K, Tso P. 1994. Synthesis and lymphatic transport of intestinal apolipoprotein A-IV in response to

graded doses of triglyceride. *J. Lipid Res.* 35:1141–51

48. Kalogeris TJ, Holden VR, Tso P. 1999. Stimulation of jejunal synthesis of apolipoprotein A-IV by ileal lipid infusion is blocked by vagotomy. *Am. J. Physiol. Gastrointest. Liver Physiol.* 277: G1081–87

49. Kalogeris TJ, Qin X, Chey WY, Tso P. 1998. PYY stimulates synthesis and secretion of intestinal apolipoprotein AIV without affecting mRNA expression. *Am. J. Physiol. Gastrointest. Liver Physiol.* 275:G668–74

50. Kalogeris TJ, Tsuchiya T, Fukagawa K, Wolf R, Tso P. 1996. Apolipoprotein A-IV synthesis in proximal jejunum is stimulated by ileal lipid infusion. *Am. J. Physiol. Gastrointest. Liver Physiol.* 270:G277–86

51. Krause BR, Sloop CH, Castle CK, Roheim PS. 1981. Mesenteric lymph apolipoproteins in control and thinyl estradiol-treated rats: a model for studying apolipoproteins of intestinal origin. *J. Lipid Res.* 22:610–19

52. Larhammar D, Söderberg C, Blomgvist AG. 1993. Evolution of the neuropeptide Y family of peptides. In *The Biology of Neuropeptide Y and Related Peptides*, ed. WF Colmers, C Wahlestadt, pp. 1–41. Totoa, NJ: Humana

53. Liao TH, Hamosh P, Hamosh M. 1984. Fat digestion by lingual lipase: mechanism of lipolysis in the stomach and upper small intestine. *Pediatr. Res.* 18:402–9

54. Lin HC, Doty JE, Reedy TJ, Meyer JH. 1990. Inhibition of gastric emptying of sodium oleate depends upon length of intestine exposed to the nutrient. *Am. J. Physiol. Gastrointest. Liver Physiol.* 259: G1031–36

55. Lundgren S, Carling T, Hjälm G, Juhlin C, Rastad J, et al. 1997. Tissue distribution of human gp330/megalin, a putative $Ca^{2+}$-sensing protein. *J. Histochem. Cytochem.* 45:383–92

56. MacFarlane A, Kinsman R, Read NW.

1983. The ileal brake: ileal fat slows small bowel transit and gastric emptying in man. *Gut* 24:471–72

57. Manganaro F, Kuksis A. 1986. Purification and preliminary characterization of 2-monoacylglycerol acyltransferase from rat intestinal villus cells. *Can. J. Biochem. Cell Biol.* 63:341–47

58. Mattson FH, Beck LW. 1956. The specificity of pancreatic lipase on the primary hydroxyl groups of glycerides. *J. Biol. Chem.* 219:735–40

59. Maylie MF, Charles M, Gache C, Desnuelle P. 1971. Isolation and partial identification of a pancreatic colipase. *Biochim. Biophys. Acta* 229:286–89

60. McHugh PR, Moran TH. 1985. The stomach: a conception of its dynamic role in satiety. *Prog. Psychobiol. Physiol. Psychol.* 11:197–232

61. Meyer JH, Elashoff JD, Doty JE, Gu YG. 1994. Disproportionate ileal digestion on canine food consumption. A possible model for satiety in pancreatic insufficiency. *Dig. Dis. Sci.* 39:1014–24

62. Morgan RGH, Barrowman J, Borgström B. 1969. The effect of sodium taurodeoxycholate and pH on the gel filtration behaviour of rat pancreatic protein and lipases. *Biochim. Biophys. Acta* 175:65–75

63. Morton NM, Emilsson V, Liu YL, Cawthorne MD. 1998. Leptin action in intestinal cells. *J. Biol. Chem.* 273:26194–201

64. Murata M, Peränen J, Schreiner R, Wieland F, Kurzchalia TV, Simons K. 1995. VIP21/caveolin is a cholesterol-binding protein. *Proc. Natl. Acad. Sci. USA* 92:10339–43

65. Nilsson A. 1968. Intestinal absorption of lecithin and lysolecithin by lymph fistula rats. *Biochim. Biophys. Acta* 152:379–90

66. Northfield TC, Hofmann AF. 1975. Biliary lipid output during three meals and an overnight fast. *Gut* 16:1–11

67. Okumura T, Fukagawa K, Tso P, Taylor IL, Pappas TN. 1994. Intracisternal injection of apolipoprotein A-IV inhibits gastric secretion in pylorus-ligated conscious rats. *Gastroenterology* 107:1861–64

68. Okumura T, Fukagawa K, Tso P, Taylor IL, Pappas TN. 1995. Mechanisms of action of intracisternal apolipoprotein A-IV in inhibiting gastric acid secretion in rats. *Gastroenterology* 109:1583–88

69. Okumura T, Fukagawa K, Tso P, Taylor IL, Pappas TN. 1996. Apolipoprotein A-IV acts in the brain to inhibit gastric emptying in the rat. *Am. J. Physiol. Gastrointest. Liver Physiol.* 270:G49–53

70. Paltauf F, Esfandi F, Holasek A. 1974. Stereospecificity of lipases. Enzymatic hydrolysis of enantiomeric alkyl diacylglycerols by lipoprotein lipase, lingual lipase, and pancreatic lipase. *FEBS Lett.* 40:119–23

71. Pappas TN, Debas HT, Chang AM, Taylor IL. 1986. Peptide YY release by fatty acids is sufficient to inhibit gastric emptying in dogs. *Gastroenterology* 91:1386–89

72. Pappas TN, Debas HT, Taylor IL. 1985. Peptide YY: metabolism and effect pancreatic secretion in dogs. *Gastroenterology* 89:1387–92

73. Pappas TN, Debas HT, Taylor IL. 1986. Enterogastrone-like effect of peptide YY is vagally mediated in the dog. *J. Clin. Invest.* 77:49–53

74. Plaisancie P, Dumoulin V, Chayvialle JA, Cuber JC. 1996. Luminal peptide YY-releasing factors in the isolated vascularly perfused rat colon. *J. Endocrinol.* 151:421–29

75. Qin X, Swertfeger DK, Zheng S, Hui DY, Tso P. 1998. Apolipoprotein AIV: a potent endogenous inhibitor of lipid oxidation. *Am. J. Physiol.* 274:H1836–40. *Heart Circ. Physiol.*

76. Roberts IM, Montgomery RK, Carey MC. 1984. Rat lingual lipase: partial purification, hydrolytic properties and comparison with pancreatic lipase. *Am. J. Physiol. Gastrointest. Liver Physiol.* 247:G385–93

77. Rodriguez MD, Kalogeris TJ, Wang XL, Wolf R, Tso P. 1997. Rapid synthesis and secretion of intestinal apolipoprotein A-IV after gastric fat loading in rats. *Am. J. Physiol. Regulatory Integrative Comp. Physiol.* 272:R1170–77

78. Rosenzweig SA, Miller LJ, Jamieson JD. 1983. Identification and localization of cholecystokinin-binding sites on rat pancreatic plasma membranes and acinar cells: a biochemical and autoradiographic study. *J. Cell Biol.* 96:1288–97

79. Savage AP, Adrian TE, Carolan G, Chattarjee VK, Bloom SR. 1987. Effects of peptide YY (PYY) on mouth to caecum intestinal transit time and on the rate of gastric emptying in healthy volunteers. *Gut* 28:166–70

80. Senior JR. 1964. Intestinal absorption of fats. *J. Lipid Res.* 5:495–521

81. Simmonds WJ. 1972. Fat absorption and chylomicron formation. In *Blood Lipids and Lipoproteins: Quantitation, Composition and Metabolism*, ed. GJ Nelson, pp. 705–43. New York: Wiley Intersci.

82. Solomon TE. 1994. Control of exocrine pancreatic secretion. In *Physiology of the Gastrointestinal Tract*, ed. LR Johnson, pp. 1173–207. New York: Raven. 3rd ed.

83. Spiller RC, Trotman IF, Higgens BE, Ghatel MA, Grimble GK, et al. 1984. The ileal brake-inhibition of jejunal motility after ileal fat perfusion in man. *Gut* 25:365–74

84. Stahl A, Hirsch DJ, Gimeno RE, Punreddy S, Ge P, et al. 1999. Identification of the major intestinal fatty acid transport protein. *Mol. Cell.* 4:299–308

85. Stein O, Stein Y, Lefevre M, Roheim P. 1986. The role of apolipoprotein A-IV in reverse cholesterol transport studied with cultured cells and lipsomes derived from an ether analog of phosphatidylcholine. *Biochim. Biophys. Acta* 878:7–13

86. Stremmel W. 1988. Uptake of fatty acids by jejunal mucosal cells is mediated by a fatty acid binding membrane protein. *J. Clin. Invest.* 82:2001–10

87. Stremmel W, Strohmeyer G, Borchard F, Kochwa S, Berk PD. 1985. Isolation and partial characterization of a fatty acid binding protein in rat liver plasma membranes. *Proc. Natl. Acad. Sci. USA* 82:4–8

88. Swaney JB, Braithewaite F, Eden HA. 1977. Characterization of the apolipoproteins of rat plasma lipoproteins. *Biochemistry* 16:271–78

89. Tatemoto K. 1982. Isolation and characterization of peptide YY (PYY), a candidate gut hormone that inhibits pancreatic exocrine secretion. *Proc. Natl. Acad. Sci. USA* 79:2514–18

90. Taylor CB, Gould RG. 1967. A review of human cholesterol metabolism. *Arch. Pathol.* 84:2–14

91. Taylor IL. 1985. Distribution and release of peptide YY in dog measured by specific radioimmunoassay. *Gastroenterology* 88:731–37

92. Tso P, Balint JA, Bishop MB, Rodgers JB. 1981. Acute inhibition of intestinal lipid transport by Pluronic L-81 in the rat. *Am. J. Physiol.* 241:G487–97

93. Tso P, Balint JA, Rodgers JB. 1980. Effect of hydrophobic surfactant (Pluronic L-81) on lymphatic lipid transport in the rat. *Am. J. Physiol. Gastrointest. Liver Physiol.* 239:G348–53

94. Tso P, Drake DS, Black DD, Sabesin SM. 1984. Evidence for separate pathways of chylomicron and very low-density lipoprotein assembly and transport by rat small intestine. *Am. J. Physiol. Gastrointest. Liver Physiol.* 247:G599–610

95. Vu MK, Verkijk M, Muller ES, Biemond I, Lamers CB, Masclee AA. 1999. Medium chain triglycerides activate distal but not proximal gut hormones. *Clin. Nutr.* 18:359–63

96. Warwick ZS, Bowen KJ, Synowski SJ. 1997. Learned suppression of intake based on anticipated calories: cross-nutrient comparisons. *Physiol. Behav.* 62:1319–24

97. Weinberg RB, Dantzker C, Patton CS.

1990. Sensitivity of serum apolipoprotein A-IV levels to changes in dietary fat content. *Gastroenterology* 98:17–24

98. Weinberg RB, Spector MS. 1985. The self-association of human apolipoprotein A-IV. Evidence for an in vivo circulating dimeric form. *J. Biol. Chem.* 260:14279–86

99. Welch I, Saunders K, Read NW. 1985. Effect of ileal and intravenous infusions of fat emulsions on feeding and satiety in human volunteers. *Gastroenterology* 89: 1293–97

100. West DB, York B. 1998. Dietary fat, genetic predisposition, and obesity: lessons from animal models. *Am. J. Clin. Nutr.* 67:505–12S

101. Willnow TE, Goldstein JL, Orth K, Brown MS, Herz J. 1992. Low density lipoprotein receptor-related protein and gp330 bind similar ligands, including plasminogen activator-inhibitor complexes and lactoferrin, an inhibitor of chylomicron remnant clearance. *J. Biol. Chem.* 267:26172–80

102. Woods SC, Seeley RJ, Porte DJ, Schwartz MW. 1998. Signals that regulate food intake and energy homeostasis. *Science* 280:1378–83

103. Zhang Y, Proenca R, Maffei M, Barone M, Leopold L, Friedman JM. 1994. Positional cloning of the mouse obese gene and its human homologue. *Nature* 372:425–32

Annu. Rev. Nutr. 2001. 21:255–82

# NEW PERSPECTIVES ON FOLATE CATABOLISM

## Jae Rin Suh, A Katherine Herbig, and Patrick J Stover
*Cornell University, Division of Nutritional Sciences, Ithaca, New York 14853;
e-mail: JRS22@cornell.edu; AKH5@cornell.edu; PJS13@cornell.edu*

**Key Words**   ferritin, iron, one-carbon metabolism, pregnancy, cancer

■ **Abstract**   Folate catabolism has been assumed to result from the nonenzymatic oxidative degradation of labile folate cofactors. Increased rates of folate catabolism and simultaneous folate deficiency occur in several physiological states, including pregnancy, cancer, and when anticonvulsant drugs are used. These studies have introduced the possibility that folate catabolism may be a regulated cellular process that influences intracellular folate concentrations. Recent studies have demonstrated that the iron storage protein ferritin can catabolize folate in vitro and in vivo, and increased heavy-chain ferritin synthesis decreases intracellular folate concentrations independent of exogenous folate levels in cell culture models. Ferritin levels are elevated in most physiological states associated with increased folate catabolism. Therefore, folate catabolism is emerging as an important component in the regulation of intracellular folate concentrations and whole-body folate status.

## CONTENTS

# INTRODUCTION

The importance of folate-mediated one-carbon metabolism in fundamental metabolic and cellular processes, including DNA synthesis and methylation, has been recognized since the 1940s. Almost immediately following the discovery of folate as a metabolic cofactor, folate analogs or antifolates were developed that proved to be effective antimicrobial and antineoplastic agents. More recent studies have established a role for folate in disease prevention. Epidemiological, genetic, and biochemical data are revealing that impairments in folate metabolism are partially determinant in the initiation and progression of certain cancers, birth defects, and cardiovascular disease. Alterations of folate metabolism can result not only from folate deficiency but also from pharmaceutical therapies, genetic predisposition including single nucleotide polymorphisms, and certain physiological states. With respect to the latter, studies have identified individuals with adequate folate intake who nonetheless display symptomatic folate deficiency. Therefore, elucidating the biochemical mechanisms that regulate intracellular folate concentrations is critical to understanding the complex relationship between folate status, folate metabolism, and disease. This review focuses on the role of folate catabolism and turnover in regulating intracellular folate concentrations and on recent biochemical evidence that indicates folate catabolism may be a regulated, enzyme-mediated process.

# PHYSIOLOGICAL FUNCTIONS OF FOLATE

Folate is present in cells as a family of structurally related derivatives comprised of 2-amino-4-hydroxypteridine linked through a methylene carbon to p-aminobenzoylpolyglutamate (Figure 1). Reduced tetrahydrofolates serve as cofactors that carry one-carbon units at three different oxidation levels from methanol to formate. The one-carbons are carried on the N-5 and/or N-10 of tetrahydrofolate, and these one-carbon forms can be enzymatically interconverted. While serum folates contain a single glutamate residue, intracellular folates contain a polyglutamate peptide usually consisting of 5–8 glutamate residues that are polymerized through unusual γ-linked peptide bonds (111). The polyglutamate moiety increases the affinity of folate for folate-dependent enzymes, aids in sequestering folate within the cell, and may serve as a swinging arm that permits metabolic channeling of the cofactor among folate-dependent enzymes (103, 111). Folate

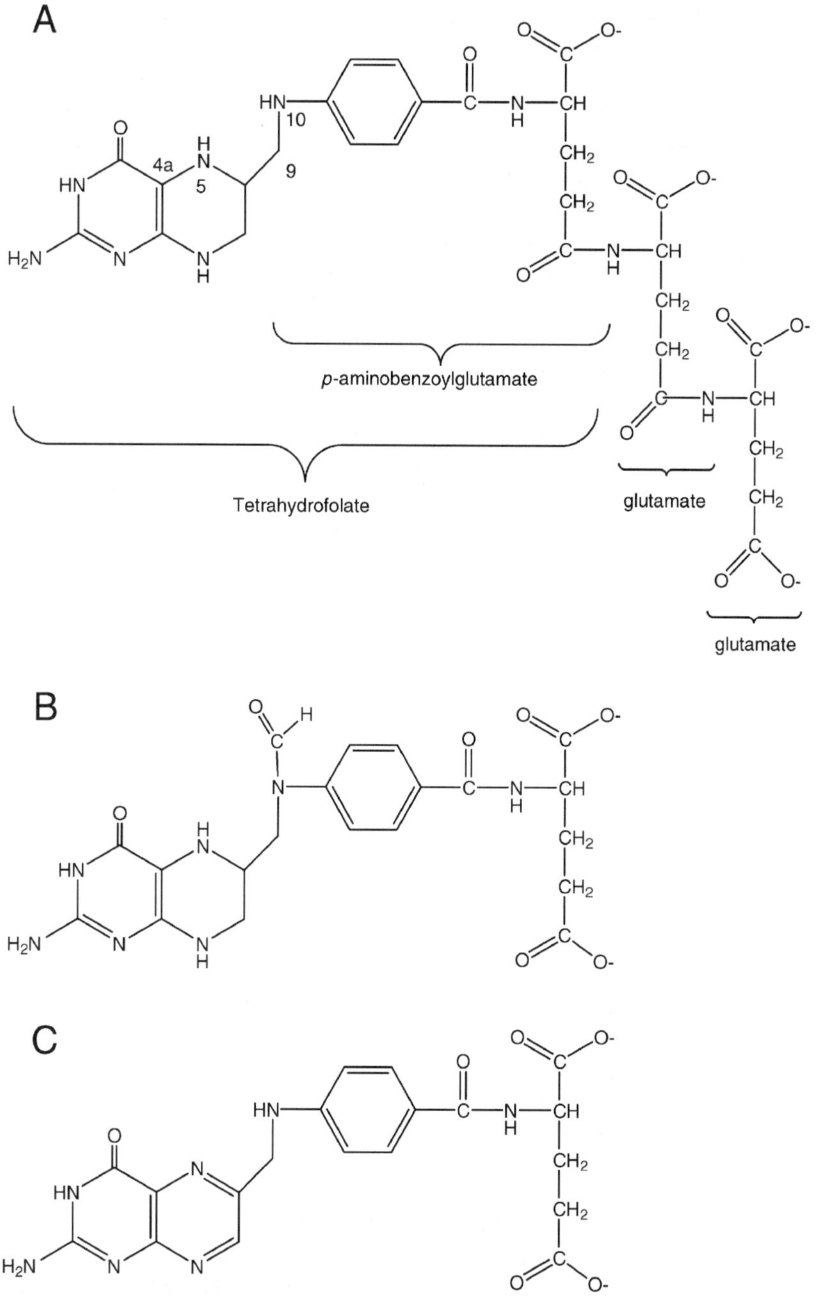

**Figure 1** Structure of folates. (*A*) Structure of tetrahydrofolate triglutamate; (*B*) structure of a one-carbon substituted folate, 10-formyltetrahydrofolate monoglutamate; (*C*) structure of synthetic folic acid.

polyglutamates are coenzymes that donate or accept one-carbon units in a set of reactions characterized as one-carbon metabolism, which occurs both in the mitochondria and the cytoplasm (130). One-carbon metabolism in the cytoplasm is necessary for the de novo synthesis of purines and thymidylate, and for the remethylation of homocysteine to methionine. Methionine can be adenylated to form S-adenosylmethionine (SAM), which is a cofactor and one-carbon donor for numerous other methylation reactions (130). Increasing evidence suggests that the primary role of mitochondrial one-carbon metabolism is to generate glycine and formate from serine. Mitochondria-derived formate traverses to the cytoplasm, where it is a major source of one-carbon units for cytoplasmic one-carbon metabolism (4).

Unlike most bacteria and yeast, mammals cannot synthesize folates de novo and, therefore, require folates in the diet. Naturally occurring dietary folates have a reduced pteridine ring and a polyglutamate polypeptide that must be hydrolyzed in the intestinal lumen to a monoglutamate form before being absorbed by the intestinal cell (40). Fully oxidized folic acid is a synthetic form of folate and is found only in food that has been fortified with it. Once the pteridine ring of folic acid is reduced in the cell to the active tetrahydrofolate form, it is considered to be folate and serves the same biological functions (111).

## CELLULAR COMPARTMENTATION OF FOLATE

Most cellular folate is compartmentalized, with up to half of the folate residing in the mitochondria and the remainder in the cytoplasm (51, 72). Folate is also present in other organelles, including the nucleus, although this folate does not make significant contributions to total cellular folate concentrations. Several studies have indicated that most cellular folate is protein bound. Initial work (143) estimated that approximately 60% of cytoplasmic folate and 20% of mitochondrial folate is tightly bound to proteins in rat liver. Subsequent studies of cell culture systems indicated that the cellular concentrations of non–protein-bound or free folate cofactor are very low or negligible (80, 81, 120) when the concentrations of all folate-binding proteins, not just the tight-binding proteins, are considered. The overall concentration of folate-binding proteins in liver might exceed the concentration of folate by as much as 5- to 10-fold (60). Considering that folate polyglutamates bind to many of these enzymes with high affinity ($K_d$ in the 100 nM range) and that the concentration of folate in liver is 25–35 $\mu$M (20, 51), it is likely that in vivo, most liver folate is protein bound. The major intracellular folate tight-binding proteins present in rat liver are the mitochondrial sarcosine and dimethylglycine dehydrogenases (136), cytoplasmic glycine N-methyltransferase (140), and 10-formyltetrahydrofolate dehydrogenase (90). These proteins are highly enriched or exclusively expressed in liver, an organ that may contain half of total body folate (42). Also consistent with the notion that most folates are protein bound, studies have demonstrated that tissue folate concentrations in rats do not increase proportionally with folate intake (21, 42, 56). Collectively, these studies indicate that intracellular folate concentrations are saturable and independent of excess exogenous folate supply, and that the threshold for intracellular folate accumulation is limited by the folate-binding capacity of the cell.

## Consequences of Impaired Folate Status

Inadequate folate status has been reported in many population groups (102). Clinically, impaired folate status is associated with gastrointestinal disorders, smoking, alcohol consumption, antiepileptic drug use. In addition, certain dietary factors can interfere with folate bioavailability (40, 102). Biochemical indices of folate status are serum and red blood cell (RBC) folate levels. Serum folate represents circulating folate, which can change quickly and is influenced by diet, whereas RBC folate levels represent intracellular folate status (40, 102). RBC folate levels are a good indicator of long-term status because cellular folate stores that accumulate during erythropoiesis are retained throughout the cell's life span and correlate strongly with hepatic concentrations (74). Therefore, in the absence of pernicious anemia, RBC folate is most representative of body stores (74).

Although cells may not accumulate excess folate relative to their binding capacity, mild folate deficiency at both the cellular and organismal levels disrupts folate-requiring anabolic pathways and leads to identifiable pathologies. Both homocysteine remethylation and thymidylate synthesis are sensitive to folate deficiency. Plasma homocysteine is considered a sensitive marker of folate status (128), but it can also be influenced by vitamin $B_6$ and $B_{12}$ status as well as by age (110). Biochemically, elevated cellular homocysteine can result from impaired methionine synthesis and lead to elevations in intracellular S-adenosylhomocysteine, a potent inhibitor of SAM-dependent reactions (141). Therefore, SAM-dependent reactions, including DNA and protein methylation, are sensitive to impairments in homocysteine remethylation. Clinically, elevated serum homocysteine is positively correlated with neural tube defects (NTDs), cardiovascular disease (7, 35, 128), and certain types of cancer (64). The relationship between folate status and NTDs is well established, with folic acid supplementation preventing three out of four cases of human NTDs (107). Furthermore, supplemental folic acid can prevent neural tube defects in *Pax3* (32) and *CartI* (144) mouse mutants, whereas methionine, but not folic acid, can lower the frequency of NTDs in *Axd* mutants (30). An independent role for folate in cardiovascular disease has also been reported (100). Studies in humans (10) and animal models (52) have demonstrated an inverse association between folate status and uracil content in DNA, presumably because of impaired thymidylate synthesis and subsequent misincorporation of dUTP into DNA (10). For example, cancerous cells, which often display cellular folate deficiency, contain increased uracil content in DNA (64). Mice with the *Pax3* mutation display impaired thymidylate synthesis, and thymidine supplementation alone can replace folate in ameliorating NTDs in these mice, indicating that folate is critical for efficient DNA synthesis in neural tube formation (32). The effect of folate deficiency on DNA synthesis is also evidenced by its morphological presentation in megaloblastic anemia and hypersegmented polymorphonuclear neutrophils (74).

# BIOCHEMICAL MECHANISMS FOR ACCUMULATION AND RETENTION OF FOLATE

## Transport of Folate

Folate monoglutamates are hydrophilic, bivalent anions present in serum at nano-molar concentrations and therefore require concentrative transport systems to meet cellular demand (116). Folate transport is required not only for cellular uptake but also for intracellular compartmentation of the cofactor (3). There are three physiological mechanisms for the transport of folates into cells (Figure 2). One route is through a family of folate-binding proteins/folate receptors (FR), which are membrane-bound receptors that mediate the unidirectional transport of folate into the cell (1). There is strong evidence that membrane-bound FRs may act via receptor-mediated endocytosis (1, 3). Alternatively, folates can be transported by reduced folate carriers, mobile carrier-mediated folate transport systems that fa-cilitate internalization of folates across membranes (116). Unlike FR-mediated transport, this process is capable of bidirectional flux. Although different carrier-mediated systems exist in different cells, they do have universal properties (116). The reduced folate carrier cDNA and gene (*RFC-1*) have been cloned, and tissue-specific alternatively spliced variants have been identified (116). There is some evidence that the reduced folate transporter may act as an anion exchanger to concentrate intracellular folate (116). Carrier-mediated systems have been doc-umented in absorptive cells and in subcellular organelles, specifically lysosomes and mitochondria (116). Recently, the gene encoding a novel mitochondrial fo-late transporter, unrelated to *RFC1*, was reported (126). Although receptor- and carrier-mediated systems may occur together in some cell types, the contribution of each to net translocation is unclear and depends on the expression level of the genes involved (116). Carrier-mediated processes are known to be much more efficient than receptor-mediated transport (48, 54). Finally, passive diffusion has been proposed to occur across cell membranes at pharmacological and possibly physiological levels of folate (1, 49). For all transport mechanisms, net accumu-lation of folate is dependent on the activity of multidrug-resistant ATPases. These proteins facilitate the removal of folate monoglutamate species and perhaps folate degradation products from various mammalian cell types (116).

## The Role of Folylpoly-$\gamma$-Glutamate Synthetase

Because newly transported folate contains a single glutamate moiety, it is ineffi-cient as a cofactor and can efflux from the cell. The active, coenzyme forms of folate are folylpolyglutamates, which contain a glutamate polypeptide attached to the *p*-aminobenzoylglutamate (*p*ABG) ring (111). The enzyme folylpoly-$\gamma$-glutamate synthetase (FPGS) can sequentially add up to eight L-glutamic acid residues to folate monoglutamates via a $\gamma$-carboxyl peptide linkage. Polyglutamy-lation of folates by FPGS is necessary to sequester folates, which need to be at least

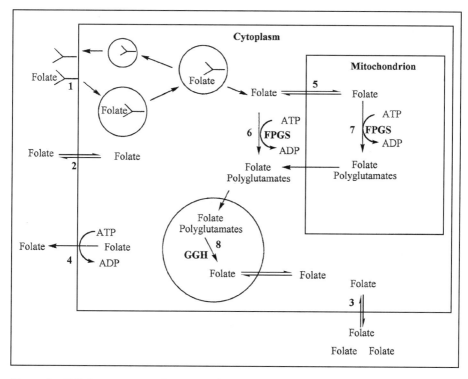

**Figure 2**  Cellular transport and accumulation of folates. Folate monoglutamates can be internalized by receptors (FR) on the cellular membrane and delivered into the cell through receptor-mediated endocytosis (1). Alternatively, folate monoglutamates can be transported through reduced folate carrier-mediated systems in addition to or exclusive of FRs (2). It has also been proposed that folate monoglutamates at high extracellular concentrations can enter the cell through passive diffusion (3). Intracellular folate monoglutamate concentrations are regulated in part by ATP-dependent exporters (4). Transport into mitochondria is limited to reduced folate monoglutamates (5) whereas both folate mono- and polyglutamates can exit, but the mechanism for the exit of folate polyglutamates has not been identified. Folate monoglutamates that enter the cytoplasm or the mitochondrion are converted to folate polyglutamates by the action of folylpoly-$\gamma$-glutamate synthetase (FPGS) (6, 7). Folate polyglutamates can enter the lysosome through a carrier-mediated system and be converted to folate monoglutamates by the action of $\gamma$-glutamyl hydrolase (GGH) (8). The mechanism for exit of folate monoglutamates from components of the endocytic pathway or from lysosomes has not been identified.

triglutamates to avoid efflux by folate exporters (94). FPGS isozymes function in both the cytosol and mitochondria of mammalian cells (72, 73). Cytosolic FPGS is necessary to maintain normal cytosolic folate pools whereas the mitochondrial isozyme is necessary for accumulation of folates in the mitochondria (17). Increased cellular FPGS activity lengthens folate polyglutamate chain length whereas increased import of folate monoglutamates lowers overall folate polyglutamate chain lengths because of substrate competition (111). Additionally, mitochondrial FPGS is necessary to avoid glycine auxotrophy (73). Polygluta-mates are not transported into the mitochondria (72), but they can be effluxed into the cytoplasm from the mitochondria without prior hydrolysis (61, 62, 73). FPGS activity can be detected in most mammalian tissues, although the highest activity is found in the liver (94).

## The Role of Folylpoly-$\gamma$-Glutamate Hydrolase

Retention of folates is also influenced by the hydrolytic action of folylpolygluta-mate hydrolase [$\gamma$-glutamyl hydrolase (GGH)]. This enzyme catalyzes the removal of the polyglutamate peptide from intracellular folate generating folate monogluta-mate, which can then exit the cell. GGH is widely distributed in tissues and primar-ily localized in the lysosomes. Its catalytic activity is specific to the $\gamma$-glutamyl peptide bond of polyglutamates (83) and acts as either an exo-peptidase or an endo-peptidase, depending on the source from which it is derived (83). It has low specificity for the pteroyl portion of the molecule and can remove the polyglutamate polypeptide from the folate degradation product $p$-aminobenzoylypolyglutamate (83). Protein-bound polyglutamates are not hydrolyzed, which accounts for the increased half-life of cellular folate polyglutamates compared with monogluta-mates (132). The role of GGH activity in regulating intracellular folate concen-trations has never been directly explored.

## FOLATE TURNOVER

Although folate transport and polyglutamylation are critical for delivering and sequestering folate within the cell, and disruption of these processes impairs folate accumulation, there is no evidence that these processes fully determine intracellular folate concentrations. Some studies have indicated that the expression and activity of the reduced folate carriers may respond to intracellular folate concentrations (53, 79, 120, 137), but definitive biochemical mechanisms for this regulation have not been established. Expression and localization of membrane-associated FRs may also be regulated by extracellular folate concentrations (55). Nonetheless, there is no direct experimental evidence that the regulation of transport processes alone can set or maintain intracellular folate concentrations at subsaturation levels in the presence of exogenous folate. Therefore, the role of folate catabolism and turnover in regulating intracellular folate concentrations must be considered.

## Rates of Folate Turnover

Consistent with the complexity of biochemical pathways that regulate folate im-port and accumulation in mammalian cells, analyses of human whole-body folate turnover have revealed the presence of several kinetically distinguishable turnover pools (69, 101, 118, 129). Biochemically, the fast-turnover pools have a half-life of hours and probably reflect newly absorbed folate that escapes cellular import or extensive polyglutamylation, whereas the slow-turnover pools reflect turnover of folate polyglutamate cofactors (69, 129). Recent kinetic modeling of folate turnover in normal human males supplemented with physiologic levels of folate revealed that the long-lived folate pools have a mean residence time of greater than or equal to 100 days (118). This study made provisions for, without directly measuring, fecal folate excretion and catabolites, which may account for nearly 50% of folate turnover (69, 118). Fecal excretion of endogenous folate cannot be measured easily because of the presence of folate from bacteria residing in the gut (118). However, fecal excretion of folate and its degradation products has been found to be an important excretory process in humans and rats (9, 69, 109).

## Chemical Stability of Folate In Vitro

The reduced forms of folate are unstable in vitro and readily undergo oxidative degradation. At pH 7.0, tetrahydrofolate has a solution half-life of about 40 min (99) but can be stabilized in vitro by the addition of reduced thiols or antioxidants, including ascorbate. Oxidation has been proposed to occur by at least two distinct irreversible mechanisms (Figure 3). The pteridine ring can be sequentially oxidized to dihydrofolate and then to folic acid through a quininoid dihydrofolate intermediate (18, 99). This mechanism is similar to that elucidated for tetrahydropterin oxidation (5, 92), which proceeds through a 4a-carbinolamine intermediate. Reduced thiols protect reduced folates from oxidation (142), presumably by forming transient 4a adducts. Alternatively, reduced folates can undergo oxidative scission at the C9-N10 bond, after which folate is no longer a viable metabolic cofactor. It has been proposed that electron loss at N10 results in the formation of an N10 nitrenium ion intermediate that rapidly converts to a more stable C9-N10 Schiff base (99). However, there is no evidence for oxidation occurring directly at N10. Hydrolysis of the Schiff base yields the scission products 6-formyltetrahydropterin (or 6-formyldihydropterin in the case of dihydrofolate catabolism) and pABG (99). One-carbon substitution at the N5 or N10 position can alter the sensitivity of reduced folates to oxidative degradation (71, 78). 5-Formyltetrahydrofolate is the most stable derivative of tetrahydrofolate, in part due to steric protection of the C4a oxidation site.

## In Vivo Catabolism of Folate

Intracellular folate turnover can occur by at least three mechanisms. Newly transported folate monoglutamate species that escape polyglutamylation can efflux from the cell. Folate polyglutamates can undergo hydrolysis of the polyglutamate peptide by GGH, resulting in their conversion to folate monoglutamate species, which then efflux from the cell. Lastly, folates can be catabolized to yield inactive degradation products. Folates are stabilized when they are protein bound. During folate deficiency in rats, free folate is depleted to a greater extent than is

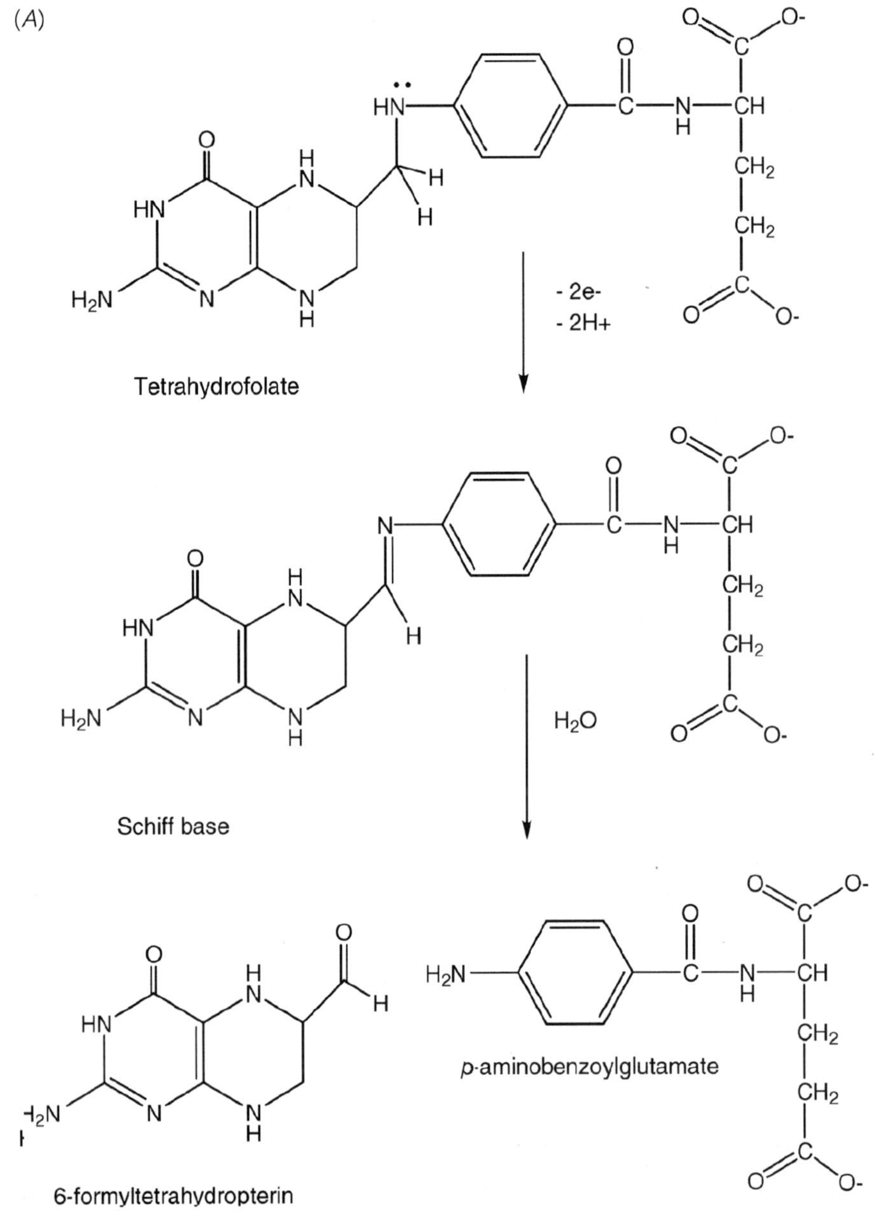

**Figure 3** Oxidation of tetrahydrofolate in vitro. Reduced folate cofactors are susceptible to oxidation by two independent pathways. (*A*) Oxidation can result in the formation of a C9-N10 Schiff base that undergoes hydrolysis to yield inactive degradation products. (*B*) The reduced pterin ring can be oxidized to form dihydrofolate, which can undergo further oxidation to produce scission products.

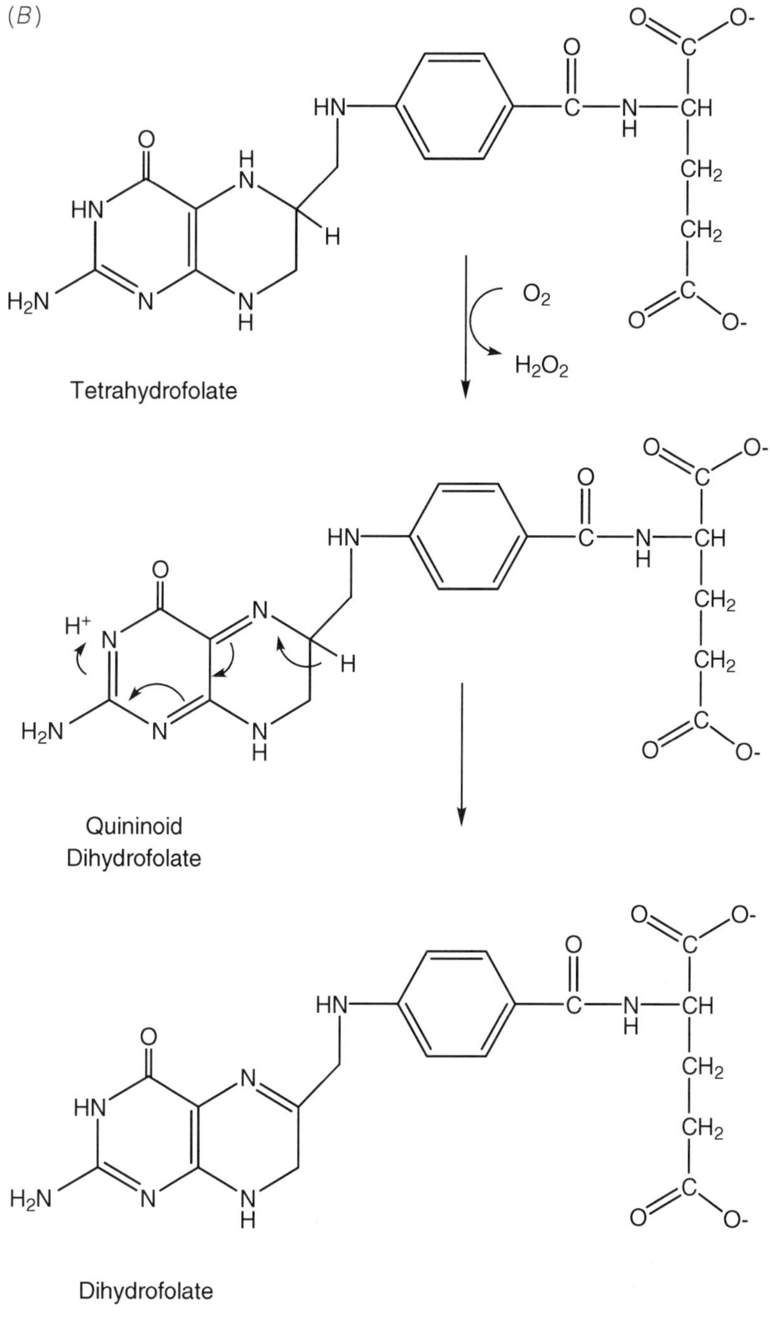

(B)

Tetrahydrofolate

$O_2$

$H_2O_2$

Quininoid
Dihydrofolate

Dihydrofolate

**Figure 3** (*Continued*)

protein-bound folate (142). In humans, early observations indicated that the amount of folate in the diet is at least 10-fold greater than that found excreted intact in urine (12, 24). This discrepancy is not accounted for by stool folate (11). Dinning et al (26) were the first to observe in vivo cleavage of folate resulting in the formation of primary aromatic, diazotizable amines in rat urine following administration of both 5-formyltetrahydrofolate and folic acid. The formation of these catabolites was determined to be a major excretory process associated with folate turnover. These amines were later identified as pABG and its acetylated derivative, acetamidobenzoylglutamate (ApABG) (68). Similarly, these folate catabolites were also identified in urine of human subjects (68, 69).

The products of folate catabolism undergo different fates. Following folate cleavage, the export of pABG polyglutamates is facilitated by removal of the polyglutamate polypeptide by GGH, and pABG is likely acetylated in the cytosol by arylamine N-acetyltransferases to produce ApABG (91), which represents >80% of total pABG excretion in humans (42, 86). ApABG does not accumulate in cells and is rapidly excreted in the urine (95). Geoghegan et al (34) suggest that the presence of free pABG in urine is not due to incomplete acetylation in vivo but rather to nonspecific extracellular degradation of intact labile folates in the circulation or bladder, or to degradation during urine collection. Pterin aldehydes generated by folate catabolism through cleavage at the C9-N10 bond are further metabolized, retained in the liver, and slowly released (69, 98).

Mechanisms of folate turnover have been validated in rodent models. Labeled folic acid becomes fully equilibrated into tissue folate polyglutamate pools within 2–3 days in rats (59). Following equilibration, one study found only cleaved folates in the urine (59) whereas another found low levels of reduced folate monoglutamates (34, 96, 109) in addition to cleaved products in urine up to 12 days postdose. It is interesting to note that, in this animal model, folate turnover rates displayed tissue-specific variations. Turnover rates of folate in the liver and kidney were very slow relative to heart, spleen, testes, and hind leg muscle at 32 days following a single administration of labeled folic acid (109). The increased stability of folates in the liver may be accounted for by its high concentration of folate tight-binding proteins.

## Mechanism of Folate Catabolism

In vivo folate catabolism has been assumed to result from random, nonregulated, nonenzymatic degradation of labile folate cofactors, in particular dihydrofolate and 10-formyltetrahydrofolate (77, 85). Both are particularly sensitive to oxidative degradation, and cellular accumulation of these folate derivatives is associated with decreases in cellular folate concentrations. The enzyme 10-formyltetrahydrofolate dehydrogenase (FDH) regulates 10-formyltetrahydrofolate levels by catalyzing the oxidative cleavage of the N10 formyl group of 10-formyltetrahydrofolate, resulting in the formation of $CO_2$ and tetrahydrofolate (15). Homozygous deletion of the gene encoding FDH in mice results in the accumulation of hepatic

10-formyltetrahydrofolate and a 30% decrease in intracellular folate concentrations when the animals are maintained on a standard chow diet (15). Similarly, intracellular folate concentrations and FDH levels positively correlate in regions of rat brain, which supports the hypothesis that 10-formyltetrahydrofolate accumulation impairs folate accumulation (77). However, there is no direct evidence that cellular accumulation of 10-formyltetrahydrofolate results in the catabolism of this folate derivative by either enzymatic or nonenzymatic mechanisms.

Cellular accumulation of dihydrofolate does result in increased folate catabolism in prokaryotes (97). Bacteria exposed to the dihydrofolate reductase inhibitor methotrexate display rapid accumulation of both dihydrofolate and $p$ABG, with subsequent folate deficiency. In mammals, increased rates of folate catabolism are associated with increased rates of cell division, presumably resulting from robust thymidylate synthesis and therefore dihydrofolate formation (85). Nonenzymatic catabolism of dihydrofolate is the assumed, but not proven, biochemical mechanism for turnover (85).

Recently, a protein was purified from rat tissue that generated $p$ABG from 5-formyltetrahydrofolate (121). The purified protein was identified as ferritin, the major iron-storage protein in the body [as reviewed by Harrison & Arosio (47)]. Ferritins are 24mers that form a hollow protein shell with a $M_r \approx 500,000$ and can store up to 4500 atoms of $Fe^{3+}$ (33, 47). In vertebrates, ferritin is primarily localized to the cytoplasm and is comprised of varying proportions of heavy-chain (HCF) and light-chain (LCF) subunits (47). Both cell type and iron status determine the relative proportions of HCF and LCF.

Ferritin-mediated folate catabolism exhibits less than a single turnover per ferritin monomeric subunit and therefore is not a catalytic event in vitro (121). The $K_m$ of 5-formyltetrahydrofolate for ferritin is in the millimolar range; the affinity for other forms of folate was not determined in this study, including the more-labile reduced folates (121). If the more oxidatively labile folates are the best substrates for ferritin-mediated catabolism, their accumulation may result in low cellular folate concentrations. Previous attempts to purify an enzyme from mammalian tissue that catalyzed the oxidative cleavage of folates to $p$ABG had not been successful (106). These attempts utilized the more-labile forms of reduced folates and, therefore, suffered from high background rates of nonenzymatic degradation, or utilized oxidized synthetic folic acid, which is not a substrate for ferritin-mediated catabolism.

Expression of rat HCF two- to fourfold over endogenous concentrations in Chinese hamster ovary cells increases rates of folate turnover nearly proportionally and reduces intracellular folate concentrations by 15% relative to control cells when cultured in the presence of pharmacological concentrations of folic acid (121). The same cells cultured in the absence of folate for 48 h display up to a 40% decrease in intracellular folate concentrations. Folates were shown to be less susceptible to ferritin-mediated catabolism with increased residency time in the cell, indicating that ferritin preferentially scavenges non–protein-bound folates that lack longer glutamate polypeptides (121). Therefore, folate turnover can regulate intracellular folate concentrations independent of exogenous folic acid concentrations, and folate catabolism may play a key role in regulating intracellular folate concentrations.

# PHYSIOLOGICAL STATES ASSOCIATED WITH ALTERED FOLATE STATUS AND INCREASED RATES OF FOLATE CATABOLISM

## Folate Nutriture and Status

The presence of A$p$ABG in urine is indicative of folate catabolism, and its concentration in urine is considered a reliable indicator of folate status (131) and turnover (34) in rats. Total urinary $p$ABG excretion exceeded that of folate excretion in rats fed diets containing a range of folic acid from deficient to adequate (131). In this study, urinary $p$ABG and hepatic folate increased linearly with increases in dietary folate (131). Total urinary A$p$ABG excretion also greatly exceeded that of intact folates (most of which was 5-methyltetrahydrofolate) in nonpregnant women under conditions of controlled dietary intake (41). However, in this study, urinary folate, but not A$p$ABG, increased with increasing folic acid intake (41), a finding that was attributed to small sample size. Larger, related studies from the same laboratory did observe increased urinary A$p$ABG, $p$ABG, as well as intact folate as a function of folate intake. Therefore, folate intake likely influences the rate of folate turnover and catabolism in humans (14).

Folate supplementation at pharmacological levels also influences the urinary excretion of folate and total $p$ABG in humans. One study found that folic acid supplementation caused large increases in urinary folate concentration but only small ones in total $p$ABG (68). Both reduced folates and oxidized folic acid were found in urine, indicating that not all the administered folic acid was processed to reduced cellular polyglutamate cofactors. Similarly, McPartlin et al (88) did not observe any significant change in total $p$ABG with supplementation of folic acid at levels more than 10 times the recommended daily allowance over the course of 3 days, but this may have been due to the shorter supplementation period (68). In conclusion, the increases in total $p$ABG associated with increased folate intake and status are consistent with the idea that folate catabolism is necessary to maintain low intracellular folate concentrations during periods of increased folate intake.

## Pregnancy and Neonatal Growth

Pregnancy imposes stress on folate stores (84) due to increased needs for growth of the fetus, the placenta, and maternal tissues (2). Increased folate is also required for uterine enlargement and expansion of blood volume, which necessitates increased red cell production (84). This increased need for folate does not come at the expense of the fetus, as newborns have significantly higher plasma and RBC folate levels compared with maternal values (14, 28, 36). Inadequate folate status is common in pregnancy (6) and is associated with increased incidence of maternal megaloblastic anemia, low-birth-weight babies (102), and preterm delivery (105).

In pregnant women, the need for folate exceeds that of the calculated total fetal and placental folate content at term, indicating that increased folate turnover may occur during pregnancy (87). Studies of rat models have demonstrated not only increased need for folate cofactors and increased one-carbon metabolism during pregnancy but also elevated rates of folate catabolism. Urinary ApABG production was shown to be higher in pregnant dams relative to nonpregnant control dams when free-fed or pair-fed on a purified, folate-free diet (84). Although some of the increase in ApABG excretion was accounted for by weight gain and therefore was independent of pregnancy, there was an authentic effect of pregnancy on folate turnover. In this study, urinary ApABG excretion increased from day 2 of gestation and peaked at day 18 to levels of up to three times that of nonpregnant rats and then fell off significantly despite increasing weight gain until day 21, the day of parturition (84). The authors of this study noted that within the rat placenta, DNA content does not change after day 17 of gestation, and growth becomes hypertrophic whereas fetal growth is almost entirely hyperplastic. Therefore, elevated ApABG excretion may represent the increasing needs for folate for DNA synthesis by the fetal and placental tissues, whereas the decrease in excretion corresponds to decreased needs as the placental tissue switches to hypertrophic growth (84). Elevated rates of folate catabolism continue during growth of weanling rats (85). Using a catch-up growth model, urinary ApABG excretion was shown to increase with hyperplastic growth. This suggests that the rate of folate catabolism is related to folate utilization in cell division, presumably resulting from increased generation of oxidatively labile dihydrofolate during DNA synthesis (85). These studies indicate a paradox: Folate catabolism increases during periods of increased physiological needs for folate in rats.

Results from studies of human folate catabolism during pregnancy are conflicting. An initial pilot study of six healthy nonpregnant women and six age-matched pregnant women demonstrated that urinary excretion of pABG and ApABG increased during the second ($\sim$200%) and third ($\sim$150%) trimesters in pregnant women compared with total pABG excretion of pregnant women during the first trimester and compared with nonpregnant controls (87). A larger subsequent study by the same laboratory, including 24 healthy gravid women and 25 nonpregnant controls, supported the pilot study, as evidenced by increased urinary ApABG during pregnancy, with maximal rates of folate catabolism occurring during the third trimester (50). At this time, rates of folate catabolism were elevated by more than twofold relative to nonpregnant controls. From this study, it was estimated that folate requirements during pregnancy are increased by 200–300 $\mu$g per day to offset losses from catabolism. In contrast, compared with nonpregnant controls, Caudill et al (14) did not find increased catabolism in the second trimester for pregnant women in either week 14 or week 26 of gestation. In contradiction with other studies, results from this study indicated that folate catabolic rates actually decrease during pregnancy. Excretion of ApABG at week 26 of gestation was significantly lower than in nonpregnant controls when women were given 450 $\mu$g of folate per day, although this effect was not seen with a folate intake of 850 $\mu$g per day. The disparate results between these two studies have been attributed to different analytical procedures used to measure ApABG and various aspects of the patient treatment protocol, including the duration of controlled dietary intake (14, 87).

Pregnancy is also associated with elevated ferritin expression. Recently, HCF message levels were found to be markedly elevated during the implantation stage of pregnancy in rats (145). Compared with minimal levels of HCF mRNA normally found in the uteri of nonpregnant (estrous cycle) rats, HCF mRNA increased 8- to 10-fold in pregnant rats. The HCF mRNA and protein expression profiles parallel progesterone concentrations, which are low in the estrous cycle, surge after fertilization and remain high until parturition, when they drop sharply. HCF mRNA also declines rapidly after parturition (145). Increased HCF expression during pregnancy was localized primarily in the cytoplasm of endometrial stromal cells whereas LCF mRNA expression did not change appreciably. Progesterone alone can induce HCF message levels and antiprogestins abolish elevations in HCF protein and mRNA when administered in early pregnancy. Likewise, progesterone treatment of ovariectomized animals results in a 25-fold increase in HCF message in the uterus. Estrogen priming can enhance the effect of progesterone in ovariectomized rats, whereas estrogen, glucocorticoid, or androgen treatment alone cannot influence expression of HCF (145).

During pregnancy, fetal iron requirements are greatest in the third trimester (70). In general, maternal serum ferritin levels decline with gestation as a result of haemodilution occurring in early pregnancy and as a result of heavy demands for iron (38, 96). Maternal serum ferritin concentrations are lowest during the third trimester of pregnancy (104), with mean levels approximating those of iron-deficiency anemia, and they decline despite the use of iron supplements (96). Failure of serum ferritin levels to decline in the third trimester is associated with iron-deficiency anemia, anemia, and lower levels of serum and RBC folate during pregnancy. High maternal serum ferritin is also a marker for maternal infection (123). Furthermore, in the third trimester, both high ferritin levels and low RBC folate are associated with preterm and very preterm delivery. High ferritin levels in the second trimester are also a predictor for preterm birth (38, 123). It is possible that low maternal ferritin levels during periods of high fetal iron requirements may occur in order to spare folate by decreasing catabolism. Although serum ferritin levels are not considered reliable indicators of tissue ferritin levels, well-designed animal studies investigating the effects of elevated maternal ferritin on folate catabolism, folate status, and pregnancy outcome are clearly warranted.

## Oral Contraceptive Use

The use of oral contraceptive agents (OCA) has been associated with low serum and RBC folate levels in women 20–44 years of age (74). Long-term use has also been associated with folate deficiency (16). The relationship between OCA use and folate status was first described in 1968 (115), but whether or not OCA use has a detrimental effect on folate status is still controversial (39). In a rat model, OCA treatment led to decreased plasma and RBC folate associated with moderate hyperhomocysteinemia (27). In addition, women who reported using OCAs regularly before pregnancy had lower RBC folate in the first trimester than did nonusers (127). Women's mean serum and RBC folate concentrations were significantly lower in users than nonusers (114), but serum and RBC folate levels were similar to those of controls in adolescent females using OCAs (39). Although some studies did not detect systemic folate deficiency, they did show localized megaloblastic changes in Papanicolaou smears from uterine cervix cells in patients taking OCAs. Cervical cells reverted to normal after folic acid therapy (75). Although several mechanisms have been proposed to explain the possible influence of OCAs on blood folate levels, two of direct relevance to this review are (*a*) the increased serum clearance and urinary excretion of folate (114) and (*b*) the increased hepatic catabolism of folates (82). The latter may be accounted for, in part, by increased ferritin synthesis associated with hormonal contraceptive use (124).

## Cancer

Rapidly proliferating cancer cells have accelerated DNA synthesis and therefore an increased requirement for folate (64). Cancerous tumor cells exhibit increased rates of folate uptake (31). Large doses of folate in well-established cancers lead to accelerated proliferation whereas folate deprivation leads to reduced or delayed growth (64). Tumor cells also display increased rates of folate catabolism. The presence of ascitic tumors in mice results in a 50% increased rate of folate catabolism, as measured by the urinary catabolites, [$^3$H]*p*ABG and [$^3$H]*N*-A*p*ABG (58). Cancer patients with active, untreated, or metastatic malignancies exhibit folate deficiency without evidence of malnourishment, malabsorption, or increased intact folate excretion (43). In the absence of significantly low serum or RBC folate concentrations, localized tissue deficiency has been observed in patients with colorectal adenoma whose normal mucosa have significantly lower folate levels in comparison to patients with nonneoplastic polyps (63). The folate content of neoplastic cells is significantly lower than the adjacent normal cells, and folate levels in normal cells from patients and controls were not significantly different (89).

Increased folate catabolism in cancerous tissue may be at least partly due to altered ferritin levels. Ferritin is increased in both cancerous tissue and in serum of afflicted patients. Because elevated serum ferritin is associated with malignant disorders (66), liver disease (23), infection, total body iron stores, and inflammation (45, 47), tissue expression is likely a better marker for carcinogenic processes. Increased generation of intracellular ferritin has been detected in leukemic cells (135), kidney cancer (65), and mammary carcinomas (76) relative to normal tissue. Patients with malignant breast carcinoma showed a sevenfold increase in tissue cytosol ferritin compared with those with benign breast disease. These differences in tissue ferritin were observed without detectable differences in serum ferritin levels (45). In a related study, ferritin concentration was elevated sixfold in malignant versus benign mammary tissue, with high cytosolic concentrations correlating with poor prognosis and dedifferentiation (134).

Increased ferritin levels in cancer cells may be influenced by expression of the oncogene c-*myc*. Using a subtraction-enhanced display technique, both HCF and c-myc were identified as mRNAs that are overexpressed in chemically induced hepatocellular carcinoma in rats. In this same model, the expression of HCF increased 10-fold as the tumor progressed (138). The relationship between c-myc and ferritin expression was validated in cell culture. Transfection of nontumorigenic clones with the c-myc cDNA increased expression of HCF mRNA in clones that acquired a tumorigenic phenotype (93). Wu et al (139) found increased HCF mRNA expression in patients with hepatocellular carcinoma, but not in patients with benign tumors (adenomas) or cirrhosis, and not in healthy patients. HCF mRNA levels were 2- to 12-fold higher in tumors compared with adjacent non-tumor tissues in 70% of patients and were highly correlated with c-myc mRNA levels in most of the patients (139). There have been no studies relating ferritin levels and folate concentrations in cancer cells.

## Anticonvulsant Drug Use

The effects of anticonvulsants on folate status have been recently reviewed (40). Although only 1% of patients treated with anticonvulsants manifest megaloblastic anemia, a greater proportion manifest macrocytosis as well as reduced serum and RBC folate, which may indicate an increased turnover or catabolism of folate (16). There is a negative dose response between carbamazepine and RBC folate levels in patients, with RBC folate levels declining further in patients taking more than one drug (37). Compared with phenobarbital, primidone, carbamazepine, and valproate, phenytoin has the greatest impact on tissue folate concentrations in rats. Chronic phenytoin treatment reduces total liver and brain folate concentrations by 66% and 25%, respectively, in rats without affecting plasma folate concentrations (13, 44). Rats treated with diphenylhydantoin had increased excretion of total *p*ABG by 80%–100% compared with control and phenobarbitone-treated rats (59), indicating a role for enhanced folate catabolism in the lowering of tissue folate by diphenylhydantoin. Both the mean daily excretion and the cumulative excretion of total *p*ABG increased as a function of increased phenytoin administration (59). This result is in accordance with clinical observations, which suggest that folate deficiency is more highly associated with phenytoin administration than with phenobarbitone. In addition to increasing folate catabolism, anticonvulsants also can directly alter folate-dependent reactions (13). For instance, valproic acid can inhibit mitochondrial folate metabolism and is also associated with increased incidence of NTDs (133). The effects of anticonvulsant drugs on ferritin levels are unknown.

## Thyroid Hormone

Purported relationships between thyroid hormone status and folate status have been conflicting, and there have been no direct studies on the effects of thyroid hormone on folate catabolism. Some studies demonstrate that hyperthyroid patients have low serum folate levels and abnormally rapid clearance of folic acid from plasma (25, 74). In contrast, other studies have indicated that serum and RBC folate levels are significantly higher in hyperthyroidic patients compared to when these same patients became euthyroidic, although these changes occurred within the reference range (33). The differences in these studies may be accounted for by lack of control for dietary intake and by the severity of the disease. Thyroid-stimulating hormone increases HCF mRNA levels in rat thyroid cells, possibly by increasing HCF transcription (22). Additionally, erythropoietin, thyrotropin-releasing hormone, and thyroid hormone all regulate ferritin translational rates (125). In rats, hyperthyroidism also decreases hepatic FDH by 65%. Both increased ferritin and decreased FDH activity would be expected to lower cellular folate concentrations.

## Alcohol

It is well-known that chronic alcoholism is associated with impaired folate status and that excess ethanol is often associated with folate deficiency (46). Ethanol-related folate deficiency can develop because of dietary inadequacy, intestinal malabsorption, altered hepatobiliary metabolism, increased renal excretion, and possibly increased folate catabolism (46). It has been proposed that ethanol may directly enhance oxidation of folate. Acetaldehyde, a metabolite of ethanol via alcohol dehydrogenase, and aldehyde oxidase may produce reactive oxygen species in the presence of free iron (12). Incubation of folate (5-methyltetrahydrofolate, 5-formyltetrahydrofolate, and folic acid) with acetaldehyde, xanthine oxidase, and iron results in $p$ABG formation (13). Cleavage of 5-methyltetrahydrofolate by ethanol was inhibited by superoxide dismutase, 4-methylpyrazole (inhibitor of alcohol dehydrogenase), and desferrioxamine (tight chelator of iron) and enhanced by the addition of ferritin and free $Fe^{2+}$ (13). Another similar in vitro study suggested free radical oxidant species target oxidation at the pteridine ring (122). However, an in vivo animal study did not find any differences in the rate of urinary folate catabolite excretion between control animals and mice after either a chronic period of or acute alcohol ingestion (57), indicating that the effects of ethanol on folate status are independent of catabolism.

## CONCLUSIONS

The studies outlined in this review suggest that folate catabolism is a regulated, enzyme-mediated event that may play a central role in regulating intracellular folate concentrations. Although the act of destroying a valuable and required nutrient seems counterintuitive, catabolism-mediated maintenance of intracellular folate at low or perhaps subsaturation levels may be necessary for effective one-carbon metabolism and may facilitate several regulatory mechanisms associated with folate metabolism. First, numerous studies have indicated that folate coenzymes are directly channeled among folate-dependent enzymes (103). Direct transfer of a folate cofactor between a donor and acceptor enzyme necessitates that the acceptor enzyme be unliganded. Therefore, metabolic channeling of folate cofactors can only occur under subsaturation conditions, and loss of channeling resulting from excess folate cofactors has been demonstrated in an in vitro reconstitution metabolic system (119). Secondly, maintenance of subsaturation levels of folate permits autotranslational regulation of thymidylate synthase and dihydrofolate reductase expression. Both dihydrofolate reductase and thymidylate synthase can bind to their respective transcripts and may inhibit translation (19, 29, 67). Thymidylate synthase can also bind to other mRNA species, including c-myc, and p53. These enzymes competitively bind mRNA and folates at the same site on the protein. Therefore, autotranslational inhibition of dihydrofolate reductase and thymidylate synthase synthesis can only function when the enzymes are unliganded. Finally, low intracellular folate permits competition between folate-dependent metabolic pathways (108). It has been proposed that purine biosynthesis, thymidylate biosynthesis, and homocysteine remethylation vie for a limited pool of folate-activated one-carbon units (108). This competition between nucleotide biosynthesis and methionine synthesis may be a regulatory mechanism that permits increased SAM-dependent methylation when synthesis of nucleotides is depressed.

A definitive role for folate degradation products in cellular function has yet to be established. There is some evidence that pABG may compete with folic acid for folate-binding proteins (8) and may assist the binding of folate to 5,10-methylenetetrahydrofolate dehydrogenase (106). In vitro studies demonstrated that pterin aldehyde acts as a substrate for xanthine oxidase, and the product, pterin-6-carboxylic acid, can act as a weak inhibitor of this enzyme (117). However, there is no evidence that pterin species generated from folate catabolism function as biological cofactors.

Collectively, the studies outlined in this review strongly implicate an important role for folate catabolism in determining intracellular folate concentrations. Additionally, the identification of physiological states associated with increased folate catabolism indicate that folate catabolism is regulated. Although the role of ferritin in facilitating folate catabolism requires further validation, initial studies indicate a complex relationship among iron status, ferritin, and folate catabolism and status. Catabolism-mediated regulation of intracellular folate concentrations may be largely independent of serum folate availability and may impact folate-mediated one-carbon metabolism much more effectively than does regulation of folate transport. Therefore, folate catabolism is implicated not only in influencing DNA synthesis and cellular homocysteine concentrations, but also in the metabolic regulation of DNA methylation and in the subsequent effects on gene expression. Elucidating the biochemical mechanisms underlying the regulation of folate catabolism and its effects on intracellular folate concentrations will be required to understand the relationships between folate status and its associated pathologies.

## ACKNOWLEDGMENTS

Our research in this review is supported by the National Institutes of Health, grant HD35678. We would like to thank Montserrat Anguera and Denise Stover for their assistance in preparing this manuscript.

**Visit the Annual Reviews home page at www.AnnualReviews.org**

## LITERATURE CITED

1. Antony AC. 1992. The biological chemistry of folate receptors. *Blood* 79:2807–20
2. Antony AC 1995. Megaloblastic anemias. In *Hematology: Basic Principles and Practice*, ed. R Hoffman, EJ Benz, SJ Shattil, B Furie, HJ Cohen, LE Silberstein, pp. 552–86. New York: Churchill Livingstone. 2nd ed.
3. Antony AC. 1996. Folate receptors. *Annu. Rev. Nutr.* 16:501–21
4. Appling DR. 1991. Compartmentation of folate-mediated one-carbon metabolism in eukaryotes. *FASEB J.* 5:2645–51
5. Archer MC, Vonderschmitt DT, Scrimgeour KG. 1972. Mechanism of oxidation of tetrahydropterins. *Can. J. Biochem.* 50:1174–82
6. Bailey LB. 1995. Folate requirements and dietary recommendations. See Ref. 96a, pp. 256–76
7. Bailey LB, Gregory JF. 1999. Polymorphisms of methylenetetrahydrofolate reductase and other enzymes: metabolic significance, risks and impact on folate requirement. *J. Nutr.* 129:779–82
8. Beck JT, Ullman B. 1989. Affinity labeling of the folate methotrexate transporter from Leishmania-Donovani. *Biochemistry* 28:6931–37
9. Bhandari SD, Gregory JF. 1992. Folic acid, 5-methyltetrahydrofolate and 5-formyltetrahydrofolate exhibit equivalent intestinal absorption, metabolism and in vivo kinetics in rats. *J. Nutr.* 122:1847–54
9a. Blakley RL, Benkovic SJ, eds. 1984. *Folates and Pterins.* New York: Wiley
10. Blount BC, Mack MM, Wher CM, MacGregor JT, Hiatt RA, et al. 1997. Folate deficiency causes uracil misincorporation into human DNA and chromosome breakage: implications for cancer and neuronal damage. *Proc. Natl. Acad. Sci. USA* 94:3290–95
11. Butterworth CE, Baugh CM, Krumdieck CL. 1969. A study of folate absorption and metabolism in man utilizing carbon-14 labeled polyglutamates synthesized by the solid phase method. *J. Clin. Invest.* 48:1131–42
12. Butterworth CE, Santini R, Frommeyer WB. 1963. The pteroylglutamate components of American diets as determined by chromatographic fractionation. *J. Clin. Invest.* 42:1929–39
13. Carl GF, Smith DB. 1983. The effect of chronic phenytoin treatment on tissue folate concentrations and the activities of the methyl synthetic enzymes in the rat. *J. Nutr.* 113:2368–74
14. Caudill MA, Gregory JF, Hutson AD, Bailey LB. 1998. Folate catabolism in pregnant and nonpregnant women with controlled folate intakes. *J. Nutr.* 128:204–8
15. Champion KM, Cook RJ, Tollaksen SL,

Giometti CS. 1994. Identification of a heritable deficiency of the folate-dependent enzyme 10-formyltetrahydrofolate dehydrogenase in mice. *Proc. Natl. Acad. Sci. USA* 91:11338–42

16. Chanarin I. 1979. *The Megalobastic Amemias.* Oxford/London: Blackwell Sci. 2nd ed.

17. Chen L, Qi H, Korenberg J, Garrow TA, Choi Y-J, Shane B. 1996. Purification and properties of human cytosolic folylpoly-γ-glutamate synthetase and organization, localization, and differential splicing of its gene. *J. Biol. Chem.* 271:13077–87

18. Chippel D, Scrimgeour KG. 1970. Oxidative degradation of dihydrofolate and tetrahydrofolate. *Can. J. Biochem.* 48:999–1009

19. Chu E, Allegra CJ. 1996. The role of thymidylate synthase as an RNA binding protein. *BioEssays* 18:191–98

20. Cichowicz DJ, Shane B. 1987. Mammalian folyl-γ-polyglutamate synthetase. 1. Purification and general properties of the hog liver enzyme. *Biochemistry* 26:504–12

21. Clifford AJ, Heid MK, Muller HG, Bills ND. 1990. Tissue distribution and prediction of total body folate of rats. *J. Nutr.* 120: 1633–39

22. Colucci-D'Amato LG, Ursini MV, Colletta G, Cirafici A, De Francisis V. 1989. Thyrotropin stimulates transcription from the ferritin heavy chain promoter. *Biochem. Biophys. Res. Commun.* 165:506–11

23. Cook JD, Skikne BS, Baynes RD. 1993. Serum transferrin receptors. *Annu. Rev. Med.* 44:63–74

24. Cooperman JM, Pesci-Bourel A, Luhby AL. 1970. Urinary excretion of folic acid activity in man. *Clin. Chem.* 16:375–81

25. Das KC, Mukherjee M, Sarkar TK, Dash RJ, Rastogi GK. 1975. Erythropoiesis and erythropoietin in hypothyriodism and hyperthyroidism. *J. Clin. Endocrinol. Metab.* 40:211–20

26. Dinning JS, Sime JT, Work PS, Allen B, Day PL. 1957. The metabolic conversion of folic acid and citrovorum factor to a diazotizable amine. *Arch. Biochem. Biophys.* 66:114–19

27. Durand P, Prost M, Blache D. 1997. Folic acid deficiency enhances oral contraceptive-induced platelet activity. *Arterioscler. Thromb. Vas. Biol.* 17:1939–46

28. Ek J, Magnus EM. 1981. Plasma and red blood cell folate during normal pregnancies. *Acta Obstet. Gynecol. Scand.* 60:247–51

29. Ercikan-Abali EA, Banerjee D, Waltham MC, Skacel N, Scotto KW, Bertino JR. 1997. Dihydrofolate reductase protein inhibits its own translation by binding to dihydrofolate reductase mRNA sequences within the coding region. *J. Biol. Chem.* 36:12317–22

30. Essien FB, Wannberg SL. 1993. Methionine but not folinic acid or vitamin B-12 alters the frequency of neural tube defects in *Axd* mutant mice. *J. Nutr.* 123:27–34

31. Fernandes DJ, Sur P, Kute TE, Capizzi RL. 1988. Proliferation-dependent cytotoxicity of methotrexate in murine L5178Y leukemia. *Cancer Res.* 48:5638–44

32. Fleming A, Copp AJ. 1998. Embryonic folate metabolism and mouse neural tube defects. *Science* 280:2107–9

33. Ford HC, Carter JM, Rendle MA. 1989. Serum and red cell folate and serum vitamin B-12 levels in hyperthyroidism. *Am. J. Hematol.* 31:233–36

34. Geoghegan FL, McPartlin JM, Weir DG, Scott JM. 1995. Para-acetamidobenzoylglutamate is a suitable indicator of folate status in rats. *J. Nutr.* 125:2563–70

35. Gerhard GT, Duell PB. 1999. Homocysteine and atherosclerosis. *Curr. Opin. Lipidol.* 10:417–28

36. Giles C. 1996. An account of 335 cases of megaloblastic anemia of pregnancy and the puerpium. *J. Clin. Pathol.* 19:1–11

37. Goggin T, Gough H, Bissessar A, Crowley M, Baker M, Callaghan N. 1987. A

comparative study of the relative effects of anticonvulsant drugs and dietary folate on the red cell folate status of patients with epilepsy. *Q. J. Med.* 65:911–19

38. Goldenberg RL, Tamura T, Dubard M, Johnston KE, Copper RL, Neggers Y. 1996. Plasma ferritin, premature rupture of membranes, and pregnancy outcome. *Am. J. Obstet. Gynecol.* 175:1356–59

39. Green TJ, Houghton LA, Donovan U, Gibson RS, O'Connor DL. 1998. Oral contraceptives did not affect biochemical folate indices and homocysteine concentrations in adolescent females. *J. Am. Diet. Assoc.* 98:49–55

40. Gregory JF. 1995. The bioavailability of folate. See Ref. 96a, pp. 195–235

41. Gregory JF, Williamson J, Bailey LB, Toth JP. 1998. Urinary excretion of [$^2$H$_4$]-folate by nonpregnant women following a single oral dose of [$^2$H$_4$]folic acid is a functional index of folate nutritional status. *J. Nutr.* 128:1907–12

42. Gregory JF, Williamson J, Liao J-F, Bailey LB, Toth JP. 1998. Kinetic model of folate metabolism in nonpregnant women consuming [$^2$H$_2$]folic acid: isotopic labeling of urinary folate and the catabolite para-acetamidobenzoylglutamate indicates slow, intake-dependent, turnover pools. *J. Nutr.* 128:1896–906

43. Gruner BA, Weitman SD. 1999. The folate receptor as a potential therapeutic anticancer target. *Invest. New Drug.* 16:205–19

44. Guest AE, Saleh AM, Pheasant AE, Blair JA. 1983. Effects of phenobarbitone and phenytoin on folate catabolism in the rat. *Biochem. Pharmacol.* 32:3179–82

45. Guner G, Kirkali G, Yenisey C, Tore IR. 1992. Cytosol and serum ferritin in breast carcinoma. *Cancer Lett.* 67:103–12

46. Halsted CH. 1995. Alcohol and folate interactions: clinical implications. See Ref. 96a, pp. 313–28

47. Harrison PM, Arosio P. 1996. The ferritins: molecular properties, iron storage function

and cellular regulation. *Biochim. Biophys. Acta* 1275:161–203

48. Henderson GB, Tsuji JM, Kumar HP. 1988. Mediated uptake of folate by a high-affinity binding protein in sublines of L1210 cells adapted to nanomolar concentrations of folate. *J. Membr. Biol.* 101:247–58

49. Henderson GI, Perez T, Schenker S, Mackins J, Antony AC. 1995. Maternal-to-fetal transfer of 5-methyltetrahydrofolate by the perfused human placental cotyledon: evidence for a concentrative role by placental folate receptors in fetal folate delivery. *J. Lab. Clin. Med.* 126:184–203

50. Higgins JR, Quinlivan E, McPartlin J, Scott JM, Weir DG, Darling MR. 2000. The relationship between increased folate catabolism and the increased requirement for folate in pregnancy. *Br. J. Obstet. Gynecol.* 107:1149–54

51. Horne DW, Patterson D, Cook RJ. 1989. Effect of nitrous oxide inactivation of vitamin B-12-dependent methionine synthase on the subcellular distribution of folate coenzymes in rat liver. *Arch. Biochem. Biophys.* 270:729–33

52. James SJ, Miller BJ, Basnakian AG, Pogribna IP, Pogribna M, Muskhelishvili L. 1997. Apoptosis and proliferation under conditions of deoxynucleotide pool imbalance in liver of folate/methyl deficient rats. *Carcinogenesis* 18:287–93

53. Jansen G, Westerhof GR, Jarmuszewski JA, Kathmann I, Rijksen G, Schornagel JH. 1990. Methotrexate transport in variant human CCRF-CEM leukemia cells with elevated levels of the reduced folate carrier, selective effect on carrier-mediated transport of physiological concentrations of reduced folates. *J. Biol. Chem.* 265:18272–77

54. Kamen BA, Capdevila A. 1986. Receptor-mediated accumulation is regulated by the cellular folate content. *Proc. Natl. Acad. Sci. USA* 83:5983–87

55. Kane MA, Elwood PC, Portillo RM,

Antony AC, Najfeld V, et al. 1988. Influence on immunoreactive folate-binding proteins of extracellular folate concentration in cultured human cells. *J. Clin. Invest.* 81:1398–406

56. Keagy PM. 1982. Integrated saturation model for tissue micronutrient concentrations applied to liver folacin. *J. Nutr.* 112:377–86
57. Kelly D, Reed B, Weir DG, Scott JM. 1981. Effect of acute chronic alcohol ingestion on the rate of folate catabolism and hepatic enzyme induction in mice. *Clin. Sci.* 60:221–24
58. Kelly D, Scott JM, Weir DG. 1983. Increased folate catabolism in mice with ascitic tumours. *Clin. Sci.* 65:303–5
59. Kelly D, Weir D, Reed B, Scott J. 1979. Effect of anticonvulsant drugs on the rate of folate catabolism in mice. *J. Clin. Invest.* 64:1089–96
60. Kim DW, Huang T, Schirch D, Schirch V. 1996. Properties of tetrahydropteroylpentaglutamate bound to 10-formyltetrahydrofolate dehydrogenase. *Biochemistry* 35:15772–83
61. Kim JS, Lowe KE, Shane B. 1993. Regulation of one-carbon metabolism in mammalian cells. *J. Biol. Chem.* 268:21680–85
62. Kim JS, Shane B. 1994. Role of folylpolyglutamate synthetase in the metabolism and cytotoxicity of 5-deazacyclotetrahydrofolate, an antipurine drug. *J. Biol. Chem.* 269:9714–20
63. Kim YI, Fawaz K, Knox T, Lee YM, Norton R, et al. 1998. Colonic mucosal concentrations of folate correlate well with blood measurements of folate status in persons with colorectal polyps. *Am. J. Clin. Nutr.* 68:866–72
64. Kim YI. 1999. Folate and cancer: a new medical application of folate beyond hyperhomocysteinemia and neural tube defects. *Nutr. Rev.* 57:314–21
65. Kirkali Z, Esen A, Kirkali G, Guner G. 1995. Ferritin: a tumor marker expressed by renal cell carcinoma. *Eur. Urol.* 28:131–34
66. Kirkali Z, Guzelsoy M, Mugan MU, Kirkali G, Yorukoglu K. 1999. Serum ferritin is a clinical marker for renal cell carcinoma: influence of tumor size and volume. *Urol. Int.* 62:21–25
67. Kitchens ME, Forsthoefel AM, Rafique Z, Spencer HT, Berger FG. 1999. Ligand-mediated induction of thymidylate synthase occurs by enzyme stabilization. *J. Biol. Chem.* 274:12544–47
68. Kownacki-Brown PA, Wang C, Bailey LB, Toth JP, Gregory JF III. 1993. Urinary excretion of deuterium-labeled folate and the metabolite *p*-aminobenzoylglutamate in humans. *J. Nutr.* 123:1101–8
69. Krumdieck CL, Fukushima K, Fukushima T, Shiota T, Butterworth CE Jr. 1978. A long-term study of the excretion of folate and pterins in a human subject after ingestion of $^{14}C$ folic acid, with observations on the effect of diphenylhydantoin administration. *Am. J. Clin. Nutr.* 31:88–93
70. Letsky EA. 1995. Erythropoiesis in pregnancy. *J. Perinat. Med.* 23:39–45
71. Lewis GP, Rowe PB. 1979. Oxidative and reductive cleavage of folates—a critical appraisal. *Anal. Biochem.* 93:91–97
72. Lin B-F, Huang R-FS, Shane B. 1993. Regulation of folate and one carbon metabolism in mammalian cells. 3. Role of mitochondrial folylpolyglutamate synthetase. *J. Biol. Chem.* 268:21674–79
73. Lin B-L, Shane B. 1994. Expression of *Escherichia coli* folylpolyglutamate synthetase in the Chinese hamster ovary cell mitochondrian. *J. Biol. Chem.* 269:9705–13
74. Lindenbaum J, Allen RH. 1995. Clinical spectrum and diagnosis of folate deficiency. See Ref. 96a, pp. 43–74
75. Lindenbaum J, Whitehead N, Reyner F. 1975. Oral contraceptive, hormones, folate metabolism and the cervical epithelium. *Am. J. Clin. Nutr.* 28:346–53
76. Marcus DM, Zinberg N. 1974. Isolation of

ferritin from human mammary and pancreatic carcinomas by means of antibody immunoabsorbents. *Arch. Biochem. Biophys.* 162:493–501

77. Martinasevic MK, Rios GR, Miller MW, Tephly TR. 1999. Folate and folate dependent enzymes associated with rat CNS development. *Dev. Neurosci.* 21:29–35

78. Maruyama T, Shiota T, Krumdieck CL. 1978. The oxidative cleavage of folates. *Anal. Biochem.* 84:277–95

79. Matherly LH, Czajkowski CA, Angeles SM. 1991. Identification of a highly glycosylated methotrexate membrane carrier in K562 human erythroleukemia cells up-regulated for tetrahydrofolate cofactor and methotrexate transport. *Cancer Res.* 51:3420–26

80. Matherly LH, Czajkowski CA, Muench SP, Psiakis JT. 1990. Role for cytosolic folate binding proteins in the compartmentation of endogenous tetrahydrofolates and the 5-formyltetrahydrofolate-mediated enhancement of 5-fluoro-2′-deoxyuridine antitumor activity in vitro. *Cancer Res.* 50:3262–69

81. Matherly LH, Muench SP. 1990. Evidence for localized conversion of endogenous tetrahydrofolate cofactors to dihydrofolate as an important element in antifolate action in murine leukemia cells. *Biochem. Pharmacol.* 39:2005–14

82. Maxwell JD, Hunter J, Stewart DA, Ardeman S, Williams R. 1972. Folate deficiency after anticonvulsant drugs: an effect of hepatic enzyme induction? *Br. Med. J.* 1:297–99

83. McGuire JJ, Coward JK. 1984. Pteroylpolyglutamates: biosynthesis, degradation and function. See Ref. 9a, pp. 135–90

84. McNulty H, McPartlin JM, Weir DG, Scott JM. 1993. Folate catabolism is increased during pregnancy in rats. *J. Nutr.* 123:1089–93

85. McNulty H, McPartlin JM, Weir DG, Scott JM. 1995. Folate catabolism is related to growth rate in weanling rats. *J. Nutr.* 125:99–103

86. McPartlin J, Courtney G, McNulty H, Weir D, Scott J. 1992. The quantitative analysis of endogenous folate catabolites in human urine. *Anal. Biochem.* 206:256–61

87. McPartlin J, Hallagan A, Scott JM, Darling M, Weir DG. 1993. Accelerated folate breakdown in pregnancy. *Lancet* 341:148–49

88. McPartlin J, Weir DG, Courtney G, McNulty H, Scott JM. 1986. The level of folate catabolism in normal populations, suggesting that the current level of RDA for folate is excessive. In *Chemistry and Biology of Pteridines*, ed. BA Cooper, VM Whitehead, pp. 513–16. Berlin/New York: Gruyter

89. Meenan J, O'Halliman E, Scott J, Weir DG. 1997. Epithelial cell folate depletion occurs in neoplastic but not adjacent normal colon mucosa. *Gastroenterology* 112:1163–68

90. Min H, Shane B, Stokstad ELR. 1988. Identification of 10-formyltetrahydrofolate dehydrogenase-hydrolase as a major folate binding protein in liver cytosol. *Biochim. Biophys. Acta* 967:348–53

91. Minchin RF. 1995. Acetylation of *p*-aminobenzoylglutamate, a folate catabolite, by recombinant human arylamine N-acetyltransferase in U937 cells. *Biochem. J.* 307:1–3

92. Moad G, Luthy CL, Benkovic SJ. 1978. The mechanism of oxidation of 6-methyl-5-carba-5-deazatetrahydropterin. Evidence for the involvement of a 4a-adduct in the oxidation of tetrahydropterins. *Tetrahedron Lett.* 26:2271–74

93. Modjtahedi N, Frebourg T, Fossar N, Lavialle C, Cremisi C, Brison O. 1992. Increased expression of cytokeratin and ferritin H genes in tumorigenic clones of the SW 613-S human colon carcinoma cell line. *Exp. Cell. Res.* 201:74–82

94. Moran RG. 1999. Roles of folylpoly-$\gamma$-glutamate synthetase in therapeutics

with tetrahydrofolate antimetabolites: an overview. *Semin. Oncol.* 26:24–32

95. Murphy M, Keating M, Boyle P, Weir DG, Scott JM. 1976. The elucidation of the mechanism of folate catabolism in the rat. *Biochem. Biophys. Res. Commun.* 71: 1017–24

96. Murphy M, Scott JM. 1979. The turnover/catabolism and excretion of folate administered at physiological concentrations in the rat. *Biochim. Biophys. Acta* 583:535–39

96a. Picciano MF, Stokstad ELR, Gregory JF, eds. 1995. *Folic Acid Metabolism in Health and Disease.* New York: Wiley-Liss

97. Quinlivan E, McPartlin J, Weir DG, Scott J. 2000. Mechanism of the antimicrobial drug trimethoprim revisited. *FASEB J.* 14:2519–24

98. Reed B, Weir DG, Scott JM. 1978. The occurrence of folate derived pteridines in rat liver. *Clin. Sci. Mol. Med.* 54:355–60

99. Reed LS, Archer MC. 1980. Oxidation of tetrahydrofolic acid by air. *J. Agric. Food Chem.* 28:801–5

100. Rimm EB, Willett WC, Hu FB, Sampson L, Colditz GA, et al. 1998. Folate and vitamin B6 from diet and supplements in relation to risk of coronary heart disease among women. *JAMA* 279:359–64

101. Russell RM, Rosenberg IH, Wilson PD, Iber FL, Oaks EB, et al. 1983. Increased urinary excretion and prolonged turnover time of folic acid during ethanol ingestion. *Am. J. Clin. Nutr.* 38:64–70

102. Sauberlich HE. 1995. Folate status of U. S. population groups. See Ref. 96a, pp. 171–94

103. Schirch V, Strong W. 1989. Interaction of folylpolyglutamates with enzymes in one-carbon metabolism. *Arch. Biochem. Biophys.* 269:371–80

104. Scholl TO. 1998. High third-trimester ferritin concentration: associations with very preterm delivery, infection and maternal nutritional status. *Obstet. Gynecol.* 92:161–66

105. Scholl TO, Johnson WG. 2000. Folic acid: influence on the outcome of pregnancy. *Am. J. Clin. Nutr.* 71:1295–1303S

106. Scott JM. 1984. Catabolism of folates. See Ref. 9a, pp. 307–27

107. Scott JM, Weir DG, Kirke PN. 1995. Folate and neural tube defects. See Ref. 96a, pp. 329–60

108. Scott JM, Wilson P, Dinn JJ, Weir DG. 1981. Pathogenesis of subacute combined degeneration: a result of methyl group deficiency. *Lancet.* 8242:337–40

109. Scott KC, Gregory JF. 1996. The fate of [$^3$H] folic acid in folate adequate rats. *J. Nutr. Biochem.* 7:261–69

110. Selhub J, Jacques PF, Wilson PW, Rush D, Rosenberg IH. 1993. Vitamin status and intake as primary determinants of homocysteinemia in an elderly population. *JAMA* 270:2693–98

111. Shane B. 1995. Folate chemistry and metabolism. See Ref. 96a, pp. 1–22

112. Shaw S, Jayatilleke E. 1990. Ethanol-induced iron mobilization: role of acetaldehyde-aldehyde oxidase generated superoxide. *Free Radic. Biol. Med.* 9:11–17

113. Shaw S, Jayatilleke E, Herbert V, Colman N. 1989. Cleavage of folates during ethanol metabolism. *Biochem. J.* 257:277–80

114. Shojania AM. 1975. The effect of oral contraceptives on folate metabolism. Part 3: Plasma clearance and urinary folate excretion. *J. Lab. Clin. Med.* 85:185–90

115. Shojania AM, Hornady G, Barnes PH. 1968. Oral contraceptives and serum folate level in woman. *Lancet* 1:1376–77

116. Sirotnak FM, Tolner B. 1999. Carrier-mediated membrane transport of folates in mammalian cells. *Annu. Rev. Nutr.* 19:92–122

117. Spector T, Ferone R. 1984. Folic acid does not inactivate xanthine oxidase. *J. Biol. Chem.* 259:10784–86

118. Stites TE, Bailey LB, Scott KC, Toth JP, Fisher WP, Gregory JF. 1997. Kinetic

modeling of folate metabolism through the use of chronic administration of deuterium-labeled folic acid in men. *Am. J. Clin. Nutr.* 65:53–60

119. Strong WB, Schirch V. 1989. In vitro conversion of formate to serine. Effect of tetrahydropteroylpolyglutamates and serine hydroxymethyltransferase on the rate of 10-formyltetrahydrofolate synthetase. *Biochemistry* 28:9430–39

120. Strong WB, Tendler SJ, Seither RL, Goldman ID, Schirch V. 1990. Purification and properties of serine hydroxymethyltransferase and C1-tetrahydrofolate synthase from L1210 cells. *J. Biol. Chem.* 265:12149–55

121. Suh J-R, Oppenheim EW, Girgis S, Stover PJ. 2000. Purification and properties of a folate catabolizing enzyme. *J. Biol. Chem.* 275:35646–55

122. Taber MM, Lakshmaiah N. 1987. Studies on hydroperoxide-dependent folic acid degradation by hemin. *Arch. Biochem. Biophys.* 257:100–6

123. Tamura T, Goldenberg RL, Johnston KE, Cliver SP, Hickey CA. 1996. Serum ferritin: a predictor of early spontaneous preterm delivery. *Obstet. Gynecol.* 87:360–65

124. Task Force Epidemiol. Res. Reprod. Health. 1998. Effects of contraceptives on hemoglobin and ferritin. *Contraception* 58:261–73

125. Thomson AM, Rogers JT, Leedman PJ. 1999. Iron-regulatory proteins, iron responsive elements and ferritin mRNA translation. *Int. J. Biochem. Cell Biol.* 31:1139–52

126. Titus SA, Moran RG. 2000. Retrovirally mediated complementation of the glyB phenotype: cloning of a human gene encoding the carrier for entry of folates into mitochondria. *J. Biol. Chem.* 275:36811–17

127. Trugo NMF, Donangelo CM, Seyfarth BSP, Henriques C, Andrade LP. 1996. Folate and iron status of nonanemic women during pregnancy: effect of routine folate and iron supplementation and relation of erythrocyte folate with iron stores. *Nutr. Res.* 16:1267–76

128. Van der Put NMJ, van den Heuvel LP, Steegers-Theunissen RPM, Trijbels FJM, Eskes KAB, et al. 1996. Decreased methylene tetrahydrofolate reductase activity due to the 677C-T mutation in families with spina bifida offspring. *J. Mol. Med.* 74:691–94

129. Von der Porten AE, Gregory JF, Toth JP, Cerda JJ, Curry SH, Bailey LB. 1992. In vivo folate kinetics during chronic supplementation of human subjects with deuterium-labeled folic acid. *J. Nutr.* 122:1293–99

130. Wagner C. 1995. Biochemical role of folate in cellular metabolism. See Ref. 96a, pp. 23–42

131. Wang C, Song S, Bailey LB, Gregory JF. 1994. Relationship between urinary excretion of *p*-aminobenzoylglutamate and folate status of the growing rat. *Nutr. Res.* 14:875–84

132. Wang Y, Nimec Z, Ryan TJ, Dias JA, Galivan J. 1993. The properties of the secreted gamma-glutamyl hydrolases from H35 hepatoma cells. *Biochim. Biophys. Acta* 1164:227–35

133. Wegner C, Nau H. 1992. Alteration of embryonic folate metabolism by valproic acid during organogenesis: implications for mechanism of teratogenesis. *Neurology* 42:17–24

134. Weinstein RE, Bond BH, Silberberg BK, Vaughn CB, Subbaiah P, Pieper DR. 1989. Tissue ferritin concentration and prognosis in carcinoma of the breast. *Breast Cancer Res. Treatment* 14:349–53

135. White GP, Worwood M, Parry DH, Jacobs A. 1974. Ferritin synthesis in normal and leukemic leukocytes. *Nature* 250:584–86

136. Wittwer AJ, Wagner C. 1981. Identification of the folate binding proteins of rat liver mitochondria as dimethylglycine

dehydrogenase and sarcosine dehydrogenase. Purification and folate binding characteristics. *J. Biol. Chem.* 256:4102–8

137. Wong SC, Zhang L, Proefke SA, Hukku B, Matherly L. 1998. Gene amplification and increased expression of the reduced folate carrier in transport elevated K562 cells. *Biochem. Pharmacol.* 55:1135–38

138. Wu CG, Groenink M, Bosma A, Reitsma PH, van Deventer SJH, Chamuleau RAFM. 1997. Rat ferritin-H: cDNA cloning, differential expression and localization during hepatocarcinogenesis. *Carcinogenesis* 18:47–52

139. Wu CG, Habib NA, Mitry RR, Reitsma PH, van Deventer SJH, Chamuleau RAFM. 1997. Increased hepatic ferritin-H messenger RNA levels correlate with those of c-myc in human hepatocellular carcinoma. *Int. J. Oncol.* 11:187–92

140. Yeo EJ, Briggs WT, Wagner C. 1999. Inhibition of glycine *N*-methyltransferase by 5-methyltetrahydrofolatepentaglutamate. *J. Biol. Chem.* 274:37559–64

141. Yi P, Melnyk S, Pogribna M, Pogribny IP, Hime RJ, James SJ. 2000. Increase in plasma homocysteine associated with parallel increases in plasma *S*-adenosylhomocysteine and lymphocyte DNA hypomethylation. *J. Biol. Chem.* 275:29318–23

142. Zakrzewski SF. 1966. Evidence for the chemical interaction between 2-mercaptoethanol and tetrahydrofolate. *J. Biol. Chem.* 241:2957–61

143. Zamierowski MM, Wagner C. 1977. Effect of folacin deficiency on folacin binding proteins in the rat. *J. Nutr.* 107:1937–45

144. Zhao Q, Behringer RR, de Crombrugghe B. 1996. Prenatal folic acid treatment suppresses acrania and meroanencephaly in mice mutant for the Cart1 homeobox gene. *Nat. Genet.* 13:275–82

145. Zhu L, Bagchi MK, Bagchi I. 1995. Ferritin heavy chain is a progesterone-inducible marker in the uterus during pregnancy. *Endocrinology* 136:4106–15

Annu. Rev. Nutr. 2001. 21:283–95

# Dietary and Genetic Effects on Low-Density Lipoprotein Heterogeneity

## Ronald M Krauss

*Lawrence Berkeley National Laboratory, Department of Molecular Medicine, University of California, Berkeley, California 94720; e-mail: Rmkrauss@lbl.gov*

**Key Words** LDL, genetics, diet, subclasses, coronary disease

■ **Abstract** We have tested whether differences in distribution and dietary responsiveness of low-density lipoprotein (LDL) subclasses contribute to the variability in the magnitude of LDL-cholesterol reduction induced by diets low in total and saturated fat and high in carbohydrate. Our studies have focused on a common, genetically influenced metabolic profile, characterized by a predominance of small, dense LDL particles (subclass pattern B), that is associated with a two- to threefold increase in risk for coronary artery disease. We have found that healthy normolipidemic individuals with this trait show a greater reduction in LDL cholesterol and particle number in response to low-fat, high-carbohydrate diets than do unaffected individuals (subclass pattern A). Moreover, such diets result in reduced LDL particle size, with induction of pattern B in a substantial proportion of pattern A men. Recent studies have indicated that this response is under genetic influence. Future identification of the specific genes involved may lead to improved targeting of dietary therapies aimed at reducing cardiovascular disease risk.

## CONTENTS

## INTRODUCTION

Reduction of LDL cholesterol by limitation of saturated fat intake is one of the keystones of dietary regimens aimed at reducing risk for coronary heart disease (43, 45). In conjunction with this goal, current dietary guidelines also advocate limitation of total fat intake, with substitution of carbohydrate. The principal mechanism by which reduced saturated fat intake can lower LDL cholesterol is via increased LDL receptor activity, which in turn leads to increased hepatic clearance and excretion of cholesterol (63). However, the metabolic effects of low-fat, high-carbohydrate diets are complex and may include increased triglycerides and very-low-density lipoproteins (VLDLs), reduced high-density lipoproteins (HDLs), and increased insulin (23), a constellation of factors associated with increased atherosclerosis risk (57). Moreover, because VLDLs are the metabolic precursors of LDLs, increased LDL production from VLDL may attenuate the reductions of LDL cholesterol achieved by saturated fat restriction.

Another factor to be considered in population-wide dietary approaches to coronary risk reduction is the considerable interindividual variability that has been demonstrated in the lipoprotein response to modification of dietary fat intake (14, 61). A portion of this variability has been attributed to genetic factors, but only a small number of specific genes have been reported to be related to lipoprotein responsiveness to dietary fat change (31, 55). Among common genetic variants, the strongest effects on plasma LDL cholesterol, and to a lesser extent on LDL response to dietary fat and cholesterol change, have been observed for the E4 variant of the apolipoprotein (apo) E gene, found in approximately 14% of the population (27, 31, 55, 60, 67).

LDL is known to be heterogeneous, comprising a number of distinct subpopulations (41). This review describes recent evidence that improved understanding of dietary and genetic influences on LDL may result from consideration of the macromolecular heterogeneity of this class of lipoproteins.

## LDL HETEROGENEITY

LDL subpopulations have been defined on the basis of a number of characteristics, including particle density, size, charge, and chemical composition (41). The distribution of mass among LDL subclasses in plasma is reflected by the particle diameter and buoyant density of the predominant LDL species. Particle diameter is most often assessed by nondenaturing gradient gel electrophoresis, which can identify as many as seven distinct electrophoretic components based on variations in particle size and shape. Density gradient and analytical ultracentrifugation are used to assess LDL buoyant density and flotation rate, respectively (41). Plasma triglyceride and VLDL levels are strongly correlated with increasing density and decreasing size of the predominant LDL species (46, 47). These LDL characteristics in turn are inversely related to levels of plasma HDL, particularly the $HDL_2$ subclass species (46, 47).

Although there is not yet a detailed understanding of the metabolic bases for these relationships, evidence indicates that heparin-releasable lipase activities may be intimately involved. Postheparin plasma lipoprotein lipase activity is associated with levels of both larger LDL (40) and HDL (39), and this may be due, at least in part, to transfer of surface lipids and apos in the course of chylomicron and

VLDL triglyceride hydrolysis. In a group of 43 healthy normolipidemic men, we found significant inverse relationships of postheparin lipoprotein lipase activity with plasma levels of triglyceride, apoB, large VLDL mass, and small, dense LDL (LDL3) (18).

Hepatic lipase, an enzyme that catalyzes degradation of HDL lipids, is also involved in the clearance of intermediate-density lipoproteins and the production of small, dense LDL from more buoyant precursors (56). Heparin-released hepatic lipase activity has been correlated with levels of LDL3 (18), and absence of small, dense LDL has been reported in humans (12) and mice (56) with genetic deficiency of hepatic lipase.

## SMALL, DENSE LDL SUBCLASS PHENOTYPE

A distinct LDL subclass pattern characterized by a predominance of small, dense LDL particles (principally LDL3) has been identified using both nondenaturing gradient gel electrophoresis (7, 41) and analytic ultracentrifugation (41, 52). The prevalence of this trait, which has been designated LDL subclass pattern B, is 30%–35% in adult men, but it is much lower in males <20 years of age and in premenopausal women (5%–10%) (7) and is intermediate (15%–25%) in post-menopausal women (17, 62). Evidence from several studies for major gene determinants of this phenotype (8) has been summarized previously (2). More recently, two additional studies using complex segregation analysis have confirmed major gene effects on LDL diameter as a quantitative trait (6, 16). The data have been most consistent with an autosomal dominant or codominant model for inheritance of the pattern B phenotype with varying additive and polygenic effects. Linkage of pattern B to the region of the LDL receptor gene locus on chromosome 19p (54) has been confirmed using quantitative sibling-pair linkage analysis of LDL particle size in 25 kindreds ascertained on the basis of two affected members with coronary artery disease (59). In these families, preliminary evidence was also obtained for linkage to regions near three other genetic loci: the apoAI/CIII/AIV cluster on chromosome 11, the CETP locus on chromosome 16, and the manganese super-oxide dismutase gene on chromosome 6. Recent analyses, however, have failed to demonstrate linkage to these candidate loci in hyperlipidemic kindreds (9). Finally, in a group of dizygotic female twins, there was significant linkage of peak LDL particle size to the apoB gene locus (10), although earlier studies had indicated significant nonlinkage of LDL subclass B to this locus in healthy families (48) and in families with familial combined hyperlipidemia (11). Taken together, these studies suggest that multiple genes may contribute to determination of particle size of the major LDL subclass in plasma, and that the responsible genetic mechanisms may differ among affected families.

Estimates of heritability of LDL particle size based on twin studies have ranged from approximately 30% to 50% (2), indicating the importance of nongenetic and environmental influences. In view of the close relationship between change in plasma triglyceride levels and change in LDL particle size (47, 51), and in view of the metabolic relationships described above, it is likely that both genetic and non-genetic determinants of pattern B involve coordinate effects on plasma triglyceride and LDL subclass metabolism. In addition to effects from age and gender, LDL particle size and density distribution have been shown to be affected by abdominal adiposity (66), oral contraceptive use (25), and the hypertriglyceridemia of AIDS (33). As described below, variation in dietary fat and carbohydrate can also strongly influence expression of the small, dense LDL phenotype and can contribute to the variations in LDL particle size distribution that are observed among individuals and population groups.

Another important metabolic correlate of the pattern B lipoprotein profile is insulin resistance, manifest as relative elevations in fasting and postglucose insulin levels (58, 62), fasting glucose levels (58), and increased steady state plasma glucose levels (58). The metabolic syndrome associated with insulin resistance has been shown to include raised triglyceride and reduced HDL levels, and the relationships of these variables to LDL particle size appear to account for correlations of smaller LDL diameter with parameters of insulin resistance (58). Insulin resistance has also been related to a tendency toward increased blood pressure, which has also been demonstrated in pattern B subjects with this syndrome (58, 62). A high prevalence of the small, dense LDL trait has been demonstrated in patients with type 2 diabetes mellitus (13, 32), and it is likely that this reflects, in large measure, the insulin resistance found in the majority of patients with this disease. A relative increase in LDL3 has also been reported in well-controlled patients with insulin-dependent diabetes mellitus in conjunction with increased levels of intermediate density lipoproteins (IDL) (50).

Thus, the occurrence of the small, dense LDL phenotype may result from interaction of multiple genetic and environmental determinants, and the trait can be viewed as a marker for the mechanisms underlying these effects. In particular, the prevalence of pattern B characteristically denotes triglyceride levels greater than 140–160 mg/dl and is uncommonly found in association with triglyceride levels below 100–110 mg/dl (7, 52). Candidate mechanisms thus include those that result in overproduction and/or impaired clearance of triglyceride-rich lipoproteins.

## LDL HETEROGENEITY AND RISK OF CORONARY ARTERY DISEASE

The plasma lipoprotein profile accompanying a predominance of small, dense LDL particles (specifically LDL3) is associated with a two- to threefold increased risk of coronary artery disease. This has been demonstrated in case-control studies of myocardial infarction (3), and of angiographically documented coronary disease (19, 22, 24). More recently, nested case-control analyses in prospective studies of three population cohorts have all demonstrated that reduced LDL particle size at baseline was a significant predictor for the development of coronary heart disease (34, 49, 64). In most, but not all, studies to date, the disease risk associated with small, dense LDL was no longer significant after adjusting for triglyceride (3, 22, 24, 64) or other risk factors (19, 34). The high degree of intercorrelation between LDL size, triglyceride, and HDL cholesterol, and the resulting multiple colinearity, confound efforts to determine the extent to which small, dense LDL is independently related to coronary disease risk. In this regard, it is likely that multiple features of the phenotype contribute to atherosclerosis and its cardiovascular manifestations. However, enhanced atherogenicity of smaller vs larger LDL is suggested by evidence of that smaller LDLs are taken up less readily by LDL receptors (53), penetrate more readily into arterial tissue (15), bind more tightly to arterial proteoglycans (1), and are oxidized more rapidly than larger LDL particles (21).

Further evidence for clinically important atherogenicity of small, dense LDL derives from analyses of the effects of lipid-altering therapy on progression of coronary artery disease, as assessed by quantitative coronary angiography. In one study involving a multiple risk factor intervention protocol including lipid-lowering drugs, reduced coronary angiographic progression with treatment was observed only in the subgroup of subjects with a predominance of small, dense LDL (45% of the total) but not in those with more buoyant LDL, despite comparable LDL cholesterol lowering in the two groups (52). More recently, in subjects with a familial history of atherosclerosis and elevated plasma apoB levels, change in coronary artery stenosis with lipid-lowering drugs was found to be most strongly related to change in LDL density, independent of changes in other risk factors (70).

It is noteworthy that a predominance of small, dense LDL is commonly found in conjunction with familial disorders of lipoprotein metabolism that are associated with increased risk of premature coronary artery disease. These include familial combined hyperlipidemia (4, 5, 36–38), as well as hyperapobetalipoproteinemia (65) and hypoalphalipoproteinemia (35). There is evidence that the inheritance of familial combined hyperlipidemia involves at least two major gene loci: one responsible for increased plasma apoB levels and one for LDL subclass pattern B (38). Such interactions of the genes underlying pattern B with other genes or environmental factors, such as diet, may contribute to related dyslipidemic syndromes, and it is likely that a portion of coronary disease risk in these syndromes is mediated by the metabolic changes responsible for the small, dense LDL phenotype.

## DIETARY EFFECTS ON LDL SUBCLASSES

Cross-sectional population analyses have suggested an association of reduced LDL particle size with relatively reduced dietary animal fat intake, and increased consumption of carbohydrates (20). Dietary effects on levels of LDL were evaluated directly in a study of 105 healthy, middle-aged men who consumed a high-fat diet (46% fat, 34% carbohydrate) for 6 weeks and a low-fat diet (24% fat, 56% carbohydrate) for 6 weeks in a randomized crossover design (26, 44). Saturated and polyunsaturated fat diets were reduced in parallel to achieve a constant polyunsaturated/saturated ratio (0.7), and intake of monounsaturated fat, cholesterol, protein, and dietary fiber were similar on the two diets.

Men with a predominance of small, dense LDL (pattern B) on the high-fat diet ($n = 18$) exhibited a twofold greater reduction in LDL cholesterol than did pattern A men. This was associated with significantly greater reductions in mass of midsized (LDL2) and small (LDL3) LDL subfractions measured by analytic ultracentrifugation. Furthermore, only pattern B subjects showed significant reductions in plasma apoB, and in LDL relative to HDL cholesterol levels. Of the 87 men with pattern A on the high-fat diet, 36 converted to pattern B on the low-fat diet. In these men, there was a shift in LDL particle mass from larger, lipid-enriched (LDL1 and -2) to smaller, lipid-depleted (LDL3 and -4) subfractions, which suggests a change in LDL composition with minimal change in particle number, and which is consistent with the observation of reduced plasma LDL cholesterol without reduced apoB (44). The group differences in LDL and apoB response could not be attributed to differences in plasma lipid levels, body mass index (which was held constant), or apoE phenotypes. Taken together, these results indicate that in the majority of healthy normolipidemic men, the reduction in LDL cholesterol seen on a low-fat, high-carbohydrate diet is due in large measure to a shift from larger, more cholesterol-enriched LDL to smaller, cholesterol-depleted LDL, whereas much greater reductions in LDL cholesterol and a reduction in the number of smaller LDL particles are achieved in individuals with a predominance of small, dense LDL on a high-fat diet (Figure 1). It should be noted that these studies were performed using isocaloric diets designed to maintain stable body weight. Because weight loss has been shown to result in reduction of small dense LDL and a shift to larger, more buoyant particles, this could attenuate the effects of low-fat, high-carbohydrate diets described here (68, 69).

Recent studies have been extended to examine the effects on LDL subclass phenotypes of further restriction in dietary fat to levels as low as 10% of calories

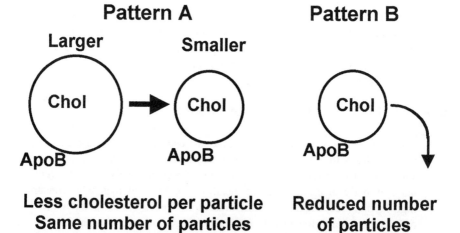

**Figure 1**   Different mechanisms underlying reductions in low-density lipoprotein (LDL) cholesterol (chol) in men with LDL subclass patterns A and B. Apo, apolipoprotein.

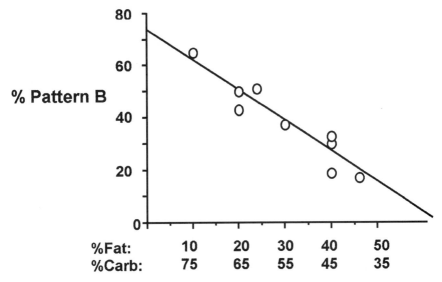

**Figure 2**  Prevalence of low-density lipoprotein subclass pattern B as a function of dietary fat and carbohydrate content. Data are derived from five studies involving a total of 596 healthy, nonobese, normolipidemic men (updated from Reference 29). The data points fit the relationship: % pattern $B = -1.16$ (% dietary fat) $+74$ ($r = -0.94, p < 0.0001$).

(29). The results have indicated that the prevalence of LDL subclass phenotype B in men increases in direct proportion to the degree to which dietary fat is replaced by carbohydrate in the diet (Figure 2). With 30% of calories as fat, approximately one third of men express the B trait, a figure that approximates the prevalence of this trait in the general population, whereas with short-term challenge of a 10% fat diet, the estimated prevalence of phenotype B in men increases to an estimated two thirds of the population. A hypothesis that has been put forward to explain these results is that genetic predisposition to phenotype is expressed with greater penetrance as dietary fat is reduced to lower levels and replaced by carbohydrate.

A possible genetic basis for the differential effects of low-fat diets on LDL levels in pattern B subjects was examined in 72 premenopausal women who were switched from their basal diet (mean 35% fat) to an outpatient low-fat (20%) diet for 8 weeks (28). Because of the low expression of pattern B in premenopausal women, genetic predisposition for pattern B was assessed by parental LDL subclass pattern. In the daughters, decreases in plasma levels of LDL cholesterol and IDL mass, as well as increases in plasma triglyceride, were significantly related to the number of pattern B parents and could not be explained by the daughters' adherence to the diet or baseline characteristics, including initial lipoprotein profile. Thus, in premenopausal women, genetic and metabolic factors responsible for LDL subclass pattern B may result in enhanced LDL responsiveness to reductions in dietary fat even though the trait is largely unexpressed because of low penetrance.

We also tested for a heritable basis for differences in LDL subclass response to low-fat diets by studying responses to a short-term challenge with a very-low-fat diet in a group of 50 children (mean age 14) according to parental LDL subclass patterns on a low-fat diet (30). Offspring of two pattern B parents had smaller LDL peak particle diameter, greater prevalence of pattern B, and higher LDL cholesterol and triglycerides than did offspring of two pattern A parents. Diet-induced reductions in LDL size and the proportion of subjects shifting from pattern A to pattern B were also greater in children of two pattern B parents. These findings suggest that parental LDL subclass patterns are informative in determining which children may be genetically susceptible to expression of subclass pattern B and related metabolic changes with consumption of a low-fat, high-carbohydrate challenge diet. Whether parental subclass pattern affects the response to longer-term consumption of less extreme diets remains to be determined.

These studies suggest that genetic factors underlying predisposition to LDL subclass phenotype B influence the lipoprotein response to low-fat diets and, in particular, determine the propensity to express phenotype B on a low-fat diet. This hypothesis is currently under investigation in studies employing pairs of siblings to test whether LDL subclass response to low-fat diets is linked to candidate genes that have been linked to LDL particle profiles in previous studies. Preliminary results of these studies have indicated that induction of pattern B by a low-fat, high-carbohydrate diet is linked to the LDL receptor gene locus on chromosome 19p (42).

Earlier studies had tested whether variants of the apoE gene influenced LDL subclass response to dietary fat restriction. Although apoE variants have significant effects on LDL levels, a strong relationship of the apoE gene to LDL subclass phenotypes has not been demonstrated. We have, however, demonstrated a significant effect of the E4 allele on LDL subclass response to reduced fat intake in men (27). This did not involve a significant difference in response of small LDL, which increased modestly in all apoE isoform groups (apoE, 2/3; apoE, 3/3; and apoE, 4/3 + 4/4). Rather, the 14% of men who were either heterozygous or homozygous for apoE4 demonstrated a significantly greater reduction in mass of large LDL than did men with apoE 3/3 (the most common genotype). Although the mechanism for this finding is not known, it may relate to the observation that larger LDL particles have greater content of apoE, and it is thus possible that the LDL elevations associated with the apoE4 allele on high-fat diets are primarily related to an effect on these larger LDL.

## CONCLUSION

Genetic factors underlying susceptibility to an increased proportion of small, dense LDL particles in plasma (subclass phenotype B) may also influence the LDL response to replacement of dietary fat by carbohydrate. The minority of healthy individuals who express this trait on a high-fat diet achieve a significantly greater

LDL cholesterol reduction with dietary fat reduction than do subjects with larger LDL (phenotype A). The reduction of small, dense LDL particles in these individuals would be predicted to achieve a reduction in the increased coronary disease risk associated with this trait. In contrast, a substantial subset of healthy, nonobese men with phenotype A exhibit a metabolic response to dietary fat restriction that results in a shift from larger to smaller LDL and expression of phenotype B with minimal change in particle number. In these men, LDL cholesterol reductions largely represent reduced cholesterol content of LDL particles and, hence, would not be expected to result in reduced risk of coronary heart disease. A genetic basis for the LDL subclass response, and the conversion from phenotype A to B, is suggested by recent studies with families. The apoE gene, which is not linked to LDL subclass phenotype B, appears to influence levels of large, but not small, LDL. Improved understanding of genetic factors influencing LDL subclass levels may provide further information regarding the basis for the marked interindividual variability in LDL response to variation in dietary fat intake.

## ACKNOWLEDGMENTS

This work was supported by the National Institutes of Health Program Project grant HL 18574 from the National Heart, Lung, and Blood Institute and by a grant from the National Dairy Promotion and Research Board that was administered in cooperation with the National Dairy Council. This work was conducted at the Ernest Orlando Lawrence Berkeley National Laboratory through the US Department of Energy under contract no. DE-AC03-76SF000. This review is also being published in modified form in *World Review of Nutrition and Dietetics* (in press, 2001).

**Visit the Annual Reviews home page at www.AnnualReviews.org**

## LITERATURE CITED

1. Anber V, Millar JS, McConnell M, Shepherd J, Packard CJ. 1997. Interaction of very-low-density, intermediate-density, and low-density lipoproteins with human arterial wall proteoglycans. *Arterioscler. Thromb. Vasc. Biol.* 17:2507–14
2. Austin MA. 1992. Genetic epidemiology of low-density lipoprotein subclass phenotypes. *Ann. Med.* 24:477–81
3. Austin MA, Breslow JL, Hennekens CH, Buring JE, Willett WC, Krauss RM. 1988. Low-density lipoprotein subclass patterns and risk of myocardial infarction. *JAMA* 260:1917–21
4. Austin MA, Brunzell JD, Fitch WL, Krauss

RM. 1990. Inheritance of low density lipoprotein subclass patterns in familial combined hyperlipidemia. *Arteriosclerosis* 10:520–30
5. Austin MA, Horowitz H, Wijsman E, Krauss RM, Brunzell J. 1992. Bimodality of plasma apolipoprotein B levels in familial combined hyperlipidemia. *Atherosclerosis* 92:67–77
6. Austin MA, Jarvik GP, Hokanson JE, Edwards K. 1993. Complex segregation analysis of LDL peak particle diameter. *Genet. Epidemiol.* 10:599–604
7. Austin MA, King MC, Vranizan KM, Krauss RM. 1990. Atherogenic lipoprotein phenotype. A proposed genetic marker

for coronary heart disease risk. *Circulation* 82:495–506

8. Austin MA, King MC, Vranizan KM, Newman B, Krauss RM. 1988. Inheritance of low-density lipoprotein subclass patterns: results of complex segregation analysis. *Am. J. Hum. Genet.* 43:838–46

9. Austin MA, Stephens K, Walden CE, Wijsman E. 1999. Linkage analysis of candidate genes and the small, dense low-density lipoprotein phenotype. *Atherosclerosis* 142:79–87

10. Austin MA, Talmud PJ, Luong LA, Haddad L, Day IN, et al. 1998. Candidate-gene studies of the atherogenic lipoprotein phenotype: a sib-pair linkage analysis of DZ women twins. *Am. J. Hum. Genet.* 62:406–19

11. Austin MA, Wijsman E, Guo SW, Krauss RM, Brunzell JD, Deeb S. 1991. Lack of evidence for linkage between low-density lipoprotein subclass phenotypes and the apolipoprotein B locus in familial combined hyperlipidemia. *Genet. Epidemiol.* 8:287–97

12. Auwerx JH, Marzetta CA, Hokanson JE, Brunzell JD. 1989. Large buoyant LDL-like particles in hepatic lipase deficiency. *Arteriosclerosis* 9:319–25

13. Barakat HA, McLendon VD, Marks R, Pories W, Heath J, Carpenter JW. 1992. Influence of morbid obesity and noninsulin-dependent diabetes mellitus on high-density lipoprotein composition and subpopulation distribution. *Metabolism* 41:37–41

14. Beynen AC, Katan MB, Van Zutphen LF. 1987. Hypo- and hyperresponders: individual differences in the response of serum cholesterol concentration to changes in diet. *Adv. Lipid Res.* 22:115–71

15. Bjornheden T, Babyi A, Bondjers G, Wiklund O. 1996. Accumulation of lipoprotein fractions and subfractions in the arterial wall, determined in an in vitro perfusion system. *Atherosclerosis* 123:43–56

16. Bu X, Krauss RM, Puppione D. 1992. Ma-

jor gene control of atherogenic lipoprotein phenotype (ALP): a quantitative segregation analysis in 20 coronary artery disease (CAD) pedigrees. *Am. J. Hum. Genet.* 51(4):A336

17. Campos H, Blijlevens E, McNamara JR, Ordovas JM, Posner BM, et al. 1992. LDL particle size distribution. Results from the Framingham Offspring Study. *Arterioscler. Thromb.* 12:1410–19

18. Campos H, Dreon DM, Krauss RM. 1995. Associations of hepatic and lipoprotein lipase activities with changes in dietary composition and low density lipoprotein subclasses. *J. Lipid Res.* 36:462–72

19. Campos H, Genest JJ Jr, Blijlevens E, McNamara JR, Jenner JL, et al. 1992. Low density lipoprotein particle size and coronary artery disease. *Arterioscler. Thromb.* 12:187–95

20. Campos H, Willett WC, Peterson RM, Siles X, Bailey SM, et al. 1991. Nutrient intake comparisons between Framingham and rural and urban Puriscal, Costa Rica. Associations with lipoproteins, apolipoproteins, and low density lipoprotein particle size. *Arterioscler. Thromb.* 11:1089–99

21. Chait A, Brazg RL, Tribble DL, Krauss RM. 1993. Susceptibility of small, dense, low-density lipoproteins to oxidative modification in subjects with the atherogenic lipoprotein phenotype, pattern B. *Am. J. Med.* 94:350–56

22. Coresh J, Kwiterovich PO Jr, Smith HH, Bachorik PS. 1993. Association of plasma triglyceride concentration and LDL particle diameter, density, and chemical composition with premature coronary artery disease in men and women. *J. Lipid Res.* 34:1687–97

23. Coulston AM, Liu GC, Reaven GM. 1983. Plasma glucose, insulin and lipid responses to high-carbohydrate low-fat diets in normal humans. *Metabolism* 32:52–56

24. Crouse JR, Parks JS, Schey HM, Kahl FR. 1985. Studies of low density lipoprotein molecular weight in human beings

with coronary artery disease. *J. Lipid Res.* 26:566–74

25. de Graaf J, Swinkels DW, Demacker PN, de Haan AF, Stalenhoef AF. 1993. Differences in the low density lipoprotein subfraction profile between oral contraceptive users and controls. *J. Clin. Endocrinol. Metab.* 76:197–202

26. Dreon DM, Fernstrom HA, Miller B, Krauss RM. 1994. Low-density lipoprotein subclass patterns and lipoprotein response to a reduced-fat diet in men. *FASEB J.* 8:121–26

27. Dreon DM, Fernstrom HA, Miller B, Krauss RM. 1995. Apolipoprotein E isoform phenotype and LDL subclass response to a reduced-fat diet. *Arterioscler. Thromb. Vasc. Biol.* 15:105–11

28. Dreon DM, Fernstrom HA, Williams PT, Krauss RM. 1997. LDL subclass patterns and lipoprotein response to a low-fat, high-carbohydrate diet in women. *Arterioscler. Thromb. Vasc. Biol.* 17:707–14

29. Dreon DM, Fernstrom HA, Williams PT, Krauss RM. 1999. A very low-fat diet is not associated with improved lipoprotein profiles in men with a predominance of large, low-density lipoproteins. *Am. J. Clin. Nutr.* 69:411–18

30. Dreon DM, Fernstrom HA, Williams PT, Krauss RM. 2000. Reduced LDL particle size in children consuming a very-low-fat diet is related to parental LDL-subclass patterns. *Am. J. Clin. Nutr.* 71:1611–16

31. Dreon DM, Krauss RM. 1997. Diet-gene interactions in human lipoprotein metabolism. *J. Am. Coll. Nutr.* 16:313–24

32. Feingold KR, Grunfeld C, Pang M, Doerrler W, Krauss RM. 1992. LDL subclass phenotypes and triglyceride metabolism in noninsulin-dependent diabetes. *Arterioscler. Thromb.* 12:1496–502

33. Feingold KR, Krauss RM, Pang M, Doerrler W, Jensen P, Grunfeld C. 1993. The hypertriglyceridemia of acquired immunodeficiency syndrome is associated with an increased prevalence of low density

lipoprotein subclass pattern B. *J. Clin. Endocrinol. Metab.* 76:1423–27

34. Gardner CD, Fortmann SP, Krauss RM. 1996. Association of small low-density lipoprotein particles with the incidence of coronary artery disease in men and women. *JAMA* 276:875–81

35. Genest J Jr, Bard JM, Fruchart JC, Ordovas JM, Schaefer EJ. 1993. Familial hypoalphalipoproteinemia in premature coronary artery disease. *Arterioscler. Thromb.* 13:1728–37

36. Hokanson JE, Austin MA, Zambon A, Brunzell JD. 1993. Plasma triglyceride and LDL heterogeneity in familial combined hyperlipidemia. *Arterioscler. Thromb.* 13:427–34

37. Hokanson JE, Krauss RM, Albers JJ, Austin MA, Brunzell JD. 1995. LDL physical and chemical properties in familial combined hyperlipidemia. *Arterioscler. Thromb. Vasc. Biol.* 15:452–59

38. Jarvik GP, Brunzell JD, Austin MA, Krauss RM, Motulsky AG, Wijsman E. 1994. Genetic predictors of FCHL in four large pedigrees. Influence of ApoB level major locus predicted genotype and LDL subclass phenotype. *Arterioscler. Thromb.* 14:1687–94

39. Johansson J, Nilsson-Ehle P, Carlson LA, Hamsten A. 1991. The association of lipoprotein and hepatic lipase activities with high density lipoprotein subclass levels in men with myocardial infarction at a young age. *Atherosclerosis* 86:111–22

40. Karpe F, Tornvall P, Olivecrona T, Steiner G, Carlson LA, Hamsten A. 1993. Composition of human low density lipoprotein: effects of postprandial triglyceride-rich lipoproteins, lipoprotein lipase, hepatic lipase and cholesteryl ester transfer protein. *Atherosclerosis* 98:33–49

41. Krauss RM, Blanche PJ. 1992. Detection and quantitation of LDL subfractions. *Curr. Opin. Lipidol.* 3:377–83

42. Krauss RM, Cantor RM, Holl LG, Blanche PJ, Rithaporn RS, et al. 1999. Linkage of LDL subclass phenotypes to the LDL

receptor gene locus on high-fat and low-fat diets. *Circulation* 100(18):I659

43. Krauss RM, Deckelbaum RJ, Ernst N, Fisher E, Howard BV, et al. 1996. Dietary guidelines for healthy American adults. A statement for health professionals from the Nutrition Committee, American Heart Association. *Circulation* 94:1795–800

44. Krauss RM, Dreon DM. 1995. Low-density-lipoprotein subclasses and response to a low-fat diet in healthy men. *Am. J. Clin. Nutr.* 62:478–87S

45. Krauss RM, Eckel RH, Howard BV, Appel LJ, Kris-Etherton P, et al. 2000. AHA Dietary Guidelines Revision 2000: a statement for healthcare professionals from the Nutrition Committee of the American Heart Association. *Circulation* 102:2296–311

46. Krauss RM, Lindgren FT, Ray RM. 1980. Interrelationships among subgroups of serum lipoproteins in normal human subjects. *Clin. Chim. Acta* 104:275–90

47. Krauss RM, Williams PT, Lindgren FT, Wood PD. 1988. Coordinate changes in levels of human serum low and high density lipoprotein subclasses in healthy men. *Arteriosclerosis* 8:155–62

48. LaBelle M, Austin MA, Rubin E, Krauss RM. 1991. Linkage analysis of low-density lipoprotein subclass phenotypes and the apolipoprotein B gene. *Genet. Epidemiol.* 8:269–75

49. Lamarche B, Tchernof A, Moorjani S, Cantin B, Dagenais GR, et al. 1997. Small, dense low-density lipoprotein particles as a predictor of the risk of ischemic heart disease in men. Prospective results from the Quebec Cardiovascular Study. *Circulation* 95:69–75

50. Manzato E, Zambon A, Zambon S, Nosadini R, Doria A, et al. 1993. Lipoprotein compositional abnormalities in type 1 (insulin-dependent) diabetic patients. *Acta Diabetol.* 30:11–16

51. McNamara JR, Jenner JL, Li Z, Wilson PWF, Schaefer EJ. 1992. Change in LDL particle size is associated with change in plasma triglyceride concentration. *Arterioscler. Thromb.* 12:1284–90

52. Miller BD, Alderman EL, Haskell WL, Fair JM, Krauss RM. 1996. Predominance of dense low-density lipoprotein particles predicts angiographic benefit of therapy in the Stanford Coronary Risk Intervention Project. *Circulation* 94:2146–53

53. Nigon F, Lesnik P, Rouis M, Chapman MJ. 1991. Discrete subspecies of human low density lipoproteins are heterogeneous in their interaction with the cellular LDL receptor. *J. Lipid Res.* 32:1741–53

54. Nishina PM, Johnson JP, Naggert JK, Krauss RM. 1992. Linkage of atherogenic lipoprotein phenotype to the low density lipoprotein receptor locus on the short arm of chromosome 19. *Proc. Natl. Acad. Sci. USA* 89:708–12

55. Ordovas JM, Schaefer EJ. 1999. Genes, variation of cholesterol and fat intake and serum lipids. *Curr. Opin. Lipidol.* 10:15–22

56. Qiu SQ, Bergeron N, Kotite L, Krauss RM, Bensadoun A, Havel RJ. 1998. Metabolism of lipoproteins containing apolipoprotein B in hepatic lipase-deficient mice. *J. Lipid Res.* 39:1661–68

57. Reaven GM. 1994. Syndrome X: 6 years later. *J. Int. Med. Suppl.* 736:13–22

58. Reaven GM, Chen YD, Jeppesen J, Maheux P, Krauss RM. 1993. Insulin resistance and hyperinsulinemia in individuals with small, dense low density lipoprotein particles. *J. Clin. Invest.* 92:141–46

59. Rotter JI, Bu X, Cantor RM, Warden CH, Brown J, et al. 1996. Multilocus genetic determinants of LDL particle size in coronary artery disease families. *Am. J. Hum. Genet.* 58:585–94

60. Savolainen MJ, Rantala M, Kervinen K, Jarvi L, Suvanto K, et al. 1991. Magnitude of dietary effects on plasma cholesterol concentration: role of sex and apolipoprotein E phenotype. *Atherosclerosis* 86:145–52

61. Schaefer EJ, Lamon-Fava S, Ausman LM, Ordovas JM, Clevidence BA, et al. 1997. Individual variability in lipoprotein cholesterol response to National Cholesterol Education Program Step 2 diets. *Am. J. Clin. Nutr.* 65:823–30

62. Selby JV, Austin MA, Newman B, Zhang D, Quesenberry CP Jr, et al. 1993. LDL subclass phenotypes and the insulin resistance syndrome in women. *Circulation* 88:381–87

63. Spady DK, Woollett LA, Dietschy JM. 1993. Regulation of plasma LDL-cholesterol levels by dietary cholesterol and fatty acids. *Annu. Rev. Nutr.* 13:355–81

64. Stampfer MJ, Krauss RM, Ma J, Blanche PJ, Holl LG, et al. 1996. A prospective study of triglyceride level, low-density lipoprotein particle diameter, and risk of myocardial infarction. *JAMA* 276:882–88

65. Teng B, Thompson GR, Sniderman AD, Forte TM, Krauss RM, Kwiterovich PO Jr. 1983. Composition and distribution of low density lipoprotein fractions in hyperapobetalipoproteinemia, normolipidemia, and familial hypercholesterolemia. *Proc. Natl. Acad. Sci. USA* 80:6662–66

66. Terry RB, Wood PD, Haskell WL, Stefanick ML, Krauss RM. 1989. Regional adiposity patterns in relation to lipids, lipoprotein cholesterol, and lipoprotein subfraction mass in men. *J. Clin. Endocrinol. Metab.* 68:191–99

67. Tikkanen MJ, Huttunen JK, Ehnholm C, Pietinen P. 1990. Apolipoprotein E4 homozygosity predisposes to serum cholesterol elevation during high fat diet. *Arteriosclerosis* 10:285–88

68. Williams PT, Krauss RM, Vranizan KM, Albers JJ, Terry RB, Wood PD. 1989. Effects of exercise-induced weight loss on low density lipoprotein subfractions in healthy men. *Arteriosclerosis* 9:623–32

69. Williams PT, Krauss RM, Vranizan KM, Wood PD. 1990. Changes in lipoprotein subfractions during diet-induced and exercise-induced weight loss in moderately overweight men. *Circulation* 81:1293–304

70. Zambon A, Hokanson JE, Brown BG, Brunzell JD. 1999. Evidence for a new pathophysiological mechanism for coronary artery disease regression: hepatic lipase-mediated changes in LDL density. *Circulation* 99:1959–64

Annu. Rev. Nutr. 2001. 21:297–321

# GASTROINTESTINAL NEMATODES, NUTRITION AND IMMUNITY: Breaking the Negative Spiral

## Kristine G Koski[1] and Marilyn E Scott[2]

[1]School of Dietetics and Human Nutrition and [2]Institute of Parasitology, Macdonald Campus of McGill University, Ste-Anne de Bellevue, Quebec H9X 3V9 Canada, e-mail: koski@macdonald.mcgill.ca; marilyn@parasit.lan.mcgill.ca

**Key Words** malnutrition, nematodes, immunity

■ **Abstract** Nutritionists have long understood that intestinal nematode parasites have deleterious effects on host nutritional status, but only recently has the importance of malnutrition as a predisposing factor to intestinal nematodes been recognized. Here we review experimental and field studies on the effects of protein, energy, zinc, vitamin A, and iron deficiencies on gastrointestinal (GI) nematodes of humans, livestock, and laboratory rodents, and draw certain conclusions about the state of our current understanding. In general, malnutrition promotes the establishment, survival, and fecundity of these parasites, but the magnitude of the effect depends on factors such as host species, parasite species, particular infection protocol used, magnitude of the infection, severity of the nutritional deficiency, and presence of single or multiple infections and single or multiple nutritional deficiencies. We highlight the Th2 arm of the immune system as a component of primary importance in the association between malnutrition and GI nematode infections. We summarize what is known about underlying mechanisms that may account for the observed patterns. Finally, we suggest future research directions.

CONTENTS

0199-9885/01/0715-0297$14.00

# GASTROINTESTINAL NEMATODES AND MALNUTRITION

## Their Place in Our World

Gastrointestinal nematodes are chronic pervasive infections that contribute to widespread morbidity and mortality worldwide. Estimated to infect over one quarter of the world's population, the four most common human gastrointestinal (GI) nematodes, *Ascaris lumbricoides*, *Trichuris trichiura*, *Necator americana*, and *Ancylostoma duodenale*, are responsible for an annual mortality of 18,000 people and for over 4 million years of life lost per annum due to premature death or disability (164). In livestock, related parasites are such an important cause of morbidity and mortality that producers use millions of dollars worth of anthelmintic drugs each year despite the full knowledge that such practices lead rapidly to drug resistance in the parasites (115). Family pets are tested regularly for intestinal nematodes and wild animal populations are host to a variety of similar parasites. All GI nematodes discussed in this review have a direct life cycle involving a single host in which adult worms mature and reproduce in the GI tract, and with one exception (*Trichinella spiralis*), all release eggs or larvae into the environment through the host feces.

## Reasons to Postulate Causal Associations Between Malnutrition and Infection

The association between undernutrition and GI nematode infection has been recognized for many decades by veterinarians and health care workers who have observed that malnutrition and intestinal parasitism share a similar geographical distribution, with the same individuals experiencing both disease states simultaneously (104). The co-existence between undernutrition and nematode infections has been explained by invoking two causal pathways: Infection leads to malnutrition and alternatively malnutrition increases susceptibility to infection (122, 133, 136, 157). However, because both pathways occur concurrently it is often difficult to resolve whether the malnutrition preceded or resulted from the parasitic infection. Intestinal nematodes may lead to malnutrition because they cause anorexia and a variety of pathophysiological responses in the GI tract (vomiting, diarrhea, malabsorption) that directly affect the ability of the host to gain nutriture from the diet; these effects can account for observations that more heavily infected individuals suffer from more severe malnutrition (132). On the other hand, one can explain the concurrent presence of high infection rates and severe malnutrition in the same individuals by citing the now classical literature that describes how malnutrition impairs immunity and that impaired immunity, in turn, increases susceptibility to infection (24, 123).

We envisage the interactions between malnutrition and infection as a negative spiral whereby malnutrition promotes infection, and infection leads to malnutrition. This construct of a negative spiral raises important questions when managing these two interacting conditions. Can and should treatment of intestinal nematodes be used as an indirect means of improving nutritional status? Can nutrient supplements be used as a means of indirectly reducing infection? Should drug treatment be given before, concurrent with, or after nutritional interventions? An understanding of the dominant pathway may be critical when proposing intervention strategies, especially in an epidemiological setting where multiple factors influence both nutritional status and infection and may modify the interaction between the two. The strength (and even the direction) of the association between infection and malnutrition depends on the parasite species (54, 152), the age and sex of the individual (102, 104), concurrent infections (119), and on factors that themselves are associated both with malnutrition and infection such as family income and level of education (118). Over time, the importance of measuring potential environmental and social confounders has influenced design of epidemiological studies on nematodes and undernutrition, but still most studies ignore multiple nutritional deficiencies and concurrent helminth, protozoa, viral, and bacterial infections.

In this review, we explore our understanding of the interactions between nutritional deficiencies and intestinal nematode infections, the nutritional factors that influence host immunity to GI nematodes, the implications for control, and areas in need of further research. Because of the number of excellent reviews on the effect of GI nematode infections on nutritional status (87, 132, 136, 157), more focus is directed toward the effects of malnutrition on GI nematodes.

# EVIDENCE THAT NUTRIENT DEFICIENCIES PROMOTE NEMATODE SURVIVAL

## Macronutrient Deficiencies: Protein-Energy Malnutrition

Combined protein-energy malnutrition (PEM) remains the most widely studied nutrient deficiency associated with infectious disease and acquired immunosuppression. There is extensive literature on the consequences of PEM on immunity (69, 100), but a much smaller body of literature on protein, energy, or combined PEM and their association with immunosuppression during GI nematode infections

(16, 100). Furthermore, even though energy, and not protein, is now considered the most prevalent nutritional deficiency worldwide (82), most studies have not distinguished between the two despite a growing body of evidence suggesting that protein and energy deficits modify host defense mechanisms differently.

***Epidemiological Studies in Human Populations***    Attempts to use epidemiological approaches to unravel cause/effect relationships between PEM and GI nematode infection explore either the causal pathway that malnutrition leads to high infection rates or the other directional pathway that presumes that high infection rates lead to malnutrition. Neither approach presents uniform findings. A study of children in rural Nigeria found that protein intakes were inversely proportional to the number of co-existing intestinal parasitic infections (116), whereas an Indonesian study that stratified children by intensity of *Trichuris* or *Ascaris* showed stunting to be positively associated with *Trichuris*, but not *Ascaris*, burden (54). The alternative approach, assessing risk of infection across variable degrees of malnutrition, has shown severely malnourished Ghanian children to have a tenfold greater prevalence of *Strongyloides stercoralis* than moderately malnourished children (100) and Zairean children with kwashiorkor to have higher *Trichuris* infection than normal, stunted, or wasted children (152). However, the outcomes with *Ascaris* differed. Two reports (54, 100) showed that *Ascaris* infection was independent of nutritional status and in Zaire (152), kwashiorkor was negatively, not positively, associated with infection intensity. One of the few observations on energy per se (90) reported a strong relationship in two-year-old children between infectious disease and a lifetime of low energy but not protein intake.

Cause-effect relationships between malnutrition and GI nematodes may be investigated using controlled interventions. Two common experimental interventions—drugs and diet—have been attempted, but each intervention presumes one unidirectional causal pathway. Evidence exists for and against both interventions modifying GI nematodes during PEM. Anthelmintic intervention studies often measure short-term growth (57) under the premise that removal of GI nematode infections will facilitate catch-up growth, perhaps because of improved protein digestibility (20, 64). Although drug treatment alone does not always result in catch-up growth, perhaps because of low infection levels (44), marginal malnutrition (53), or small sample sizes (20, 57), many studies have reported consistent improvements in growth following drug treatment of *Ascaris*, *Trichuris*, and hookworm (3, 54, 55, 91, 134, 135, 137–139, 149). Unfortunately, very few dietary intervention studies that target PEM monitor impact on intestinal nematodes. Despite nutritional repletion following 29 weeks of high-protein diets resulting in improved serum albumin, hookworm egg production did not change relative to baseline levels in 12 malnourished adults with heavy hookworm infestations, leading the authors to conclude that hookworms were unaffected by improvements in host protein status (151). Later, Gupta et al (52) reported that nutritional status was unimproved by supplementary feeding of preschool children in India unless they also received anthelmintic treatment. This latter investigation is one of very few human studies using both protein supplements and anthelmintics simultaneously.

*Field and Experimental Studies in Livestock*    Much research on GI nematode-PEM interactions is described within the literature on parasitic infections in livestock, where producers and researchers have long recognized that GI nematodes impair productivity of cattle, sheep, and pigs as a result of parasite-induced reduction in feed intake, poor digestibility and absorption of feed, and pathophysiological defects in epithelial processes such as intestinal leakage of plasma proteins (13, 26, 157). Considerable attention has been directed toward demonstrating the deleterious impact of intestinal parasites on nitrogen utilization and livestock performance, but the reciprocal relationship, that well-nourished animals resist intestinal parasitism better than those less adequately fed, is gaining increasing prominence as investigators recognize that prolonged parasitism in protein-deficient animals can be reversed by protein supplementation (26, 113, 156, 157). Studies in lambs have demonstrated that high-protein diets enhance the development of immunity against *Haemonchus contortus* (1), *Trichostrongylus colubriformis* (66), and *Ostertagia circumcincta* (27). The long-term ability of sheep to control their GI nematode infections under natural grazing conditions has been shown to be directly proportional to the protein content during the post-weaning diet (33). Recently, Knox & Steel (77) reported improved resilience to infection in sheep given urea supplements. In fact, when given the choice of diets, infected sheep selected the diet with the higher protein concentration (79, 80). Protein, rather than energy, was identified as the major factor limiting the ability of *T. colubriformis*–infected lambs to utilize feed (17) because of a speculated parasite-induced loss of endogenous protein. Only one study has directly examined the consequences of energy restriction; energy-restricted sheep infected with nematodes have increased mortality (51). Taken together, these studies indicate that infection with GI nematodes in livestock increases the protein needs of the host or reduces the effectiveness of the immune response. However, the contribution of energy restriction requires further investigation.

*Laboratory Studies in Rodents*    In both humans and livestock, infection is a continuous process where the host is constantly exposed to parasite eggs or larvae. Certainly in human studies, it is very difficult, if not impossible, to distinguish between susceptibility to incoming infections and clearance of existing infections. In laboratory models, researchers are able to separate these two processes by controlled infection protocols. Most GI nematodes used in laboratory rodents elicit a protective immune response that eliminates the parasites within 2–3 weeks of the first infection in well-nourished hosts. Is this protective response lost during protein deficiency? In rats fed a low-protein diet (5–10% versus 30%), the initial establishment and short-term survival of *Nippostrongylus brasiliensis* was unaffected, but the protein-deficient rats had increased worm survival (15, 30). Similarly, in both *Trichinella spiralis*-infected mice (47) and in *Trichuris muris*-infected mice

(92, 93), 4% protein deficiency delayed expulsion of adult worms. However, studies using the mouse–*Heligmosomoides polygyrus* model are less conclusive. Worm survival was unaffected when mice were fed a 2% casein diet, despite reduced body weight gain and overt hypoalbuminemia (18), whereas worm survival was prolonged when mice were fed both marginal (7%) and low (3%) protein diets (16) despite absence of hypoalbuminemia. The discrepancy among findings may be explained in part by differences in diet composition, but it is more likely a consequence of differences in protective immunity. Primary infections with *N. brasiliensis*, *T. spiralis*, and *T. muris* induce strong protective immunity whereas a primary *H. polygyrus* infection normally invokes a weak host immune response, due to the immunosuppressive action of adult worms (35, 97), that promotes long-lasting chronic infections.

Repeated infection ("challenge") protocols with *H. polygyrus* normally stimulate strong protective immunity upon re-infection, and all studies using these infection protocols support the hypothesis that restriction of dietary protein enhances GI nematode survival. Several studies using a challenge infection protocol have shown that a 2–3% protein diet increased worm survival, suggesting that protein deficiency impaired the capacity for acquired host resistance in previously immunized mice (16, 61, 71, 130). In repeated infection protocols, *H. polygyrus*–infected mice fed 2–3% protein accumulated worms in proportion to the intensity of exposure, whereas worm accumulation in mice fed 8–16% protein actually declined at higher infection doses (71, 129). Under semi-natural infection conditions in which a group of susceptible animals was continuously exposed to *H. polygyrus*, a 2% protein diet increased the rate at which uninfected mice acquired the parasites and also increased the survival of adult worms (129). Effects on parasite reproduction have been less consistent. Worm fecundity was unaffected by the 2–3% protein diets in some studies (16, 130) but was elevated in the malnourished mice in other studies (71, 129). Thus, severe protein deficiency prolongs survival of GI nematodes in rodents, and in all cases where elimination of the parasite is normally immunologically mediated, the data strongly suggest that the mechanism underlying the prolonged parasite survival is perturbed host immunity.

A few studies have directly examined the effects of energy restriction independent of protein deficiency in laboratory models and the results strongly suggest that the effects of energy restriction during GI nematodes infections are independent of protein restriction. Lunn et al (88) demonstrated prolonged *N. brasiliensis* survival in energy-restricted rats that was accompanied with hypoalbuminemia, which the authors attributed to protein leakage into the intestine through parasite-induced lesions. Recent work in our laboratory successfully produced a mild to moderate energy deficit that was not accompanied by any signs of protein deficiency. We showed that a 20% or 25% reduction in energy intake, independent of any alteration in protein status, exerted dramatic effects on survival of *H. polygyrus* in mice (78). What was particularly striking about this observation was that, in this host-parasite model, a smaller energy deficit than protein restriction produced comparable changes in parasite numbers; furthermore, there were contrasting differences in host immunity between the energy and protein restrictions demonstrating independent effects of dietary deprivations (61, 78).

## Micronutrient Deficiencies

As with macronutrients, studies on the association between micronutrient deficiencies and intestinal nematode infections reveal the complexity of the interrelationship. Although beneficial effects of potassium, molybdenum, and cobalt, but not selenium and copper, have been reported against GI nematodes in livestock (157), most research on trace elements and GI nematode infection in humans and in laboratory models focuses on deficiencies of zinc, vitamin A, or iron, which are among the most pervasive nutritional deficiencies in humans worldwide.

*Zinc*    The first study to suggest a relationship between zinc deficiency and increased nematode infections was a cross-sectional survey of Jamaican children (21) that showed a weak but significant negative correlation between plasma zinc levels and numbers of *Trichuris*. A later randomized, double-blind clinical trial of Guatemalan children reported contrasting results with no effect of zinc supplementation on re-infection with GI nematodes following drug treatment (49). This absence of effect was attributed to the lack of pre-existing zinc deficiency in these Guatemalan children. In addition to effects on parasite numbers, an intriguing association between refeeding of severely malnourished infants and parasite reproduction emerged when Bundy & Golden (21) noted a transient increase in *Ascaris* egg production during refeeding that was attributed to a decrease in plasma zinc. This relationship highlights a possible unexpected consequence of refeeding programs and we suggest that this temporary decline in plasma zinc may lead to further immunosuppression releasing the parasite from immunologically induced constraints in egg production (126).

Data are now accumulating in rodent models to show a graded response depending on the magnitude of the dietary zinc restriction. In primary *H. polygyrus* infections where immunity is not normally stimulated, moderate (3 mg/kg) (16) and severe (0.75 mg/kg) (126) dietary zinc restriction prolonged *H. polygyrus* survival whereas a marginal deficiency (5 mg/kg) did not (95). This pattern correlated well with biochemical and physiological indicators of tissue, but not plasma, zinc deficiency, and with host immune effectors. Investigators have also examined several infection models where immunity is fully functional and have confirmed a relationship between zinc deficiency and increased worm burdens. Fenwick et al (41) reported delayed expulsion and higher burdens of *T. spiralis* in rats fed a moderately deficient diet (3 mg/kg) compared with control animals, whereas intake of 3 mg zinc/kg diet had no effect on the number or size of *N. brasiliensis* in rats but increased total egg output (38). When rats were infected with *Strongyloides ratti*, the 3 mg/kg dietary zinc delayed but did not abolish the ability to eliminate intestinal worms by day 28 pi (40). Similarly, a diet of 3 mg/kg zinc during challenge infection with *H. polygyrus* (16) had no effect on *H. polygyrus* worm burdens whereas a more severe deficiency (0.75 mg/kg) profoundly impaired the immune response and facilitated *H. polygyrus* survival (126, 127). Interestingly, data from repletion studies (40, 41) using both *S. ratti* and *T. spiralis* hint that repletion actually improves ability to control infection over that of the well-nourished control animals, supporting the therapeutic use of zinc.

A complication associated with laboratory models of zinc deficiency is the reduced food intake that accompanies zinc-deficiency. Whereas concurrent energy restriction appeared to have no effect on *N. brasiliensis*, *T. spiralis*, or *S. ratti* infections, many of the effects attributed to zinc deficiency in *H. polygyrus* were a consequence, at least in part, of the concurrent energy restriction (125–127. The greater number of worms and higher per capita egg production in zinc-deficient mice after challenge infection were also detected in pair-fed control mice, indicating effects of both zinc and energy restriction (126, 127). Parasites developed more rapidly in energy-restricted mice during a primary infection and even more so in zinc-deficient mice, perhaps reflecting zinc- and energy-dependent changes in worm migrational habits, local inflammatory response to the larval stage, and/or GI physiology such as gut transit time or intestinal contractility. Zinc deficiency and energy restriction produced opposite effects on position of worms during a primary infection: In zinc-deficient mice, adults moved posteriorad whereas in energy-restricted mice, fourth stage larvae were more anteriorad (126). The parasites themselves were not zinc deficient (126), suggesting that the negative impacts of zinc deficiency on worm survival, development, and migration were likely mediated through perturbations on the host immune response. During both primary and challenge infections, *H. polygyrus* were more sensitive to dietary protein deficiency (3%) than to zinc restriction (3 mg/kg) (16). Furthermore, each nutrient deficit was independent of the other, suggesting that each had a different physiological effect on the host immune system.

***Vitamin A***    Several studies suggest an association between vitamin A and *Ascaris* infection, with the strong implication that *Ascaris* leads to malabsorption of vitamin A (136, 147, 148). However, this area remains controversial. Ahmed et al (4) were unable to demonstrate impaired vitamin A absorption in *Ascaris*-infected children, yet Curtale et al (31) reported that *Ascaris* was a significant risk factor for xerophthalmia in Nepal. Vitamin A supplementation had a stronger effect on vitamin A status than treatment of *Ascaris* in Indonesian children (146), yet vitamin A status improved following treatment for *Ascaris* in other studies (63, 89, 108). Very few studies have examined the effects of vitamin A deficiency on host resistance to GI nematode infections in animal models. During primary infection with *T. spiralis*, vitamin A deficiency did not alter the number of larvae in the intestine or muscle, the worm expulsion rate, or the level of egg output despite induction of multiple systemic and gut-associated immunological defects in mice (23). Both numbers and egg production of *H. polygyrus* were elevated in vitamin A–deficient mice (45).

*Iron*  Iron deficiency and anemia have been frequently observed in patients with hookworm infection in a dose-dependent relationship such that individuals with higher levels of infection have greater risk for lower hemoglobin status (5, 58, 102, 140, 141). Hookworms derive their nutrients from host blood and tissue and as a result can induce significant iron losses in the intestine (140). Human studies have shown that high levels of iron intake do not lower prevalence of infection (83, 151) and have led to the conclusion that hookworm infection causes iron deficiency, rather than iron deficiency predisposing to infection. This generalization appears not to be true under controlled experimental conditions. Iron deficiency increased larval establishment and adult survival of *N. brasiliensis* in rats (15). Repletion of iron did not fully restore hemoglobin values but was effective in accelerating parasite expulsion (15). During challenge infection with *N. brasiliensis*, Duncombe et al (37) observed higher worm burdens in rats fed a iron-free diet compared with well-fed controls, suggesting that acquired resistance to secondary nematode infections is dependent on adequate iron nutriture. More research is required on effects of iron deficiency on other GI nematodes, particularly those causing chronic infections, before one can make definitive comments of the role of dietary iron in development and control of intestinal parasitism.

*Conclusion*   PEM as well as poor vitamin A, zinc, and iron intakes predispose to GI nematode infections, which in turn exacerbate the nutritional deficiencies and further prolong nematode survival in human, livestock, and rodent models. Interestingly, the degree of deficiency required to increase worm burdens differs for each nutrient, and for protein and energy, changes in worm burdens occurred without overt signs of compromised nutritional status. This suggests that the changes in host defense mechanisms occurred before biochemical signs of clinical deficiency for protein and energy, whereas for vitamin A and zinc, severe dietary deficiencies that were accompanied by declines in serum and/or tissue concentrations were required before effects on host defenses were noted.

# IMMUNOLOGICAL MECHANISMS UNDERLYING NUTRITION-INFECTION INTERACTIONS

## Th1 versus Th2 and Nematode Immunity

Immune responses to infectious organisms involve two categories of T helper (Th) cells: type I Th (Th1) cells are responsible for cell-mediated immunity against bacterial, protozoal, viral infections, and intracellular parasites whereas type 2 Th (Th2) cells mediate antibody-dependent immunity against extracellular parasites including GI nematodes. Each response phenotype produces a dominant pattern of cytokine and immune effectors. Moreover, each phenotypic profile (Th1 versus Th2) is antagonistic to the differentiation and activity of effectors belonging to the reciprocal phenotype (98). Primed Th2 cells secrete interleukin (IL)-4, IL-5,

IL-9, and IL-10, which promote the proliferation and activation of Th2-associated effectors such as IgE or IgG1 secreting plasma cells, eosinophils, and mucosal mast cells (MMC) (28) whereas Th1 cells produce IL-2 and IFN-$\gamma$ and interact with APCs to synthesize IL-12. Th1-associated cytokines are important in macrophage activity and isotype selection for IgG2a, IgG2b, and IgG3, which mediate responses against bacterial and viral infections (86). The distinction between these two arms is not complete, however. Both Th cell types secrete IL-3, tumor necrosis factor-$\alpha$, and granulocyte-macrophage colony stimulating factor (98). Furthermore, each cytokine has pleiotropic effects on multiple types of lymphoid cells, and there is much duplication of function among the different cytokines.

Experimental studies show that functional immunity to GI nematodes involves systemic Th2-type cytokines and effectors and, with rare exception (84), that IL-4 is a requirement for the Th2 cell response. In humans infected with helminth parasites, serum IgE and IgG1 levels are directly proportional to parasite-induced IL-4 production and inversely related to IFN-$\gamma$ synthesis (74) where IgE-mediated eosinophil and mast cell activities are associated with effective resolution of helminth infections (6). The role of IL-4 has been clearly demonstrated in laboratory studies with *H. polygyrus* where anti-IL-4 antibodies and anti-IL-4 receptor antibodies block immunological control (154, 155). Consistent with these data, mice infected with *N. brasiliensis* and deficient in the signal transducer and transcriptional activator of IL-4, secreted lower amounts of Th2-dependent antibodies (145), but not Th1-dependent antibodies (128).

## Evidence that Nutrient Deficits Impair Systemic Th1 and Th2 Immunity

In immunology, a working theory is that the reciprocal cross-regulation of Th1 and Th2 cytokines and their effectors produce a dominant immunological phenotype, which for GI nematodes is represented by the Th2 phenotype. It has been proposed that nutritional deficiencies may prevent the expression of the dominant Th2 phenotypes and that energy deficits (78), vitamin A deficits (23), and protein deficits (61) result in the overexpression of the Th1 cytokine IFN-$\gamma$ and the down-regulation of essential Th2 cytokines. The absence of Th2 cytokines and their effectors results in prolonged survival of GI nematodes. Recently, we have shown that down-regulation of IL-4 and other Th2 cytokines and effectors occurred during zinc deficiency (121), protein deficiency (61), and energy restriction (78) and was associated in all cases with prolonged survival of *H. polygyrus*. However, energy restriction lowered both Th1 and Th2 cytokines (78), whereas protein malnutrition decreased Th2 and increased Th1 cytokine profiles (61). Vitamin A deficiency also failed to support the hypothesis of an up-regulation of a Th1 during *H. polygyrus* infection (45); however, during *T. spiralis* more IFN-$\gamma$ was secreted by spenocytes in the vitamin A–deficient mice (23). Taken together, these results demonstrate important mechanistic differences between nutrients in their ability to modify the reciprocal relationship between Th1 and Th2 phenotypes and would further suggest that immunopathology could result from defects in specific pathways, not simply a result of dysregulation in Th1 versus Th2 phenotypes.

# The Importance of Intestinal Immunity to Nematode Infections

The GI tract is one of the largest immunological organs in the body and serves as the first line of defense against GI nematodes. Cells in the gut-associated lymphoid tissue (GALT) respond to intestinal pathogens by processing antigens for recognition by lymphocytes, by initiating a cascade of specialized Th2 immune responses to parasite-specific antigens at intestinal and systemic sites, by regulating the trafficking of immune mediators from the periphery back to the infected gut, and by participating directly in cytotoxic activities that limit parasite establishment and survival (19, 39, 109, 111, 153, 159). The GALT is categorized into two anatomically and functionally distinct compartments: the afferent limb [Peyer's patches, isolated lymphatic follicles, and mesenteric lymph nodes (MLN)] where antigen is presented to naïve lymphocytes (14, 81), and the efferent limb (intraepithelium and lamina propria of intestinal microvilli) where antigen-specific effectors mediate their anthelmintic effects (9). MMC progenitors, basophils, and eosinophils are drawn by chemotaxis to the intraepithelium and lamina propria, as seen for example in *N. brasiliensis* infection (7, 25, 67, 94). There they bind to IgE and parasite antigens (7, 103, 131), which leads to degranulation and release of histamine and serine proteases (75, 161) that are associated with worm expulsion. These events occur rapidly after infection. For example, infection with *T. spiralis* results in transport of IgE into the intestinal lumen within 24 hours of infection (110, 143). Previous studies have documented the early synthesis, production and uptake of Th2 cytokines by GALT (2, 12, 43, 65, 99, 114, 120). A further indication of the unique immune responses in the mucosa is the large percentage of T cells with gamma delta receptors that provide a contact signal for isotype switching to IgE production in the presence of IL-4 (42, 46, 68, 162). These observations have led to the conclusion that mucosal cells residing in the gut are the most important source of local cytokines during early parasitic infection (111).

# Evidence that Intestinal Immunity is Perturbed by Nutrient Deficits During Nematode Infections

Studies comparing responses of intestinal with peripheral lymphoid sites in the infected, malnourished host have been recently completed in our laboratories using the *H. polygyrus* model. We have demonstrated important differential responses in both the pattern and timing of host immunity in these two lymphoid compartments during protein (61), energy (78), and vitamin A deficiency (45). We found that protein malnutrition was more detrimental to gut-associated than to systemic IL-4 production: Deficient MLN cells secreted less IL-4 and more IFN-$\gamma$ shortly after challenge whereas deficient spleen cells secreted more IFN-$\gamma$ only at 2 weeks post-challenge infection (pci). Adequate protein intake was necessary for mRNA expression and protein synthesis of IL-4 in GALT but did not affect IL-5 or IL-10 production. Thus based on our protein results, decreased IL-4 combined with increased IFN-$\gamma$ contributed to reduced levels of IgE, MMC, and gut eosinophils and to prolonged parasite survival, supporting the hypothesis that protein malnutrition increased the survival of a nematode parasite by decreasing gut-associated Th2 cytokines and effectors and increasing INF-$\gamma$(61).

However, neither vitamin A nor energy deficits support this classical theory that postulates down-regulation of Th2 and simultaneous up-regulation of Th1 cytokines. Energy deficits suppressed both Th1 (IFN-$\gamma$) and Th2 profiles (IL-4, IL-5, IgE, IgG1, and eosinophils) in both the gut and splenic lymphoid tissues (78). From our study we concluded that a surge in IL-4 production is required by both the systemic and GALT immune systems early during first exposure to a nematode infection, and that energy restriction prevents this. Similarly, in vitamin A–deficient mice (45), both IL-4 and IFN-$\gamma$ decreased in MLN, whereas the expected up-regulation of IFN-$\gamma$ associated with the corresponding down-regulation of IL-4, which is observed in *T. spiralis*–infected vitamin A–deficient mice (23), was only observed in the systemic response to a challenge infection in vitamin A–deficient mice infected with *H. polygyrus*.

***Conclusion***    Current evidence shows that the immune system during nematode infections in malnourished hosts (protein, energy, zinc, and vitamin A) is characterized by declines in several Th2 immune effectors: IgE (16, 45, 61, 78, 125), parasite-specific IgG1 (16, 23, 45, 78, 125), and eosinophils (16, 45, 61, 78, 125). Additional evidence has been provided that both zinc and energy alter the functioning of specific cellular components, in particular T-cell and APCs (127), pointing to specific cellular defects resulting from nutritional deficiencies. Importantly, no single nutrient deficiency suppressed all immune responses nor did all immune responses respond similarly to each nutrient. Our studies on single deficiencies of protein, energy, and vitamin A in the *H. polygyrus*–infected mouse model provide evidence that each nutrient has a distinct role in modifying Th1/Th2 profiles during GI nematode infections, and that responses differ significantly by gut versus systemic tissue.

## MALNUTRITION, INFECTION, AND IMMUNITY—A CO-EVOLUTIONARY PARADIGM

The concept of a co-evolutionary trade-off between host protective immunity and parasitic infection is not new (11, 96). GI nematodes have evolved a finely tuned ability to recognize biochemical and physiological cues of the host in order to initiate their establishment (142). Host resistance to GI nematodes is a heritable trait tied directly to the expression of host immunity (11, 96, 160), with a phenotypic spectrum ranging from exaggerated susceptibility to rapid clearance of infection (50). Because helminth infections in general do not induce long-lasting immunity, the most effective immune strategy may not be to completely clear an existing infection, but to support a chronic low-level infection that provides continual antigenic stimulation.

On an evolutionary time scale, the co-evolution between host and parasite most likely occurred in undernourished individuals. This co-evolutionary environment raises important questions. As nutritional conditions improved, did the host evolve to invest the additional resources into growth, reproduction, and tissue maintenance, or into mounting a more vigorous immune response? The answer may be seen by contrasting what occurs today in developed versus developing countries. Developed countries are characterized by abundant food, excellent sanitation, adequate health care, and pharmaceutical interventions, and dramatically reduced prevalence of GI nematodes, yet increasing incidence of food allergies. In contrast, developing countries are characterized by malnutrition, GI nematode infections, yet remarkably little allergy (6). Some evolutionary biologists have suggested that intestinal parasites have exerted a strong selective force for a specific Th2 immune phenotype in GALT (34, 144). The GALT is considered to be the most primitive immune organ in vertebrates, and there is considerable support for the idea that the pathological consequences of Th2 response (i.e. food allergy) are an evolutionary hangover from a time when hosts needed a strong Th2 response to protect against parasites (107). If these observations are indeed true, then we could argue that the increased incidence of allergy arises not only from reduced exposure to nematode infections but also from improved availability of nutrients.

It is unlikely that links between host-parasite co-evolution and nutritional status end with host immunity. Recent studies in the viral literature highlight a need for sensitivity to how nutritional status may affect the parasites directly. Beck & Levander (10) have found that not only is the virulence of a benign strain of the Coxsackievirus B3 higher in selenium-deficient hosts, but also that the virus retains its virulent state when passaged into a well-nourished host. This suggests the possibility that parasitic organisms quickly co-evolve within their present nutritional environment. Therefore, issues such as the possible effects of nutritional status on the biology of the parasite, genetic heterogeneity in the host population with regard to resistance and susceptibility to infection, and the role of improved nutritional status not only in reducing infection but perhaps in increasing immunopathologies, may need to be considered when planning intervention programs that target nutritional deficiencies, GI nematodes, or both.

## BREAKING THE NEGATIVE SPIRAL

Three main types of interventions are envisioned to directly attack the nutrition-infection-immunity triad: improved nutritional status, prevention or treatment of infection, and improved immunocompetence. Each intervention can be achieved in many ways, and each should in theory have beneficial repercussions on the other conditions. However, in a system as complex as a human community, such "simple" solutions may not be a panacea.

## Nutritional Interventions

Although we presume that hosts are better able to control their helminth infections when well-nourished, there is a surprising lack of field studies in human populations where the benefits of nutritional improvement on helminth infection have been examined. Even in clinical trials with vitamin A supplementation where the outcome on infectious diseases has been monitored, helminth infections have largely been ignored (8). In free-grazing sheep, supplementary feeding with sunflower meal was shown to be more beneficial, but also more expensive, than slow-release anthelmintics in reducing production losses due to GI nematodes (156). The cost was reduced when urea-molasses blocks were used as nutritional supplements; these enhance the ability of ruminants to withstand GI infection (76). In the laboratory, repletion after zinc-deficient diets were fed restored the ability of the host to control *T. spiralis* infections (40, 41) and refeeding protein-deficient rats with methionine improved their ability to control *N. brasiliensis* (29). These studies indicate that improved nutritional status will reduce infection or infection-induced pathology.

The laboratory studies and much of the speculations about livestock and human infections focus on the benefit to an individual of improved nutritional status and consequent improved resistance to infection. However, the host population or community consists of a broad spectrum of individuals who differ in their genetically determined propensity to resist infections and who may differ in their response to supplementation. Three paradigms exist. If the effects of malnutrition are subtle relative to genetically determined resistance to infection, then nutrition interventions may not change the overall prevalence of infection, but may be beneficial only to those heavily infected individuals who have high need of nutrients for tissue repair. If nutritional deficiency acts in a synergistic manner in the genetically susceptible individuals, then nutrition will be very important for them, but will have little impact on the genetically resistant individual who is protected from infection despite being malnourished. This would be expected, for example, in ruminant parasites where protein deficiency does not completely abolish the capacity for antibody or eosinophil responses in resistant strains (26, 62). If malnutrition inhibits the development of resistance then nutrition interventions will be helpful in restoring the capacity of the genetically resistant individuals to control infection but may also increase their risk of immunopathology. Nutritional interventions may also be beneficial if the dietary constituents themselves have anthelmintic properties. Primates (60), pre-historic man (22), and present day (59, 105) appear to selectively ingest plants with medicinal properties as a natural means to manage helminth infections. Studies in livestock demonstrate anthelmintic properties of indigenous plants (56, 101), and much attention is being paid to the value of allelochemicals against human helminth infections (163). Thus interventions that promote use of a variety of indigenous plants may have both nutritional and antiparasite benefits, assuming plant products are selected wisely.

## Anthelmintics

Drug efficacy itself is also affected by nutritional status. The ability of benzimidazole drugs to eliminate *N. brasiliensis* is significantly impaired in rats fed a diet deficient in iron and protein alone (37) or in combination (36), compared with well-nourished rats, presumably because of the reduced uptake of drug by the parasite (106). A variety of mechanisms may account for this observation, including the fact that nutritional status may affect drug absorption, drug metabolism, and drug uptake by the parasite. Malnutrition can reduce the success of drug interventions and the reduced efficacy is likely to promote selection of drug-resistant parasites (106), further limiting chemotherapeutic control of GI nematode infections. We might conclude therefore that nutritional intervention should precede drug treatments to ensure maximal drug effectiveness during intervention programs. However, parasitic infections may in turn reduce the absorption of nutrients and therefore the efficacy of nutritional intervention may be improved if parasites are eliminated first. Studies are urgently needed to evaluate the relative benefits of drug treatments before, during, or after nutritional interventions so as to achieve the goal of maximized benefits of such integrated approaches.

## Enhanced Immunocompetence

GI nematodes do not induce life-long immunity, perhaps because they fail to stimulate long-lived IgE$^+$ B cells responsible for memory, as reported for *N. brasiliensis*–infected rats (85). A consequence of the incomplete protective response is the need to carefully consider when a nematode vaccine should be administered so as to attain maximum protection from the vaccine. Most clinical problems associated with GI nematodes occur in young animals, in children, or during pregnancy—that is, at times when malnutrition may be a problem. It is well known from the microparasite vaccination experience that vaccination is ineffective in malnourished children (78, 117) and the same problem could arise when vaccines become available for use against GI nematodes. Other forms of immune enhancements have been under consideration including injections of plasmids containing genes that express key cytokines (72, 112) and administration of probiotics (32) to stimulate Th1 response in the gut. The implication of such interventions for GI nematodes infections must not be ignored.

## CONCLUSION

In reviewing the body of literature relating malnutrition, nematode infection and immunity, a few key points have become very clear. Despite the very large number of studies, a central dogma has yet to emerge in this interdisciplinary area of research. We know many facts, often about very specific effects of deficits of a certain nutrient on a receptor molecule or on levels of a specific cytokine, and there are large numbers of field studies that repeatedly show that malnutrition and infection occur together. Yet more and more it is becoming clear that generalizations cannot be made about the effects of different nutrients on the various components of the immune response and that lack of understanding of the basis of functional immunity against nematodes makes it very difficult to pinpoint the nutrient deficiencies that should be of most concern. There remains a very large gap between the science of the molecular biologists and that of the public health sector, although both share the common objective of improved understanding of nutrition-infection-immunity interactions with the goal of reducing morbidity and mortality in human and livestock populations. We need gradually to move to greater cooperation and integration of research questions so that those mechanisms that will be of critical importance in making public health decisions emerge. For example, as energy deficiency is a dominant nutritional problem in the world, and as modest deficits in energy appear to have dramatic influences on the host immune response to GI nematode infections, more research should be directed toward energy deficiency, infection, and immunity. Such work would be of tremendous benefit to the large-scale interventions that are now in progress, but that target infection and vitamin and mineral deficiencies (48, 150). In addition, a better understanding of the relationship between malnutrition and drug efficacy in the nematode-infected host is required. Focus must be centred on the intestine; it is the site of nutrient absorption, it is the home of the majority of parasitic organisms, and it is arguably the largest immunological organ in the body. Breaking out of the negative spiral requires cooperation between immunologists, parasitologists, and nutritionists, between molecular biologists and public health workers. It is the communication among these groups that will uncover those research questions, the answers to which will best lead us to appropriate management of these important health problems.

## ACKNOWLEDGMENTS

We appreciate the thoughtful discussions with our former graduate students, especially R. Ing.

**Visit the Annual Reviews home page at www.AnnualReviews.org**

## LITERATURE CITED

1. Abbott EM, Parkins JJ, Holmes PH. 1988. Influence of dietary protein on the pathophysiology of haemonchosis in lambs given continuous infections. *Res. Vet. Sci.* 45:41–49

2. Abitorabi MA, Mackay CR, Jerome EH, Osorio O, Butcher EC, Erle DJ. 1996. Differential expression of homing molecules on recirculating lymphocytes from sheep gut,

peripheral, and lung lymph. *J. Immunol.* 156:3111–17

3. Adams EJ, Stephenson LS, Latham MC, Kinoti SN. 1994. Physical activity and growth of Kenyan school children with hookworm, *Trichuris trichiura* and *Ascaris lumbricoides* infections are improved after treatment with albendazole. *J. Nutr.* 124:1199–206

4. Ahmed F, Mohiduzzaman M, Jackson AA. 1993. Vitamin A absorption in children with ascariasis. *Br. J. Nutr.* 69:817–25

5. Albonico M, Stoltzfus RJ, Savioli L, Tielsch JM, Chwaya HM, et al. 1998. Epidemiological evidence for a differential effect of hookworm species, *Ancylostoma duodenale* or *Necator americanus*, on iron status of children. *Int. J. Epidemiol.* 27(3):530–37

6. Allen JE, Maizels RM. 1996. Immunology of human helminth infection. *Int. Arch. Allergy Immunol.* 109(1):3–10

7. Arizono N, Yamada M, Tegoshi T, Okada M, Uchikawa R, Matsuda S. 1994. Mucosal mast cell proliferation following normal and heterotopic infections of the nematode *Nippostrongylus brasiliensis* in rats. *APMIS* 102:589–96

8. Beagley KW, Elson CO. 1992. Cells and cytokines in mucosal immunity and inflammation. *Gastroenterol. Clin. N.A.* 21:347-66

9. Beaton GH, Martorell R, Aronson KJ, Edmonston B, McCabe G et al. 1993. *Effectiveness of vitamin A supplementation in the control of young child morbidity and mortality in developing countries.* UN Admin. Comm. Coord./Subcomm. Nutr. (ACC/SCN) State-of-the-Art Ser. Nutr. Policy Discuss. Pap. No. 13, WHO. 119 pp.

10. Beck MA, Levander OA. 2000. Host nutritional status and its effect on a viral pathogen. *J. Infect. Dis.* 182(Suppl.):93–96

11. Behnke JM, Barnard CJ, Wakelin D. 1992. Understanding chronic nematode infections: evolutionary considerations, current hypotheses and the way forward. *Int. J. Parasitol.* 22:861–907

12. Berlin C, Berg EL, Briskin MJ, Andrew DP, Kilshaw PJ, et al. 1993. $\alpha 4\beta 7$ integrin mediates lymphocyte binding to the mucosal vascular addressin MAdCAM-1. *Cell* 74:185–95

13. Blackburn H, Rocha J, Figueiredo EP, Berne ME, Viera LS et al. 1991. Interaction of parasitism and nutrition and their effects on production and clinical parameter in goats. *Vet. Parasitol.* 40:99–112

14. Bogen SA, Weinberg DS, Abbas AK. 1991. Histologic analysis of T lymphocyte activation in reactive lymph nodes. *J. Immunol.* 147:1537–41

15. Bolin TD, Davis AE, Cummins AG, Duncombe VM, Kelly JD. 1977. Effect of iron and protein deficiency on the expulsion of *Nippostronglyus brasiliensis* from the small intestine of the rat. *Gut* 18:182–86

16. Boulay M, Scott ME, Conly SL, Stevenson MM, Koski KG. 1998. Dietary protein and zinc restrictions independently modify a *Heligmosomoides polygyrus* (Nematoda) infection in mice. *Parasitology* 116:449–62

17. Bown MD, Poppi DP, Sykes AR. 1991. The effect of post-ruminal infusion of protein or energy on the pathophysiology of *Trichostrongylus colubriformis* infection and body composition in lambs. *Aust. J. Agric. Res.* 42:253–67

18. Brailsford TJ, Mapes CJ. 1987. Comparisons of *Heligmosomoides polygyrus* primary infection in protein-deficient and well-nourished mice. *Parasitology* 95:311–21

19. Brandtzaeg P. 1998. Development and basic mechanisms of human gut immunity. *Nutr. Rev.* 56(Suppl.):5–18

20. Brown KH, Gilman RH, Khatun M, Ahmet G. 1980. Absorption of macronutrients from a rice-vegetable diet before and after treatment of ascariasis in children. *Am. J. Clin. Nutr.* 33:1975–82

21. Bundy DAP, Golden MHN. 1987. The impact of host nutrition on gastrointestinal helminth populations. *Parasitology* 95:623–35

22. Capasso L. 1998. 5300 years ago, the Ice Man used natural laxatives and antibiotics. *Lancet* 352(9143):1864

23. Carman JA, Pond L, Nashold F, Wassom DL, Hayes CE. 1992. Immunity to

*Trichinella spiralis* infection in Vitamin A-deficient mice. *J. Exp. Med.* 175:111–20

24. Chandra RK. 1983. Nutrition, immunity and infection: present knowledge and future directions. *Lancet* 1:688–91

25. Chen XJ, Enerback L. 1996. Immune response to a *Nippostrongylus brasiliensis* infection in athymic and euthymic rats: surface expression of IgE receptors, IgE occupancy and secretory ability of mast cells. *Int. Arch. Allergy Immunol.* 109:250–57

26. Coop RL, Holmes PH. 1996. Nutrition and parasite interaction. *Int. J. Parasitol.* 26:951–62

27. Coop RL, Huntley JF, Smith WD. 1995. Effect of dietary protein supplementation on the development of immunity to *Ostertagia circumcincta* in growing lambs. *Res. Vet. Sci.* 59(1):24–29

28. Cox FEG, Liew EY. 1992. T-cell subsets and cytokines in parasitic infections. *Parasitol. Today* 8:371–74

29. Cummins AG, Bolin TD, Duncombe VM, Davis AE. 1986. The effect of methionine and protein deficiency in delaying expulsion of *Nippostronglyus brasiliensis* in the rat. *Am. J. Clin. Nutr.* 44:857–62

30. Cummins AG, Duncombe VM, Bolin TD, Davis AE, Kelly JD. 1978. Suppression of rejection of *Nippostronglyus brasiliensis* in iron and protein deficient rats: effect of syngeneic lymphocyte transfer. *Gut* 19:823–26

31. Curtale F, Pokhrel RP, Tilden RL, Higashi G. 1995. Intestinal helminths and xerophthalmia in Nepal. A case-control study. *J. Trop. Ped.* 41:334–37

32. D'Angelo G, Angeletti C, Catassi C, Coppa GV. 1998. Probiotics in childhood. *Minerva Pediatr.* 50(5):163–73

33. Datta FU, Nolan JV Rowe JB, Gray GD, Crook BJ. 1999. Long-term effects of short-term provision of protein-enriched diets on resistance to nematode infection, and live-weight gain and wool growth in sheep. *Int. J. Parasitol.* 29:479–88

34. Daynes RA, Araneo BA, Dowell TA,

Huang K Dudley D. 1990. Regulation of murine lymphokine production in vivo. III. The lymphoid tissue microenvironment exerts regulatory influences over T helper cell function. *J. Exp. Med.* 171:979–96

35. Dehlawi MS, Wakelin D. 1988. Suppression of mucosal mastocytosis by *Nematospiroides dubius* results from an adult worm-mediated effect upon host lymphocytes. *Parasite Immunol.* 10:85–95

36. Duncombe VM, Bolin TD, Davis EA, Kelly JD. 1977. *Nippostrongylus brasiliensis* infection in the rat: effect of iron and protein deficiency and dexamethasone on the efficacy of benzimidazole anthelmintics. *Gut* 18:892–96

37. Duncombe VM, Bolin TD, Davis A, Kelly JD. 1979. The effect of iron and protein deficiency on the development of acquired resistance to reinfection with *Nippostrongylus brasiliensis* in rats. *Am. J. Clin. Nutr.* 32:553–58

38. El-Hag HMA, Macdonald DC, Fenwick P, Aggett PJ, Wakelin D. 1989. Kinetics of *Nippostrongylus brasiliensis* infection in the zinc-deficient rat. *J. Nutr.* 119:1506–12

39. Ernst PB, Song F, Klimpel GR, Haeberle H, Bamford KB, et al. 1999. Regulation of the mucosal immune response. *Am. J. Trop. Med. Hyg.* 60(Suppl.):2–9

40. Fenwick PK, Aggett PJ, Macdonald D, Huber C, Wakelin D. 1990. Zinc deficiency and zinc repletion: effect on the response of rats to infection with *Strongyloides ratti. Am. J. Clin. Nutr.* 52:173–77

41. Fenwick PK, Aggett PJ, Macdonald D, Huber C, Wakelin D. 1990. Zinc deficiency and zinc repletion: effect on the response of rats to infection with *Trichinella spiralis. Am. J. Clin. Nutr.* 52:166–72

42. Ferrick DA, Schrenzel MD, Mulvania T, Hsieh B, Ferlin WG, Lepper H. 1995. Differential production of interferon-$\gamma$ and interleukin-4 in response to Th1- and Th2-stimulating pathogens by $\gamma\delta$ T cells in vivo. *Nature* 373:255–57

43. Flo J, Massouh E. 1997. Age-related

changes of naive and memory CD4 rat lymphocyte subsets in mucosal and systemic lymphoid organs. *Dev. Comp. Immunol.* 21:443–53

44. Freij L, Meeuwisse GW, Berg NO, Wall S, Gebre-Medhin M. 1979. Ascariasis and malnutrition. A study in urban Ethiopian children. *Am. J. Clin. Nutr.* 32:1545–53

45. Gagnon CMA, Koski KG, Conly S, Scott ME, Stevenson MM. 1996. Dietary vitamin A deficiency alters Th2 cytokine profiles in mice infected with a gastrointestinal (GI) nematode. *FASEB J.* 9:A480

46. Gascan H, Aversa GG, Gauchat JF, Van Vlasselaer P, Roncarolo MG, et al. 1992. Membranes of activated CD4$^+$ T cells expressing T cell receptor (TcR) alpha beta or TcR gamma delta induce IgE synthesis by human B cells in the presence of interleukin-4. *Eur. J. Immunol.* 22:1133–41

47. Gbakima AA. 1993. The effect of dietary protein on *Trichinella spiralis* infection and inflammatory reactions in the tongue in CD1 mice. *Nutr. Res.* 13:787–800

48. Gopaldas T. 1996. More nutrients, fewer parasites, better learning. *World Hlth. Forum* 17:367–68

49. Grazioso CF, Isalgué M, de Ramírez I, Ruz M, Solomons NW. 1993. The effect of zinc supplementation on parasitic reinfestation of Guatemalan schoolchildren. *Am. J. Clin. Nutr.* 57:673–78

50. Grencis RK. 1996. T cell and cytokine basis of host variability in response to intestinal nematode infections. *Parasitology* 112(Suppl.):31–37

51. Gulland FMD. 1992. The role of nematode parasites in Soay sheep (*Ovis aries* L.) mortality during a population crash. *Parasitology* 105:493–503

52. Gupta MC, Arora KL, Mithal S, Tandon BN. 1977. Effect of periodic deworming on nutritional status of *Ascaris*-infested preschool children receiving supplementary food. *Lancet* 2(8029):108–10

53. Hadidjaja P, Bonang E, Suyardi MA, Abidin SAN, Ismid IS, Margono SS. 1998. The effect of intervention methods on nutritional status and cognitive function of primary school children infected with *Ascaris lumbricoides. Am. J. Trop. Med. Hyg.* 59:791–95

54. Hadju V, Abadi K, Stephenson LS, Noor NN, Mohammed HO, Bowman DD. 1995. Intestinal helminthiasis, nutritional status, and their relationship; a cross-sectional study in urban slum school children in Indonesia. *Southeast Asian J. Trop. Med. Public Health* 26:719–29

55. Hadju V, Stephenson LS, Abadi K, Mohammed HO, Bowman DD, Parker RS. 1996. Improvements in appetite and growth in helminth-infected schoolboys three and seven weeks after a single dose of pyrantel pamoate. *Parasitology* 113:497–504

56. Hammond JA, Fielding D, Bishop SC. 1997. Prospects for plant anthelmintics in tropical veterinary medicine. *Vet. Res. Commun.* 21:213–28

57. Hlaing T. 1993. Ascariasis and childhood malnutrition. *Parasitology* 107 (Suppl.):125–36

57a. Holland CV, Taren DL, Crompton DWT, Nesheim MC, Sanjur D, et al. 1988. Intestinal helminthiases in relation to the socioeconomic environment of Panamanian children. *Soc. Sci. Med.* 26(2):209–13

58. Hopkins RM, Gracey MS, Hobbs RP, Sargo RM, Yates M, Thompson RCA. 1997. The prevalence of hookworm infection, iron deficiency and anaemia in an Aboriginal community in north-west Australia. *Med. J. Aust.* 166(5):241–44

59. Huang KC, ed. 1999. *The Pharmacology of Chinese Herbs.* Boca Raton, FL: CRC. 512 pp. 2nd ed.

60. Huffman MA, Gotoh S, Turner LA, Hamai M, Yoshida K. 1997. Seasonal trends in intestinal nematode infection and medicinal plant use among chimpanzees in the Mahale mountains, Tanzania. *Primates* 38:111–25

61. Ing R, Su Z, Scott ME, Koski KG. 2000. Suppressed T helper 2 immunity and prolonged survival of a nematode parasite in protein-malnourished mice. *Proc. Natl. Acad. Sci. USA* 97(13):7078–83

62. Israf DA, Coop RL, Stevenson LM, Jones DG, Jackson F, et al. 1996. Dietary protein influences upon immunity to *Nematodirus battus* infection in lambs. *Vet. Parasitol.* 61:273–86

63. Jalal F, Nesheim MC, Agus Z, Sanjur D, Habicht JP. 1998. Serum retinol concentrations in children are affected by food sources of beta-carotene, fat intake, and anthelmintic drug treatment. *Am. J. Clin. Nutr.* 68(3):623–29

64. Jin SJ, Hwang WI, Ryu TG, Oh SH. 1981. Protein absorption of adult men with intestinal helminthic parasites. *Food Nutr. Bull.* 5(Suppl.):131–38

65. Joel DD, Chanana AD. 1985. Comparison of pulmonary and intestinal lymphocyte migrational patterns in sheep. *Ann. NY Acad. Sci.* 459:56–66

66. Kambara T, McFarlane RG, Abell TJ, McAnulty RW, Sykes AR. 1993. The effect of age and dietary protein on immunity and resistance in lambs vaccinated with *Trichostrongylus colubriformis*. *Int. J. Parasitol.* 23(4):471–76

67. Kasugai T, Tei H, Okada M, Hirota S, Morimoto M, et al. 1995. Infection with *Nippostrongylus brasiliensis* induces invasion of mast cell precursors from peripheral blood to small intestine. *Blood* 85:1334–40

68. Kaufmann SH. 1996. Gamma/delta and other unconventional T lymphocytes: What do they see and what do they do? *Proc. Natl. Acad. Sci. USA* 93:2272–79

69. Keith ME, Jeejeebhoy KN. 1997. Immunonutrition. *Baillieres Clin. Endocrinol. Metabol.* 11(4):709–38

70. Keusch GT. 1991. Nutritional effects on response of children in developing countries to respiratory tract pathogens: implications for vaccine development. *Rev. Infect. Dis.* 13(Suppl. 6):486–91

71. Keymer AE, Tarlton AB. 1991. The population dynamics of acquired immunity to *Heligmosomoides polygyrus* in the laboratory mouse: strain, diet and exposure. *Parasitology* 103:121–26

72. Kim JJ, Maguire HC Jr, Nottingham LK, Morrison LD, Tsai A, et al. 1998. Coadministration of IL-12 or IL-10 expression cassettes drives immune responses toward a Th1 phenotype. *J. Interferon Cytokine Res.* 18(7):537–47

73. King CL, Low CC, Nutman TB. 1993. IgE production in human helminth infection: reciprocal interrelationship between IL-4 and IFN-$\gamma$. *J. Immunol.* 150:1873–80

74. King CL, Nutman TB. 1993. IgE and IgG subclass regulation by IL-4 and IFN-$\gamma$ in human helminth infections: assessment by B cell precursor frequencies. *J. Immunol.* 151:458–65

75. King SJ, Miller HR. 1984. Anaphylactic release of mucosal mast cell protease and its relationship to gut permeability in *Nippostrongylus*-primed rats. *Immunology* 51:653–60

76. Knox MR. 1996. Integrated control programs using medicated blocks. In *Sustainable Parasite Control in Small Ruminants: An International Workshop*, ed. LeJambre LF, Knox MR, pp. 141–45. Canberra: Aust. Cent. Int. Agric. Res. (ACIAR)

77. Knox MR, Steel JW. 1999. The effects of urea supplementation on production and parasitological responses of sheep infected with *Haemonchus contortus* and *Trichostrongylus colubriformis*. *Vet. Parasitol.* 83:123–35

78. Koski KG, Su Z, Scott ME. 1999. Energy deficits suppress both systemic and gut immunity during infection. *Biochem. Biophys. Res. Commun.* 264:796–801

79. Kyriazakis I, Anderson DH, Oldham JD, Coop RL, Jackson F. 1996. Long-term subclinical infection with *Trichostrongylus colubriformis*: effects on food intake, diet selection and performance of growing lambs. *Vet. Parasitol.* 61:297–313

80. Kyriazakis I, Oldham JD, Coop RL, Jackson F. 1994. The effect of subclinical intestinal nematode infection on the diet selection of growing sheep. *Br. J. Nutr.* 72:665–77

81. Laissue JA, Chappuis BB, Muller C, Reubi JC, Gebbers JO. 1993. The intestinal immune system and its relation to disease. *Dig. Dis.* 11:298–312

82. Latham MC. 1990. Protein-energy malnutrition: its epidemiology and control. *J. Environ. Pathol. Toxicol. Oncol.* 10:168–80

83. Latham MC, Stephenson LS, Hall A, Wolgemuth JC, Elliot TC, Crompton DW. 1983. Parasitic infections, anaemia and nutritional status: a study of their interrelationships and the effect of prophylaxis and treatment on workers in Kwale District, Kenya. *Trans. R. Soc. Trop. Med. Hyg.* 77:41–48

84. Lawrence RA, Gray CA, Osborne J, Maizels RM. 1996. *Nippostrongylus brasiliensis*: cytokine responses and nematode expulsion in normal and IL-4-deficient mice. *Exp. Parasitol.* 84(1):65–73

85. Le Gros G, Schultze N, Walti S, Einsle K, Finkelman F, et al. 1996. The development of IgE$^+$ memory B cells following primary IgE immune responses. *Eur. J. Immunol.* 26(12):3042–47

86. Locksley RM. 1994. Th2 cells: help for helminths. *J. Exp. Med.* 179:1405–7

87. Lunn PG, Northrop CA, Wainwright M. 1988. Hypoalbuminemia in energy-malnourished rats infected with *Nippostrongylus brasiliensis* (Nematoda). *J. Nutr.* 118:121–27

88. Lunn PG, Northrop-Clewes CA. 1993. The impact of gastrointestinal parasites on protein-energy malnutrition in man. *Proc. Nutr. Soc.* 52:101–11

89. Marinho HA, Shrimpton R, Giugliano R, Burini RC. 1991. Influence of enteral parasites on the blood vitamin A levels in preschool children orally supplemented with retinol and/or zinc. *Eur. J. Clin. Nutr.* 45:539–44

90. Mata LJ, Kromal RA, Urrutia JJ, Garcia B. 1977. Effect of infection on food intake and the nutritional state: perspectives as viewed from the village. *Am. J. Clin. Nutr.* 30:1215–27

91. McGarvey ST, Aligui G, Graham KK, Peters P, Olds GR, et al. 1996. *Schistosomiasis japonica* and childhood nutritional status in northeastern Leyte, the Philippines: a randomized trial of praziquantel versus placebo. *Am. J. Trop. Med. Hyg.* 54:498–502

92. Michael E, Bundy DAP. 1991. The effect of the protein content of CBA/Ca mouse diet on the population dynamics of *Trichuris muris* (Nematoda) in primary infection. *Parasitology* 103:403–11

93. Michael E, Bundy DAP. 1992. Nutrition, immunity and helminth infection: effect of dietary protein on the dynamics of the primary antibody response to *Trichuris muris* (Nematoda) in CBA/Ca mice. *Parasite Immunol.* 14:169–83

94. Miller HR, Jarrett WF. 1971. Immune reactions in mucous membranes. I. Intestinal mast cell response during helminth expulsion in the rat. *Immunology* 20:277–88

95. Minkus TM, Koski KG, Scott ME. 1992. Marginal zinc deficiency has no effect on primary or challenge infections in mice with *Heligmosomoides polygyrus* (Nematoda). *J. Nutr.* 122:570–79

96. Mitchell GF. 1991. Co-evolution of parasites and adaptive immune responses. *Immunol. Today* 12:A2–5

97. Monroy FG, Enriquez FJ. 1992. *Heligmosomoides polygyrus*: a model for chronic gastrointestinal helminthiasis. *Parasitol. Today* 8:49–54

98. Mosmann TR, Sad S. 1996. The expanding universe of T-cell subsets: Th1, Th2 and more. *Immunol. Today* 17:138–46

99. Nakache M, Berg EL, Streeter PR, Butcher EC. 1989. The mucosal vascular addressin is a tissue-specific endothelial cell adhesion molecule for circulating lymphocytes. *Nature* 337:179–81

100. Neuman CG, Lawlor GJ, Stiehm ER, Swendseid ME, Newton C, et al. 1975. Immunologic responses in malnourished children. *Am. J. Clin. Nutr.* 28:89–104

101. Nfi A, Ndi C, Bayemi PH, Njwe R, Tchoumboue J, et al. 1999. The anthelmintic efficacy of some indigenous plants in the Northwest province of Cameroon. *Rev. Élev. Méd. Vét. Pays Trop.* 52:103–6

102. Olsen A, Magnussen P, Ouma JH, Andreassen J, Friis H. 1998. The contribution of hookworm and other parasitic infections to haemoglobin and iron status among children and adults in western Kenya. *Trans. R. Soc. Trop. Med. Hyg.* 92(6):643–49

103. Pearce FL, Befus AD, Gauldie J, Bienenstock J. 1982. Mucosal mast cells. II. Effects of anti-allergic compounds on histamine secretion by isolated intestinal mast cells. *J. Immunol.* 128:2481–86

104. Pelletier DL. 1994. The potentiating effects of malnutrition on child mortality: epidemiologic evidence and policy implications. *Nutr. Rev.* 52(12):409–15

105. Peng WD, Zhou XM, Crompton DW. 1998. Ascariasis in China. *Adv. Parasitol.* 41:109–48

106. Prichard RK, Kelly JD, Bolin TD, Duncombe VM, Fagan MR. 1981. The effect of iron and protein deficiency on plasma levels and parasite uptake of [$^{14}$C] fenbendazole in rats infected with *Nippostrongylus brasiliensis*. *Aust. J. Exp. Biol. Med. Sci.* 59:567–73

107. Pritchard DI, Hewitt C, Moqbel R. 1997. The relationship between immunological responsiveness controlled by T-helper 2 lymphocytes and infections with parasitic helminths. *Parasitology* 115(Suppl.):33–44

108. Rai Shiba K, Nakanishi M, Upadhyay MP, Hirai K, Ohno Y, et al. 2000. Effect of intestinal helminth infection on retinol and beta-carotene status among rural Nepalese. *Nutr. Res.* 20(1):15–23

109. Ramaswamy K, Goodman RE, Bell RG. 1994. Cytokine profile of protective anti-*Trichinella spiralis* CD4$^+$ OX22– and non-protective CD4$^+$ OX22$^+$ thoracic duct cells in rats: secretion of IL-4 alone does not determine protective capacity. *Parasite Immunol.* 16:435–45

110. Ramaswamy K, Hakimi J, Bell RG. 1994. Evidence for an interleukin 4-inducible immunoglobulin E uptake and transport mechanism in the intestine. *J. Exp. Med.* 180:1793–803

111. Ramaswamy K, Negrao-Correa D, Bell RG. 1996. Local intestinal immune responses to infections with *Trichinella spiralis*. Real-time, continuous assay of cytokines in the intestinal (afferent) and efferent thoracic duct lymph of rats. *J. Immunol* 156:4328–37

112. Raz E, Tighe H, Sato Y, Corr M, Dudler JA, et al. 1996. Preferential induction of a Th1 immune response and inhibition of specific IgE antibody formation by plasmid DNA immunization. *Proc. Natl. Acad. Sci. USA* 93(10):5141–45

113. Roberts JA, Adams DB. 1990. The effect of level of nutrition on the development of resistance to *Haemonchus contortus* in sheep. *Aust. Vet. J.* 67:89–91

114. Roberts K, Kilshaw PJ. 1993. The mucosal T cell integrin $\alpha$-M290-$\beta$-7 recognizes a ligand on mucosal epithelial cell lines. *Eur. J. Immunol.* 23:1630–35

115. Roos MH. 1997. The role of drugs in the control of parasitic nematode infections: must we do without? *Parasitology* 114(Suppl.):137–44

116. Rosenberg IH, Bowman BB. 1984. Impact of intestinal parasites on digestive function in humans. *Fed. Proc.* 43:246–50

117. Sanders AB, How SJ, Lloyd DH, Hill R. 1991. The effect of malnutrition on vaccination against *Dermatophilus congolensis* infection in ruminants. *J. Comp. Pathol.* 105(1):37–48

118. Deleted in proof

119. Sawaya AL, Amigo H, Sigulem D. 1990. The risk approach in preschool children suffering malnutrition and intestinal parasitic infection in the city of Sao Paulo, Brazil. *J. Trop. Ped.* 36(4):184–88

120. Schweighoffer T, Tanaka Y, Tidswell M, Erle DJ, Horgan KJ, et al. 1993. Selective expression of integrin $\alpha 4\beta 7$ on a subset of human CD4$^+$ memory T cells with hallmarks of gut-trophism. *J. Immunol.* 151:717–29

121. Scott ME, Koski KG. 2000. Zinc deficiency impairs immune responses against parasitic nematode infections at intestinal and systemic sites. *J. Nutr.* 130(Suppl.):1412–20

121a. Scott ME, Smith G, eds. 1994. *Parasitic and Infectious Diseases: Epidemiology and Ecology.* San Diego: Academic Press. 398 pp.

122. Scrimshaw NS, San Giovanni JP. 1997. Synergism of nutrition, infection and immunity: an overview. *Am. J. Clin. Nutr.* 66(Suppl.):464–77

123. Scrimshaw NS, Taylor CE, Gordon JE. 1968. *Interactions of Nutrition and Infection.* Geneva: World Health Organization

124. Shetty PS, Shetty N. 1993. Parasitic infection and chronic energy deficiency in adults. *Parasitology* 107(Suppl.):159–67

125. Shi HN, Koski KG, Stevenson MM, Scott ME. 1997. Zinc deficiency and energy restriction modify immune responses in mice during both primary and challenge infection with *Heligmosomoides polygyrus* (Nematoda). *Parasite Immunol.* 19:363–73

126. Shi HN, Scott ME, Koski KG, Boulay M, Stevenson MM. 1995. Energy restriction and severe zinc deficiency influence growth, survival and reproduction of *Heligmosomoides polygyrus* (Nematoda) during primary and challenge infections in mice. *Parasitology* 110:599–609

127. Shi HN, Scott ME, Stevenson MM, Koski KG. 1998. Energy restriction and zinc deficiency impair the functions of murine T cells and antigen-presenting cells during gastrointestinal nematode infection. *J. Nutr.* 128:20–27

128. Shimoda K, van Deursen J, Sangster MY, Sarawar SR, Carson RT, et al. 1996. Lack of IL-4–induced Th2 response and IgE class switching in mice with disrupted Stat6 gene. *Nature* 380:630–33

129. Slater AFG, Keymer AE. 1986. *Heligmosomoides polygyrus* (Nematoda): the influence of dietary protein on the dynamics of repeated infection. *Proc. R. Soc. London.* B229:69–83

130. Slater AFG, Keymer AE. 1988. The influence of protein deficiency on immunity to *Heligmosomoides polygyrus* (Nematoda) in mice. *Parasite Immunol.* 10:507–22

131. Smith TJ, Weis JH. 1996. Mucosal T cells and mast cells share common adhesion receptors. *Immunol. Today* 17:60–63

132. Solomons NW. 1993. Pathways to the impairment of human nutritional status by gastrointestinal pathogens. *Parasitology* 107(Suppl.):19–35

133. Solomons NW, Scott ME. 1994. Nutritional status of host populations influences parasitic infections. In *Parasitic and Infectious Diseases, Epidemiology and Ecology,* ed. ME Scott, G Smith, ch. 9, pp. 101–14. San Diego: Academic. 398 pp.

134. Stephenson LS, Crompton DWT, Latham MC, Nesheim MC, Schulpen TWJ. 1979. The effects of *Ascaris* infection on growth of malnourished preschool children. *East Afr. Med. J.* 56:142

135. Stephenson LS, Crompton DWT, Latham MC, Schulpen TWJ, Nesheim MC, Jansen AA. 1980. Relationships between *Ascaris* infection and growth of malnourished preschool children in Kenya. *Am. J. Clin. Nutr.* 33:1165–72

136. Stephenson LS, ed. 1987. *The Impact of*

*Helminth Infections on Human Nutrition.* London: Taylor Francis Ltd. 233 pp.

137. Stephenson LS, Latham MC, Adams EJ, Kinoti SN, Pertet A. 1993. Weight gain of Kenyan school children infected with hookworm, *Trichuris trichiura* and *Ascaris lumbricoides* is improved following once- or twice-yearly treatment with albendazole. *J. Nutr.* 123:656–65

138. Stephenson LS, Latham MC, Kurz KM, Kinoti SN, Brigham H. 1989. Treatment with a single dose of albendazole improves growth of Kenyan schoolchildren with hookworm, *Trichuris trichiura* and *Ascaris lumbricoides* infections. *Am. J. Trop. Med. Hyg.* 41:78–87

139. Stephenson LS, Latham MC, Kinoti SN, Kurz KM, Brigham H. 1990. Improvements in physical fitness of Kenyan schoolboys infected with hookworm, *Trichuris trichiura* and *Ascaris lumbricoides* following a single dose of albendazole. *Trans. R. Soc. Trop. Med. Hyg.* 84:277–82

140. Stoltzfus RJ, Albonico M, Chwaya HM, Savioli L, Tielsch J, et al. 1996. Hemoquant determination of hookworm-related blood loss and its role in iron deficiency in African children. *Am. J. Trop. Med. Hyg.* 55:399–404

141. Stoltzfus RJ, Chwaya HM, Tielsch JM, Schulze KJ, Albonico M, Savioli L. 1997. Epidemiology of iron deficiency anemia in Zanzibari schoolchildren: the importance of hookworms. *Am. J. Clin. Nutr.* 65(1):153–59

142. Sukhdeo MVK, Sukhdeo SC. 1994. Optimal habitat selection by helminths within the host environment. *Parasitology* 109(Suppl.):41–55

143. Svetic A, Madden KB, Zhou X, Lu P, Katona IM, et al. 1993. A primary intestinal helminthic infection rapidly induces a gut-associated elevation of Th2–associated cytokines and Il-3. *J. Immunol.* 150:3434–41

144. Taguchi T, McGhee JR, Coffman RL, Beagley KW, Eldridge JH et al. 1990. Analysis of Th1 and Th2 cells in murine gut-associated tissues. Frequencies of $CD4^+$ and $CD8^+$ T cells that secrete IFN-$\gamma$ and IL-5. *J. Immunol.* 145:68–77

145. Takeda K, Tanaka T, Shi W, Matsumoto M, Minami M, et al. 1996. Essential role of Stat6 in Il-4 signalling. *Nature* 380:627–30

146. Tanumihardjo SA, Permaesih D, Muherdiyantiningsih, Rustan E, Rusmil K, et al. 1996. Vitamin A status of Indonesian children infected with *Ascaris lumbricoides* after dosing with vitamin A supplements and albendazole. *J. Nutr.* 126:451–57

147. Taren DL, Nesheim MC, Crompton DW, Holland CV, Barbeau I, et al. 1987. Contributions of ascariasis to poor nutritional status in children from Chiriqui Province, Republic of Panama. *Parasitology* 95(3):603–13

148. Taren DL, Sanjur D, Rivera G, Crompton DWT, Nesheim M, et al. 1992. The nutritional status of Guaymi Indians living in Chiriqui province, Republic of Panama. *Archiv. Latinoam. Nutr.* 42(2):118–26

149. Thein-Hlaing, Thane-Toe, Than-Saw, Myat-Lay-Kyin, Myint-Lwin. 1991. A controlled chemotherapeutic intervention trial on the relationship between *Ascaris lumbricoides* infection and malnutrition in children. *Trans. R. Soc. Trop. Med. Hyg.* 85:523–28

150. The Partnership for Child Development. 2000. http://www.child-development.org

151. Tripathy K, Garcia FT, Lotero H. 1971. Effect of nutritional repletion on human hookworm infection. *Am J. Trop. Med. Hyg.* 20:219–23

152. Tshikuka J-G, Gray-Donald K, Scott M, Olea KN. 1997. Relationship of childhood protein-energy malnutrition and parasite infections in an urban African setting. *Trop. Med. Int. Hlth* 2:374–82

153. Uchikawa R, Yamada M, Matsuda S,

Kuroda A, Arizono N. 1994. IgE antibody production is associated with suppressed interferon-$\gamma$ levels in mesenteric lymph nodes of rats infected with the nematode *Nippostrongylus brasiliensis*. *Immunology* 82:427–32

154. Urban JF, Katona IM, Paul WE, Finkelman FD. 1991. Interleukin 4 is important in protective immunity to a gastrointestinal nematode infection in mice. *Proc. Natl. Acad. Sci USA* 88:5513–17

155. Urban JF, Madden KB, Svetic A, Cheever A, Trotta PP, et al. 1992. The importance of Th2 cytokines in protective immunity to nematodes. *Immunol. Rev.* 127:205–20

156. van Houtert MFJ, Barger IA, Steel JW. 1995. Dietary protein for young grazing sheep: interactions with gastrointestinal parasitism. *Vet. Parasitol.* 60:283–95

157. van Houtert MFJ, Sykes AR. 1996. Implications of nutrition for the ability of ruminants to withstand gastrointestinal nematode infections. *Int. J. Parasitol.* 26:1151–68

158. Villamor E, Fawzi WW. 2000. Vitamin A supplementation: implications for morbidity and mortality in children. *J. Infect. Dis.* 182(Suppl.):122–33

159. Wahid FN, Behnke JM, Grencis RK, Else KJ, Ben-Smith AW. 1994. Immunological relationships during primary infection with *Heligmosomoides polygyrus*: Th2 cytokines and primary response phenotype. *Parasitology* 108:461–71

160. Wakelin D. 1994. Host populations: genetics and immunity. In *Parasitic and Infectious Diseases, Epidemiology and Ecology*, ed. ME Scott, G Smith, ch. 8, pp. 83–100. San Diego: Academic. 398pp.

161. Wastling JM, Scudamore CL, Thornton EM, Newlands GF, Miller HR. 1997. Constitutive expression of mouse mast cell protease-1 in normal BALB/c mice and its up-regulation during intestinal nematode infection. *Immunology* 90:308–13

162. Wen L, Pao W, Wong FS, Peng Q, Craft J, et al. 1996. Germinal center formation, immunoglobulin class switching, and autoantibody production driven by "non-$\alpha\beta$" T cells. *J. Exp. Med.* 183:2271–82

163. Whitfield PJ. 1996. Novel anthelmintic compounds and molluscicides from medicinal plants. *Trans. R. Soc. Trop. Med. Hyg.* 90:596–600

164. WHO. 1999. *The World Health Report 1999: Making a Difference*. Geneva. 122 pp.

Annu. Rev. Nutr. 2001. 21:323–41

# SUCCESSFUL WEIGHT LOSS MAINTENANCE

## Rena R Wing[1] and James O Hill[2]

[1]The Miriam Hospital, Brown University, Providence, Rhode Island 02906, and
[2]Center for Human Nutrition, University of Colorado Health Sciences Center, Denver, Colorado 80262; e-mail: Rwing@Lifespan.org, James.Hill@uchsc.edu

**Key Words**   reduced-obese, obesity treatment, diet, exercise, obesity

■ **Abstract**   Obesity is now recognized as a serious chronic disease, but there is pessimism about how successful treatment can be. A general perception is that almost no one succeeds in long-term maintenance of weight loss. To define long-term weight loss success, we need an accepted definition. We propose defining successful long-term weight loss maintenance as intentionally losing at least 10% of initial body weight and keeping it off for at least 1 year. According to this definition, the picture is much more optimistic, with perhaps greater than 20% of overweight/obese persons able to achieve success. We found that in the National Weight Control Registry, successful long-term weight loss maintainers (average weight loss of 30 kg for an average of 5.5 years) share common behavioral strategies, including eating a diet low in fat, frequent self-monitoring of body weight and food intake, and high levels of regular physical activity. Weight loss maintenance may get easier over time. Once these successful maintainers have maintained a weight loss for 2–5 years, the chances of longer-term success greatly increase.

## CONTENTS

0199-9885/01/0715-0323$14.00                                                                    **323**

# INTRODUCTION

Obesity is a major health problem in the United States, with over 50% of Americans classified as overweight or obese. Many of these individuals are attempting to lose weight (39). However, the perception of the general public is that long-term reduction in body weight is difficult to achieve. The goal of this chapter is to summarize the information available on successful weight loss maintenance. How many achieve this goal? How do they do it? What are the consequences? In describing successful weight loss maintainers, we draw heavily on findings from the National Weight Control Registry (NWCR), a registry of individuals who have been extremely successful at long-term weight loss maintenance.

# PREVALENCE OF WEIGHT LOSS MAINTENANCE

Currently, few data are available on the prevalence of successful weight loss maintenance. One limit is the lack of a consistent criterion to define "success" and another is the difficulty of distinguishing intentional from unintentional weight loss. We therefore propose to define success in weight loss maintenance as achieving an intentional weight loss of at least 10% of initial body weight and maintaining this weight loss for at least one year. We could not find sufficient data, collected in a systematic fashion, to provide reliable information on predictors of weight loss for longer periods.

Overall there is a feeling of pessimism regarding long-term weight loss success (18). This pessimism started with a study by Stunkard & McLaren-Hume (42), who followed 100 obese individuals referred to a nutritional weight loss program and found that 2 years after treatment, only 2% maintained a weight loss of at least 20 lb. This finding was instrumental in creating the perception, perpetuated in the popular media, that hardly anyone succeeds in long-term maintenance of weight loss.

Recent studies of clinical programs are more positive. Every year for 4 years, Kramer et al (24) followed up on 114 men and 38 women who had participated in a behavioral weight loss program. Using a strict criterion of maintaining 100% of one's weight loss, they found that only 0.9% of men and 5.3% of women were consistently successful (i.e. maintaining this criterion all of the 4 years). However, looking only at year 4, cross-sectional data showed that 2.6% of men and 28.9% of women had maintained 100% of their weight loss. Several studies have used 5 kg or greater weight loss as a criterion of success. With this criterion, 13% (51) to 22% (41) of participants are successful 5 years after treatment.

These studies may underestimate the true prevalence of weight loss maintenance because they are based on only one episode of weight loss and may not be representative of the general population. Most people who lose weight do so on their own, without participation in formal programs (5, 6); thus, data from clinical research programs may reflect "hard core" dieters, who may be most resistant to successful weight loss maintenance. Bartlett et al (4) reviewed eight studies that examined the prevalence of successful weight loss in community samples; they were unable to reach conclusions regarding prevalence because these studies lacked consistent definitions of successful weight loss and many failed to use nationally representative samples. Moreover, most of the studies assessed weight loss, not weight loss maintenance.

McGuire et al (27) recently reported results of a random-digit-dial telephone survey in a nationally representative sample of 500 adults in the United States. Weight loss maintainers were defined as those who at the time of the survey had maintained a weight loss of $\geq 10\%$ of their maximum weight for at least 1 year. Of particular interest are those who reported being overweight [body mass index (BMI) $\geq 27$ kg/m$^2$] at their maximum weight ($N = 228$). Of these, 62% indicated that at some point in their life they had lost 10% of their maximum weight, and 38% reported that they were currently 10% below their maximum weight. Of the 228 reporting having been overweight, 69 (30.3%) had maintained this 10% weight loss for at least 1 year. These 69 individuals had on average maintained a weight loss of 42 lb for 7 years.

This survey included a question about whether the weight loss was intentional. Of the 228 overweight individuals in the survey, 47 (20.6%) reported that they had intentionally lost weight and had maintained a weight loss of 10% for at least 1 year. Of these individuals, 28 had reduced to normal weight (BMI < 27).

# HOW TO DEFINE SUCCESS IN WEIGHT LOSS MAINTENANCE?

It is important to adopt a consistent definition of successful weight loss maintenance. The definition must include criterion for magnitude of weight loss and duration of maintenance. Weight losses of 5%–10% of initial body weight can lead to substantial improvement in risk factors for diabetes and heart disease and can lead to reductions in or discontinuations of medications for these conditions (31). Thus, if the focus is on overall health, achieving and maintaining a 10% weight loss should be considered successful, even though for many obese individuals this weight loss may not return them to a nonobese state. Successful weight loss maintenance may involve some weight regain. For example, an individual who lost 20% of initial body weight but regained half of the lost weight would still be 10% below initial body weight, would presumably still have overall improved health, and thus should be considered "successful."

In defining successful weight loss, it is important that the loss be intentional. Several recent studies suggest that unintentional weight loss occurs frequently in the population. Because the causes and consequences of unintentional weight loss are likely to differ from those associated with intentional weight loss, it is important to distinguish between the two.

Finally, we propose that 1 year of maintenance be the minimum criterion, in keeping with the Institute of Medicine (IOM) definition. A 5-year duration might be a stricter criterion, but we believe research would be stimulated by first adopting the 1-year criterion and then studying the factors that help those individuals who have succeeded for 1 year sustain their success through 5 years.

Thus, we propose that individuals who have intentionally lost at least 10% of their body weight and have kept it off at least 1 year be considered "successful weight loss maintainers." By this definition, according to our data, 21% of overweight/obese persons may be successes.

## THE NATIONAL WEIGHT CONTROL REGISTRY

Much of the information about successful weight loss maintenance comes from the National Weight Control Registry (NWCR), founded in 1994 to study weight loss and weight maintenance strategies of successful weight loss maintainers. To be eligible for the NWCR, individuals must have maintained at least a 30-lb weight loss for at least 1 year. On recruitment, all subjects sign an informed consent form and then are sent several questionnaires to complete. These questionnaires seek information about weight loss and weight maintenance behaviors, as well as weight history, quality of life, and demographic information. All participants are asked to complete additional follow-up questionnaires on an annual basis.

There are currently over 3000 subjects in the NWCR. They average 45 years of age and are 80% women, 97% Caucasian, and 67% married. The average weight loss reported by NWCR participants is 30 kg, and the average duration of weight maintenance is 5.5 years. These subjects maintain a body weight that is, on average, 10 BMI units lower than their pre–weight loss BMI (from 35–25 kg/m$^2$).

About half (46%) of NWCR subjects report having been overweight as children. Many report a strong family history of obesity, with 46% reporting one parent as overweight or obese and 27% reporting both parents as overweight or obese.

Almost all NWCR subjects (90%) have experienced previous unsuccessful attempts at weight loss. No obvious factor or factors distinguish this successful weight loss from previous failures other than registry participants noting a greater commitment, stricter dieting, and a greater role of exercise.

Clearly, a negative energy balance is needed to produce weight loss. A negative energy balance can be achieved by either decreasing intake or increasing expenditure. Research studies consistently show that successful weight loss maintainers change both their intake and their expenditure in order to lose weight and maintain their losses. In the NWCR, 89% of participants reported modifying both diet and exercise to achieve their successful weight loss (22). In subjects who reported modifying food intake to lose weight, the most commonly reported methods were restricting intake of certain types or classes of foods (88%), limiting quantity

(44%), and counting calories (44%). However, there was marked variability in how they made these changes. About half of the registry participants (45%), but 63% of the men, reported losing on their own whereas the remainder of the registrants (55%), and 60% of the women, used a formal (e.g. commercial) weight loss program (22).

Although most health professionals recommend changes in both diet and physical activity for weight loss, many popular weight loss plans emphasize diet more than physical activity. It is worth noting that very few of these successful weight loss maintainers used diet alone to lose weight.

## STRATEGIES FOR MAINTENANCE OF WEIGHT LOSS

Although the approaches to weight loss differed widely among NWCR subjects, we found much more similarity in the strategies used for maintenance of weight loss. The three strategies that were common to a large proportion of NWCR participants include (a) eating a diet low in fat and high in carbohydrate, (b) frequent self-monitoring, and (c) regular physical activity.

### Diet

To determine current dietary intake, registry members were asked on entry into the registry to complete the Block Food Frequency questionnaire. On average, participants reported consuming 1381 kcal/day (5778 ± 2200 kJ/day), with 24% of calories from fat, 19% from protein, and 56% from carbohydrates (22). There were no differences in the quality of the diet reported by participants who lost weight on their own compared with those who used weight loss programs (40). Both groups ate a diet that satisfied the Daily Reference Intakes for calcium, vitamin C, vitamin A, and vitamin E.

Recently, because some popular diets recommend restricting carbohydrates to lose weight, data from registry participants were analyzed to determine carbohydrate intake (57). Only 7.6% of registry members reported eating fewer than 90 g of carbohydrate/day; for many of these individuals, total daily energy intake appeared unreasonably low. Additional analyses were done to determine the proportion of subjects eating diets with <24% carbohydrates (1500 calories/≤90 g of carbohydrate). Less than 1% of registry participants consumed such low-carbohydrate diets. Compared with registry members who had higher carbohydrate intake, those ingesting <24% carbohydrates maintained their weight loss for less time and were less physically active. Thus, the low-fat, high-carbohydrate, low-calorie–eating pattern appears to be what characterizes the majority of registry participants.

Registry members reported eating on average 4.87 meals or snacks/day, with few eating less often than twice a day (22). On average, they ate at fast food restaurants approximately once a week (0.74 times/week) and had 2.5 meals/week in other types of restaurants. Thus, although the majority of meals were eaten at home, these individuals maintained their weight loss while enjoying meals at restaurants.

As part of the random-digit-dialing survey described above, successful weight loss maintainers (those who intentionally lost ≥10% of their maximum weight and maintained it for at least 1 year) were compared with regainers (those who lost at least 10% of their body weight but gained it back) and controls (those whose weight had never been ≥10% above their current level and who were weight stable) (29). These individuals were all asked to complete the Food Habits Questionnaire. This questionnaire examines strategies used to restrict fat intake and has been shown to relate to fat intake. Weight loss maintainers reported greater avoidance of fried foods and more substitution of low-fat for high-fat foods than either regainers or controls. Again, these findings suggest the importance of low-fat eating in the maintenance of weight loss.

Other studies have shown that successful weight loss maintenance is associated with changes in both the quantity and quality of foods consumed. Clinic-based studies have examined the association between self-reported dietary intake and weight loss after either 12 or 18 months of treatment. These studies indicate that individuals who are most successful at weight loss maintenance report lower caloric intake (19), reduced portion sizes (17), reduced frequency of snacks, and, perhaps most consistently, reduction in the percentage of calories from fat (11, 55).

Several studies have identified decreased consumption of specific foods as being associated with weight loss maintenance. French et al (8) found that decreased consumption of french fries, dairy products, sweets, and meat was positively associated with weight loss maintenance. Holden et al (15) present data on 118 patients who were followed for 3 years after ending a very-low-calorie diet. Those who reported that they consumed cheese, butter, high-fat snacks, fried foods, and desserts less than once a week were more successful at long-term weight control. Eating "healthy" foods at least once/week was unrelated to weight loss.

## Self-Monitoring Weight and Behaviors Related to Weight

Registry members were asked how frequently they monitored their weight. Over 44% reported weighing themselves at least once a day, and 31% reported weighing themselves at least once a week (22). Few other studies have examined weighing as a component of long-term weight loss maintenance. However, monitoring dietary intake is frequently associated with weight loss success. Guare et al (10) completed a 1-year follow-up on 106 participants in behavioral weight loss programs. Those participants who at 1 year most frequently monitored their intake maintained a weight loss of 18 kg compared with the approximately 5-kg weight loss maintained by those who monitored their intake less often. Other studies have likewise found that consistent self-monitoring is related to weight loss (3). This is not surprising. Frequent monitoring of weight allows one to detect weight regain in its early stages and to initiate strategies to reverse the trend and avoid a major relapse.

Self-monitoring may be viewed as one component of the more general construct of cognitive restraint (i.e. the degree of conscious control one exerts over eating behaviors). On the Three Factor Eating Scale, registry members report high levels of dietary restraint (mean = 7.1), similar to the levels reported by patients who have recently completed treatment for obesity, though not nearly as high as the levels seen in eating-disordered patients (23). These data suggest that successful maintainers continue long-term to use behavior-change strategies taught in weight loss programs. However, why some individuals can persist in conscious control of intake whereas others revert back to old habits is unclear.

## Physical Activity

Regular physical activity has been found in many studies to be associated with long-term weight loss maintenance (20, 37). Most subjects in the NWCR report engaging in regular physical activity to lose weight as well as to maintain the weight loss. Only 9% of registry subjects report maintaining weight loss without regular physical activity. Using the Paffenbarger Physical Activity Questionnaire (33), we determined current levels of physical activity. Women in the registry report expending an average of 2545 kcal on physical activity per week and men report an average of 3293 kcal/week. This amount of physical activity is comparable to about 1 h of moderate intensity physical activity, such as brisk walking, per day. This is much higher than physical activity recommendations for the general public. The Surgeon General recommends that adults engage in 30 min of moderate intensity physical activity at least 3 days/week (46). Among registry subjects, 52% expend more than 1000 kcal and 72% more than 2000 kcal on physical activity per week.

Physical activity experts now recommend that rather than only planned exercise, people increase "lifestyle physical activity," which involves being more active in daily life (e.g. increase walking, taking stairs, etc) (46). Most registry subjects report efforts to increase both lifestyle activity and regular planned exercise. As noted above, only 9% report that they do no physical activity for weight loss maintenance. Among registry members, 49% report using a combination of walking and another form of regular exercise, 28% report only walking, and 14% report only another form of regular exercise. Thus, the combination of lifestyle and programmed exercise is used by almost half the participants, and walking is an important aspect of the exercise for over 75%.

Table 1 shows the six most frequently reported physical activities of subjects in the registry (45). It is interesting that a high proportion of subjects report weight lifting. In the registry, 24% of men and 20% of women regularly engage in weight lifting. A representative national population, the National Health Interview Survey, conducted in 1991, reported that 20% of men but only 9% of women regularly engage in weight lifting. Thus, women in the registry engage in weight lifting to a much greater extent than do women in the general population. The extent to which this contributes to their success in weight loss maintenance is not clear.

**TABLE 1**   The six most common activities reported by
National Weight Control Registry subjects

| Activity | % Reporting engaging in activity |
| --- | --- |
| Walking | 76.6 |
| Cycling | 20.6 |
| Weight lifting | 20.3 |
| Aerobics | 17.8 |
| Running | 10.5 |
| Stair climbing | 9.3 |

# METABOLIC AND BEHAVIORAL FACTORS IN WEIGHT LOSS MAINTENANCE

It is not clear to what extent metabolic versus behavioral factors contribute to the low success rate in long-term weight loss maintenance. It could be that there is a physiological set-point for weight and that reducing weight below this level leads to physiological compensation. Alternatively, the difficulty in maintaining a weight loss could be due to the difficulty in making permanent changes in diet and physical activity behaviors.

## The Metabolic State of the Reduced-Obese

The difficulty in long-term weight maintenance could have metabolic causes. It is possible that weight loss creates a metabolic state favoring weight regain in order to return body weight to some optimal or regulated level. This metabolic state could be due to one or more of the following causes: (*a*) a resting metabolic rate lower than expected for the new, lower body weight; (*b*) a reduced ability to oxidize fat, thus favoring positive fat balance and fat gain; (*c*) increased insulin sensitivity; and/or (*d*) relatively low leptin levels.

*Low Resting Metabolic Rate in the Reduced-Obese State*    Resting metabolic rate (RMR) declines with weight loss, but the question is whether this decline leaves the reduced-obese with an inappropriately low RMR or whether the decline in RMR is appropriate for the new, lower body mass. During the acute phase of weight loss, RMR appears to decline because of both food restriction and loss of body mass (35, 50). This is why is it important to measure RMR after a period of weight stabilization following weight loss. In the long-term, the decline in RMR would be expected to be proportional to the decline in fat-free mass (FFM) because fat loss produces only very small declines in RMR (35).

Some reports indicate that RMR declines with weight loss to a much greater extent than the decline in FFM, whereas other reports indicate that the decline in RMR with weight loss is appropriate for the reduction of FFM. In favor of a greater-than-expected drop in RMR with weight loss, Leibel et al (26) reported a reduction in resting metabolic rate of 12.6–16.7 kJ/kg of FFM lost in obese subjects maintaining a 10% reduction in body weight. Others (9, 38, 50) have found that the reduction in RMR with weight loss, over the long-term, is appropriate for the reduction in body mass. Astrup et al (2) recently published a meta-analysis of RMR in reduced-obese subjects. They reviewed 12 published studies and obtained individual data on 124 reduced-obese subjects and 121 control subjects from 15 different published studies. Using traditional meta-analysis, they found that RMR was about 5% lower in reduced-obese subjects than in control subjects. However, the more interesting analysis was a comparison of the 124 reduced-obese with the 121 control subjects. In this comparison, RMR was not significantly lower in the reduced-obese ($P < 0.09$). Furthermore, the 3%–5% reduction in RMR seen in the reduced-obese group was explained entirely by 15% of the reduced-obese subjects. They suggested that although a low RMR might characterize some reduced-obese subjects, this is not the norm.

We examined RMR in relation to FFM in 50 NWCR subjects and in 50 matched control subjects (56). In both groups, RMR was appropriate for body composition and there was no evidence of a lower-than-expected RMR in NWCR subjects. The regression line relating FFM and RMR was not different for the two groups, which suggests that RMR in our reduced-obese subjects was not inappropriately low.

It is possible that the extremely high levels of physical activity seen in NWCR subjects may be masking a low RMR. Van Dale et al (48) found that subjects who engaged in regular exercise during and following weight loss had a "normal" RMR relative to body mass, whereas those who did not exercise had a lower-than-predicted RMR relative to body mass. It should be noted, however, that in our study (56), the matched control subjects were reporting high levels of physical activity, similar to those reported by NWCR subjects.

The controversy in this area continues. In NWCR subjects, we failed to find any evidence of a greater "metabolic efficiency" or a "metabolic impairment." Although increased metabolic efficiency might occur in some subjects, it does not seem to be an obligatory consequence of weight loss. It is possible that some of the differences between studies may reflect heterogeneity between reduced-obese subjects. It is also likely that other methodological issues contribute to different results. We know little, for example, about how the method of weight reduction (large versus small deficit, exercise versus no exercise), the amount of weight loss, or the duration of weight loss maintenance affect the metabolic state of the reduced-obese individual. Part of the problem has been getting access to enough long-term successes to study how these factors impact metabolism after weight loss.

***Fat Oxidation in the Reduced-Obese State***    Because achieving body weight maintenance requires achieving fat balance, an alteration in the ability to use fat as a fuel could be a factor in predisposing reduced-obese subjects to regain weight. Given that it is affected by many dietary factors and by physical activity, assessment of substrate oxidation is not easy. Several investigators have reported that reduced-obese subjects may have a higher respiratory quotient (RQ), indicative of a lower rate of fat oxidation, than do control subjects. Larson et al (25) reported a higher adjusted 24-h RQ in formerly obese subjects than in matched control subjects who had not lost weight. Astrup et al (1) found lower rates of fat oxidation in formerly obese subjects compared with controls while both groups were consuming high-fat diets.

In the NWCR we found registry members had a slightly higher (0.807 versus 0.791, $P = 0.05$) fasting RQ than a control group of nonreduced individuals (56). However, the usual diet NWCR subjects reported consuming was lower in fat than that of the control subjects. Because usual fat oxidation is positively correlated with usual fat intake, it is not clear whether the lower fat oxidation seen in NWCR subjects reflects an altered metabolic state or simply an altered diet.

Thus, although there are consistent reports of a higher RQ (i.e. lower fat oxidation) in reduced-obese subjects, the question remains as to whether this indicates an impairment in or a reduced capacity for fat oxidation. It remains a distinct possibility, however, that a low rate of fat oxidation in reduced-obese subjects could predispose them to weight gain, especially when they consume high-fat diets.

***Insulin Resistance as a Contributor to Weight Regain***    The role of insulin resistance in weight gain is also controversial. Several studies have shown that within a population, those who are most insulin sensitive at baseline will gain the most weight (13, 43, 47), although this finding is not consistent across all populations (14). Similarly, there are inconsistent findings related to whether insulin sensitivity predicts weight regain. Yost et al (59) reported that in 10 moderately obese women, changes in insulin sensitivity (determined using a euglycemic clamp) following a 3-month period of weight loss and a 3-month period of weight maintenance were positively correlated with subsequent weight gain at 12 and 18 months. The authors hypothesized that the increased insulin sensitivity produced a decrease in skeletal muscle lipid oxidation, directing lipid toward storage in adipose tissue. In contrast, Wing (53) examined this relationship in two groups of subjects who participated in a 3- to 6-month weight loss program. In 125 nondiabetic subjects, changes in neither fasting insulin nor insulin levels in response to a glucose load were significantly related to subsequent weight regain. Similarly, insulin sensitivity measured using Bergman's minimal model was not related to subsequent weight regain in 33 diabetic subjects. The inconsistency across studies may relate to differences in study population, methods of assessing insulin sensitivity, and/or duration of the weight maintenance phase. Furthermore, all the studies reported changes in body weight (rather than fat mass), and none reported changes in physical activity levels, an important determinant of insulin sensitivity. Thus, whether insulin sensitivity plays a role in weight regain following a period of weight loss remains to be determined. Studies of rats provided with an obesity-producing diet have not, in general, found insulin sensitivity to predict weight gain (34). Currently we have no data on insulin sensitivity among NWCR subjects.

*Low Leptin as a Factor in Weight Regain*   It has recently been suggested that low leptin levels may exist in reduced-obese subjects and may be a factor in propensity to regain weight (7). In this study, leptin levels were positively correlated with body fat mass in a group of eight reduced-obese and eight control subjects. However, leptin levels were lower in the reduced-obese subjects. Reduced-obese subjects also had a lower rate of fat oxidation than did the control subjects. Nagy et al (30), however, found the leptin levels were not related to weight regain over a 4-year period in 14 postmenopausal women. Furthermore, Wing et al (55) reported that leptin levels decreased along with body weight during obesity treatment and that neither baseline levels nor changes in serum leptin predicted weight regain. Leptin levels drop with weight loss, and the initial drop may be greater than the drop in fat mass (36). The important question for weight loss maintenance is whether the relationship between circulating leptin levels and body fat mass is altered significantly from baseline after weight loss and weight stabilization. It is important to point out that the question can only be answered if a period of weight stabilization precedes measurements. We are currently collecting data on circulating leptin levels in NWCR subjects.

## The Metabolic State of NWCR Subjects

In summary, we have not been able to document a clear metabolic state consistent with the notion of increased "metabolic efficiency" in reduced-obese subjects. It is certainly possible that the high levels of physical activity seen in NWCR subjects may be "masking" this metabolic predisposition to regain weight. Alternatively, it is possible that NWCR subjects do not exhibit such a metabolic predisposition and that their success is due to permanent behavior changes of the kind generally recommended in weight loss programs.

## Behavioral Factors in Long-Term Weight Loss Maintenance

Although we have not clearly identified metabolic factors important for long-term weight loss maintenance, we have identified behavioral factors that seem to predict success. These include eating a diet low in fat, self-monitoring body weight and food intake, and engaging in high levels of physical activity. We believe that the current population recommendations to reduce dietary fat are consistent with success in weight loss maintenance. Our subjects report 24% of total energy from fat, and many recommendations to the public are to reduce dietary fat below 30%. It is possible that a recommendation of 25% of energy from fat would be a better recommendation for persons maintaining a weight loss, but insufficient data exist to support such a public health recommendation. Our data would, however, argue strongly against any increases in the amount of dietary fat recommended to the public.

Self-monitoring has been recognized as a useful behavior during weight loss, and data obtained from the NWCR suggests that this is a useful behavior to continue during weight maintenance.

Finally, high levels of physical activity seem to be associated with long-term weight maintenance. Although the exact way in which physical activity helps with successful weight loss maintenance is not fully understood, it does seem that a high degree of regular physical activity is a key to the success of the subjects in the registry. Data from the NWCR suggest that the optimal amount of physical activity to maintain weight loss may be about 1 h/day, or an expenditure of approximately 2500–3000 kcal/week. Others have reported results similar to these. Schoeller et al (37) found that the relationship between the amount of physical activity and the prevention of weight regain was not linear. They found that a threshold value of 11 kcal/kg of body weight was necessary to prevent weight regain. This value roughly translates into the addition of 1.3 h of such moderate activity as brisk walking per day, or 0.6 h of vigorous activity per day. More recently, Jakicic et al (16) found that after weight loss, 200 min or more of physical activity per week was associated with continued weight maintenance, whereas less physical activity was associated with weight gain in a dose-dependent fashion.

Taken together, this body of literature in obese-reduced subjects suggests that our physical activity goals for weight management programs may need to be substantially higher than the physical activity recommendations to the general population. It is important to realize that the current physical activity guidelines for the population were developed to optimize cardiovascular health and were not based on prevention of weight gain. Although we have substantial data to suggest that regular physical activity protects against weight gain in nonobese individuals (12), we do not have a good database on which to develop specific physical activity guidelines to prevent weight gain. Developing such a database should be a high priority.

## PSYCHOLOGICAL CONSEQUENCES OF SUCCESSFUL WEIGHT LOSS MAINTENANCE

Concern has been raised that weight loss, and the vigilance required to maintain weight loss long-term, may be associated with increased risk of eating disorders or depression symptomatology. This concern stems in large part from the study by Keys et al (21) of semistarvation in normal-weight young men. In their study, weight losses of approximately 25% of initial weight were achieved in these normal-weight individuals. Such weight losses were associated with extreme negative psychological reactions and, in a subgroup, short periods of binge eating. The important question is whether the more-modest weight losses (10% of body weight) that typically occur in overweight persons produce such negative effects. This literature was recently reviewed by the National Task Force on the Prevention and Treatment of Obesity (32). They concluded that participants in behavioral weight loss programs typically experience improvements in symptoms of depression or anxiety with weight loss, regardless of whether the weight loss is produced by moderate diets, very-low-calorie diets, or weight loss medications.

Before weight loss programs, participants typically report levels of dysphoria in the nondepressed range; these levels are further reduced with weight loss. Binge eaters, who enter treatment with higher levels of depressive symptomatology, experience greater improvements with weight loss. Likewise, both binge eaters and nonbinge eaters who participate in weight loss programs that utilize a balanced diet with moderate caloric restriction experience reduction in binge eating episodes. Rather than precipitating binge eating (a common concern), such programs appear to ameliorate this problem. Three studies (44, 49, 58) have evaluated the effect of very-low-calorie diets and subsequent refeeding on binge eating. In two of the three (49, 58), there was no adverse effect of the very-low-calorie diet on binge eating, but the third study did suggest a temporary increase in binge eating in those who were nonbingers at baseline (44). Methodological issues related to the assessment of binge eating in this study make it difficult to interpret the results.

Likewise, no adverse psychological effects of weight loss have been observed in the NWCR (23). At entry into the registry, members are asked to complete the Center for Epidemiologic Studies Depression Scale (CES-D), the Symptom-Checklist-90-R, and selected questions from the Eating Disorders Examination related to binge eating and purging. Scores on these assessments were compared with findings in the literature for relevant comparison groups (including those with psychiatric disorders, obese patients, nondieting control subjects, and random samples of the US population).

Registry participants reported an average CES-D score of 9.2 (range 0–52); 18% of registry participants scored >16, the cutoff used to distinguish "cases" for nondepressed individuals. These findings are similar to nondepressed community control subjects (who have mean CES-D scores of 4.1–10.4, with 21% of individuals reporting scores >16). In contrast, studies of clinically depressed patients have mean scores of 13–38 on the CES-D, with over 70% of individuals scoring >16. Registry participants also appear similar to obese and nonobese community samples on the Global Symptoms Index of the SCL-90-R.

Rates of binge eating and vomiting were also very low in registry members; 8% reported four or more binges/month, and only 1.8% reported any episodes in the preceding month of vomiting for weight loss purposes. These results are strikingly lower than what is observed in eating-disordered populations.

In addition, participants in the registry are asked to indicate whether weight loss has resulted in improvement, worsening, or no change in various aspects of their life (22). As shown in Table 2, the vast majority of individuals report positive changes in all aspects. Over 90% of the sample reported improvement in their overall quality of life, level of energy, mobility, general mood, and self-confidence.

There are only two areas where any substantial worsening due to weight loss was noted. Fourteen percent of registry members reported worsening in time spent thinking about food (49% reported improvement in this regard) and 20% reported worsening in time spent thinking about their weight (51% reported improvement in this regard). Thus overall weight loss maintenance appears to produce marked improvements in quality of life for the majority of individuals.

**TABLE 2**    Effect of weight loss on other areas of life[a]

| Determinant | Improved | No difference | Worse |
|---|---|---|---|
| Quality of life | 95.3 | 4.3 | 0.4 |
| Level of energy | 92.4 | 6.7 | 0.9 |
| Mobility | 92.3 | 7.1 | 0.6 |
| General mood | 91.4 | 6.9 | 1.6 |
| Self-confidence | 90.9 | 9.0 | 0.1 |
| Physical health | 85.8 | 12.9 | 1.3 |
| Interactions with | | | |
|    opposite sex | 65.2 | 32.9 | 0.9 |
|    same sex | 50.2 | 46.8 | 0.4 |
|    strangers | 69.5 | 30.4 | 0.1 |
| Time spent interacting with | | | |
|    others | 59.1 | 39.6 | 1.3 |
| Job performance | 54.5 | 45.0 | 0.6 |
| Other hobbies | 49.1 | 36.7 | 0.4 |
| Interactions with | | | |
|    parents | 32.8 | 65.0 | 2.2 |
| Interactions with | | | |
|    spouse | 56.3 | 37.3 | 5.9 |
| Time spent thinking about | | | |
|    food | 49.1 | 36.7 | 14.2 |
|    weight | 51.0 | 28.6 | 20.4 |

[a]$N = 784$. Results indicate percentage.

## FACTORS ASSOCIATED WITH WEIGHT REGAIN

Registry members are followed over time to try to identify variables related to continued success (28). Over 1 year of follow-up, 35% of registry participants regained 5 lbs or more, 59% maintained their weight loss, and 6% lost additional weight. Baseline characteristics that increased the risk of regain included more recent weight loss (fewer than 2 years versus more than 2 years), larger weight losses (>30% of maximum weight versus <30%), and higher levels of depression, disinhibition, and binge eating at entry into the registry. These findings are of interest, particularly the duration effect. It appears that the first few years after weight loss are the most vulnerable period for weight regain. Maintaining ones weight loss for 2–5 years decreased the risk of subsequent regain by 50%. Thus, individuals who succeed in maintaining their weight loss for more than 2 years have a markedly improved chance of continuing to maintain it long-term.

Regainers were also characterized by several key behavior changes that occurred over the year of follow-up and distinguished them from maintainers. Gainers increased their fat intake, whereas maintainers kept theirs consistent. Both groups reported decreases in physical activity, but the regainers had greater decreases: expending approximately 800 fewer kcal/week compared with 400 kcal/week in the maintainers. Gainers also reported decreases in their level of dietary restraint and increases in disinhibition (i.e. loss of control while eating). These findings confirm the importance of the behavior changes described in earlier sections of this chapter for the long-term maintenance of weight loss.

## SUMMARY

It is important that a consensus be reached on a definition for successful weight loss maintenance. Our recommendation is that an intentional weight loss of greater than or equal to 10% of initial body weight that is maintained at least 1 year be considered success. According to this definition, approximately 20% or more of individuals who attempt weight loss would be "successful." Although the NWCR does not provide information about how many people achieve long-term weight loss success, it does provide information about strategies used to achieve and maintain a weight loss. With regard to weight loss, the most obvious conclusion from the NWCR is that weight loss should include both changing diet and increasing physical activity. We do not, however, see any particular type of diet modification to achieve the weight loss that is common to these successful weight loss maintainers.

We believe that strategies for weight loss maintenance may be the key to long-term weight management success. We find three behaviors in a vast majority of NWCR subjects. First, these subjects engage in high levels of physical activity. The amount of physical activity that facilitates successful weight loss maintenance may be closer to 1 h/day rather than the 30 min three times per week suggested in recommendations to the general public. Consequently, we may need to increase our physical activity goals in obesity treatment programs. Second, these subjects report eating a diet low in fat and high in carbohydrate. We believe this is important information given the oscillating nature of popular diet books regarding optimum macronutrient composition for weight loss. Third, these subjects report regular self-monitoring of weight. Maintaining a substantial weight loss may be a long-term challenge, and it may be important to have access to information about success. This may be particularly important in terms of initiating early strategies to stop weight regain. Currently, the data seem to suggest that differences in behavior are stronger predictors of weight regain than the differences in physiology or metabolism. Further research with frequent assessments of behavior and metabolic parameters may be helpful in determining which set of factors is most strongly related to long-term maintenance of weight loss.

Part of the reasons for developing the NWCR was to counter the belief that "no one succeeds long-term at weight loss." We believe the subjects in the NWCR show that you can achieve and maintain substantial amounts of weight loss. Furthermore, we have found that these subjects live "normal" lives after weight loss and consistently report that life is better after weight loss. Our subjects tell us that their success requires substantial effort but that it is worth it. Finally, our data suggest that over time, it does get easier to maintain weight loss. It may be a lifelong struggle, but once you have maintained a weight loss for 2–5 years, the chances of longer-term success greatly increase.

## ACKNOWLEDGMENTS

We express our gratitude to Drs. Mary Lou Klem, Maureen McGuire, Holly Wyatt, and Helen Seagle for assistance in these studies. The work described here was supported in part by NIH grants DK42529 (JOH), DK48520 (JOH), and HL41330 (RRW).

**Visit the Annual Reviews home page at www.AnnualReviews.org**

## LITERATURE CITED

1. Astrup A, Buemann B, Christensen NJ, Toubro S. 1994. Failure to increase lipid oxidation in response to increasing dietary fat content in formerly obese women. *Am. J. Physiol.* 266:E592–99

2. Astrup A, Gotzsch PC, van de Werken K, Ranneries C, Toubro S, et al. 1999. Meta-analysis of resting metabolic rate in formerly obese subjects. *Am. J. Clin. Nutr.* 69:1117–22

3. Baker RC, Kirschenbaum DS. 1993. Self-monitoring may be necessary for successful weight control. *Behav. Ther.* 24:377–94

4. Bartlett SJ, Faith MS, Fontaine KR, Cheskin LJ, Allison DB. 1999. Is the prevalence of successful weight loss and maintenance higher in the general community than the research clinic? *Obes. Res.* 7:407–13

5. Brownell KD. 1993. Whether obesity should be treated. *Health Psychol.* 12:339–41

6. Brownell KD, Rodin J. 1994. Medical, metabolic, and psychological effects of weight cycling. *Arch. Int. Med.* 154:1325–30

7. Filozof CM, Murua C, Sanchez MP, Brailovsky C, Perman M, et al. 2000. Low plasma leptin concentrations and low rate of fat oxidation in weight-stable post-obese subjects. *Obes. Res.* 8:205–10

8. French SA, Jeffery RW, Forster JL, McGovern PG, Kelder SH, Baxter J. 1994. Predictors of weight change over two years among a population of working adults: The Healthy Worker Project. *Int. J. Obes.* 18:145–54

9. Goran MI, Shewchuk R, Gower BA, Nagy TR, Carpenter WH, Johnson RK. 1998. Longitudinal changes in fatness in white children: no effect of childhood energy expenditure. *Am. J. Clin. Nutr.* 67:309–16

10. Guare JC, Wing RR, Marcus MD, Epstein LH, Burton LR, Gooding WE. 1989. Analysis of changes in eating behavior and weight loss in type II diabetic patients. *Diabetes Care* 12:500–3

11. Harris JK, French SA, Jeffery RW, McGovern PG, Wing RR. 1994. Dietary and physical activity correlates of long-term weight loss. *Obes. Res.* 2:307–13

12. Hill JO, Melanson E. 1995. Overview of the determinants of overweight and obesity: current evidence and research issues. *Med. Sci. Sports Exerc.* 31:S515–21

13. Hoag S, Marshall JA, Jones RH, Hamman RF. 1995. High fasting insulin levels associated with lower rates of weight gain in persons with normal glucose tolerance: the San Luis Valley Diabetes Study. *Int. J. Obes.* 19:175–80

14. Hodge AM, Dowse GK, Alberti KG, Tuomilehto J, Gareeboo H, Zimmet PZ. 1996. Relationship of insulin resistance to weight gain in nondiabetic Asian Indian, Creole, and Chinese Mauritians. Mauritius Non-Communicable Disease Study Group. *Metabolism* 45:627–33

15. Holden JH, Darga LL, Olson SM, Stettner DC, Ardito EA, Lucas CP. 1992. Long-term follow-up of patients attending a combination very-low calorie diet and behaviour therapy weight loss programme. *Int. J. Obes.* 16:605–13

16. Jakicic JM, Winters C, Lang W, Wing RR. 1999. Effects of intermittent exercise and use of home exercise equipment on adherence, weight loss, and fitness in overweight women: a randomized trial. *JAMA* 282:1554–60

17. Jeffery RW, Bjornson-Benson WM, Rosenthal BS, Kurth CL, Dunn MM. 1984. Effectiveness of monetary contracts with two repayment schedules on weight reduction in men and women from self-referred and population samples. *Prev. Med.* 15:273–79

18. Kassirer J, Angell M. 1998. Losing weight: an ill-fated New Year's resolution. *N. Engl. J. Med.* 338:52

19. Katahn M, Pleas J, Thackery M, Wallston KA. 1982. Relationship of eating and activity self-reports to follow-up weight maintenance in the massively obese. *Behav. Ther.* 13:521–28

20. Kayman S, Bruvold W, Stern JS. 1990. Maintenance and relapse after weight loss in women: behavioral aspects. *Am. J. Clin. Nutr.* 52:800–7

21. Keys A, Brozek J, Henschel A, Mickelsen O, Taylor HL. 1950. *The Biology of Human Starvation.* Minneapolis: Univ. Minn. Press

22. Klem ML, Wing RR, McGuire MT, Seagle HM, Hill JO. 1997. A descriptive study of individuals successful at long-term maintenance of substantial weight loss. *Am. J. Clin. Nutr.* 66:239–46

23. Klem ML, Wing RR, McGuire MT, Seagle HM, Hill JO. 1998. Psychological symptoms in individuals successful at long-term maintenance of weight loss. *Health Psychol.* 17:336–45

24. Kramer FM, Jeffery RW, Forster JL, Snell MK. 1989. Long-term follow-up of behavioral treatment for obesity: patterns of weight regain among men and women. *Int. J. Obes.* 13:123–36

25. Larson DE, Ferraro RT, Robertson DS, Ravussin E. 1995. Energy metabolism in weight-stable postobese individuals. *Am. J. Clin. Nutr.* 62:735–39

26. Leibel RL, Rosenbaum M, Hirsch J. 1995. Changes in energy expenditure resulting from altered body weight. *N. Engl. J. Med.* 332:621–28

27. McGuire M, Wing R, Hill J. 1999. The prevalence of weight loss maintenance among American adults. *Int. J. Obes.* 23:1314–19

28. McGuire MT, Wing RR, Klem ML, Lang W, Hill JO. 1999. What predicts weight regain among a group of successful weight losers? *J. Consult. Clin. Psychol.* 67:177–85

29. McGuire MT, Wing RR, Klem ML, Hill JO. 1999. Behavioral strategies of individuals who have maintained long-term weight losses. *Obes. Res.* 7:334–41

30. Nagy TR, Davies SL, Hunter GR, Darnell B, Weinsier RL. 1998. Serum leptin concentrations and weight gain in postobese postmenopausal women. *Obes. Res.* 6:257–61

31. Natl. Inst. Health, Natl. Heart Lung Blood Inst. 1998. Clinical guidelines on the identification, evaluation and treatment of overweight and obesity in adults—the evidence report. *Obes. Res.* 6:51–209S

32. Natl. Taskforce Prev. Treat. Obes. 2000. Dieting and the development of eating disorders in overweight and obese adults. *Arch. Int. Med.* 160:2581–89

33. Paffenbarger RS Jr, Wing AL, Hyde RT. 1978. Physical activity as an index of heart attack risk in college alumni. *Am. J. Epidemiol.* 108:161–75

34. Pagliassotti MJ, Gayles EC, Hill JO. 1997. Dietary fat and energy balance. *Ann. NY Acad. Sci.* 827:431–48

35. Ravusssin E, Lillioja S, Anderson TE, Christin L, Bogardus C. 1986. Determinants of 24-hour energy expenditure in man: methods and results using a respiratory chamber. *J. Clin. Invest.* 78:1568–78

36. Rosenbaum M, Nicolson M, Hirsch J, Murphy E, Chu F, Leibel R. 1997. Effects of weight change on plasma leptin concentrations and energy expenditure. *J. Clin. Endocrinol. Metab.* 82:3647–54

37. Schoeller DA, Shay K, Kushner RF. 1997. How much physical activity is needed to minimize weight gain in previously obese women? *Am. J. Clin. Nutr.* 66:551–56

38. Seidell JC, Muller DC, Sorkin JD, Andres R. 1992. Fasting respiratory exchange ratio and resting metabolic rate as predictors of weight gain: the Baltimore Longitudinal Study on Aging. *Int. J. Obes.* 16:667–74

39. Serdula MK, Mokdad AH, Williamson DF, Galuska DA, Mendlein JM, Heath GW. 1999. Prevalence of attempting weight loss and strategies for controlling weight. *JAMA* 282:1353–58

40. Shick SM, Wing RR, Klem ML, McGuire MT, Hill JO, Seagle HM. 1998. Persons successful at long-term weight loss and maintenance continue to consume a low-energy, low-fat diet. *J. Am. Diet. Assoc.* 98:408–13

41. Stalonas PM, Kirschenbaum DS. 1985. Behavioral treatment for obesity: eating habits revisited. *Behav. Ther.* 16:1–14

42. Stunkard AJ, McLaren-Hume M. 1959. The results of treatment for obesity. *Arch. Int. Med.* 103:79–85

43. Swinburn BA, Nyomba BL, Saad MF, Zurlo F, Raz I, et al. 1991. Insulin resistance associated with lower rates of weight gain in Pima Indians. *J. Clin. Invest.* 88:168–73

44. Telch CF, Agras WS. 1993. The effects of a very low calorie diet on binge eating. *Behav. Ther.* 24:177–93

45. Thompson HR, Bear SL, Seagle HM, Klem ML, McGuire MT, et al. 1997. Exercise behaviors in reduced-obese subjects in the National Weight Control Registry. *Obes. Res.* 5:84S (Abstr.)

46. US Dep. Health Hum. Serv. 1996. *Physical Activity and Health: A Report of the Surgeon General.* Atlanta, GA: US Dep. Health Hum. Serv., Cent. Dis. Control Prev., Natl. Cent. Chronic Dis. Prev. Promot.

47. Valdez R, Mitchell BD, Haffner SM, Hazuda HP, Morales PA, et al. 1994. Predictors of weight change in a bi-ethnic population. The San Antonio Heart Study. *Int. J. Obes.* 18:85–91

48. Van Dale D, Saris WHM, Ten Hoor F. 1990. Weight maintenance and restring metabolic rate 18–40 months after a diet-exercise treatment. *Int. J. Obes.* 14:347–59

49. Wadden TA, Foster GD, Letizia KA. 1994. One-year behavioral treatment of obesity: comparison of moderate and severe caloric restriction and the effects of weight maintenance therapy. *J. Consult. Clin. Psychol.* 62:165–71

50. Wadden TA, Foster GD, Letizia KA, Mullen JL. 1990. Long-term effects of dieting on resting metabolic rate in obese outpatients. *JAMA* 264:707–11

51. Wadden TA, Sternberg JA, Letizia KA, Stunkard AJ, Foster GD. 1989. Treatment of obesity by very low calorie diet, behaviour therapy, and their combination: a five-year perspective. *Int. J. Obes.* 13:39–46

52. Weinsier RL, Nelson KM, Hensrud DD, Darnell BE, Hunter GR, Schutz Y. 1995 Metabolic predictors of obesity. Contribution of resting energy expenditure, thermic effect of food, and fuel utilization to four-year weight gain of post-obese and never-obese women. *J. Clin. Invest.* 95:980–85

53. Wing RR. 1997. Insulin sensitivity as a predictor of weight regain. *Obes. Res.* 5:24–29

54. Wing RR, Epstein LH. 1981. Prescribed level of caloric restriction in behavioral weight loss programs. *Addict. Behav.* 6:139–44

55. Wing RR, Sinha M, Considine R, Lang W, Caro J. 1996. Relationship between weight loss maintenance and changes in serum leptin levels. *Horm. Metab. Res.* 28:698–703

56. Wyatt HR, Grunwald GK, Seagle HM, Klem ML, McGuire MT, et al. 1999. Resting energy expenditure in reduced-obese subjects in the National Weight Control Registry. *Am. J. Clin. Nutr.* 69:1189–93

57. Wyatt HR, Seagle HM, Grunwald GK, Bell ML, Klem ML, et al. 2000. Long-term weight and very low carbohydrate diets in the National Weight Control Registry. *Obes. Res.* 8:87S (Abstr.)

58. Yanovski SZ, Gormally JF, Leser MS, Gwirtsman HE, Yanovski JA. 1994. Binge eating disorder affects outcome of comprehensive very-low-calorie diet treatment. *Obes. Res.* 2:205–12

59. Yost TJ, Jensen DR, Eckel RH. 1995. Weight regain following sustained weight reduction is predicted by relative insulin sensitivity. *Obes. Res.* 3:583–87

Annu. Rev. Nutr. 2001. 21:343–79

# NUTRITIONAL MANAGEMENT OF MAINTENANCE DIALYSIS PATIENTS: Why Aren't We Doing Better?

Rajnish Mehrotra[1] and Joel D Kopple[2]

[1,2]*Division of Nephrology and Hypertension, Harbor-UCLA Medical Center and Research and Education Institute, Torrance, California 90509, UCLA School of Medicine and [2]UCLA School of Public Health, University of California, Los Angeles, California 90024; e-mail: rmehrotra@rei.edu, jkopple@rei.edu*

**Key Words**  protein-energy malnutrition, anorexia, chronic renal failure, comorbidity, inflammation

■ **Abstract**  About 40% of patients undergoing maintenance dialysis suffer from varying degrees of protein-energy malnutrition. This is a problem of substantial importance because many measures of nutritional status correlate with the risk of morbidity and mortality. There are many causes of protein-energy malnutrition in maintenance dialysis patients. Evidence indicates that nutritional decline begins even when the reduction in glomerular filtration rate is modest, and it is likely that the observed decrease in dietary protein and energy intake plays an important role. The nutrient intake of patients receiving maintenance dialysis also is often inadequate, and several lines of evidence suggest that toxins that accumulate with renal failure suppress appetite and contribute to nutritional decline once patients are on maintenance dialysis. Recent epidemiologic studies have suggested that both increased serum levels of leptin and inflammation may reduce nutrient intake and contribute to the development of protein-energy malnutrition. It is likely that associated illnesses, which are highly prevalent, contribute to malnutrition in maintenance dialysis patients. Recent data from the United States Renal Data System registry suggest that in the United States, the mortality rate of dialysis patients is improving. However, it remains high. We offer suggestions for predialysis and dialysis care of these patients that can result in improvement in their nutritional status. Whether this improvement will result in a decrease in patient morbidity and mortality is unknown.

## CONTENTS

## INTRODUCTION

In the United States, over the past decade the number of patients undergoing maintenance dialysis (MD) has increased progressively (231). The vast majority of these patients are treated by in-center maintenance hemodialysis (MHD), while about 15% receive chronic peritoneal dialysis (CPD). Even though there has been a progressive decline in the annual mortality rate of these patients, it remains inordinately high: The adjusted first-year mortality rate for MD patients who commenced dialysis in 1997 was 18.4 per 100 patient years (231). The high prevalence of protein-energy malnutrition (PEM) and its association with poor patient outcome was recognized almost two decades ago and has been reaffirmed in numerous studies since then. Although PEM is most widely recognized and studied, it should be pointed out that many MD patients may have deficiencies of vitamins and minerals, and malnutrition of these nutrients may have adverse clinical ramifications as well. In this review, we focus on some of the key factors that contribute to PEM in MD patients and suggest some reasons why we are not doing better at preventing or treating this disorder.

## Prevalence of Protein-Energy Malnutrition in Maintenance Dialysis Patients

Numerous surveys of MD patients in the United States and elsewhere have demonstrated a high prevalence of PEM. The estimates of prevalence vary, but the average is about 40% (4, 35, 76a, 91, 128, 139, 163, 174, 177, 185, 190, 237, 246). The majority of these patients have mild to moderate malnutrition, with about 6%–8% having severe malnutrition. At first glance, it may appear that the prevalence rates of various measures of PEM have remained unchanged over the past two decades. However, the patients on dialysis today are, on average, older and sicker (e.g. from diabetes mellitus, vascular disease) than they were even 5 years ago (231), which may explain the finding that the prevalence of PEM remains high.

## Relationship Between Malnutrition and Patient Morbidity and Mortality

In MHD patients, nutritional parameters that have been independently correlated with increased mortality and morbidity include low visceral protein concentrations (e.g. low predialysis serum albumin) (7, 34, 38, 39, 57, 88, 90, 117, 128, 132, 172,

227), reduced muscle protein mass (indicated by low predialysis serum creatinine concentrations) (7, 30, 39, 128), decreased nutrient intake (low urea nitrogen appearance rates—i.e. net urea generation, an indicator of dietary protein intake) (1, 43, 178), low predialysis serum cholesterol concentrations (7, 43, 57, 128), and low total body nitrogen (5, 185). Furthermore, in direct contrast to findings in the general population, body size is inversely correlated with patient outcome in MHD patients (43, 48, 113, 117, 240). Similarly, in CPD patients, low serum albumin levels (6, 7, 20, 28, 42, 74, 140, 192, 208, 220), reduced urea nitrogen appearances (52, 143, 220), decreased edema-free/fat-free mass (33, 143), low serum creatinine (6, 7) and creatinine appearance rates (182), poorer overall protein and energy nutritional status as assessed by subjective global assessment (33, 143), or decreased total body nitrogen content (52, 185) also are associated with high morbidity and mortality. Hence, understanding the mechanisms that lead to malnutrition and how they contribute to the excess morbidity and mortality are critical for improving the outcomes for these patients.

# ETIOLOGY OF PROTEIN-ENERGY MALNUTRITION IN MAINTENANCE DIALYSIS PATIENTS

MD patients constitute a highly heterogeneous group of individuals, and the etiology of PEM in these patients is likely to be multifactorial. The proposed causes are summarized in Table 1. It is likely that in a given patient, varying combinations of these causes result in PEM, and the relative contributions of some or all of these factors vary widely between patients. A detailed analysis of each of these etiologies is beyond the scope of this discussion, and a brief overview of the key factors is presented in the following sections before discussion of the key question: Why are we not doing better?

# FACTORS LIMITING IMPROVEMENT IN NUTRITIONAL STATUS

## Nutrition in the Predialysis Phase of Chronic Renal Failure

Evidence of nutritional decline begins long before patients with progressive chronic renal failure (CRF) develop end-stage renal disease. Several single- and multicenter studies from various parts of the world have demonstrated the presence of PEM in a significant proportion of patients with decreased renal function (i.e. predialysis patients) or in those who have just commenced MD therapy (28, 153, 176, 210, 218, 242). Between 1995 and 1997, over 60% of all incident MD patients in the United States were classified as hypoalbuminemic (168). During the screening (baseline) phase of the Modification of Diet in Renal Disease (MDRD) Study, a cross-sectional assessment of 1785 clinically stable patients

**TABLE 1**    Causes of protein-energy malnutrition in patients
with end-stage renal disease

---

Low nutrient intake
    Inadequate solute clearances
    Impaired gastric emptying
    Increased leptin levels
    Comorbidity
    Intraperitoneal instillation of dialysate

Comorbidity

Inflammation

Endocrine disorders of uremia
    Resistance to insulin
    Resistance to insulin-like growth factor-1 and growth hormone
    Hyperparathyroidism
    Hyperglucagonemia

Nutrient losses during dialysis

Blood loss
    Occult gastrointestinal bleeding
    Venipuncture
    Sequestration in hemodialyzer

Metabolic acidosis

---

with moderate to advanced CRF [mean $\pm$ standard deviation glomerular filtration rate (GFR): 39.8 $\pm$ 21.1 ml/min/1.73 m$^2$] demonstrated a high prevalence of measures of nutritional decline (153). It must be pointed out that the vast majority of patients studied were not malnourished. Of the patients, 11%–16% had a dietary protein intake (DPI) of <0.75 g/kg/day, 10% had a body weight <90% of standard, 19% had a serum albumin of <3.8 g/dl, 30% had a serum transferrin level of <250 mg/dl, and 9% had a serum cholesterol of <160 mg/dl; the mean of these and other nutritional parameters declined as the GFR decreased (153). Moreover, there was a direct association between various anthropometric and serum markers of nutritional status with GFR in this and one other study (84, 153). Because the MDRD Study screened only clinically stable patients, it is likely that the magnitude of undernutrition among patients with moderate to advanced CRF is significantly higher than was determined during the baseline phase for this study. These findings are of particular importance because nutritional parameters at the time of initiation of dialysis are strong predictors of subsequent patient outcome (12, 33, 34, 90, 143, 192, 227), and the predictive value persists for at least 5 years (117).

    The causes for this nutritional decline is probably multifactorial; the decrease in protein and energy intake plays a particularly important role. Several cross-sectional studies have demonstrated a progressive decline in DPI with decreasing

GFR (110, 148, 153, 186); this observation has been confirmed in longitudinal studies as well (84, 197). The mean dietary energy intake in the baseline phase of the MDRD Study was ~29 kcal/kg/day, a value substantially lower than that recommended for healthy adults (216) and for those with CRF (161); these abnormally low energy intakes were evident even for patients with a GFR > 50 ml/min/1.73 m$^2$ (153). Because DPI and various nutritional markers covary with GFR and energy intakes are abnormally low even at modest declines in GFR, it has been postulated that low nutrient intake contributes to the nutritional decline observed during the predialysis phase. Until recently, this hypothesis remained untested. In a recent analysis of the baseline phase of the MDRD study, the association of GFR with several of the anthropometric and biochemical and nutritional parameters was either attenuated or eliminated after controlling for protein and energy intakes (153). These epidemiological studies suggest that a low nutrient intake may indeed contribute to the nutritional decline in CRF patients. Because the reduction in dietary energy intake—as opposed to the apparent energy needs—is greater than the inadequacy of dietary protein intake, it is likely that inadequate energy intake is the more important contributor to the development of PEM in these patients. Indeed, in short-term studies in nondialyzed CRF patients, an increase in energy intake resulted in an improvement in various nutritional parameters (111).

Thus, there is strong evidence that the nutritional decline begins early in CRF, and a key strategy for preventing PEM or improving the nutritional status of patients as they approach MD therapy requires intervention regarding nutritional intake long before they present for dialysis. However, almost one third of CRF patients in the United States are referred to a nephrologist <1 month prior to commencing MD and almost one half have never seen a dietitian (228). Only about one third of all incident patients starting MD have seen a dietitian on two or more occasions (228). Hence, the vast majority of the incident MD patients receive suboptimal nutritional care prior to initiation of dialysis. The causes for this problem are beyond the scope of this discussion, but this remains a serious problem that requires attention.

## Low Nutrient Intake in Maintenance Dialysis Patients

The relationships between nutritional status and dietary nutrient intake in MD has largely been studied using measurements of dietary protein intake (DPI) derived from urea kinetic modeling. In clinically stable MD patients, the rate of urea nitrogen appearance (UNA) in the dialysate and urine is assumed to closely reflect the DPI and is called the protein equivalent of nitrogen appearance (PNA). Whereas in MHD patients the PNA is derived from sophisticated computer modeling, in CPD patients the PNA is estimated by direct measurement of urea nitrogen in dialysate and urine. This PNA, in grams per day, may then be normalized to a standardized body weight (nPNA), which, in turn, is derived from equations based on age, gender, actual body weight, and height. However, it has been argued that this normalization may be misleading because malnourished patients with reduced edema-free/fat-free masses may appear to have an adequate or high protein intake even though the intake is low in relation to their requirements (67). This may be the principal reason why several investigators have been unable to demonstrate any relationship between nPNA and various measures of nutritional status (65, 99, 244) or patient outcome (21). In two recent studies, normalizing PNA to a desirable body weight or to an edema-free/fat-free mass yielded significant correlations with measures of nutritional status whereas normalizing to actual body weight did not (105, 188), leading some investigators to suggest that PNA should be normalized to edema-free/fat-free mass (29). Thus, data indicate that low nutrient intake is a major determinant of the nutritional status of MD patients, and a critical assessment of the method for normalizing PNA is necessary before concluding otherwise. Convenient, reliable, and inexpensive methods for assessing the energy intake in a large number of MD patients would also be of great value for examining this matter.

## Protein and Energy Requirements in Maintenance Dialysis Patients

The ideal study design to determine the protein and energy requirements for MD patients would be to conduct a prospective, controlled trial using patients who are randomized to receive different levels of energy and protein intake and to study the impact on nutritional status, morbidity, and mortality. However, it is unlikely that such a trial will be conducted in the near future in the United States, and hence, we are obliged to depend on such surrogate measures as metabolic balance studies to determine the requirements. The rigorous methodology used in these studies permits an accurate estimation of protein and energy requirements, and therefore, they usually involve small numbers of patients studied at clinical research centers. It is unclear what denominator should be used to normalize the energy and protein requirements of these patients. Rather than current body weight, it has been suggested that standard body weight, based upon patient age, gender, height, and frame size, derived from the Second National Health and Nutrition Evaluation Survey should be used to calculate the dietary requirements. The body composition of MD patients, particularly those receiving CPD, is significantly different than in healthy adults, and some investigators have suggested that desirable body weight should be computed from edema-free/fat-free body mass, which in turn could be determined from dialysate and urine creatinine appearance (232). Even though these arguments have merit, we should await outcome-based studies before making any fundamental changes to our approach in dealing with this issue.

*Energy Requirements for Maintenance Hemodialysis Patients*    To maintain neutral energy balance, energy intake should equal energy expenditure. Several studies have demonstrated that the energy expenditure in MHD patients is identical to that of healthy adults under a variety of conditions (Table 2) (155, 201, 217); only one study demonstrated a higher resting energy expenditure by 7.3% (86). The effect of hemodialysis (HD) procedures remains uncertain because the two

**TABLE 2**    Energy requirements of maintenance hemodialysis patients

| Energy Expenditure | Requirement (reference) |
| --- | --- |
| Lying | Normal (155, 201, 217); 7.3% increase (86) |
| Sitting | Normal (155) |
| Postprandial | Normal (155) |
| Exercise | Normal (155) |
| Hemodialysis | Same as resting (170); 20% greater than resting (86) |

| Nutrition Parameter[a] | Energy Intake[a] (kcal/kg of desirable body weight) |
| --- | --- |
| Body weight (kg) | 32.4 |
| Nitrogen balance (g/day) | 31.1 |
| Nitrogen balance minus unmeasured losses (g/day) | 38.5 |
| Midarm circumference (cm) | 34.1 |
| Midarm muscle area (cm$^2$) | 33 |
| Body fat (%) | 32 |

[a]From Reference 206.

studies that addressed this issue came to conflicting conclusions (86, 170). In the study by Ikizler et al, which demonstrated a 20% increase in energy expenditure during HD (86), patients had eaten shortly before the onset of the dialysis procedure. This increase in energy expenditure may actually reflect the specific dynamic action of food.

Studies of nitrogen balances and a variety of anthropometric parameters have been used to determine the energy intake necessary to maintain a stable nutritional status in MHD patients consuming an average of 1.13 g of protein/kg/day (Table 2) (206). These analyses suggest such that such an energy intake should be between 31.1–38.5 kcal/kg/day (Table 2).

Based upon these studies, the National Kidney Foundation-Kidney Dialysis Outcome Quality Initiative (NKF-KDOQI) suggests a dietary energy intake of 35 kcal/kg/day for MHD patients younger than 65 years of age and an intake between 30–35 kcal/kg/day for patients older than 65 years of age (161). There are no studies available to determine energy requirements in elderly MHD patients.

***Energy Requirements for Chronic Peritoneal Dialysis Patients***    Energy intake of patients on peritoneal dialysis (PD) represents a sum of dietary intake and absorption of glucose from the dialysate. At least three published studies have addressed the issue of energy requirements in CPD patients (15, 70, 232). The resting energy expenditure of CPD patients is similar to that of healthy, normal adults (70). Metabolic balance studies of patients on chronic ambulatory peritoneal dialysis (CAPD) eating their usual diets showed a strong correlation between total energy intake and nitrogen balance, irrespective of the duration for which the patients were on dialysis (15). Based upon these studies, the NKF-KDOQI suggests a dietary energy intake of 35 kcal/kg/day for CPD patients younger than 65 years of age and an intake between 30–35 kcal/kg/day for patients older than 65 years of age (161). In a recent study, Uribarri et al demonstrated stable total body weight, edema-free/fat-free mass, and anthropometric parameters in 49 CPD patients on a total energy intake of ~29 kcal/kg/day and a DPI of ~1 g/kg/day over a 6-month period (232). However, the CPD patients were relatively obese for their height, and when adjusted for the patients' overweight condition, energy intake rose to recommended levels.

***Protein Requirements for Maintenance Hemodialysis Patients***   Most healthy adults and nondialyzed patients with CRF are able to maintain neutral nitrogen balance while eating a diet containing about 0.60 g of protein/kg/day as long as adequate energy is provided and most of the proteins are of high biological value. However, the dietary protein requirements of MHD patients are increased above these values by an amount that is greater than can be accounted for by the obligatory amino acid and protein losses. To our knowledge, there are six published studies that have evaluated nitrogen balance in MHD patients (Table 3) (25, 54, 112, 121, 189, 206). In addition, several observational studies demonstrated a relationship between DPI and morbidity and mortality (1, 43, 66, 178) that others were unable to reproduce (158, 159). Based upon currently available data, the NKF-KDOQI on nutrition in CRF (161) suggests that a DPI of 1.2 g/kg/day is necessary to ensure neutral or positive nitrogen balance in most clinically stable MHD patients; at least 50% of the DPI should be of high biological value.

***Protein Requirements for Chronic Peritoneal Dialysis Patients***   To our knowledge, three nitrogen balance studies have been conducted using CPD patients (Table 4) (15, 23, 56). These studies indicate that a DPI of 1.2 g/kg/day or greater is almost always associated with neutral or positive nitrogen balance. Moreover, several studies have shown a relationship between DPI, as determined by the normalized protein equivalent of total nitrogen appearance, the serum albumin and total body protein balance (15, 23, 56), and mortality (28). Based on currently available data, the NKF-KDOQI recommended a DPI of 1.2–1.3 g/kg/day for clinically stable CPD patients (161). There are no studies available for patients receiving automated peritoneal dialysis (APD). However, there is no reason to believe that their requirements will be materially different from those undergoing CAPD. Hence, the recommendations should be applicable to patients undergoing APD as well.

**TABLE 3**  Dietary protein requirements, as determined by nitrogen balance, in maintenance hemodialysis patients[a]

| Author (reference) | No. | Age Range | Diabetics | Study Duration (days) | Dialysis Regimen (times/week) | Energy Intake (kcal/kg/day) | Protein Intake (g/kg/day) | Mean N-Balance (g/day) |
|---|---|---|---|---|---|---|---|---|
| Ginn et al (54) | 4 | 17–22 | None | 7–32 | 2 | 50–55 | 0.4–1.48 HBV<br><br>0.14–0.95 LBV | Neutral/+ at ≥0.75 g/kg HBV protein<br>Negative at 0.95 LBV protein |
| Kopple et al (112) | 3 | | None | 21–28 | 2 | 35–45 | 0.75 (0.63 HBV)<br>1.25 (0.88 HBV) | Neutral<br>Neutral |
| Borah et al (25) | 5 | 35–65 | None | 7 | 3 | 20.5–30.9 | 0.5 (37% HBV)<br>1.4 (77% HBV) | −1.98<br>+0.95 |
| Lim et al (121)[b] | 6 | 20–59 | None | 9 | 3 | 29.5 ± 1.5 | 0.87 ± 0.06 | 0.37 ± 1.0 |
| Slomowitz et al (206) | 6 | 24–64 | None | 21–23 | 3 | 37.3 ± 2.1 | 1.13 ± 0.2 | 0.57 ± 0.42 (0/+ 4/6) (neutral/positive in 4 of 6 patients) |
| Rao et al (189)[c] | 15 | 18–55 | None | 7 | 3 | 33 ± 6.5<br>32.8 ± 6.7 | 0.61 ± 0.1<br>1.06 ± 0.18 | 0.17<br>4.03 |

[a]N-balance was not adjusted for unmeasured losses through the skin, hair, and nail growth, sweat, and flatus.  HBV, high biological value; LBV, low biological value.

[b]Energy intake was not constant from patient to patient.

[c]All nitrogen output was estimated and not measured directly.

**TABLE 4**   Dietary protein requirements, as determined by nitrogen balance, in chronic peritoneal dialysis patients[a]

| Author | No. | Age Range | Diabetics | Study Duration (days) | Dialysis Regimen | Protein Intake (g/kg/day) | Total Energy Intake (kcal/kg/day) | N-Balance (g/day) |
|---|---|---|---|---|---|---|---|---|
| Giordano et al (56) | 8 | 25–73 | None | 14 | CAPD | 1.2 | 39.6–44.9 | 0/+ in 7/8 |
| Blumenkrantz et al (23) | 8 | 27–59 | None | 14–33 | CAPD | 0.98 ± 0.03<br>1.44 ± 0.02 | 41.3 ± 1.9<br>42.1 ± 1.2 | +0.35 ± 0.83<br>+2.94 ± 0.54 |
| Bergstrom et al (15) | 12 | 27–62 | None | 6–11 | CAPD | 0.76–2.09 | 28–50 | +correlation with DPI |
|  | 9 | 27–62 | None | 6–11 | CAPD | 0.64–1.69 | 25–51 | No correlation with DPI |

[a]CAPD, Chronic ambulatory peritoneal dialysis; DPI, dietary protein intake.

## Spontaneous Protein and Energy Intake in Maintenance Dialysis Patients

Some of the studies that have examined the spontaneous dietary energy and protein intake in MD patients are summarized in Table 5. As is evident, the mean intakes of both energy and protein in MD patients are substantially lower than their reported nutritional needs; the decrement in the energy intake is greater than the decrement in protein intake. There is evidence that energy intake is more important than protein intake in determining the nutritional status of MD patients. An insufficient energy intake, even in the face of adequate protein intake, can result in a negative nitrogen balance in CRF patients (111, 198, 206). In the nitrogen balance studies by Bergstrom et al using CPD patients (15), dietary energy intake correlated significantly with nitrogen balance in all studies, whereas the DPI correlated with nitrogen balance only among patients who had recently started dialysis. Finally, in studies by Pollock et al, using both MHD and CPD patients, total body protein as measured by neutron activation analysis correlated with estimated energy intake rather than protein intake (185).

## Causes of Anorexia in Maintenance Dialysis Patients

There are probably several causes for anorexia in MD patients. In this section, we present an overview of some of the key factors suspected to play a role. More recently, the potential contribution of inflammation to PEM in MD patients has been investigated; the potential role of comorbidity in inducing anorexia is discussed below, as is the role of inflammation in suppressing appetite.

***Inadequate Solute Clearances***   Anorexia is a cardinal uremic manifestation in patients with progressive CRF that tends to improve over several days or weeks after initiation of MD. Based upon these observations, it has been proposed that uremic toxins exist that accumulate during the progressive decline of renal function and that they are removed, to varying degrees, by dialysis. This hypothesis was initially tested in cross-sectional studies: The dose of dialysis was expressed

**TABLE 5**  Spontaneous dietary protein and energy intake in maintenance dialysis patients[a]

| Author (reference) | Dietary Energy Intake | Dietary and Peritoneal Energy Intake | Dietary Protein Intake |
|---|---|---|---|
| MHD | | | |
| Blumenkrantz et al (22) | 29 | | 1.01 |
| Schonfeld et al (202) | 23.6 | | 0.95 |
| Wolfson et al (241) | 26.4 | | 1 |
| Stewart et al (214) | 24.9 | | 1.02 |
| Lorenzo et al (126) | 26.8 | | 1.02 |
| HEMO Study (221) | 22.8 | | 0.94 |
| CAPD | | | |
| Baeyer et al (8) | 23 | 30 | 0.83 |
| Heide et al (73) | | 29–33 | 1.0–1.4 |
| Guarnieri et al (62) | 23.9 | | 1.03 |
| Schilling et al (199) | 24 | | 0.98 |
| Pollock et al (184) | 24 | | 0.98 |

[a]MHD, Maintenance hemodialysis; CAPD, chronic automated peritoneal dialysis.

as Kt/V, an index of urea removal, and nPNA, an index of DPI derived from UNA appearance. These analyses demonstrated a significant relationship between measures of small solute removal (Kt/V) and DPI (nPNA) in both MHD and CPD patients (14, 15, 58, 124, 130, 167). This led to the assumption that there are small-molecular-weight uremic toxins that are responsible for anorexia in CRF patients. It was soon pointed out that part of this relationship was secondary to mathematical coupling (68, 226), as both indices are derived from the terms utilized to calculate the rate of UNA and are normalized to the volume of distribution of urea. However, several investigators have demonstrated a relationship between the dose of urea removal and DPI, calculated from dietary records and interviews (15, 68), and hence, this relationship may be statistically significant, even when the dose of urea and creatinine removal is not normalized to body size (15, 167).

Three lines of evidence suggest that an increase in solute clearances will lead to an increase in DPI. First, initiation of dialysis in uremic CRF patients usually results in an increase in DPI; this effect has been demonstrated for both MHD (146, 179, 186) and CPD patients (143, 186). Second, several longitudinal studies over the past few years lend support to the notion that an increase in solute clearances may result in a rise in dietary intake of nutrients. At least one randomized, controlled trial demonstrated that an increase in the dose of dialysis for MHD patients with a DPI < 1.0 g/kg/day resulted in an increase in DPI over the 3-month follow-up period (123). A more recent, uncontrolled study came to the same conclusion (142). A more definitive answer to this question for MHD patients is likely to be available once the ongoing HD adequacy study (HEMO), funded by the National Institutes of Health, is completed. At least three uncontrolled studies have shown that in CPD patients, there is an increase in DPI with a rise in small solute clearances (41, 55, 135). More recently, a prospective, randomized trial confirmed the beneficial effect of an increase in dialytic clearances on the DPI in CPD patients (133). The only study unable to demonstrate a relationship between an increase in dialysis volumes and DPI in CPD patients was unable to achieve any increase in total clearances, which were below the currently acceptable minimum standards for adequacy of PD (69). Third, uncontrolled observations of small numbers of patients have shown that a new approach to dialysis therapy, daily treatment with nocturnal HD, which results in substantial increases in solute clearances, results in significant increases in DPI (145, 171, 183). To our knowledge, no published study has evaluated the influence of increased clearances on total energy intake for either MHD or CPD patients.

Significant progress has been made in elucidating the nature of uremic toxins that result in anorexia in uremic patients. Early observations suggested that for the same level of small solute clearances by dialysis, CPD patients had a higher DPI than did MHD patients dialyzed with low-flux membranes (14). In MHD patients hemodialyzed with high-flux membranes, the DPI for a given level of small solute clearance was demonstrated to be higher than in patients dialyzed with low-flux membranes (124). Because high-flux hemodialyzer membranes remove more molecules of a higher molecular weight, and because PD seems to remove more of the larger molecules than does HD, it was inferred that this improvement in DPI may be related to the removal, by dialysis, of substances of larger molecular weight, the so-called middle molecules. Recent experimental data suggest that middle molecule fractions, in the 1- to 5-kDa range, isolated from both the dialyzer ultrafiltrate of plasma and from normal urine inhibit food intake in rats in a dose-dependent manner (3). It is likely that these middle molecule fractions act in the splanchnic region and/or brain to inhibit food intake and that the effect is specific for ingestive behavior (138). However, a recent study was unable to demonstrate an increase in DPI when the middle molecule clearances were presumably increased by transferring MHD patients from a low-flux to a high-flux dialyzer (141). The HEMO study may provide additional information as to whether HD with high-flux characteristics (i.e. with a greater propensity to remove larger middle molecules) will increase DPI, dietary energy intake, and nutritional status.

***Delayed Gastric Emptying***    Gastroparesis is a well-known complication of diabetes mellitus and probably contributes to the low nutrient intake in this subgroup of patients. Gastroparesis may also occur not uncommonly in nondiabetic MD patients. Several studies have shown an impairment in gastric motility in MHD and CPD patients using both radionuclide studies (19, 60, 96) and electric gastrography (106, 119). In a recently published study using electric gastrography, over 50% of MHD and CPD patients demonstrated abnormal gastric emptying (119). However, it should be pointed out that not all investigators have demonstrated abnormalities in gastric emptying in MD patients (207, 243). Nevertheless, it is possible that occult gastroparesis contributes to the pathogenesis of PEM in some nondiabetic

MD patients; administration of erythromycin to hypoalbuminemic nondiabetic MHD patients with occult gastroparesis results in improvement in gastric emptying accompanied by an increase in serum albumin (193). The etiology of this gastroparesis remains unclear, although it has been postulated that derangements in the endocrine system of the gut may play a pathogenic role. In CPD patients, instillation of dialysate into the peritoneal cavity may contribute to abnormal gastric electrical activity (119) as well as to the prolongation in gastric emptying time (102).

*Increased Serum Leptin Levels*    Leptin is a polypeptide that is encoded by the *ob* gene. In rodents, leptin acts on the hypothalamus to regulate food intake and energy expenditure (27, 64, 180) and, hence, plays a key role in regulating body weight. The role of leptin in regulating body weight in humans is less clear. Several investigators have demonstrated elevated serum leptin levels in MD patients (75, 80, 93, 150, 165, 169, 204, 213, 247). Hence, elevated leptin levels may play a role in determining the nutritional status of MD patients. Several cross-sectional studies have shown an inverse correlation between serum leptin levels and DPI (93, 247). Others have been unable to demonstrate a relationship between recent weight change or other nutritional measures and serum leptin levels (150). However, three recent longitudinal studies have demonstrated that increased serum leptin levels are associated with weight loss in MHD (169) and CPD patients (75, 213).

The etiology of hyperleptinemia in MD patients is likely to be multifactorial. Leptin is metabolized, at least in part, in the kidney and, hence, accumulates in progressive renal failure (151, 204). Moreover, insulin stimulates leptin synthesis (109, 136), and the hyperinsulinemia associated with CRF may contribute to hyperleptinemia. Finally, activation of the acute-phase response (APR) may result in increased leptin levels; a recent study using CPD patients demonstrated a significant direct correlation between C-reactive protein and serum leptin levels in CPD patients (213).

*Intraperitoneal Instillation of Dialysate*    Clinical experience suggests that CPD patients are more likely to report early satiety or feelings of fullness. A study of the eating behavior of CPD patients indicates that compared with MHD patients, they have a lower food intake (82), which is associated with a constant feeling of fullness, a lower ranking of palatability of food, and a lower eating drive than in the predialysis state (83). An impairment in gastric emptying, as discussed above, may contribute to this abnormality. At least two other probable explanations have been offered to explain the suppression of appetite in CPD patients.

The abdominal distention produced either by intraperitoneal instillation of large volumes of dialysate or large ultrafiltration induced by the PD solutions, which are hyperosmolar, may have a direct inhibitory effect on appetite, independent of the absorption of nutrients, as has been demonstrated in a rabbit model of PD (9). If this hypothesis is true, the suppression of appetite should be uniform for all kinds of nutrients. In a PD model designed to study the ingestive behavior of rats, instillation of glucose-based dialysate resulted in a dose-dependent suppression of carbohydrate intake only, whereas the instillation of an amino acid-based dialysate resulted in a dose-dependent suppression of both carbohydrate and protein intake (137). This suggests that the inhibition of appetite caused by PD solutions is specific for various nutritional constituents of the diet and is not simply an effect of hyperosmolality or large filling volumes. This observation is highly relevant because the PD solutions available commercially use glucose as an osmotic agent, and up to 70% of instilled glucose is absorbed, accounting for 20%–30% of the total energy intake in CPD patients (59).

## Impact of Comorbidity on Nutritional Status

In the United States, MD patients have a high incidence and prevalence of co-morbidity (231). Over 50% of the patients who commence MD are over the age of 65 years and almost half are diabetic (231). There is a high prevalence of cardiovascular disease at the time of initiating MD—almost a third have a history of congestive heart failure and almost a quarter have a history of ischemic heart disease (231). Almost 50% of new patients have three or more comorbid conditions when they initiate MD (231). Moreover, this high prevalence of comorbidity is generally acknowledged to be an underestimate of the true burden; a more rigorous review of a sample of the national cohort demonstrated a significantly higher prevalence of associated diseases than are reported in the national registry (230). Each year, 10%–15% of prevalent MD patients are diagnosed with atherosclerotic heart disease, congestive heart failure, peripheral vascular disease, and/or cerebrovascular disease (231). In 1998 in the United States, the average number of hospital admissions was 1.5 times per MD patient, with each spending an average of 13–15 days per year in the hospital (231). There is also a high incidence of complications resulting from dialysis vascular accesses or peritoneal catheters used in MD and CPD patients (i.e. infectious complications, vascular access thromboses), which may not require hospitalization but which add to the disease burden of these individuals. These comorbidities are responsible for a substantial proportion of the medicines prescribed on an average day. During 1996–1997, the median number of medications consumed per day by MD patients ranged from 8 to 10 (229); in addition, 26%–30% were prescribed proton pump inhibitors and 13% an agent that promotes gastrointestinal motility (229).

It is likely that the associated comorbidities, intercurrent illnesses, and medications consumed by MD patients contribute not only to the high prevalence of PEM but also to the association between malnutrition and high mortality in MD patients. The presence of comorbid illnesses has been shown to increase the mortality risk in MHD and CPD patients (101, 215). Older age, the presence of diabetes mellitus, and the presence of cardiac disease are each associated with an increased risk of death for MD patients (231) as well as with a worse nutritional status (20, 118, 188). It truly is the question of what came first, the chicken or the egg. On the one hand, in some epidemiological analyses that adjust for the presence of comorbid illnesses, such measures of PEM as serum albumin lose their value as predictors of mortality for MD patients (101). On the other hand, the excess risk of death associated with diabetes mellitus is eliminated when the analyses are adjusted for predialysis serum albumin, creatinine, and urea (129).

Associated illnesses may both increase morbidity and mortality and cause malnutrition in ways in which the malnutrition makes little or no contribution to the elevated mortality. Alternatively, a comorbid illness might cause an increase in morbidity and mortality in part by lowering nutrient intake or by impairing intestinal absorption of nutrients. Associated illnesses may also result in the activation of the APR; some studies have reported that elevated serum levels of acute-phase proteins are restricted to older MD patients (188), who in turn are likely to have greater comorbidities. Finally, inadequate nutrient intake due to anorexia, e.g. caused by chronic uremia, may predispose to many illnesses, thereby increasing morbidity and mortality.

## Inflammation

Over the past 5 years, several studies have suggested a role for inflammation both in CRF patients not on dialysis and in MD patients.

### Markers of Inflammation and Renal Failure

Tissue injury, inflammation, or infection initiates an acute-phase response (APR). The first step results in the activation of monocytes and/or macrophages, which, in turn, release the two major cytokines that are the proximate initiators of the APR: interleukin (IL)-1 (45) and tumor necrosis factor alpha (TNF-$\alpha$) (17). Both of these cytokines stimulate the release of IL-6, which amplifies this APR. These cytokines, in turn, stimulate or inhibit the synthesis of a variety of proteins in the liver, the so-called acute-phase proteins (APPs): namely, C-reactive protein (CRP), serum amyloid A (SAA), C3 component of complement, $\alpha$-acid glycoprotein, fibrinogen, haptoglobin, and $\alpha$-chymotrypsin (156, 209). The hepatic synthesis of the visceral proteins, albumin (10, 157), prealbumin (11, 53), and transferrin, which are traditionally considered markers of nutritional status, are reciprocally inhibited by these cytokines. The short-term activation of the APR is considered to be a key protective mechanism; however, its activation in a wide variety of chronic illnesses in humans is potentially maladaptive.

Activation of each of these levels of the APR has been documented in CRF and MD patients. Elevated levels of IL-1 (18, 44, 77, 125, 181), TNF-$\alpha$ (32, 44, 77, 181), IL-6 (24, 31, 78, 95), and hepatocyte growth factor (134) have been demonstrated in the predialysis blood of MHD patients or the steady state blood of CPD patients (44, 120, 181). However, not all investigators have been able to demonstrate an elevated concentration of these cytokines (40, 187). The differences might, in part, be related to the relative short half-life of these cytokines and the transient, rather than continuous, nature of the inflammatory response in some patients (98). The serum concentrations of several positive APPs [CRP

(47, 65, 71, 85, 89, 100, 144, 173, 188, 224, 244, 248), SAA (100, 244, 248), and fibrinogen (108, 188, 223, 234)] have also been elevated in variable proportions of MD patients. The most frequently studied serum APP, CRP, is reported to be elevated in 22%–53% of MHD patients in cross-sectional studies. In summary, there is overwhelming evidence that the APR is activated in a significant proportion of MD patients.

### Acute-Phase Response and Malnutrition

Studies of cachexia associated with cancer and chronic infections have shed light on the relationship between the markers of the APR and malnutrition. It appears that much of the adverse nutritional impact of the APR is mediated by the cytokines, primarily IL-6. The cytokine cascade outlined above has been implicated in anorexia as well as in the depletion of somatic proteins by both a catabolic and an antianabolic effect and in depletion of visceral proteins by an antianabolic effect. Anorexia and, hence, inadequate dietary protein and energy intake are likely to exacerbate this depletion of protein stores.

Cytokines, especially TNF-$\alpha$, may suppress appetite (104). It is also likely that this anorectic effect is modulated by prostaglandins because antiinflammatory agents blunt the anorectic effects of cytokines (46). Also, these cytokines induce muscle catabolism with release of amino acids and inhibition of muscle protein synthesis (13, 154, 238). Specifically, intravenous administration of TNF-$\alpha$ in animals results in an increased breakdown of skeletal muscle (49). Transgenic mice with elevated levels of IL-6 have a muscle-wasting syndrome with up-regulation of ubiquitin-proteasome–mediated proteolysis, an effect abolished by the administration of IL-6 receptor antibody (225). Furthermore, there is a close association between proinflammatory cytokines and an increase in resting energy expenditure in cachectic individuals with rheumatoid arthritis (195).

The APR also engenders hypoalbuminemia by decreasing the rate of albumin synthesis (157). In vitro treatment of hepatocytes with IL-1 rapidly inhibits albumin synthesis (10); it is now known that this inhibition occurs at the transcriptional level (10). Hypocholesterolemia, another manifestation of PEM, may also be linked to the APR. Serum cholesterol concentrations tend to decrease during an APR (for example, after an acute myocardial infarction or with an infection) and increases after the APR has abated (196). A reduction of serum cholesterol has been observed during IL-2 infusions (239).

### Acute-Phase Response and PEM in MD Patients

Over the past 5 years, a compelling case has been made that APR contributes to the manifestations of PEM in MD patients, particularly with respect to hypoalbuminemia. Serum CRP has been used by many investigators as a marker for the APR; a highly significant negative correlation between serum albumin and serum CRP has been consistently demonstrated in MHD (98, 100, 173, 188) and CPD (65, 244) patients. Similar correlations have been demonstrated between serum albumin and both SAA (100, 244) and IL-6 (95). The correlation coefficient values for these relationships have generally been between 0.25 and 0.55 (65, 98, 100, 173, 188, 244, 248) and, hence, suggest that in addition to inflammation, other causes play a role in inducing hypoalbuminemia in these patients. Kinetic analyses have shown diminished albumin turnover rates in six hypoalbuminemic MHD patients (99). The serum levels of positive APPs, $\alpha$2-macroglobulin and ferritin, were significantly greater in these patients compared with six individuals with normal serum albumin levels. By multiple regression analyses, the rate of albumin synthesis was negatively correlated with $\alpha$2-macroglobulin (99); this argues for a role of APR in reducing the rate of albumin synthesis and inducing hypoalbuminemia (99). Although there are no studies correlating serum cholesterol and APPs, a negative correlation has been demonstrated between the serum cholesterol level and IL-6 levels (24).

Several studies have analyzed the relationship between measures of both the somatic protein pool and body mass with markers of the APR in MHD patients. In a study of 45 MHD patients, Kaizu et al demonstrated that IL-6 levels correlated negatively with both midarm muscle area and body weight change over 3 years (95). In the study by Qureshi et al, two thirds of MHD patients with moderate to severe malnutrition as defined by subjective global assessment had a high CRP level compared with 29% with mild malnutrition and 17% with normal nutritional status (188). The exact mechanisms by which inflammation affects the nutritional status of MD patients remain elusive. One study examined the relationship between DPI and serum CRP and SAA levels in MHD patients and was unable to demonstrate a correlation (100). This study, however, did not exclude a role for inflammation in inducing PEM in MD patients because the nutritional effects of the APR may be manifested by a decline in energy or protein intake. Furthermore, failure to demonstrate a correlation between the APR and DPI may be a result of a blunting of the APR in patients with low DPI and malnutrition, as has been observed in animal models of PEM (92). In a study using CPD patients, the serum levels of TNF-$\alpha$ were higher in patients with anorexia and were particularly high in patients with gastrointestinal symptoms (2). On the other hand, it is not known whether an increase in APP in serum of CRF or MD patients is associated with a hypercatabolic state, as no investigator has systematically studied this question.

In summary, the above evidence suggests a role for inflammation in the pathogenesis of some of the manifestations of PEM in MD patients. However, it is highly unlikely to be the sole cause because only about 50% of CRF patients with malnutrition show evidence for elevated APPs (210). Although one explanation for this may be the transient nature of the APR (98), another equally likely explanation is that PEM in MD patients is, indeed, multifactorial. Moreover, as indicated previously, PEM, by reducing host resistance, may predispose to comorbid conditions associated with inflammation. Thus, it is possible not only that inflammation contributes to PEM, but that PEM predisposes to inflammation. The PEM-inducing effects of inflammation also appear to be due to induction of anorexia. Thus, if the nutrient intake of MD patients were maintained, the adverse effects of inflammation on nutritional status might be markedly ameliorated. Finally, it should be recognized that in CRF and MD patients, the role of inflammation as cause of PEM, morbidity, and mortality is so far based on epidemiological data. There are virtually no randomized, prospective, interventional studies of CRF or MD patients that have examined whether reduction in inflammatory status (*a*) decreases the incidence, prevalence, or severity of PEM or (*b*) decreases morbidity or mortality.

## The Relationship Between Inflammation and Increased Dietary Protein Requirements in Maintenance Dialysis Patients

A clinically stable MD patient does not have a marked increase in urea nitrogen appearance compared with normal individuals ingesting similar diets providing 1.1–1.4 g of protein/kg/day. However, it has been suggested that an MD patient has, in general, a decreased ability to conserve body proteins when protein intake is reduced below the recommended levels. Indeed, the recommended dietary protein allowances for MD patients are higher (1.2–1.3 g/kg/day) than for normal, nonpregnant, nonlactating adults (161). This increase exceeds the increment in the daily protein intake that is necessary to offset the losses into the dialysate of proteins, peptides, and free amino acids (122). The finding that many MD patients may be unable to decrease their net protein degradation to maintain protein balance when the dietary intake falls below 1.0–1.2 g/kg/day suggests that MD patients may have an inability to conserve protein normally.

## Sources of Inflammation Related to the Dialysis Procedure

To maximize interventions aimed at reducing inflammation in dialysis patients, an understanding of what engenders the APR is imperative. A wide variety of mechanisms have been proposed and are summarized in Table 6.

*Bioincompatible Membranes*    A dialysis membrane that results in activation of the complement cascade is considered to be bioincompatible. Evidence that complement activation induces the APR is conflicting. Several investigators have demonstrated that HD with bioincompatible membranes, as opposed to biocompatible membranes, results in activation of APR (32, 149). Other investigators have either been unable to demonstrate elevated levels of cytokines following HD (40, 95, 187) or have demonstrated an equal activation of the APR with both kinds of membranes (79). Still others have demonstrated that contact with bioincompatible membranes results in an increase in IL-1$\beta$ and TNF-$\alpha$ mRNA transcription in mononuclear cells exiting from the dialyzer, without actual elevation in the serum concentrations of these cytokines (200). It is probable that these primed mononuclear cells require a second stimulus in order to translate the enhanced gene expression to an increase in the synthesis and release of these cytokines. Elegant experimental studies demonstrate that complement-activating membranes induce net protein catabolism (63). In a randomized control trial, the use of biocompatible membranes was associated with several manifestations of better nutritional status: namely, higher serum levels of albumin and insulin-like growth factor-1 as well as greater weight gain (179). In another study, transferring hypoalbuminemic MHD

**TABLE 6** Proposed sources of inflammation in end-stage renal disease

Related to the dialysis procedure
  Hemodialysis
    Dialyzer
      Bioincompatible membranes
      Processing of dialyzers for reuse
    Dialysate
      Endotoxins
    Vascular access
      Prosthetic arteriovenous grafts
      Percutaneous catheters
  Peritoneal dialysis
    Dialysate
      Plasticizers
      Glucose degradation product
    Access
      Peritoneal dialysis catheters
Related to chronic renal failure per se
    Uremic toxicity (oxidant and carbonyl stress)
    Volume overload
    Growth hormone resistance
    Altered intestinal bacterial flora
    Chronic subclinical infection

patients from a bioincompatible to a biocompatible membrane resulted in a small but significant increase in serum albumin (219). Overall, the evidence suggests that the use of bioincompatible membranes may have an adverse nutritional impact, possibly via the activation of the APR. However, recent studies demonstrating an increased prevalence of an activated APR were conducted using patients who had been dialyzed with biocompatible membranes (24, 98, 100, 248). Furthermore, in 1997, less than 20% of US dialysis units were still using bioincompatible membranes, further reducing the clinical importance of these membranes as a cause of inflammation (231). Hence, it is reasonable to conclude that although bioincompatible membranes may induce the APR, they are unlikely to be the predominant cause for the high incidence of inflammation in MD patients.

*Dialysate*    The dialysate that is used during the HD procedure is nonsterile and may contain small amounts of endotoxin. Endotoxin has been implicated as a cause of the APR in MHD patients (116). One in vitro study found no difference in the measures of inflammation when ultrapure dialysate was compared with nonsterile dialysate when the endotoxin concentrations were in the range usually found in dialysate (222). Kaysen et al failed to demonstrate an increase in IL-$1\beta$, SAA, or monocyte mRNAs encoding IL-$1\alpha$, IL-$1\beta$, IL-2, or TNF-$\alpha$ when pre- and postdialysis blood samples were compared (100). Nonetheless, the data from some in vivo studies are more consistent with the thesis that impure dialysate can elicit an inflammatory response (114). Therefore, whereas the use of nonsterile dialysate remains suspect, the issue remains unresolved.

With respect to the potential role of the sterile dialysate used in PD, strong evidence exists that PD solutions induce a low-grade inflammatory reaction within the peritoneal cavity (26). However, to our knowledge, no study has examined the role of peritoneal dialysate in inducing a systemic APR.

*Dialysis Vascular Access*    Several studies have demonstrated that in MHD patients, serum albumin levels are the greatest in those with native arteriovenous fistulae, are significantly lower in those who have prosthetic arteriovenous grafts, and are the lowest in those with transcutaneous venous catheters (100, 118). Although it is tempting to speculate that these differences in serum albumin are due to variations in the activation of the APR, the only study that has addressed this issue was unable to demonstrate a relationship between the elevation of serum CRP or SAA with the type of vascular access (100). It is likely that the relationship between the type of vascular access and nutritional status is confounded by comorbidity. For example, elderly or more chronically ill patients are more likely to have a prosthetic arteriovenous graft or transcutaneous catheter. Similarly, prosthetic arteriovenous grafts, and particularly the transcutaneous catheter, are more likely to induce comorbid events than are native arteriovenous fistulae.

## Sources of Inflammation Related to Chronic Renal Failure per se

Two lines of evidence strongly suggest that activation of the APR in patients with end-stage renal disease (ESRD) is independent of the dialysis procedure. First, elevated serum levels of cytokines (61, 78, 160, 181) as well as APPs (210, 211) have been consistently demonstrated in nondialyzed patients with near–end-stage renal failure. Second, recent data suggest that the elevation of APPs in patients with ESRD is intermittent and spans a period of several dialysis treatments (98), a finding that is less consistent with a dialysis-related cause of inflammation. Several hypotheses for dialysis-independent causes of inflammation have been postulated.

*Uremia-Dependent Processes*    There is compelling evidence from CRF and MD patients for an increased oxidative stress (increased levels of oxidants and decreased levels of antioxidants leading to oxidation of carbohydrates and lipids) (127) and carbonyl stress (inadequate detoxification or inactivation of reactive carbonyl compounds derived from both carbohydrates and lipids by oxidative and nonoxidative reactions) (152). It is probable that oxidative and carbonyl stress may stimulate the vascular endothelium and activate the APR (81, 94).

*Volume Overload*    Chronic congestive heart failure is associated with elevated levels of proinflammatory cytokines; this is probably caused by such factors as low tissue perfusion, hypoxia, liver congestion, and bowel wall edema. It has been suggested that proinflammatory cytokines play a pivotal role in the loss of edema-free/fat-free body mass and the development of the hypoalbuminemia of cardiac cachexia (51). Recent evidence suggests that volume overload may predispose to the transfer of endotoxin across the bowel wall and the induction of an APR (164). It has not been shown whether volume overload, which occurs commonly in MD patients, will cause the same response in these individuals.

*Altered Hormonal Milieu*    Uremia is characterized by resistance to the anabolic effects of growth hormone and insulin-like growth factor-I (50). In a highly provocative study of adult patients without renal failure but with growth hormone deficiency, treatment with recombinant growth hormone resulted in a significant decline in the levels of CRP (203). This may suggest that a functional deficiency of growth hormone, and/or insulin-like growth factor-1 may be a cause of the APR in CRF and MD patients. However, this hypotheses remains untested.

## Sources of Inflammation Related to Comorbidity

The role of comorbidity, superimposed illnesses, and medication usage was discussed above. These illnesses may engender an inflammatory response and might be an important cause of the elevated serum levels of cytokines and APPs in CRF patients.

## Is Inflammation the Link Between Malnutrition and Cardiovascular Mortality?

To date, five studies have demonstrated the relationship between elevated serum CRP concentrations and the risk of death for MHD patients (16, 89, 173, 245, 248). In all except one study (173), serum CRP was a more powerful predictor of death than was albumin. Similar relationships have been demonstrated for CPD patients (166). Furthermore, elevated serum levels of other APPs [hepatocyte growth factor (134), hyaluronan (212)] and cytokines [IL-6 (24, 103)] are associated with an increased risk of death for CRF and MD patients. Moreover, both in predialysis patients as well as in those undergoing MD, there are significant correlations between markers of inflammation and carotid atherosclerosis (134, 210). Thus, it is likely that inflammation indeed may be the link between malnutrition and cardiovascular mortality.

It is now widely accepted that atherosclerosis is an inflammatory disease (194). During the early stages of atherosclerosis, the initial endothelial dysfunction initiates an APR, which further promotes atherosclerosis, thus creating a vicious cycle. It is possible that the elevated levels of cytokines and APPs in patients with ESRD may just be a marker, rather than the cause, of the vascular process. Indeed, in a recent study using predialysis patients, the atherosclerotic burden assessed via carotid duplex ultrasonography correlated significantly with the serum CRP (210).

On the other hand, there is a large body of evidence that the APR may potentiate atherosclerosis.

Two pro-atherogenic substances, lipoprotein(a) [Lp(a)] and fibrinogen, are positive APPs, and their serum levels are elevated in patients with an activated APR. Elevated concentrations of Lp(a) have been demonstrated in MD patients (115). In normal subjects, the genetically inherited polymorphism in the size of apo(a) explains a large part of the variability in plasma Lp(a) concentrations (233), and there is evidence that this apo(a) size polymorphism is an important determinant of serum Lp(a) concentrations in patients with renal failure (211). However, these data fail to explain all the variability in plasma Lp(a) concentrations in MD patients. Plasma Lp(a) concentrations are reported to be higher in malnourished predialysis patients (211). There are two likely explanations for this association. First, IL-6 responsive motifs have been identified in the 5' flanking regulatory region on chromosome 6 of the gene for apo(a), which is a component of Lp(a) (235), and Lp(a) has been shown to have the characteristics of an acute-phase reactant (131). Several studies have now demonstrated a close relationship between plasma Lp(a) in MHD patients and markers of inflammation (97, 188, 211, 248). Second, in CPD patients, elevated serum Lp(a) levels correlate with peritoneal albumin losses (76, 236), raising the possibility that it is the hypoalbuminemia that stimulates the hepatic synthesis of Lp(a). With respect to fibrinogen, elevated serum levels of this protein are consistently demonstrated in MHD patients (107, 108, 188, 223, 234), and it is widely accepted as an APP.

The APR may not only raise the serum concentrations of proatherogenic proteins, but also reduce the protective effect of high-density lipoprotein (HDL) cholesterol. Unmodified HDL contains enzymes (PAF acetyl hydrolase and paroxanase) that destroy oxidized low-density lipoprotein, an atherogenic molecule. Apo A-1 normally comprises half of all the proteins in HDL. During the APR, SAA replaces apo A-1 on the HDL (37), and ceruloplasmin binds to HDL (162). Whereas the former process inhibits the protective activity of the HDL enzymes and reduces its ability to prevent the infiltration of monocytes into fatty streaks (162), the latter process promotes the oxidized LDL-induced stimulation of macrophage chemotactic protein-1 in the arterial wall (162). Hence, the net effect of these changes is to convert HDL from an anti- to a proatherogenic compound. There is evidence for reduced activity of paroxanase in uremic patients (175); however, the relationship between the markers of inflammation and this reduced activity have not been tested.

Hence, it is highly likely that the activated APR in MD patients contributes to the accelerated atherosclerosis and the high cardiovascular mortality seen in these patients.

## WHY ARE WE APPARENTLY NOT DOING BETTER?

There is strong evidence that in the United States, the outcome for MD patients has been progressively improving. Between 1988 and 1997, death rates for all incident MD patients in the United States have fallen 38.5% (231). This has occurred even

**TABLE 7**   Why are we not doing better?

Patient-related factors
  Increasing age
  Increasing comorbidities

Health care system–related factors
  Predialysis care
    Delayed referral to nephrologist
    Suboptimal nutritional assessment and management
    Inadequate reimbursement for dietitian services
    Delayed initiation of maintenance dialysis
  Dialysis care
    Inadequate dose of dialysis
    Inadequate reimbursement for oral, enteral, or intravenous
      nutritional supplements
    Short duration of hemodialysis treatments
    Inadequate time spent by nephrologists with patients

Expanding frontiers of our knowledge
  Uremic factors that suppress appetite
  Causes and potential role of hyperleptinemia
  Causes and potential role of inflammation

though the dialysis population has become older and has a greater proportion of individuals with diabetes mellitus and the prevalence of other comorbidities appears to be increasing (231). The time trend of the nutritional status of the US dialysis population is, however, difficult to ascertain because no systematic studies have addressed this issue. Yet, there is a sense that the prevalence rates of malnutrition have largely remained unchanged. However, as indicated above, the patient pool today is remarkably different from that of two decades ago. Hence, the unchanged prevalence rate may, in fact, reflect an improvement in the nutritional management. Moreover, MD patients with PEM are more likely to die, and the mortality rate of MD patients has fallen; these considerations also suggest that the true prevalence of PEM in MD patients may have decreased. Nonetheless, there is much room for improvement. We have summarized in Table 7 some possible causes of PEM in MD patients that, in our opinion, deserve special attention. In the following paragraphs, we present our recommendations, which may be valuable in improving the nutritional management of MD patients.

As discussed earlier, nutritional decline begins even when there is only a moderate reduction in GFR. Because prevention is usually better than cure, nutritional care should begin when patients have mild to moderate CRF. The severity of renal failure is often underestimated if one relies on measurement of serum creatinine alone (205). The creatinine clearance can be easily estimated by formulae that incorporate a patient's age, gender, body weight, and serum creatinine (36), an easy bed-side tool. The decline in energy intake in patients with progressive CRF is evident even when the GFR exceeds 50 ml/min/1.73 m$^2$ (153), a level of renal function that usually is associated with a serum creatinine in the range of 1.5–2.5 mg/dl, and the patient at that stage may be cared for by nonnephrologists. We recommend that patients with this degree of renal failure be referred to a nephrologist and managed in a multidisciplinary manner that includes the service of a dietitian. Nutritional assessment and management should be included as part of the evaluation of CRF patients. In patients with advanced CRF, if nutritional management is unable to improve the dietary protein and energy intakes to safe levels, timely initiation of MD should be considered (147, 161).

The past few years have seen an increase in the delivered dose of dialysis in the United States, and the proportions of patients who meet the adequacy standards for dialysis clearances of small solutes has progressively increased. There still remains room for improvement: In the United States, 20% of adult MHD patients between October and December 1998 (72) and 44% of adult CPD patients in 1999 (191) were underdialyzed according to current standards. The debate over the optimal length of HD treatments remains unresolved, but experience with nocturnal dialysis (145, 171, 183) and long, diurnal dialysis (87) suggests that a longer length of HD may improve patient morbidity or mortality. Recent studies also suggest that the frequency of physician visits and the total amount of time the physicians spend with MD patients is directly related to patient survival. Hence, increasing the physician time per patient may result in improved outcomes. Finally, of the techniques available for nutritional support (oral food supplements, tube feeding, intradialytic parenteral nutrition, total parenteral nutrition, intraperitoneal nutrition), there are government and third-party–payer barriers, including, arguably, unreasonable requirements for reimbursement. Prevention of PEM, thus, in MD patients with inadequate dietary energy and protein intakes remains elusive.

Aggressive treatment of associated illnesses, particularly cardiac illnesses, is also likely to pay rich dividends. The role of antioxidants to lower the oxidant stress in uremia remains untested but holds promise. In conclusion, we need to make progress on all fronts in order to improve the nutritional management of these patients.

**Visit the Annual Reviews home page at www.AnnualReviews.org**

## LITERATURE CITED

1. Acchiardo SR, Moore LW, Latour PA. 1983. Malnutrition as the main factor in morbidity and mortality of hemodialysis patients. *Kidney Int.* 24:199–203
2. Aguilera A, Codoceo R, Selgas R, Garcia P, Picornell M, et al. 1998. Anorexigen (TNF-alpha, cholecystokinin) and orexigen (neuropeptide Y) in peritoneal dialysis (PD) patients: their relationship with nutritional parameters. *Nephrol. Dial. Transplant.* 13: 1476–83
3. Anderstam BA, Mamoun AH, Sodersten P, Bergstrom J. 1996. Middle-sized uremic fractions from uremic ultrafiltrate and normal urine inhibit ingestive behavior in the rat. *J. Am. Soc. Nephrol.* 7:2453–60

4. Aparicio M, Cano N, Chauveau P, Azar R, Canaud B, et al. 1999. Nutritional status of haemodialysis patients: a French national co-operative study. *Nephrol. Dial. Transplant.* 14:1679–86

5. Arora P, Strauss BJ, Bronvnicar D, Stroud D, Atkins RC, et al. 1998. Total body nitrogen predicts long-term mortality in hemodialysis patients—a single center experience. *Nephrol. Dial. Transplant.* 13:1731–36

6. Avram MM, Glodwasser P, Erroa M, Fein PA. 1994. Predictors of survival in continuous ambulatory peritoneal dialysis patients: the importance of prealbumin and other nutritional and metabolic factors. *Am. J. Kidney Dis.* 23:91–98

7. Avram MM, Mittman N, Bonomini L, Chatopadhay J, Fein P. 1995. Markers for survival in dialysis: a seven year prospective study. *Am. J. Kidney Dis.* 26:209–19

8. Baeyer HV. 1981. In *Unexpected Alterations of Nutritional Habits in Patients Undergoing CAPD*, ed. KM Gahl GM, Nolph KD. Amsterdam: Excerpta Med.

9. Balaskas EV, Rodela H, Oreopoulos DG. 1993. Effects of intraperitoneal infusion of dextrose and amino acids on the appetite of rats. *Perit. Dial. Int.* 13:S490–98

10. Ballmer PE, McNurlan MA, Grant I, Garlick PJ. 1995. Down-regulation of albumin synthesis in the rat by human recombinant interleukin-1 beta or turpentine and the response to nutrients. *J. Parenter. Enter. Nutr.* 19:266–71

11. Banks RE, Forbes MA, Sotrr M, Higginson J, Thompson D, et al. 1995. The acute phase response in patients receiving subcutaneous IL-6. *Clin. Exp. Immunol.* 102:217–23

12. Barret BJ, Parfrey PS, Morgan J. 1997. Prediction of early death in end-stage renal disease patients starting dialysis. *Am. J. Kidney Dis.* 29:214–22

13. Beisel WR. 1995. Herman Award Lecture 1995: Infection-induced malnutrition— from cholera to cytokines. *Am. J. Clin. Nutr.* 62:813–19

14. Bergstrom J, Alvestrand A, Lindholm B, Tranaeus A. 1991. Relationship between Kt/V and protein catabolic rate (PCR) is different in continuous peritoneal dialysis and hemodialysis patients. *J. Am. Soc. Nephrol.* 2:358 (Abstr.)

15. Bergstrom J, Furst P, Alvestrand A, Lindholm B. 1993. Protein and energy intake, nitrogen balance, and nitrogen losses in patients treated with continuous ambulatory peritoneal dialysis. *Kidney Int.* 44:1048–57

16. Bergstrom J, Heimburger O, Lindholm B, Qureshi AR. 1995. Elevated serum CRP is a strong predictor of increased mortality and low serum albumin in hemodialysis patients. *J. Am. Soc. Nephrol.* 10:287A (Abstr.)

17. Beutler B, Cerami A. 1989. The biology of cachectin/TNF—a primary mediator of host response. *Annu. Rev. Immunol.* 7:625–55

18. Bingel M, Lonnemann G, Koch KM, Dinarello CA, Shaldon S. 1988. Plasma interleukin-1 activity during hemodialysis: the influence of dialysis membranes. *Nephron* 50:273–76

19. Bird NJ, Streather CP, O'Doherty MJ, Barton IK, Gaunt JI, et al. 1994. Gastric emptying in patients with chronic renal failure on continuous ambulatory peritoneal dialysis. *Nephrol. Dial. Transplant.* 9:287–90

20. Blake PG, Flowerdew G, Blake R, Oreopoulos DG. 1993. Serum albumin in patients on continuous ambulatory peritoneal dialysis—predictors and correlations with outcomes. *J. Am. Soc. Nephrol.* 3:1501–10

21. Blake PG, Somblos K, Abraham G, Weissgarten J, Pemberton R, et al. 1991. Lack of correlation between urea kinetic indices and clinical outcome. *Kidney Int.* 39:700–6

22. Blumenkrantz M, Kopple JD, Gutman RA, Chan YK, Barbour GL, et al. 1980. Methods for assessing nutritional status of patients with renal failure. *Am. J. Clin. Nutr.* 33:1567

23. Blumenkrantz MJ, Kopple JD, Moran JK, Coburn JW. 1982. Metabolic balance studies and dietary protein requirements in patients undergoing continuous ambulatory peritoneal dialysis. *Kidney Int.* 21:849–61

24. Bologa RM, Levine DM, Parker TS, Cheigh JS, Serur D, et al. 1998. Interleukin-6 predicts hypoalbuminemia, hypocholesterolemia, and mortality in hemodialysis patients. *Am. J. Kidney Dis.* 32:107–14

25. Borah MF, Schonfeld PY, Gotch FA, Sargent JA, Wolfson M, et al. 1978. Nitrogen balance during intermittent dialysis therapy of uremia. *Kidney Int.* 14:491–500

26. Breborowicz A, Oreopoulos DG. 1997. Evidence for the presence of chronic inflammation during peritoneal dialysis: therapeutic implications. *Perit. Dial. Int.* 17:S37–41

27. Campfield LA, Smith FH, Guisez Y, Devos R, Burn P. 1995. Evidence for a peripheral signal linking adiposity and central neural networks. *Science* 269:546–49

28. Canada-USA Perit. Dial. Study Group. 1996. Adequacy of dialysis and nutrition in continuous peritoneal dialysis: association with clinical outcomes. *J. Am. Soc. Nephrol.* 7:198–207

29. Canaud B, Leblanc M, Garred LJ, Bosc JY, Argiles A, et al. 1997. Protein catabolic rate over lean body mass ratio: a more rational approach to normalize the protein catabolic rate in dialysis patients. *Am. J. Kidney Dis.* 30:672–79

30. Cano N, Fernandez JP, Lacombe P, Lankester M, Pascal S, et al. 1987. Statistical selection of nutritional parameters in hemodialyzed patients. *Kidney Int.* 32:S178–80

31. Cavaillon JM, Poignet JL, Fitting C, Delons S. 1992. Serum interleukin-6 in long-term hemodialyzed patients. *Nephron* 60:307–13

32. Chollet-Martin S, Stamatakis G, Bailly S, Mery JP, Gougerot-Pocidalo MA. 1991. Induction of tumor necrosis factor-alpha during hemodialysis. Influence of membrane type. *Clin. Exp. Immunol.* 83:329–32

33. Chung SH, Lindholm B, Lee HB. 2000. Influence of initial nutritional status on continuous ambulatory peritoneal dialysis patient survival. *Perit. Dial. Int.* 20:19–26

34. Churchill DN, Taylor DW, Cook RJ, LaPlante P, Barre P, et al. 1992. Canadian hemodialysis morbidity study. *Am. J. Kidney Dis.* 19:214–34

35. Cianciaruso B, Brunori G, Kopple JD, Traverso G, Panarello G, et al. 1995. Cross-sectional comparisons of malnutrition in continuous ambulatory peritoneal dialysis and hemodialysis patients. *Am. J. Kidney Dis.* 26:475–86

36. Cockroft DW, Gault MH. 1976. Prediction of creatinine clearance from serum creatinine. *Nephron* 16:31–41

37. Coetzee GA, Strachan AF, van der Westhuyzen DR, Hoppe HC, Jeenah MS, et al. 1986. Serum amyloid A-containing human high density lipoprotein 3 density size, and apolipoprotein composition. *J. Biol. Chem.* 261:9644–51

38. Collins AJ, Ma JZ, Umen A, Keshaviah P. 1994. Urea index (Kt/V) and other predictors of hemodialysis patient survival. *Am. J. Kidney Dis.* 23:272–82

39. Culp K, Flanigan M, Lowire EG, Lew N, Zimmerman B. 1996. Modeling mortality risk in hemodialysis patients using laboratory values as time-dependent co-variates. *Am. J. Kidney Dis.* 28:741–46

40. Davenport A, Crabtree J, Andeonjna C, Will EJ, Davison AM. 1991. Tumor necrosis factor does not increase during routine cuprophan hemodialysis in healthy well-nourished patients. *Nephrol. Dial. Transplant.* 6:435–39

41. Davies SJ, Phillips L, Griffiths AM, Naish PF, Russell GI. 2000. Analysis of the effects of increasing delivered dialysis treatment to malnourished peritoneal dialysis patients. *Kidney Int.* 57:1743–54

42. Davies SJ, Russell L, Bryan J, Phillips L,

Russell GI. 1995. Comorbidity, urea kinetics, and appetite in continuous ambulatory peritoneal dialysis patients: their interrelationship and prediction of survival. *Am. J. Kidney Dis.* 26:353–61

43. Degoulet P, Legrain M, Reach I, Aime F, Devries C, et al. 1982. Mortality risk factors in patients treated by chronic hemodialysis: report of the Diaphane Collabarative Study. *Nephron* 31:103–10

44. Descamps-Latscha B, Herbelin A, Nguyen AT, Roux-Lombard P, Zingraff J, et al. 1995. Balance between IL-1 beta, TNF alpha, and their specific inhibitors in chronic renal failure and maintenance dialysis. Relationships with activation markers of T cells, B cells and monocytes. *J. Immunol.* 154:882–89

45. Dinarello CA. 1984. Mechanism of disease: interleukin-1 and the pathogenesis of the acute phase response. *N. Engl. J. Med.* 311:1413–18

46. Dinarello CA, Roubenoff RA. 1996. Mechanisms of loss of lean body mass in patients on chronic dialysis. *Blood Purif* 14:388–94

47. Docci D, Bilancioni R, Baldrati L, Capponcini C, Turci F, et al. 1990. Elevated acute-phase reactants in hemodialysis patients. *Clin. Nephrol.* 34:88–91

48. Fleischmann E, Teal N, Dudley J, May W, Bower JD, et al. 1999. Influence of excess weight on mortality and hospital stay in 1346 hemodialysis patients. *Kidney Int.* 55:1560–67

49. Flores EA, Bistrian BR, Pomposelli J, Dinarello CA, Blackburn GL, et al. 1989. Infusion of tumor necrosis factor/cachectin promotes muscle catabolism in the rat. A synergistic effect with interleukin 1. *J. Clin. Invest.* 83:1614–22

50. Fouque D, Peng SC, Kopple JD. 1995. Impaired metabolic response to recombinant insulin-like growth factor-1 in dialysis patients. *Kidney Int.* 47:876–83

51. Freeman LM, Roubenoff R. 1994. The nutrition implications of cardiac cachexia. *Nutr. Rev.* 52:340–47

52. Fung L, Pollock C, Caterson RJ, Mahony JF, Waugh DA, et al. 1996. Dialysis adequacy and nutrition determine prognosis in continuous ambulatory peritoneal dialysis patients. *J. Am. Soc. Nephrol.* 7:737–44

53. Fung WP, Thomas T, Dickson PW, Aldred AR, Milland J, et al. 1988. Structure and expression of the rat trasnthyretin (prealbumin) gene. *J. Biol. Chem.* 263:480–88

54. Ginn HE, Frost A, Lacy WW. 1968. Nitrogen balance in hemodialysis patients. *Am. J. Clin. Nutr.* 21:385–93

55. Ginsberg N, Fishbane D, Lynn R. 1996. The effect of improved dialytic efficiencies on measures of appetite in peritoneal dialysis patients. *J. Ren. Nutr.* 6:217–21

56. Giordano C, De Santo G, Pluvio M, Di La Capodicasa G, et al. 1980. Protein requirements of patients on CAPD: a study of nitrogen balance. *Int. J. Artif. Org.* 3:11–14

57. Goldwasser P, Mittman N, Antignani A, Burrell D, Collier J, et al. 1993. Predictors of mortality in hemodialysis patients. *J. Am. Soc. Nephrol.* 3:1613–22

58. Goodship TH, Passlick-Deetjen J, Ward MK, Wilkinson R. 1993. Adequacy of dialysis and nutritional status in CAPD. *Nephrol. Dial. Transplant.* 8:1366–71

59. Grodstein GP, Blumenkratz MJ, Kopple JD, Moran JK, Coburn JW. 1981. Glucose absorption during continuous ambulatory peritoneal dialysis. *Kidney Int.* 19:564–67

60. Grodstein GP, Harrison A, Roberts C, Ippoitili A, Kopple JD. 1979. Impaired gastric emptying in hemodialysis patients. *Kidney Int.* 16:952 A (Abstr.)

61. Guarnieri G, Togigo G, Fiotti N, Ciocci B, Situlin R, et al. 1997. Mechanisms of malnutrition in uremia. *Kidney Int.* 52:S41–44

62. Guarnieri G, Togigo G, Situlin R, Faccini L, Coli U, et al. 1983. Muscle biopsy studies in chronically uremic patients: evidence for malnutrition. *Kidney Int.* 24:187–93

63. Gutierrez A, Alvestrand A, Wahren J, Bergstrom J. 1990. Effect of in vivo contact between blood and dialysis membranes on

protein catabolism in humans. *Kidney Int.* 38:487–94

64. Halaas JL, Gajiwala KS, Maffei M, Cohen SL, Chait BT, et al. 1995. Weight reducing effects of the plasma protein encoded by the obese gene. *Science* 269:543–46

65. Han DS, Lee SW, Kang SW, Choi KH, Lee Hy, et al. 1996. Factors affecting low serum values of serum albumin in CAPD patients. *Adv. Perit. Dial.* 12:288–92

66. Harter HR. 1983. Review of significant findings from the National Co-operative Dialysis study and recommendations. *Kidney Int.* 24:107–12

67. Harty J, Boulton H, Curwell J, Heelis N, Uttley L, et al. 1993. Limitations of urea kinetic models as predictors of nutritional and dialysis adequacy in continuous ambulatory peritoneal dialysis patients. *Am. J. Nephrol.* 13:454–63

68. Harty J, Boulton H, Faragher B, Venning M, Gokal R. 1996. The influence of small solute clearance on dietary protein intake in continuous ambulatory peritoneal dialysis patients: a methodologic analysis based on cross-sectional and prospective studies. *Am. J. Kidney Dis.* 28:535–60

69. Harty J, Boulton H, Venning M, Gokal R. 1997. Impact of increasing dialysis volume on adequacy targets: a prospective study. *J. Am. Soc. Nephrol.* 8:1304–10

70. Harty J, Conway L, Keegan M, Curwell J, Venning M, et al. 1995. Energy metabolism during CAPD: a controlled study. *Adv. Perit. Dial.* 11:229–33

71. Haubitz M, Brunkhorst R, Wrenger E, Froese P, Schulze M, et al. 1996. Chronic induction of C-reactive protein by hemodialysis but not peritoneal dialysis therapy. *Perit. Dial. Int.* 16:158–62

72. Health Care Financ. Admin. 1999. *1999 Annual Report: End Stage Ren. Disease Clinical Performance Measures Project.* Baltimore, MD: Health Care Financ. Admin.

73. Heide B, Pierratos A, Khanna R, Pettit J, Ogilvie R, et al. 1983. Nutritional status of patients undergoing continuous ambulatory peritoneal dialysis (CAPD). *Perit. Dial. Bull.* 3:138

74. Heimburger O, Bergstrom J, Lindholm B. 1994. Albumin and aminoacid levels as markers of adequacy in continuous ambulatory peritoneal dialysis. *Perit. Dial. Int.* 14:123–32

75. Heimburger O, Lonnqvist F, Danielsson A, Nordenstrom J, Stenvinkel P. 1997. Serum immunoreactive leptin concentration and its relation to the body fat content in chronic renal failure. *J. Am. Soc. Nephrol.* 8:1423–30

76. Heimburger O, Stenvinkel P, Beglund L, Tranaeus A, Lindholm B. 1996. Increased plasma lipoprotein(a) in continuous ambulatory peritoneal dialysis is related to peritoneal transport of glucose. *Nephron* 72:135–44

76a. HEMO Study Group. 1998. The hemodialysis (HEMO) pilot study: nutrition program and participant characteristics at baseline. *J. Ren. Nutr.* 8:11–20

77. Herbelin A, Nguyen AT, Zingraff J, Urena P, Descamps-Latscha B. 1990. Influence of uremia and hemodialysis on circulating interleukin-1 and tumor necrosis factor alpha. *Kidney Int.* 37:116–25

78. Herbelin A, Urena P, Nguyen AT, Zingraff J, Descamps-Latscha B. 1991. Elevated circulating levels of interleukin-6 in patients with chronic renal failure. *Kidney Int.* 39:954–60

79. Honkanen E, Gronhagen-Riska C, Teppo AM, Maury CP, Meri S. 1991. Acute-phase proteins during hemodialysis: correlations with serum interleukin-1 beta levels and different dialysis membranes. *Nephron* 57:283–87

80. Howard JK, Load GM, Clutterbuck EJ, Ghatei MA, Pusey CD, et al. 1997. Plasma immunoreactive leptin concentration in end stage renal disease. *Clin. Sci.* 93:119–26

81. Huang YH, Ronnelid J, Frostegard J. 1995. Oxidized LDL induces enhanced

antibody formation and MCH class II-dependent INF-gamma production in lymphocytes from healthy individuals. *Arterioscler. Thromb. Vasc. Biol.* 15:1577–83

82. Hylander B, Barkeling B, Rossner S. 1992. Eating behavior in continuous ambulatory peritoneal dialysis and hemodialysis patients. *Am. J. Kidney Dis.* 20:592–97

83. Hylander B, Barkeling B, Rossner S. 1997. Changes in patients' eating behavior: in the uremic state, on continuous ambulatory peritoneal dialysis, and after transplantation. *Am. J. Kidney Dis.* 29:691

84. Ikizler TA, Greene JH, Wingard RL, Parker RA, Hakim RM. 1995. Spontaneous dietary and protein intake during progression of chronic renal failure. *J. Am. Soc. Nephrol.* 6:1386–91

85. Ikizler TA, Wingard RL, Harvell J, Shyr Y, Hakim RM. 1999. Association of morbidity with markers of nutrition and inflammation in chronic hemodialysis patients: a prospective study. *Kidney Int.* 55:1945–51

86. Ikizler TA, Wingard RL, Sun M, Harvell J, Parker RA, et al. 1996. Increased energy expenditure in hemodialysis patients. *J. Am. Soc. Nephrol.* 7:2646–53

87. Innes A, Charra B, Burden RP, Morgan AG, Laurent G. 1999. The effect of long, slow haemodialysis on patient survival. *Nephrol. Dial. Transplant.* 14:919–22

88. Iseki K, Kawazoe N, Fukiyama K. 1993. Serum albumin is a strong predictor of death in chronic dialysis patients. *Kidney Int.* 44:115–19

89. Iseki K, Tozawa M, Yoshi S, Fukiyama K. 1999. Serum C-reactive protein (CRP) and risk of death in chronic dialysis patients. *Nephrol. Dial. Transplant.* 14:1956–60

90. Iseki K, Uehara H, Nishime K, Tokuyama K, Yoshihara K, et al. 1996. Impact of the initial levels of laboratory variables on survival in chronic dialysis patients. *Am. J. Kidney Dis.* 28:541–48

91. Jacob V, Le Carpentier JE, Salzano S, Naylor V, Wild G, et al. 1990. IGF-1, a marker of undernutrition in hemodialysis patients. *Am. J. Clin. Nutr.* 52:39–44

92. Jennings G, Elia M. 1992. The acute-phase response to turpentine-induced abscess in malnourished rats at different environmental temperatures. *Met. Clin. Exp.* 41:141–47

93. Johansen KL, Mulligan K, Tai V, Schambelan M. 1998. Leptin, body composition and indices of malnutrition in patients on dialysis. *J. Am. Soc. Nephrol.* 9:1080–84

94. Jovinge S, Ares MP, Kallin B, Nilsson J. 1996. Human monocytes/macrophages release TNF alpha in response to oxidized LDL. *Arterioscler. Thromb. Vasc. Biol.* 1996:1573–79

95. Kaizu Y, Kimura M, Yoneyama T, Miyaji K, Hibi I, et al. 1998. Interleukin-6 may mediate malnutrition in chronic hemodialysis patients. *Am. J. Kidney Dis.* 31:93–100

96. Kao CH, Hsu YH, Wang SJ. 1996. Delayed gastric emptying in patients with chronic renal failure. *Nucl. Med. Commun.* 17:164–67

97. Kario K, Matsu T, Kobayashi H, Matsuo M, Asada R, et al. 1995. High lipoprotein(a) levels in chronic hemodialysis patients are closely related to the acute-phase reaction. *Thromb. Haemost.* 74:1020–24

98. Kaysen GA, Dubin JA, Muller HG, Rosales LM, Levin NM, et al. 2000. The acute-phase response varies with time and predicts serum albumin levels in hemodialysis patients. *Kidney Int.* 58:346–52

99. Kaysen GA, Rathore V, Shearer GC, Depner TA. 1995. Mechanisms of hypoalbuminemia in hemodialysis patients. *Kidney Int.* 48:510–16

100. Kaysen GA, Stevenson FT, Depner TA. 1997. Determinants of albumin concentration in hemodialysis patients. *Am. J. Kidney Dis.* 29:658–68

101. Keane WF, Collins AJ. 1994. Influence of comorbidity on mortality and

morbidity in patients treated with hemodialysis. *Am. J. Kidney Dis.* 24:1010–18

102. Kim DJ, Kang W-H, Kim HY, Lee BH, Kim B, et al. 1999. The effect of dialysate dwell on gastric emptying time in patients on continuous ambulatory peritoneal dialysis. *Perit. Dial. Int.* 19(Suppl. 2):S176–78

103. Kim H, Bologa R, Parker T, Levine D, et al. 1999. Serum IL-6 as an indicator of survival outcome in CAPD patients. *J. Am. Soc. Nephrol.* 10:246 A (Abstr.)

104. Kirschgessner TG, Uysal KT, Wiesbrock SM, Marino MW, Hotamisligil GS. 1997. Tumor necrosis factor alpha contributes to obesity-related hyperleptinemia by regulating leptin release from adipocytes. *J. Clin. Invest.* 100:2777–82

105. Kloppenburg WD, Stegman CA, de Jong PE, Huisman RM. 1999. Relating protein intake to nutritional status in hemodialysis patients: how to normalize the protein equivalent of total nitrogen appearance. *Nephrol. Dial. Transplant.* 14:2165–72

106. Ko CW, Chang CS, Wu MJ, Chen GH. 1998. Transient impact of hemodialysis on gastric myoelectrical activity of uremic patients. *Dig. Dis. Sci.* 43:1159–64

107. Koch M, Kutkuhn B, Grabensee B, Ritz E. 1997. Apolipoprotein A, fibrinogen, age, and history of stroke are predictors of death in dialysed diabetic patients: a prospective study in 412 subjects. *Nephrol. Dial. Transplant.* 12:2603–11

108. Koch M, Kutkuhn B, Trenkwalder E, Bach D, Grabensee B, et al. 1997. Apolipoprotein B, fibrinogen, HDL cholesterol, and apolipoprotein(a) phenotypes predict coronary artery disease in hemodialysis patients. *J. Am. Soc. Nephrol.* 8:1889–98

109. Kolaczynski JW, Nyce MR, Considine RV, Boden G, Nolan JJ, et al. 1996. Acute and chronic effects of insulin on leptin production in humans: studies in vivo and in vitro. *Diabetes* 45:699–701

110. Kopple JD, Berg R, Houser H, Steinman TI, Teschan P, et al. 1989. Nutritional status of patients with differing levels of chronic renal insufficiency. *Kidney Int.* 36(Suppl. 27):S184–94

111. Kopple JD, Monteon FJ, Shaib JK. 1986. Effect of energy intake on nitrogen metabolism in nondialyzed patients with chronic renal failure. *Kidney Int.* 29:734–42

112. Kopple JD, Shinaberger JH, Coburn JW, Sorensen MK, Rubini ME. 1969. Optimal dietary protein treatment during chronic hemodialysis. *Trans. Am. Soc. Artif. Int. Org.* 15:302–8

113. Kopple JD, Zhu X, Lew NL, Lowrie EG. 1999. Body weight-for-height relationships predict mortality in maintenance hemodialysis patients. *Kidney Int.* 56:1136–48

114. Krautzig S, Linnenweber S, Schindler R, Shaldon S, Koch KM, et al. 1996. New indicators to evaluate bacteriological quality of the dialysis fluid and the associated inflammatory response in ESRD patients. *Nephrol. Dial. Transplant.* 11:S87–91

115. Kronenberg F, Uutermann G, Dieplinger H. 1996. Lipoprotein(a) in renal disease. *Am. J. Kidney Dis.* 27:1–25

116. Laude-Sharp M, Caroff M, Simard L, Pusineri C, Kazatchkine M, et al. 1990. Induction of IL-1 during hemodialysis: transmembrane passage of intact endotoxin (LPS). *Kidney Int.* 38:1089–94

117. Leavey SF, Strawderman RL, Jones CA, Port FK, Held PJ. 1998. Simple nutritional indicators as independent predictors of mortality in hemodialysis patients. *Am. J. Kidney Dis.* 31:997–1006

118. Leavey SF, Strawderman RL, Young EW, Saran R, Roys E, et al. 2000. Cross-sectional and longitudinal predictors of serum albumin in hemodialysis patients. *Kidney Int.* 58:2119–28

119. Lee SW, Song JH, Kim GA, Yang HJ, Lee KJ, et al. 2000. Effect of dialysis modalities on gastric myoelectrical activity in

end-stage renal disease patients. *Am. J. Kidney Dis.* 36:566–73

120. Libetta C, De Nicola L, Rampino T, De Simone W, Memoli B. 1996. Inflammatory effects of peritoneal dialysis: evidence of systemic monocyte activation. *Kidney Int.* 49:506–11

121. Lim VS, Flanigan MJ, Zavala DC, Freeman RM. 1985. Protective adaptation of low serum triiodothyronine in patients with chronic renal failure. *Kidney Int.* 28:541–49

122. Lim VS, Kopple JD. 2000. Protein metabolism in patients with chronic renal failure: role of uremia and dialysis. *Kidney Int.* 58:1–10

123. Lindsay R, Spanner E, Heienheim P, Lefebure J, Hodsman, et al. 1992. Which comes first, Kt/V or PCR—chicken or egg? *Kidney Int.* 42(Suppl. 3):S32–37

124. Lindsay RM, Spanner E. 1989. A hypothesis: The protein catabolic rate is dependent upon the type and amount of treatment in dialyzed uremic subjects. *Am. J. Kidney Dis.* 13:382–89

125. Lonnemann G, Bingel M, Koch KM, Shaldon S, Dinarello CA. 1987. Plasma interleukin-1 activity in humans undergoing hemodialysis with regenerated cellulosic membranes. *Lymphokine Res.* 6:63–70

126. Lorenzo V, de Bonis E, Rufino M, Hernandez D, Rebollo SG, et al. 1995. Caloric rather than protein deficiency predominates in stable chronic hemodialysis patients. *Nephrol. Dial. Transplant.* 10:1885–89

127. Loughrey CM, Young IS, Lightbody JH, McMaster D, McNamee PT, et al. 1997. Oxidative stress in haemodialysis. *Q. J. Med.* 87:679–83

128. Lowrie EG, Lew N. 1990. Death risk in hemodialysis patients: the predictive value of commonly measured variables and an evaluation of death rate differences between facilities. *Am. J. Kidney Dis.* 15:458–82

129. Lowrie EG, Lew NL, Huang WH. 1992. Race and diabetes as death risk predictors in hemodialysis patients. *Kidney Int.* 42:S22–31

130. Lysaght MJ, Pollock CA, Hallet MD, Ibels LS, Farrell PC. 1989. The relevance of urea kinetic modeling to CAPD. *ASAIO Trans.* 35:784–90

131. Maeda S, Abe A, Seishima M, Makino K, Noma A, et al. 1989. Transient changes of serum lipoprotein (a) as an acute phase protein. *Atherosclerosis* 78:145–50

132. Mailloux LU, Napolitano B, Bellucci AG, Mossey RT, Vernance MA, et al. 1996. The impact of co-morbid risk factors at the start of dialysis upon the survival of ESRD patients. *ASAIO J.* 42:164–69

133. Mak S-K, Wong P-N, Lo K-Y, Tong GMW, Fung LH, et al. 2000. Randomized prospective study of the effect of increased dialytic dose on nutritional and clinical outcome in continuous ambulatory peritoneal dialysis patients. *Am. J. Kidney Dis.* 36:105–14

134. Malatino LS, Mallamaci F, Benedetto FA, Bellanuova I, Cataliotti A, et al. 2000. Hepatocyte growth factor predicts survival and relates to inflammation and intima media thickness in end-stage renal disease. *Am. J. Kidney Dis.* 36:945–52

135. Malhotra D, Tzamaloukas AH, Murata GH, Fox L, Goldman RS, et al. 1996. Serum albumin in continuous ambulatory peritoneal dialysis: its predictors and relationship to urea clearance. *Kidney Int.* 50:243–49

136. Malmstrom R, Taskien M-R, Karonen S-L, Yki-Jarvinene H. 1996. Insulin increases plasma leptin concentrations in normal subjects and patients with NIDDM. *Diabetologia* 39:993–96

137. Mamoun AH, Anderstam B, Sodersten P, Lindholm B, Bergstrom J. 1996. Influence of peritoneal dialysis solutions with glucose and amino acids on ingestive behavior in rats. *Kidney Int.* 49:1276–82

138. Mamoun AH, Sodersten P, Anderstam

B, Bergstrom J. 1999. Evidence of splanchnic-brain signaling in inhibition of ingestive behavior by middle molecules. *J. Am. Soc. Nephrol.* 10:309–14

139. Marcen R, Teruel JL, de la Cal MA, Gamez C. 1997. The impact of malnutrition in morbidity and mortality in stable hemodialysis patients. Spanish Cooperative Study of Nutrition in Hemodialysis. *Nephrol. Dial. Transplant.* 12:2324–31

140. Marcus RG, Chiange E, Dimaano F, Uribarri J. 1994. Serum albumin: associations and significance in peritoneal dialysis patients. *Adv. Perit. Dial.* 10:94–98

141. Marcus RG, Cohl E, Uribarri J. 1998. Middle molecule clearance does not influence protein intake in hemodialysis patients. *Am. J. Kidney Dis.* 31:491–94

142. Marcus RG, Cohl E, Uribarri J. 1999. Protein intake seems to respond to increases in Kt/V despite baseline Kt/V greater than 1.2. *Am. J. Nephrol.* 19:500–4

143. McCusker FX, Teehan BP, Thorpe KE, Keshaviah PR, Churchill DN, et al. 1996. How much peritoneal dialysis is necessary for maintaining a good nutritional status? *Kidney Int.* 56(Suppl.):S56–61

144. McIntyre C, Harper I, MacDougal I, Raine A, Williams A, et al. 1997. Serum C-reactive protein as a marker for infection and inflammation in regular dialysis patients. *Clin. Nephrol.* 48:371–74

145. McPhatter LL, Lockridge RS Jr, Albert J, Anderson H, Craft V, et al. 1999. Nightly home hemodialysis: improvement in nutrition and quality of life. *Adv. Ren. Rep. Ther.* 6:358–65

146. Mehrotra R, Kopple JD. 2000. Increase in serum albumin upon initiation of maintenance hemodialysis: evidence for improvement in nutritional status? *J. Am. Soc. Nephrol.* 11:287A (Abstr.)

147. Mehrotra R, Nolph KD. 1998. Argument for timely initiation of dialysis. *J. Am. Soc. Nephrol.* 9:S96–99

148. Mehrotra R, Saran R, Moore HL, Prowant

BF, Khanna R, et al. 1997. Towards targets for initiation of chronic dialysis. *Perit. Dial. Int.* 17:497–508

149. Memoli B, Postiglione L, Cianciaruso B, Bisesti V, Cimmaruta C, et al. 2000. Role of different dialysis membranes in the release of interleukin-6 soluble receptor in uremic patients. *Kidney Int.* 58:417–24

150. Merabet E, Dagago-Jack S, Coyne DW, Klein S, Santiago JV, et al. 1997. Increased plasma leptin concentration in end-stage renal disease. *J. Clin. Endocrinol. Metab.* 82:847–50

151. Meyer C, Robson D, Rackovsky N, Nadkarni V, Gerich J. 1997. Role of kidney in human leptin metabolism. *Am. J. Physiol.* 273:E903–7

152. Miyata T, van Ypersele de Strihou C, Kurokawa K, Baynes JW. 1999. Alterations in nonenzymatic biochemistry in uremia: origin and significance of "carbonyl stress" in long-term uremic complications. *Kidney Int.* 55:389–99

153. Modif. Diet Renal Dis. Study Group. 2000. Relationship between nutritional status and the glomerular filtration rate: results from the MDRD study. *Kidney Int.* 57:1688–703

154. Moldawer LL, Copeland EM. 1997. Proinflammatory cytokines, nutritional support, and the cachexia syndrome: interactions and therapeutic options. *Cancer* 79:1828–39

155. Monteon FJ, Laidlaw SA, Shaib JK, Kopple JD. 1986. Energy expenditure in patients with chronic renal failure. *Kidney Int.* 30:741–47

156. Moshage H. 1997. Cytokines and the hepatic acute phase response. *J. Pathol.* 191:257–66

157. Moshage HJ, Janssen JAM, Franssen JH, Hafkenscheid JCM, Yap SH. 1987. Study of the molecular mechanisms of decreased liver synthesis of albumin in inflammation. *J. Clin. Invest.* 79:1635–41

158. Movilli E, Filippini M, Brunori G,

Sandrini M, Costantino E, et al. 1995. Influence of protein catabolic rate on nutritional status, morbidity and mortality in elderly uraemic patients on chronic hemodialysis: a prospective 3-year follow-up study. *Nephrol. Dial. Transplant.* 10:514–18

159. Movilli E, Mombelloni S, Gaggiotti M, Maiorca R. 1993. Effect of age on protein catabolic rate, morbidity and mortality in ureamic patients with adequate dialysis. *Nephrol. Dial. Transplant.* 8:735–39

160. Nakanishi I, Moutabarrik A, Okada N, Kitamura E, Hayashi A, et al. 1994. Interleukin-8 in chronic renal failure and dialysis patients. *Nephrol. Dial. Transplant.* 9:1435–42

161. Natl. Kidney Found. I Init. K-DOQ. 2000. Clinical practice guidelines for nutrition in chronic renal failure. *Am. J. Kidney Dis.* 35:S1–140

162. Navab M, Berliner JA, Watson AD, Hama SY, Territo MC, et al. 1996. The yin and yang of oxidation in the development of the fatty streak. A review based on the 1994 George Lyman Duff Memorial Lecture. *Arteriscler. Thromb. Vasc. Res.* 16:831–42

163. Nelson EE, Hong CD, Pesce AL, Singh S, Pollak VE. 1990. Anthropometric norms for the dialysis population. *Am. J. Kidney Dis.* 16:32–37

164. Niebauer J, Volk HD, Kemp M, Dominguez M, Schumann RR, et al. 1999. Endotoxin and immune activation in chronic heart failure: a prospective cohort study. *Lancet* 353:1838–42

165. Nishizawa Y, Shoji T, Tanaka S, Yamashita M, Morita A, et al. 1998. Plasma leptin level and its relationship between body composition in hemodialysis patients. *Am. J. Kidney Dis.* 31:655–61

166. Noh H, Lee SW, Kang SW, Shin SK, Choi KH, et al. 1998. Serum C-reactive protein: a predictor of mortality in continuous ambulatory peritoneal dialysis patients. *Perit. Dial. Int.* 18:387–94

167. Nolph KD, Moore HL, Prowanat B, Meyer M, Twardowski ZJ, et al. 1993. Cross sectional assessment of weekly urea and creatinine clearances and indices of nutrition in continuous ambulatory peritoneal dialysis. *Perit. Dial. Int.* 13:178–83

168. Obrador GT, Arora P, Kausz AT, Pereira BJG. 1999. Prevalence and factors associated with sub optimal care before initiation of dialysis in United States. *J. Am. Soc. Nephrol.* 10:1793–800

169. Odamaki M, Furuya R, Yoneyama T, Nishikino M, Hibi I, et al. 1999. Association of the serum leptin concentration with weight loss in chronic hemodialysis patients. *Am. J. Kidney Dis.* 33:361–68

170. Olevitch LR, Bowers BM, DeOreo PB. 1994. Measurement of resting energy expenditure via indirect calorimetery during adult hemodialysis treatment. *J. Ren. Nutr.* 4:192–97

171. O'Sullivan DA, McCarthy JT, Kumar R, Williams AW. 1998. Improved biochemical variables, nutrient intake, and hormonal factors in slow nocturnal hemodialysis: a pilot study. *Mayo Clin. Proc.* 73:1035–45

172. Owen WF Jr, Lew NL, Liu Y, Lowrie EG, Lazarus JM. 1993. The urea reduction ratio and serum albumin concentration as predictors of mortality in patients undergoing maintenance hemodialysis. *N. Engl. J. Med.* 14:1001–6

173. Owen WF, Lowrie EG. 1998. C-reactive protein as an outcome predictor for maintenance hemodialysis patients. *Kidney Int.* 54:627–36

174. Palop L, Martinez JA. 1997. Cross-sectional assessment of nutritional and immune status in renal patients undergoing continuous ambulatory peritoneal dialysis. *Am. J. Clin. Nutr.* 66:498–503S

175. Paragh G, Asztalos L, Seres I, Balogh Z, Locsey L, et al. 1999. Serum paraxonase activity changes in uremic and kidney transplanted patients. *Nephron* 83:126–31

176. Park JS, Jung HH, Yang WS, Kim HH, Kim SB, et al. 1997. Protein intake and nutritional status in patients with pre-dialysis chronic renal failure on unre-stricted diet. *Kor. J. Int. Med.* 12:115–21

177. Park YK, Kim JH, Kim KJ, Seo AR, Kang EH, et al. 1999. A cross-sectional study comparing the nutritional status of peri-toneal dialysis and hemodialysis patients. *J. Ren. Nutr.* 9:149–56

178. Parker TF, Laird NM, Lowrie EG. 1983. Comparison of the study groups in the national cooperative dialysis study and a description of morbidity, mortality and patient withdrawal. *Kidney Int.* 23:42–49

179. Parker TF III, Wingard RL, Husni L, Ik-izler TA, Parker RA, et al. 1996. Effect of membrane biocompatibility on nutri-tional parameters in chronic hemodialysis patients. *Kidney Int.* 49:551–56

180. Pelleymounter MA, Cullen MJ, Baker MB, Hecht R, Winters D, et al. 1995. Ef-fect of the obese gene product on body weight regulation in ob/ob mice. *Science* 269:540–43

181. Pereira BJG, Shapiro L, King AJ, Falagas ME, Strom JA, et al. 1994. Plasma levels of IL-1 beta, TNF alpha, and their spe-cific inhibitors in undialyzed patients with chronic renal failure. *Kidney Int.* 45:890–96

182. Perez RA, Blake PG, Spanner E, Patel M, McMurray S, et al. 2000. High creatinine excretion ratio predicts a good outcome in peritoneal dialysis patients. *Am. J. Kidney Dis.* 36:362–67

183. Pierratos A, Ouwendyk M, Francoeur R, Vas S, Raj DS, et al. 1998. Nocturnal hemodialysis: three year experience. *J. Am. Soc. Nephrol.* 9:859–68

184. Pollock CA, Allen BJ, Warden RA, Cater-son RJ, Blagojevic N, et al. 1990. Total body nitrogen by neutron activation ana-lysis in maintenance dialysis patients. *Am. J. Kidney Dis.* 16:38–45

185. Pollock CA, Ibels LS, Ayass W, Caterson RJ, Waugh D, et al. 1995. Total body ni-trogen as a prognostic marker in mainte-nance dialysis. *J. Am. Soc. Nephrol.* 6:86–88

186. Pollock CA, Ibels LS, Zhu FY, Warnant M, Caterson RJ, et al. 1997. Protein in-take in renal disease. *J. Am. Soc. Nephrol.* 8:777–83

187. Powell AC, Bland L, Oettiger CW, MaAl-lister S, Oliver JC, et al. 1991. Lack of elevation of plasma interleukin-1beta or tumor necrosis alpha during unfavor-able hemodialysis conditions. *J. Am. Soc. Nephrol.* 2:1007–13

188. Qureshi AR, Alvestrand A, Danielsson A, Divino-Filho JC, Gutierrez A, et al. 1998. Factors predicting malnutrition in hemodialysis patients: a cross-sectional study. *Kidney Int.* 53:773–82

189. Rao M, Sharma M, Juneja R, Jacob S, Jacob CK. 2000. Calculated nitrogen bal-ance in hemodialysis patients: influence of protein intake. *Kidney Int.* 58:336–45

190. Rayner HC, Stroud DB, Salamon KM, Strauss BJ, Thompson NM, et al. 1991. Anthropometry underestimates body pro-tein depletion in hemodialysis patients. *Nephron* 59:33–34

191. Rocco M, Flanigan M, Frankenfield D, Frederick P, Prowant B, et al. 2000. CAPD adequacy data in a national cohort sample: the 1999 health care financing administration (HCFA) ESRD Peritoneal Dialysis Clinical Performance Measures (PD-CPM). *J. Am. Soc. Nephrol.* 11:217A (Abstr.)

192. Rocco MV, Jordan JR, Burkart JM. 1993. The efficacy number as a predictor of mor-bidity and mortality in peritoneal dialysis patients. *J. Am. Soc. Nephrol.* 4:1184–91

193. Ross EA, Koo LC. 1998. Improved nutri-tion after detection and treatment of oc-cult gastroparesis in nondiabetic dialysis patients. *Am. J. Kidney Dis.* 31:62–66

194. Ross R. 1999. Atherosclerosis—an in-flammatory disease. *N. Engl. J. Med.* 340:115–26

195. Roubenoff R, Roubenoff RA, Cannon JG, Kehayias JJ, Zhuang H, et al. 1994. Rheumatoid cachexia: cytokine driven hypercatabolism accompanying reduced body cell mass in chronic inflammation. *J. Clin. Invest.* 93:2379–86

196. Sammalkorpi KT, Valtonen VV, Maury CPJ. 1990. Lipoproteins and acute-phase response during acute infection. Interrelationships between C-reactive protein and serum amyloid A protein lipoproteins. *Ann. Med.* 22:397–401

197. Saran R, Moore H, Mehrotra R, Khanna R, Nolph KD. 1998. Longitudinal evaluation of renal Kt/Vurea of 2.0 as a threshold for initiation of dialysis. *ASAIO J.* 44:M677–81

198. Sargent JA, Gotch FA, Borah M, Piercy L, Spinozzi N, et al. 1978. Urea kinetics: a guide to nutritional management of renal failure. *Am. J. Clin. Nutr.* 31:1696–702

199. Schilling H, Wu G, Pettit J, Harrison J, McNeill K, et al. 1985. Nutritional status of patients on long-term CAPD. *Perit. Dial. Bull.* 5:12–18

200. Schindler R, Lonnemann G, Shaldon S, Koch KM, Dinarello CA. 1990. Transcription, not synthesis, of interleukin-1 and tumor necrosis factor by complement. *Kidney Int.* 37:85–93

201. Schneeweiss B, Graninger W, Stockenhuber F, Druml W, Ferenci P, et al. 1990. Energy metabolism in acute and chronic renal failure. *Am. J. Clin. Nutr.* 52:596–601

202. Schonfeld PY, Henry RR, Laird NM, Roxe DM. 1983. Assessment of nutritional status of the national co-operative dialysis study population. *Kidney Int.* 23:80–88

203. Sesmilo G, Biller BMK, Llevadot J, Hayden D, Hanson G, et al. 2000. Effect of growth hormone administration on inflammatory and other cardiovascular risk markers in men with growth hormone deficiency. A randomized controlled clinical trial. *Ann. Int. Med.* 133:111–22

204. Sharma K, Considine RV, Michel B, Dunn SR, Weisberg LS, et al. 1997. Plasma leptin is partly cleared by the kidney and is elevated in hemodialysis patients. *Kidney Int.* 51:1980–85

205. Shemesh O, Golbetz H, Kriss JP, Myers BD. 1985. Limitations of creatinine as a filtration marker in glomerulopathic patients. *Kidney Int.* 28:830–38

206. Slomowitz LA, Monteon FJ, Grosvenor M, Laidlaw SA, Kopple JD. 1989. Effect of energy intake on nutritional status in maintenance hemodialysis patients. *Kidney Int.* 35:704–11

207. Soffer EE, Geva B, Helman C, Avni Y, Bar-Meir S. 1987. Gastric emptying in chronic renal failure patients on hemodialysis. *J. Clin. Gastroenterol.* 9:651–53

208. Spiegel DM, Breyer JA. 1994. Serum albumin: a predictor of long-term outcome in peritoneal dialysis patients. *Am. J. Kidney Dis.* 23:283–85

209. Steel DM, Whitehead AS. 1994. The major acute-phase reactants: C-reactive protein, serum amyloid P component and serum amyloid A protein. *Immunol. Today* 15:81–88

210. Stenvinkel P, Heimburger O, Paultre F, Diczfalusky U, Wang T, et al. 1999. Strong association between malnutrition, inflammation, and atherosclerosis in chronic renal failure. *Kidney Int.* 55:1899–911

211. Stenvinkel P, Heimburger O, Tuck C, Berglund L. 1998. Apo(a)-isoform size, nutritional status and inflammatory markers in chronic renal failure. *Kidney Int.* 53:1336–42

212. Stenvinkel P, Heimburger O, Wang T, Lindholm B, Bergstrom J, et al. 1999. High serum hyaluronan indicates poor survival in renal replacement therapy. *Am. J. Kidney Dis.* 34:1083–88

213. Stenvinkel P, Lindholm B, Lonnqvist F, Katzarski K, Heimburger O. 2000. Increases in serum leptin levels during

peritoneal dialysis are associated with inflammation and a decrease in lean body mass. *J. Am. Soc. Nephrol.* 11:1303–9

214. Stewart J, Schvaneveldt NB, Christensen NK, Lauritzen GC, Stein DM. 1993. The effect of computerized dietary analysis nutrition education on nutrition knowledge, nutritional status, dietary compliance, and quality of life of hemodialysis patients. *J. Ren. Nutr.* 3:177–85

215. Strujik DG, Krediet RT, Koomen GC, Boeschoten EW, Arisz L. 1994. The effect of serum albumin at the start of continuous ambulatory peritoneal dialysis treatment on patient survival. *Perit. Dial. Int.* 14:121–26

216. Subcomm. Tenth Ed. RDAs, Food Nutr. Board, Comm. Life Sci., Natl. Res. Counc. 1989. *Recommended Dietary Allowances*. Washington, DC: Natl. Acad.

217. Tabakian A, Juillard L, Laville M, Joly MO, Laville M, et al. 1998. Effects of recombinant growth factors on energy expenditure in maintenance hemodialysis patients. *Miner. Electr. Metab.* 24:273–78

218. Tan SH, Lee E, Tay ME, Leoo BK. 2000. Protein nutritional status of adult patients starting chronic ambulatory peritoneal dialysis. *Adv. Perit. Dial.* 16:291–96

219. Tayeb JS, Provenzano R, El-Ghoroury M, Bellovich K, Khairullah Q, et al. 2000. Effect of biocompatibility of hemodialysis membranes on serum albumin levels. *Am. J. Kidney Dis.* 35:606–10

220. Teehan BP, Schleifer CR, Brown JM, Sigler MH, Raimondo J. 1990. Urea kinetic analysis and clinical outcome in CAPD: a five-year longitudinal study. *Adv. Perit. Dial.* 6:181–85

221. Deleted in proof

222. Tielemans C, Husson C, Schurmans T, Gastaldello K, Madhoun P, et al. 1996. Effects of ultrapure dialysate and non-sterile dialysate on the inflammatory response

during in vitro hemodialysis. *Kidney Int.* 49:236–43

223. Tomura S, Nakamura Y, Doi M, Ando R, Ida T, et al. 1996. Fibrinogen, coagulation factor VII, tissue plasminogen activator, plasminogen activator inhibitor-1 and lipid as cardiovascular risk factors in chronic hemodialysis and continuous ambulatory peritoneal dialysis patients. *Am. J. Kidney Dis.* 27:848–54

224. Trznadel K, Lucaik M, Paradowski M, Kubasiewicz-Ujma B. 1989. Hemodialysis and the acute-phase response in chronic uremic patients. *Int. J. Artif. Org.* 12:762–65

225. Tsujinaka T, Fujita J, Ebisui C, Yano M, Kominami E, et al. 1996. Interleukin 6 receptor antibody inhibits muscle atrophy and modulates proteolytic systems in interleukin 6 transgenic mice. *J. Clin. Invest.* 97:244–49

226. Uehlinger DE. 1996. Another look at the relationship between protein intake and dialysis dose. *J. Am. Soc. Nephrol.* 7:166–68

227. US Ren. Data Syst. 1992. Comorbid conditions and correlations with mortality among 3,399 incident hemodialysis patients. *Am. J. Kidney Dis.* 20:32–38

228. US Ren. Data Syst. 1997. USRDS 1997 Annual Data Report. Bethesda, MD: US Dep. Public Health Hum. Serv., Public Health Serv., Natl. Inst. Health

229. US Ren. Data Syst. 1998. USRDS 1998 Annual Data Report. Bethesda, MD: US Dep. Public Health Hum. Serv., Public Health Serv., Natl. Inst. Health

230. US Ren. Data Syst. 1999. USRDS 1999 Annual Data Report. Bethesda, MD: US Dep. Public Health Hum. Serv., Public Health Serv., Natl. Inst. Health

231. US Ren. Data Syst. 2000. USRDS 2000 Annual Data Report. Bethesda, MD: US Dep. Public Health Hum. Serv., Public Health Serv., Natl. Inst. Health

232. Uribarri J, Leibowtiz J, Dimaano F. 1998. Caloric intake in a group of peritoneal

dialysis patients. *Am. J. Kidney Dis.* 32:1019–22

233. Utermann G, Menzel HJ, Kraft HG, Duba HC, Kemmler HG, et al. 1987. Lp(a) glycoprotein phenotypes; inheritance and relation to Lp(a)-lipoprotein concentrations in plasma. *J. Clin. Invest.* 80:458–65

234. Vaziri ND, Gonzakes EC, Wang J, Said S. 1994. Blood coagulation, fibrinolytic, and inhibitory proteins in end-stage renal disease. *Am. J. Kidney Dis.* 23:828–35

235. Wade DP, Clarke JG, Lindahl GE, Liu AC, Zysow BR, et al. 1993. Genetic influences on lipoprotein(a) concentrations. *Biochem. Soc. Trans.* 21:499–502

236. Wanner C, Bartens W, Walz G, Nauck M, Schollmeyer P. 1995. Protein loss and genetic polymorphism of apolipoprotein(a) modulate serum lipoprotein(a) in CAPD patients. *Nephrol. Dial. Transplant.* 10:75–81

237. Williams AJ, McArley A. 1999. Body composition, treatment time, and outcome in hemodialysis. *J. Ren. Nutr.* 9:157–62

238. Wilmore DW. 1991. Catabolic illness—strategies for enhancing recovery. *N. Engl. J. Med.* 325:695–702

239. Wilson DE, Birchfield GR, Hejai JS, Ward JH, Samlowski WE. 1989. Hypocholesterolemia in patients treated with interleukin-2: appearance of remnant-like lipoproteins. *J. Clin. Oncol.* 7:1573–77

240. Wolfe RA, Ashby VB, Daugirdas JT, Agodoa LYC, Jones CA, et al. 2000. Body size, dose of dialysis and mortality. *Am. J. Kidney Dis.* 35:80–88

241. Wolfson M, Strong CJ, Minturn D, Gray DK, Kopple JD. 1984. Nutritional status and lymphocyte function in maintenance hemodialysis patients. *Am. J. Clin. Nutr.* 39:547–55

242. Woodrow G, Oldroyd B, Turney JH, Tompkins L, Brownjohn AM, et al. 1996. Whole body and regional body composition in patients with chronic renal failure. *Nephrol. Dial. Transplant.* 11:1613–18

243. Wright RA, Clemente R, Wathen R. 1984. Gastric emptying in patients with chronic renal failure receiving hemodialysis. *Arch. Intern. Med.* 144:495–96

244. Yeun JY, Kaysen GA. 1997. Acute phase proteins and peritoneal dialysate albumin loss are the main determinants of serum albumin in peritoneal dialysis patients. *Am. J. Kidney Dis.* 30:923–27

245. Yeun JY, Levine RA, Mantadilok V, Kaysen GA. 2000. C-reactive protein predicts all-cause and cardiovascular mortality in hemodialysis patients. *Am. J. Kidney Dis.* 35:469–76

246. Young GA, Kopple JD, Lindholm B, Vonesh EF, DeVicchi A, et al. 1991. Nutritional assessment of continuous ambulatory peritoneal dialysis patients. *Am. J. Kidney Dis.* 17:462–71

247. Young GA, Woodrow G, Kendall S, Oldroyd B, Turney JH, et al. 1997. Increased plasma leptin/fat ratio in patients with chronic renal failure: a cause for malnutrition? *Nephrol. Dial. Transplant.* 12:2318–23

248. Zimmerman J, Herrlinger S, Pruy A, Metzger T, Wanner C. 1999. Inflammation enhances cardiovascular risk and mortality in hemodialysis patients. *Kidney Int.* 55:648–58

Annu. Rev. Nutr. 2001. 21:381–406

# INHIBITION OF CARCINOGENESIS BY DIETARY POLYPHENOLIC COMPOUNDS

Chung S Yang, Janelle M Landau, Mou-Tuan Huang, and Harold L Newmark

*Department of Chemical Biology, College of Pharmacy, Rutgers, The State University of New Jersey, Piscataway, NJ 08854-8020; e-mail: csyang@rci.rutgers.edu*

■ **Abstract** Plants consumed by humans contain thousands of phenolic compounds. The effects of dietary polyphenols are of great current interest due to their antioxidative and possible anticarcinogenic activities. A popular belief is that dietary polyphenols are anticarcinogens because they are antioxidants, but direct evidence for this supposition is lacking. This chapter reviews the inhibition of tumorigenesis by phenolic acids and derivatives, tea and catechins, isoflavones and soy preparations, quercetin and other flavonoids, resveratrol, and lignans as well as the mechanisms involved based on studies in vivo and in vitro. Polyphenols may inhibit carcinogenesis by affecting the molecular events in the initiation, promotion, and progression stages. Isoflavones and lignans may influence tumor formation by affecting estrogen-related activities. The bioavailability of the dietary polyphenols is discussed extensively, because the tissue levels of the effective compounds determine the biological activity. Understanding the bioavailability and blood and tissue levels of polyphenols is also important in extrapolating results from studies in cell lines to animal models and humans. Epidemiological studies concerning polyphenol consumption and human cancer risk suggest the protective effects of certain food items and polyphenols, but more studies are needed for clear-cut conclusions. Perspectives on the application of dietary polyphenols for the prevention of human cancer and possible concerns on the consumption of excessive amounts of polyphenols are discussed.

## CONTENTS

# INTRODUCTION

Phenolic compounds comprise one of the largest and most ubiquitous group of plant metabolites. They are formed to protect the plant from photosynthetic stress, reactive oxygen species, wounds, and herbivores. Phenolic compounds are an important part of the human diet. The most commonly occurring ones in foods are flavonoids and phenolic acids. Early interest in polyphenols was related to their "antinutritional" effects, i.e. decreasing absorption and digestibility of food because of their ability to bind proteins and minerals. The astringency of many fruits and beverages is due to the precipitation of salivary proteins with plant polyphenols. Current interest stems from the observations that dietary polyphenolic compounds have antioxidative, antiinflammatory, and anticarcinogenic activities. This chapter discusses these activities in light of their biochemical properties and bioavailabilities, with the goal of understanding the potential of dietary polyphenolic compounds in cancer prevention.

# DIETARY SOURCES AND CHEMICAL PROPERTIES

All plant phenolic compounds arise from the common intermediate, phenylalanine, or its close precursor, shikimic acid. They can be divided into at least ten different classes based on their general chemical structures (88). The plant phenolic compounds in the human diet are numerous; we have chosen selected groups of polyphenols for discussion, with emphasis on possible applications for the prevention of cancer. Some representative structures are shown in Figure 1. Many of these compounds are usually glycosylated by sugars such as glucose, rhamnose, galactose, and arabinose.

## Phenolic Acids and Derivatives

Hydroxybenzoic acids and hydroxycinnamic acids are abundant in food and may account for about one third of the phenolic compounds in our diet. These

### Phenolic acids and derivatives

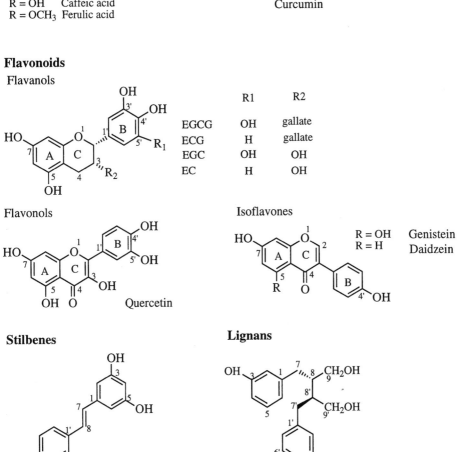

R = OH     Caffeic acid
R = OCH₃ Ferulic acid

Curcumin

### Flavonoids
Flavanols

| | R1 | R2 |
|------|-----|--------|
| EGCG | OH | gallate |
| ECG | H | gallate |
| EGC | OH | OH |
| EC | H | OH |

Flavonols

Quercetin

Isoflavones

R = OH   Genistein
R = H    Daidzein

### Stilbenes

### Lignans

Resveratrol

Enterodiol

**Figure 1** Representative structures of selected classes of dietary polyphenols. EGCG, (−)-epigallocatechin-3-gallate; ECG, (−)-epicatechin-3-gallate; EGC, (−)-epigallocatechin; EC, (−)-epicatechin.

compounds are found as esters, which are either soluble and accumulate in vacuoles or insoluble as cell-wall components. The most frequently encountered hydroxycinnamic acids are caffeic acid and ferulic acid. Caffeic acid is found in many fruits such as apple, plum, tomato, and grape. Ferulic acid is linked through ester bonds to hemicellulose of the cell wall, and is found in food sources such as wheat bran (5 mg/g). Derivatives of hydroxycinnamic acid are found in almost every plant. Those of interest include chlorogenic acid (a caffeoyl ester) and curcumin. Chlorogenic acid, which is present in many fruits and vegetables and in coffee (about 7% of the dried beans), is the key substrate for enzymatic oxidation that leads to browning, particularly in apples and pears. Curcumin, which contains two ferulic acid molecules linked by a methylene, with a $\beta$-diketone structure in a highly conjugated system, is the major yellow pigment in turmeric and mustard. It is used widely as a food preservative and yellow coloring agent for foods, drugs, and cosmetics.

## Flavonoids

Flavonoids are the largest class of phenolic compounds; over 5000 compounds have been described. They are mainly classified into flavones, flavanols (catechins), isoflavones, flavonols, flavanones, and anthocyanins. All are structurally related to the parent compound, flavone (2-phenylbenzopyrone).

*Flavanols*   The main flavanols are catechins, which are abundant in tea, red wine, and chocolate. Grape and chocolate catechins are mainly (+)-catechin and (−)-epicatechin (EC), whereas tea catechins also have galloyl esters of catechins as major components. Proanthocyanidins are polymeric flavanols (4 to 11 units) that are present in plant materials such as grape seeds (reviewed in 80a). Red wine contains more flavonoids than grape juice because the winemaking process extracts some of the flavonoids from the seeds and skins of grapes.

*Flavonols*   Quercetin is the main flavonol in the human diet, present in many fruits, vegetables, and beverages. It is particularly abundant in onions (0.3 mg/g fresh weight) and tea (10–25 mg/L). Quercetin usually occurs as $O$-glycosides, with D-glucose as the most frequent sugar residue. More than 170 different quercetin glycosides have been identified.

*Isoflavones*   Soybeans are the only significant dietary source of isoflavones. The primary isoflavones in soy are genistein and daidzein (approximately 1 mg/g dry bean), which are generally considered as phytoestrogens.

## Stilbenes

Stilbenes contain two phenyl compounds connected by a 2-carbon methylene bridge. They occur in nature in a rather restricted distribution. Most stilbenes in plants act as antifungal phytoalexins, compounds that are usually synthesized only in response to infection or injury. The most extensively studied stilbene is *trans*-resveratrol (3,5,4′-trihydroxystilbene), which is present in grapes, wine, and peanuts. Red wine contains 1.5 to 3.0 mg resveratrol/L.

## Lignans

Lignans are diphenolic compounds that contain a 2,3-dibenzylbutane structure that is formed by the dimerization of two cinnamic acid residues. Most lignans appear to pass through the intestinal tract as fiber. Dietary secoisolariciresinol diglycoside (SDG) and matairesinol, however, can be converted by intestinal microflora to the mammalian lignans, enterodiol and enterolactone, which are absorbed through enterohepatic circulation. Flaxseed meal and flour are the richest source of SDG and matairesinol.

## Dietary Intake of Phenolic Compounds

The diversity of the chemical structures and variability in foods make calculating the phenolic content in food difficult. A recent publication has confirmed the previously reported daily phenolic intake of 1 g (81). Other recent calculations of dietary intake were based on only a few specific flavonoids, which, of course, yielded much lower values. One study in Holland on flavonols and flavones estimated the average intake at 23 mg/day (27). A second group in Denmark estimated the intake of flavones, flavonols, and flavanones to be 28 mg/day (54). Another calculation indicated that vegetables (including dry legumes) might provide up to 218 mg of total phenols/day in an average US diet (102). This is likely to be an overestimation based on the use of the Folin assay, which cannot distinguish between phenolics and ascorbic acid. Fruits are usually richer in polyphenols than vegetables, with total phenolic content as high as 1–2 g/100 g fresh weight in certain fruits. Another major source of polyphenols is beverages such as red wine, coffee, tea, and fruit juices. Their consumption varies significantly among individuals. For example, tea drinkers may consume 200 to 800 mg catechins (in 1 to 4 cups of green tea) per day.

## Antioxidative Properties

Plant polyphenols are well recognized for their antioxidative activities. They scavenge free radicals, thus breaking the free radical chain reaction of lipid peroxidation. The main structural features for these activities are exemplified by the ortho-dihydroxy structure in the B-ring, 2,3 double bond in conjunction with a 4-keto function, and hydroxyl groups at positions 3 and 5 in flavonols, the di- and trihydroxyphenol structures in catechins, and the side chain double bonds in conjugation with the ortho-dihydroxyphenol structure in caffeic acid. Polyphenols also quench reactive oxygen and nitrogen species generated in biological systems. Another antioxidative mechanism is the chelation of metals such as iron and copper ions, which prevent their participation in Fenton-type reactions and the generation of highly reactive hydroxyl radicals. This ability to react with metal ions, however, also enables polyphenols to act as pro-oxidants. Using three different oxidation systems, flavonoids were shown to be potent antioxidants against peroxyl and hydroxyl radicals, but to be pro-oxidants with $Cu^{2+}$ (10). The reduction of $Cu^{2+}$ to $Cu^+$ by flavonoids may produce the initiation radical. Caffeic acid also showed pro-oxidant activity on $Cu^{2+}$-induced low-density lipoprotein oxidation during the propagation phase (107). These pro-oxidant actions of polyphenolic compounds may be important in vivo in certain situations, for example, when tissue injury causes the release of free iron or copper.

Many investigators believe that dietary polyphenols have beneficial health effects because they are strong antioxidants. The scientific basis for this thesis is weak. Many of the claimed beneficial effects have not been convincingly demonstrated. Even when the effects are demonstrated in certain animal models, the results may not be due to antioxidative activities. The bioavailability of many dietary polyphenols is rather low and their tissue concentrations may not be high enough to display the effects observed in vitro.

## ABSORPTION, BIOAVAILABILITY, AND BIOTRANSFORMATION

The bioavailability of polyphenols is an important determinant in understanding their biological activities. Lack of understanding on this issue has led to excessive claims regarding the in vivo biological activity of polyphenols based on extrapolation from studies in vitro. The bioavailability varies greatly between different polyphenols. Factors influencing bioavailability include the chemical properties of the polyphenols, deconjugation/reconjugation in the intestines, intestinal absorption, and enzymes available for metabolism.

### Absorption

The intestinal absorption is the first step to be considered. A commonly accepted concept is that the polyphenols are absorbed by passive diffusion. For this to occur, the glycosylated polyphenols need to be converted to the aglycone by glycosidases in the food or gastrointestinal mucosa, or from the colon microflora. For example, polyphenol glucosides are hydrolyzed by human $\beta$-glucosidase in the intestine, whereas polyphenol rhamnosides need to be hydrolyzed by microflora $\alpha$-rhamnosidases in the colon. There is also evidence for the direct absorption of quercetin-4′-$O$-glucoside and cyanidin-3-glucoside, which have been detected in human plasma after ingestion of food containing these compounds (3, 66). Recent studies suggest that a glucose transport system may be involved in the absorption of quercetin-3-$O$-glucoside, which was more bioavailable than quercetin was in rats (67). Quercetin 3-$O$-rutinoside (rutin) was much less bioavailable than quercetin aglycone was in this study. The bioavailability of quercetin glucoside was also much higher than was quercetin rutinoside in humans, suggesting that the glucoside is actively absorbed in the small intestine (28). Cinnamic acid is absorbed by a $Na^+$-dependent, carrier-mediated transport process in the rat jejunum (104).

Carrier-mediated transport process may be a common process in the absorption of polyphenols. The effects of certain efflux pumps, such as P-glycoprotein and multidrug-resistant associated proteins, on the bioavailability of dietary polyphenols require more investigation.

## Biotransformation

The polyphenols are readily conjugated by glucuronidation, sulfation, and methylation in the small intestine, liver, and other organs. This concept is illustrated in Figure 2, using (−)-epigallocatechin (EGC) as an example. Glucuronidation is catalyzed by microsomal UDP-glucuronosyltransferases (UGT) utilizing UDP-glucuronic acid as the cofactor. Among the isoforms of UGT, the UGT1A family is the main source of enzymes for the glucuronidation of polyphenols (81), but the UGT enzymes responsible for the conjugation of different polyphenols still need to be characterized. Sulfation is catalyzed by cytosolic sulfotransferases (SULT) with 3′-phosphoadenosine 5′-phosphosulfate (PAPS) as the sulfate donor. Although phenol SULT (SULT1A) catalyzes the sulfation of phenols, the roles of different SULT isoforms in the conjugation of different types of polyphenols require further investigation. Catechol-$O$-methyltransferase (COMT) catalyzes the transfer of a methyl group to polyphenols from S-adenosylmethionine (SAM). The polyphenol molecule provides multiple potential sites for these reactions. For example, the molecule can be methylated followed by glucuronidation or sulfation at other sites. The sequence and extent of these reactions depends on several factors: (*a*) substrate specificity of the enzyme that determines the reactivity and the position of the conjugation; (*b*) the availability of the conjugating enzymes and

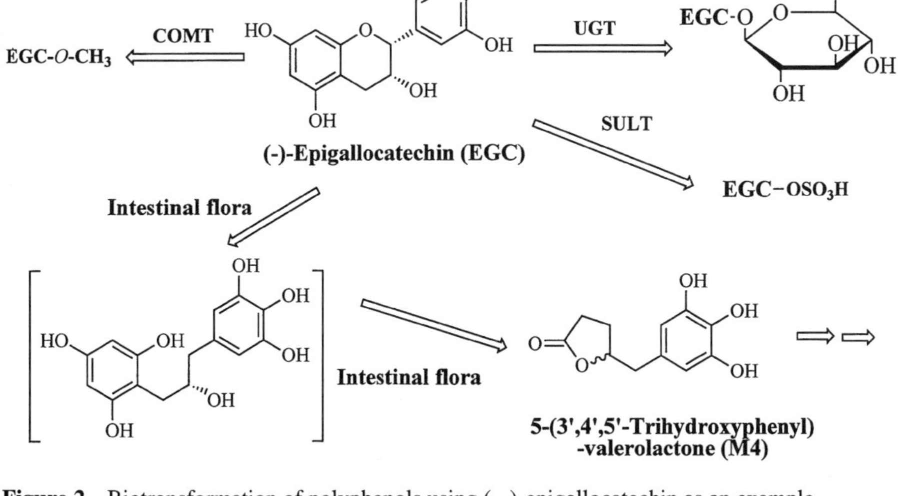

**Figure 2**   Biotransformation of polyphenols using (−)-epigallocatechin as an example.

their respective cofactors that are affected by species differences, genetic polymorphism, enzyme induction, diet, and metabolic state; (c) the doses of dietary
polyphenols and competing substrates such as medication that may saturate the
enzyme system or deplete the cofactors, and thus affect the extent of conjugation.
The extent of conjugation is dose- and time-dependent and has large individual
variabilities. Conjugation of polyphenols affects their biological fate; for example,
administration of piperine (an inhibitor of UGT) markedly increases the level of
serum curcumin in rats and humans (83).

Phase I metabolism is important for some polyphenols. Compounds containing double bonds are subject to reductive metabolism. For example, curcumin
is converted to tetrahydrocurcumin in the intestinal tract. Cytochrome P450 enzymes can oxidize and create additional phenolic groups on the ring or to catalyze
the O-demethylation of the methylated polyphenols. These reactions may take
place only with compounds having a low number of phenolic groups. Extensively
hydroxylated polyphenols may be too hydrophilic to be substrates of cytochrome
P450 enzymes.

## Microbial Degradation and Enterohepatic Circulation

Dietary polyphenols refractory to absorption in the upper gastrointestinal tract enter
into the colon. Conjugated polyphenol metabolites excreted in the bile also reach
the colon and are deconjugated by microflora hydrolases. The colon microflora
can form reductive and ring-fission metabolites, which can be absorbed. For example, dietary lignans are converted to enterodiol and enterolactone in the colon and
undergo enterohepatic circulation in which they are absorbed, transported to the
liver, and secreted in bile. Ring fission compounds of EGC such as trihydroxyphe-
nyl-$\gamma$-valerolactone (Figure 2) (55) have been found in human plasma and urine
(mostly in glucuronide and sulfate forms). Further degradation of the valerolactone
moiety to propionic acid and carboxylic acid is also expected based on the results
from (+)-catechin (30). The variability in the populations of intestinal microflora
adds to the individual and species differences in the absorption and biotransformation of dietary polyphenols.

A survey of the published bioavailability studies shows that human plasma
concentrations of intact flavonoids do not exceed 1 $\mu$M when the polyphenols
are given in doses similar to those consumed in our diets (81). Our estimation on
plasma levels of tea catechins of moderate tea drinkers agrees with this assessment.
The peak value of plasma genistein after ingesting 60 g of baked soybean powder
is reported to be 2.4 $\mu$M (103).

## INHIBITION OF TUMORIGENESIS
## AND MECHANISMS INVOLVED

Many publications have described the inhibition of tumorigenesis by plant polyphenols. With an interest on dietary prevention of cancer, we rate the evidence the
strongest if the polyphenols were given in the diet, rather than by topical application

or injection. Polyphenols that are effective when given during the postinitiation period, i.e. by inhibiting tumor promotion and progression, are believed to be more useful in preventing cancer in humans than are polyphenols, which are effective only when given before and during the carcinogen treatment. Transplanted tumor models may be more relevant to therapy than carcinogenesis. Although the inhibition of carcinogenesis by dietary polyphenols has been studied extensively, the molecular mechanisms of action and their applicability to human cancer prevention are unclear. The relevance of many of the in vitro studies is uncertain, because of the much higher concentrations of polyphenols used in comparison to the tissue levels attainable via dietary intake. For many polyphenols, bioavailability and tissue levels are key factors in determining whether the agent is effective in specific target organs. Recently, many in vitro studies have been published on the modulation of oncogenes, tumor suppressor genes, cell cycle, apoptosis, angiogenesis, and related signal transduction pathways by polyphenols. In this review, we include only mechanistic studies that are relevant to the inhibition of carcinogenesis in vivo.

## Phenolic Acids and Their Derivatives

The inhibitory effect of topically applied caffeic acid, ferulic acid, chlorogenic acid, and curcumin on tumor promotion by 12-$O$-tetradecanoylphorbol-13-acetate (TPA) has been demonstrated (37). The test compound (1–20 $\mu$mol) was applied together with 5 nmol of TPA twice weekly for 20 weeks to the skin of mice previously initiated with 7,12-dimethylbenz[a]anthracene (DMBA), and dose-dependent reduction of tumor multiplicity (number of tumors per mouse) was observed. Among these compounds curcumin was most active. Additional studies indicated that desmethoxycurcumin and caffeic acid phenethyl ester (a constituent of the propolis of honey bee hives) were also active in this model (reviewed in 15). Caffeic acid, ellagic acid, chlorogenic acid, and ferulic acid (0.02–0.05% in the diet) also inhibit 4-nitroquinoline-1-oxide (4-NQO)-induced tongue carcinogenesis in rats (93). More recent studies indicate that curcumin (0.2% and 0.6% in the diet), administered to azoxymethane (AOM)-treated rats during the promotion/progression stage, inhibited colon tumorigenesis (46). The multiplicity of both the invasive and noninvasive adenocarcinomas was lower, and the apoptosis of colonic tumor cells was higher, in the curcumin-treated group. Curcumin (0.1% in the diet) also inhibited intestinal tumorigenesis in the APC$^{min}$ mice (60). Increased enterocyte apoptosis and proliferation as well as decreased expression of the oncoprotein $\beta$-catenin were observed in the curcumin-treated group. A similar inhibitory effect was found with caffeic acid phenethyl ester (0.03% in the diet), but not with quercetin or rutin (2% in the diet).

Curcumin (0.2% in the diet) also inhibited diethylnitrosamine (DEN)-induced hepatocarcinogenesis in mice; both tumor multiplicity and tumor incidence were significantly inhibited (12). Orally administered curcumin (0.5–4% in the diet) inhibited benzo(a)pyrene-induced forestomach, $N$-ethyl-$N'$-nitro-$N$-nitrosoguanidine-induced duodenal, and AOM-induced colon tumorigenesis (33). Orally administered curcumin, however, had little or no effect on chemically induced lung and mammary carcinogenesis in mice (26, 35, 36). In DMBA-induced mammary carcinogenesis in mice and rats, inhibition was demonstrated with dibenzoylmethane (which has a $\beta$-diketone structure similar to curcumin) but not with curcumin (35*, 84). Apparently, the bioavailability of the agent to the target tissues is a major determining factor. On the other hand, 1% curcumin in the diet reduced the incidence of $\gamma$-ray-initiated and diethylstilbestrol-promoted mammary tumors in rats (40). In the rat serum, low levels of tetrahydrocurcumin (300 nM) and curcumin (16 nM) were observed; these bioavailable compounds may cause the inhibition directly or by modulating estrogen actions.

Antiinflammatory activity, due mainly to the inhibition of arachidonic acid metabolism, is thought to be a key mechanism for the anticarcinogenic action of curcumin and perhaps other polyphenolic compounds. Curcumin inhibits cyclooxygenase (COX)-2 expression in human colon epithelial cells, and the activity is proposed to be due to inhibition of NF-$\kappa$B via blocking the phosphorylation of I$\kappa$B by IKKs (76). Curcumin (5–50 $\mu$M) also down-regulates epidermal growth factor receptor (EGF-R) and inhibits its activation by ligands in human prostate cancer cell lines (21). The importance of these mechanisms in cancer prevention remains to be demonstrated in vivo.

## Tea, Catechins, and Related Compounds

The inhibitory activity of tea against carcinogenesis has been demonstrated in different animal models for organ sites such as skin, lung, esophagus, stomach, liver, small intestine, pancreas, colon, bladder, and mammary gland (reviewed in 16, 45, 111, 113, 115). Both green and black tea preparations (2–4 mg tea solids/ml), when given to mice as the sole source of drinking fluid, inhibited UVB-induced skin tumorigenesis in DMBA-treated mice and in the UVB-induced complete skin tumorigenesis model (15). In the UVB-induced complete skin tumorigenesis model, caffeine was inhibitory, but decaffeinated tea only decreased the tumor volume. Green and black tea (in drinking fluid) and EGCG (given i.p.) also inhibited the growth of established skin papillomas in mice previously treated with DMBA/TPA or UVB/TPA.

Inhibition of lung tumorigenesis by tea preparations has been demonstrated in A/J mice (reviewed in 112). Administration of decaffeinated green or black tea to mice (as the sole source of drinking fluid) for 3 weeks starting 2 weeks before the 4-(methylnitrosamine)-1-(3-pyridyl)-1 butanone (NNK) treatment, or for 15 weeks starting 1 week after the NNK treatment, markedly reduced the number of tumors formed in the mice. In mice that had already developed adenomas at 16 weeks after the NNK injection, the progression of adenomas to adenocarcinomas was significantly inhibited by the administration of black tea from weeks 16 to 52. These experiments indicate that tea has broad inhibitory activity against lung carcinogenesis, and it is effective when administered during the initiation, promotion, or progression stages of carcinogenesis. A similar conclusion for the inhibition of skin carcinogenesis is also supported by strong experimental evidence. The protective effect of tea against colon carcinogenesis in other models, however, is less conclusive. Inhibitory activity has been demonstrated in some studies but not in others. Many studies did not show a protective effect against chemically induced breast cancer formation, except when a high-fat diet was used (80).

Many authors have considered (−)-epigallocatechin gallate (EGCG) as the active component of green tea because EGCG is the most abundant catechin, and cancer inhibitory activity of EGCG has been demonstrated. The inhibition of EGCG against skin, stomach, colon, and lung carcinogenesis (13, 106, 108) as well as the growth of human prostate and breast tumors in athymic mice (56) have been reported. Other catechins, theaflavins, and caffeine may also contribute to the inhibition of carcinogenesis. Theaflavins (a mixture of theaflavin and theaflavin gallates) inhibit lung and esophageal carcinogenesis (68, 116). Based on studies in the UV light-induced complete mouse skin carcinogenesis model with green tea, decaffeinated green tea, and caffeine, Conney et al postulated that the "lowering of body fat levels," mainly by caffeine, is a key factor in the inhibition of tumorigenesis (16, 38, 57). This concept may also be applicable to other models. In the inhibition of spontaneous lung tumorigenesis in A/J mice by brewed black tea and green tea infusions, mice in the tea-treated groups had significantly lower (10–16%) body weights than the control group, and the fat-pad weights were even more dramatically decreased (53). The inhibitory action of caffeine against lung tumorigenesis has been demonstrated previously in mice (106) and in rats (13).

## Quercetin and Other Flavonoids

When 30 $\mu$mol of quercetin was applied topically to mouse skin 2 h before or 1 h after each TPA application in a DMBA-initiated two-stage skin carcinogenesis model, the multiplicity of papillomas and incidence of carcinomas were markedly decreased (100). Oral administration of quercetin, however, did not prevent UVB-induced skin carcinogenesis in mice (87). Apparently, the bioavailability of the orally administered quercetin to the target organ is a key issue. When given i.p., quercetin and apigenin inhibited melanoma cell (B16-BL6) growth and metastatic potential in syngenetic mice (9). Feeding rats with quercetin or chalcone and 2-hydroxychalcone (0.05% in the diet), during either the initiation or promotion stage, inhibited 4-NQO-induced carcinoma formation in the tongue. These compounds also decreased cell proliferation and polyamine levels (61). Dietary quercetin inhibited DMBA-induced tumorigenesis in hamster buccal pouch (4). Quercetin and ellagic acid, when given during the initiation stage, also inhibited DEN-induced lung tumorigenesis in mice (48). Inhibition of DMBA-induced mammary tumorigenesis in rats by quercetin was observed in one study (101), but not in another (75).

The effects of quercetin and rutin on intestinal carcinogenesis have been studied by many investigators but the results are not consistent. In the AOM-induced colon carcinogenesis model, inhibitory action by quercetin and rutin has been observed in mice (20), but the lack of such an inhibitory effect (22) and enhancement of colon carcinogenesis (75) have also been observed in rats. In the APC$^{min}$ mouse model, quercetin and rutin (2% in the diet) also did not inhibit intestinal tumorigenesis (60). In a medium-term multiorgan carcinogenesis model in rats, quercetin (1% in the diet) inhibited tumor promotion in the small intestine (2). Treatment of colon cancer cell lines and primary human colorectal tumors with quercetin (10 $\mu$M) reduced the level of Ras protein (79). Apigenin, fisetin, and kaempferol were less active in this experimental system. In another study, quercetin and luteolin (20 $\mu$M) inhibited the proliferation and induced apoptosis of skin cancer cell lines A431 and other cell lines (38). Inhibition of EGF mediated EGF-R tyrosine kinase activity, the phosphorylation of EGF-R and other proteins, and the secretion of matrix metalloproteinase-2 (MMP-2) and MMP-9 were also observed. Orange juice, which is rich in flavonoids, or a naringin-supplemented diet inhibited the development of mammary tumors in DMBA-treated female rats on a high-fat diet (85).

The possible enhancement of carcinogenesis by quercetin is a concern. In addition to the enhancement of colon carcinogenesis by quercetin (75) as mentioned above, promotion of nitrosomethylurea (NMU)-induced mammary tumors in rats has been suggested (5).

## Isoflavones and Soybean

Soybean is rich in genistein and daidzein, which are commonly regarded as phytoestrogens. They have weak estrogenic activity, but can be estrogen antagonists at higher concentrations. Many studies have demonstrated an inhibitory effect against mammary tumorigenesis by soybean or soybean products (reviewed in 64, 95). Daily injection of genistein (0.8 mg/day) to rats starting at 35 days of age for 6 months reduced MNU-induced mammary tumor multiplicity, but daidzein was less effective (17). Exposure to genistein neonatally or prepubertally reduced the number of terminal end buds, and this may be a major factor for the reduced mammary tumorigenesis observed in animal models (52). A recent study showed that fermented soy milk (which contains larger amounts of genistein and daidzein than unfermented soy milk) and isoflavone mixtures, given to rats starting at 7 weeks of age, inhibited mammary tumorigenesis induced by 2-amino-1-methyl-6-phenylimidazo[4,5-b]pyridine (PhIP) (72). Although genistein is an inhibitor of protein tyrosine kinase and topoisomerase in vitro, its effect on these enzymes has not been demonstrated in these animal models.

A high-isoflavone diet inhibits MNU-induced prostate-related cancer in Lobund-Wistar rats (77). A soy protein–based diet also inhibited the growth and enhanced apoptosis of transplanted LNCaP prostate adenocarcinomas in nude mice (8). Inhibition of growth and enhanced apotosis of LNCaP cells by genistein were observed in vitro with an IC$_{50}$ of 40 $\mu$M (74). This concentration was much higher than the expected levels in the prostate. Genistein injection reduced the growth of tumor implanted in the dorsolateral prostate of rats, and this effect may be due in part to the down-regulation of the expression of EGF and HER2/Neu receptors (18). Dietary genistein (50 mg/kg body weight/day), soy phytochemical concentrate (0.2% of the diet), and soy protein isolates (20% of the diet) reduced the volume of transplanted murine bladder cancer in C57BL/6 mice (118). Reduced angiogenesis and increased apoptosis by the treatment were also observed. In a separate study with seven human bladder cancer cell lines, genistein (3–20 $\mu$g/ml) caused G2-M cell cycle arrest and inhibition of cdc2 kinase activity; daidzein and biochanin-A were less effective (91). Genistein (200 $\mu$mol/kg body weight), administered orally on 10 alternative days, inhibited lung tumor nodule formation in mice injected with B16F-10 melanoma cells (63).

The effects of genistein and soybean preparations on colon tumorigenesis are uncertain (reviewed in 95). In carcinogen-treated rats, both inhibition and no effect on ACF formation have been reported. Genistein was reported to increase the noninvasive and total adenocarcinoma multiplicity, but to have no effects on the multiplicity of invasive adenocarcinoma (78). In APC$^{min}$ mice feeding on a high-fat/low-fiber/low-calcium diet, treatment with soy isolates (with high isoflavone content) had no significant effect on the incidence, multiplicity, and size of intestinal tumor (86).

These studies indicate that dietary intake of soy preparations or genistein has the potential to inhibit experimental mammary and prostate carcinogenesis, probably due to its modulation of estrogenic activity. Again the bioavailability is a problem, as the injected genistein is more effective in inhibiting transplanted tumors.

## Resveratrol and Other Grape Constituents

Because of its presence in red wine, the biological activity of resveratrol has received considerable attention. When resveratrol (1–25 $\mu$mol) was topically applied together with TPA to mice in a two-stage carcinogenesis model, marked inhibition of the tumor incidence and multiplicity was observed. Resveratrol also inhibited the development of preneoplastic lesion in DMBA-treated mouse mammary glands in culture (42). In the AOM-induced colon carcinogenesis model, resveratrol administration (200 $\mu$g/kg/day) to rats reduced ACF formation and the expression of *Bax* and p21$^{CIP}$ in the mucosa surrounding the ACF (94). Resveratrol administration (i.p., 1 mg/kg/day) to rats inhibited the growth of innoculated Yoshida AH-130 ascites hepatoma (11). Administration of an extract of the herb *Polygonum cuspidatum* (which contained 8% resveratrol and derivatives) in the diet (1.2%) inhibited AOM-induced colon tumorigenesis and DMBA-induced mammary tumorigenesis in mice (M-T Huang, unpublished). On the other hand, resveratrol (and curcumin) was not effective in inhibiting mouse lung tumorigenesis induced by benzo(a)pyrene plus NNK (26).

The mechanisms of the inhibitory activity against tumorigenesis by resveratrol are not clear. Resveratrol was reported to be an estrogen agonist and antagonist, but only the antagonist action was demonstrated in growing rats (99). Inhibition of the expression and function of the androgen receptor in LNCaP cells by resveratrol was reported, but only at concentrations of 100 $\mu$M or higher (65). The suppression of prostate-specific antigen expression by resveratrol in these cells, however, was reported to be androgen receptor-independent (31).

The antiinflammatory activity of resveratrol is likely to be important in inhibiting carcinogenesis. Inhibition of COX activity (43) and suppression of COX-2 expression by resveratrol in different cell lines have been reported (69, 92). Resveratrol (2–5 $\mu$M) suppressed the transformation of mouse epidermal JB6P+ cells and induced apoptosis via a p53-dependent pathway (32). It induced apoptosis in THP-1 human monocytic leukemia cells by a Fas-independent signaling pathway (98).

A polyphenolic fraction from grape seeds, which contain catechins, procyanidins, and procyanidin gallates, inhibited TPA-promoted skin tumorigenesis in mice previously treated with DMBA (117). A diet enriched with red wine solids (solids from 750 ml of red wine per kg diet), which contained catechins, gallic acid, and other polyphenols, delayed the onset of tumors in the HTLV-1 transgenic mouse (14).

## Lignans and Flaxseed

The effects of lignans and flaxseed on tumorigenesis have been reviewed by Thompson (95). The mammalian enterodiol and enterolactone are produced in the colon from plant precursors such as SDG. Therefore, these compounds may exert a direct effect on colon tumorigenesis. Flaxseed or defatted flaxseed (2.5% or 5% in the diet) or SDG equivalent to that in the 5% flaxseed, when given to AOM-treated rats for 100 days, lowered the number of ACF and the number of aberrant crypts per ACF (44). The results suggest that the inhibitory effect of flaxseed is partially due to SDG.

Administration of flaxseed (5% in the diet) to rats for 4 weeks prior to injection of DMBA, or continuously until sacrifice, decreased the incidence and multiplicity of mammary tumors (82). Enterodiol and enterolactone have estrogenic activities. Similar to the effect of genistein, early life exposure to lignans apparently affected the mammary gland development, which caused the reduction of tumorigenesis. When 5% flaxseed or an equivalent amount of SDG was given in the diet to dams during pregnancy and lactation, the off-springs had a reduction in the number of terminal bud structures in the mammary glands (97). Feeding of flaxseed (2.5% or 5% in the diet) for 7 weeks, beginning 13 weeks after DMBA-treatment, to rats that already developed mammary tumors (~1-cm diameter), decreased the tumor size by over 50% as well as the number and volume of new tumors formed (96). Similar effects were observed with purified SDG or flaxseed oil (rich in $\alpha$-linolenic acid) fed at levels equivalent to those in 5% flaxseed; but flaxseed oil appeared to be only effective in inhibiting the growth of preformed tumors. Feeding flaxseed (2.5%, 5%, or 10% in the diet) to mice, for two weeks before and two weeks after injection of the melanoma cell line B16B26, reduced the number of metastatic lung tumors by 32%, 34%, or 63%, respectively (109).

## STUDIES IN HUMANS

### Tea and Catechins

A major constraint in extrapolating results from cell lines and animal models to humans is the bioavailability and tissue levels of the effective components. The pharmacokinetics of tea polyphenols have been studied in humans (110). The total peak plasma concentrations of EGCG, EGC, and EC (free plus conjugated forms) were around 2 to 3 $\mu$M or lower. These are much lower than the concentrations used in many studies with cell lines (reviewed in 113). If only the nonconjugated forms of tea polyphenols are considered, the concentrations are even lower. The biological activities of glucuronide, sulfate, and methylated derivatives and ring fission metabolites remain to be determined.

Many ecological, case-control, and cohort studies have investigated the effects of tea consumption on human cancer incidence (reviewed in 6, 7, 45, 50, 114, 115). The reduction of human cancer risk by tea consumption has been demonstrated in some studies but not in others. For example, several studies in Japan and China suggest that green tea consumption is associated with lower incidence of gastric cancer, but such an association was not observed in many other studies. Studies in Saitama, Japan, have shown that women consuming more than 10 cups of tea daily are likely to have a lower risk for cancer (all sites combined), and increased tea consumption was associated with lower risk for breast cancer metastasis and recurrence (39, 70). In a case-control study in Shanghai, frequent consumption of tea (green tea) was shown to be associated with a lower incidence of esophageal cancer, especially among nonsmokers and nonalcohol-drinkers (24). On the other hand, in the Netherlands Cohort Study on Diet and Cancer, consumption of (black) tea was not found to affect the risk for colorectal, stomach, lung, and breast cancers (25). A preliminary report associated with NHANES I follow-up study (10 years) indicated a general inverse association between tea consumption ($>1.5$ cups/day) and colon cancer in both males and females (90). This potentially very important study needs to be expanded.

The quantity of tea consumed and other lifestyle-related factors such as smoking and diet are likely to be important confounding factors. The different results on tea and cancer may be due to different etiological factors involved in different populations. Tea may be only effective against certain types of cancer caused by specific etiological factors. Additional research on the mechanisms of action of tea constituents and the development of useful exposure biomarkers for human studies, such as urinary and blood levels of tea constituents, are key to our understanding of the relationship between tea consumption and human cancer risk (114).

## Dietary Flavonoids

In a 25-year follow-up study on 9959 Finnish men, dietary intake of flavonoids was inversely associated with the incidence of cancer at all sites combined (49). The association was mainly due to lung cancer, with relative risk of 0.54 (highest versus lowest quartiles), and was not attributed to the intake of vitamin E, vitamin C, $\beta$-carotene, or total calories. Of the major dietary flavonoid sources, the consumption of apples showed an inverse association with lung cancer incidence. In a population-based case-control study in Hawaii involving 582 lung cancer patients, after adjusting for smoking and intake of saturated fat and $\beta$-carotene, an inverse association was observed between lung cancer risk and the consumption of onions, apples, or white grapefruits as well as the calculated total intake of quercetin (62).

Onions and apples are the main food sources of quercetin. Since onions are also rich in organosulfur compounds and apples are rich in phenolic acids and derivatives, the involvement of nonflavonoid compounds cannot be eliminated. It would be useful if biomarkers for the dietary intake of specific flavonoids were used in future studies. An approach in this direction was made by measuring plasma and urine levels of quercetin and kaempferol after ingestion of tea and onion (19). The plasma and urinary levels were low and the variations were large; more work in this area is needed.

The bioavailability, metabolism, and excretion of quercetin have been studied. In a study in ileostomized patients, 52% of quercetin glycosides from onions, 24% of pure quercetin, and 17% of rutin were absorbed without microbial degradation (29). The rate of urinary excretion of total quercetin in these subjects was highest after ingestion of the glycosides. A recent study found that, of the ingested quercetin glucosides, approximately 50% is absorbed probably as glucosides in the small intestines and subsequently metabolized (73). In a clinical trial, quercetin was injected i.v. to human subjects (23). Inhibition of lymphocyte protein tyrosine phosphorylation was observed during the period of 1 to 16 h after quercetin administration. Renal toxicity was observed when the dosage went up to 945 mg/m$^2$ (at 1-week or 3-week intervals). Quercetin pharmacokinetics were described by a first-order two-compartment model with median $t_{1/2\alpha}$ and $t_{1/2\beta}$ of 6 and 43 min, respectively.

## Isoflavone- and Lignan-Rich Foods

Many epidemiological studies have investigated the relationship between cancer risk and the consumption of food items that are rich in isoflavones and lignans (reviewed in 1, 51, 64, 95, 105). The lower breast and prostate cancer rates in Japan and China (as compared to Western countries) have been associated with the higher levels of consumption of foods rich in isoflavones and lignans (or higher urinary excretion of metabolites of these compounds). Because these two groups of populations are also very different in other dietary practices (such as the high meat and high fat content in the Western diet) and other habits, these cross section studies should be interpreted with caution.

Case-control studies are generally more informative, but the results on breast cancer from different studies are inconsistent (reviewed in 105). In studies in Singapore and Japan, high soy intake ($\geq 55$ g/day) or frequent consumption of bean curd ($\geq 3$ time/week) was associated with reduced breast cancer risks in women, but such an association was not observed in a large study in China. Bean curd consumption was inversely associated with risk for breast cancer in both premenopausal and postmenopausal Asian-American women who were foreign born, but not in Asian-American women born in the United States. In an Australian study, the risk of breast cancer was inversely associated with urinary excretion of equol (an isoflavone metabolite) and enterolactone. In a study in China, women with high levels of urinary isoflavones appeared to be associated with lower risk for breast cancer, and the association was stronger if the urinary excretion of both isoflavones and total phenols was taken into consideration.

In a prospective study with Seventh-Day Adventist men in California, frequent consumption of soy milk was associated with a reduced risk of prostate cancer (41). Bean curd has been associated with lower risk of prostate cancer among Japanese men, of gastric cancer among Japanese men and women, and of lung cancer among Chinese men. A reduced risk for gastric cancer was also associated with consumption of soybean ($\geq$5 kg/year) in China and Japan (reviewed in 51).

One of the proposed mechanisms by which isoflavones affect mammary tumorigenesis is through their effects on estrogens. Consumption of a 36-ounce portion of soymilk (113–207 mg total isoflavones) per day, starting on day 2 of a menstrual cycle until day 2 of the next cycle, by healthy normal cycling women reduced circulating levels of $17\beta$-estradiol and progesterone, but had no effect on luteinizing hormone or follicle-stimulating hormone (58, 59). The mean menstrual cycle length did not change. The mean daily serum levels of genistein and daidzein (free and conjugated forms at 15 h after soymilk ingestion) were 3.14 and 11.37 $\mu$M, respectively. The urinary recovery of isoflavones varied from 9% to 37% of the intake among the subjects. Consumption of soymilk also increased the excretion of 2-hydroxyestrone, but not that of $16\beta$-hydroxyestrone. When 60 g of baked soybean powder (containing 112 $\mu$mol genistein and 103 $\mu$mol daidzein) was given to volunteers, plasma levels of genistein and daidzein peaked after 6 h with values of 2.44 and 1.56 $\mu$M, respectively. The half-life in the blood was 8 h for genistein and 6 h for daidzein. Most of the subjects showed 2 or 3 peaks in urinary excretion over 3 days, probably due to enterohepatic recirculation. Total recovery from urine and feces was 54.7% for daidzein and 20.1% for genistein (103).

Daily feeding of soy preparations containing 45 mg isoflavones for 16 days, or 37.4 mg genistein for 6 months, to premenopausal women has been reported to increase proliferation of breast epithelium as well as plasma estradiol levels and the volume of nipple aspirate fluid. These results are suggestive of estrogenic effects and their implications in cancer risk needs to be studied carefully. The consequence of feeding infants with soy milk, thereby exposing them to high levels of phytoestrogens (95), needs to be investigated.

After consumption of flaxseed, more than 2 days are needed for enterodiol and enterolactone to return to baseline concentrations in plasma and urine (71), apparently due to enterohepatic circulation. Feeding 10 g raw flaxseed per day for 3 months to women did not change the menstrual cycle length, but lengthened the luteal phase length. No significant changes in sex hormones were observed, except for a decreased plasma estrodiol to progesterone ratio (95). The effect of consumption of flaxseed on human cancer risk is not clear.

# PERSPECTIVES ON CANCER PREVENTION BY DIETARY POLYPHENOLS

Numerous laboratory studies have demonstrated the inhibition of carcinogenesis by polyphenols. Nevertheless, these results should be interpreted with caution in assessing the contribution of dietary polyphenols to the reduction of human cancer risk. Some polyphenols identified in animals may have direct application, limited use, or no use in cancer prevention in humans based on the following mechanistic considerations.

1. Some polyphenols are considered cancer chemopreventive agents because they inhibit carcinogen activation, commonly catalyzed by cytochrome P450 enzymes, in vivo or in vitro. If the carcinogen used in the animal model is not a human carcinogen, then the agent may not be useful in humans. General inhibitors of cytochrome P450 enzymes are not useful, because they may affect their normal physiological functions such as in steroid metabolism.

2. Many polyphenols are considered chemopreventive agents because they induce phase II enzymes. In theory, induction of phase II enzymes may facilitate the elimination of certain carcinogens or their reactive intermediates. Caution is needed, however, in applying this concept to humans. The induction of phase II enzymes is probably an adaptive response to potentially harmful agents. For example, some phase II enzymes are electrophiles or pro-oxidants; at moderate doses, the effects may be beneficial, but toxic effects may be produced at high doses. In addition, some phase II enzymes participate in the activation of certain carcinogens.

3. Certain polyphenols inhibit arachidonic acid metabolism. Metabolism of arachidonic acid (and linoleic acid) leads to the production of many pro-inflammatory or mitogenic metabolites such as certain prostaglandins and reactive oxygen species. The inhibition of phospholipase $A_2$, COX, and lipooxygenase are potentially beneficial, and have been proposed as a mechanism in the chemopreventive action of curcumin and other polyphenols. Verification of such activities in human tissues will further substantiate this concept for cancer prevention.

4. Isoflavones and lignans are phytoestrogens and have been demonstrated to modulate hormone-dependent carcinogenesis in animals. As discussed previously, the time of administration of these agents during animal development is a key factor. In human applications, the possible estrogenic activity of high doses is a concern, especially in premenopausal women and infants.

5. Modulation of different oncogenes, tumor suppressor genes, and signal transduction pathways, leading to inhibition of cell proliferation, transformation, and angiogenesis as well as to the induction of apoptosis, has been proposed by many investigators as mechanisms for the chemopreventive activities of many polyphenolic compounds. As our understanding of the signal transduction pathways and the molecular events leading to carcinogenesis increases, more results in this area will become available from studies in cell cultures. These studies should be

integrated with studies in vivo in order to evaluate the applicability of these mechanisms in cancer prevention in humans. Comparison of the effective concentration of a polyphenol in cell lines with the levels achievable in animal and human tissues is of great importance.

6. Polyphenols are well recognized for their antioxidative properties. They are considered cancer chemopreventive by some authors, because polyphenols can quench or prevent the formation of reactive oxygen and nitrogen species, which play important roles in carcinogenesis. Evidence for these mechanisms, however, has been mostly circumstantial and more investigations are needed.

As is true with many agents, excessive amounts of polyphenols can be toxic, even though they are from dietary sources. The limited absorption of most of the dietary polyphenols may be considered as a protective mechanism. Strategies to boost tissue levels by using supplements or by manipulation of absorption should be implemented with caution. Flavonoids are reported to induce cleavage in the MLL gene and may contribute to infant leukemia (89). Again, it is not known whether this in vitro study can be extrapolated to human situations, because of the dose and bioavailability issue. More research in this area is needed and this publication calls attention to the possible problems with intake of excessive amounts of flavonoids.

Evidence on the prevention of human cancers has to come from human studies; both observational epidemiological studies and intervention trials are needed. Many epidemiological studies have demonstrated that reduced cancer risk is associated with frequent consumption of vegetables and fruits in general. Certain studies have reported the association with a specific type of food item such as apple, onion, or soybean. Although these food items are rich in polyphenols, the contribution by other compounds cannot be eliminated. For more precise information on the role of dietary polyphenols in cancer prevention in humans, reliable biomarkers for the consumption of specific polyphenols are needed, in addition to the use of dietary questionnaires. The association between the consumption of a specific type of polyphenol (or food item) and lowered cancer risk needs to be observed consistently in different studies, before dietary recommendations can be made. The National Cancer Institute and other institutions are pursuing human cancer chemoprevention trials. This subject has been reviewed (47). We hope discussions in this chapter are informative to the readers and useful to researchers in this area.

## ACKNOWLEDGMENTS

We are grateful to Drs H Adlercreutz, LU Thompson, and AH Wu for sending their reprints to us. We thank Ms H Phyu, Ms D Wong, Ms JH Ju, Dr S Prabhu, and Mr J Hong for their assistance in the preparation of this manuscript. This work was supported by NIH grant CA56673.

**Visit the Annual Reviews home page at www.AnnualReviews.org**

## LITERATURE CITED

1. Adlercreutz H, Mazur W. 1997. Phyto-oestrogens and Western diseases. *Ann. Med.* 29:95–120

2. Akagi K, Hirose M, Hoshiya T, Mizoguchi Y, Ito N, Shirai T. 1995. Modulating effects of ellagic acid, vanillin and quercetin in a rat medium term multi-organ carcingoenesis model. *Cancer Lett.* 94:113–21

3. Aziz AA, Edwards CA, Lean ME, Crozier A. 1998. Absorption and excretion of conjugated flavonols, including quercetin-4′-O-beta-glucoside and isorhamnetin-4′-O-beta-glucoside by human volunteers after the consumption of onions. *Free Radic. Res.* 29:257–69

4. Balasubramanian S, Govindasamy S. 1996. Inhibitory effect of dietary flavonol quercetin on 7,12-dimethylbanz[a]anthracene-induced hamster buccal pouch carcingoenesis. *Carcinogenesis* 17:877–79

5. Barotto NN, Lopez CB, Eynard AR, Fernandez Zapico ME, Valentich MA. 1998. Quercetin enhances pretumorous lesions in the NMU model of rat pancreatic carcinogenesis. *Cancer Lett.* 129:1–6

6. Blot WJ, McLaughlin JK, Chow W-H. 1997. Cancer rates among drinkers of black tea. *Crit. Rev. Food Sci. Nutr.* 37:739–60

7. Buschman JL. 1998. Green tea and cancer in humans: a review of the literature. *Nutr. Cancer* 31:151–59

8. Bylund A, Zhang J-X, Bergh A, Damber J-E, Widmark A, et al. 2000. Rye bran and soy protein delay growth and increase apoptosis of human LNCaP prostate adenocarcinoma in nude mice. *Prostate* 42:304–14

9. Caltagirone S, Rossi C, Poggi A, Ranelletti FO, Natali PG, et al. 2000. Flavonoids apigenin and quercetin inhibit melanoma growth and metastatic potential. *Int. J. Cancer* 87:595–600

10. Cao G, Sofic E, Prior RL. 1997. An-tioxidant and pro-oxidant behavior of flavonoids: structure-activity relationships. *Free Radic. Biol. Med.* 22:749–60

11. Carbo N, Costelli P, Baccino FM, Lopez-Soriano FJ, Argiles JM. 1999. Resveratrol, a natural product present in wine, decreases tumour growth in a rat tumour model. *Biochem. Biophys. Res. Commun.* 254:739–43

12. Chuang SE, Kuo ML, Hsu CH, Chen CR, Lin JK, et al. 2000. Curcumin-containing diet inhibits diethylnitrosamine-induced murine hepatocarcinogenesis. *Carcinogenesis* 21:331–35

13. Chung F-L, Wang M, Rivenson A, Iatropoulos MJ, Reinhardt JC, et al. 1998. Inhibition of lung carcinogenesis by black tea in Fischer rats treated with a tobacco-specific carcinogen: caffeine as an important constituent. *Cancer Res.* 58:4096–101

14. Clifford AJ, Ebeler SE, Ebeler JD, Bills ND, Hinrichs SH, et al. 1996. Delayed tumor onset in transgenic mice fed an amino acid-based diet supplemented with red wine solids. *Am. J. Clin. Nutr.* 64:748–56

15. Conney AH, Lou YR, Xie JG, Osawa T, Newmark HL, et al. 1997. Some perspectives on dietary inhibition of carcinogenesis: studies with curcumin and tea. *Proc. Soc. Exp. Biol. Med.* 216:234–45

16. Conney AH, Lu Y-P, Lou Y-R, Xie J-G, Huang M-T. 1999. Inhibitory effect of green and black tea on tumor growth. *Proc. Soc. Exp. Biol. Med.* 220:229–33

17. Constantinou AI, Mehta RG, Vaughan A. 1996. Inhibition of *N*-methyl-*N*-nitorosourea-induced mammary tumors in rats by the soybean isoflavones. *Anticancer Res.* 16:3293–98

18. Dalu A, Haskell JF, Coulard L, Lamartiniere CA. 1998. Genistein, a component of soy, inhibits the expression of the EGF

and ErbB2/Neu receptors in the rat dorsolateral prostate. *Prostate* 37:36–43

19. de Vries JH, Hollman PC, Meyboom S, Buysman MN, Zock PL, et al. 1998. Plasma concentrations and urinary excretion of the antioxidant flavonols quercetin and kaempferol as biomarkers for dietary intake. *Am. J. Clin. Nutr.* 68:60–65

20. Deschner EE, Ruperto J, Wong G, Newmark HL. 1991. Quercetin and rutin as inhibitors of azoxymethane-induced colonic neoplasia. *Carcinogenesis* 12:1193–96

21. Dorai T, Gehani N, Katz A. 2000. Therapeutic potential of curcumin in human prostate cancer. II. Curcumin inhibits tyrosine kinase activity of epidermal growth factor receptor and depletes the protein. *Mol. Urol.* 4:1–6

22. Exon JH, Magnuson BA, South EH, Hendrix K. 1998. Dietary quercetin, immune functions and colonic carcinogenesis in rats. *Immunopharmacol. Immunotoxicol.* 20:173–90

23. Ferry DR, Smith A, Malkhandi J, Fyfe DW, deTakats PG, et al. 1996. Phase I clinical trial of the flavonoid quercetin: pharmacokinetics and evidence for *in vivo* tyrosine kinase inhibition. *Clin. Cancer Res.* 2:659–68

24. Gao YT, McLaughlin JK, Blot WJ, Ji BT, Dai Q, Fraumeni JJ. 1994. Reduced risk of esophageal cancer associated with green tea consumption. *J. Natl. Cancer Inst.* 86:855–58

25. Goldbohm RA, Hertog MGL, Brants HAM, van Poppel G, van den Brandt PA. 1996. Consumption of black tea and cancer risk: a prospective cohort study. *J. Natl. Cancer Inst.* 88:93–100

26. Hecht SS, Kenney PM, Wang M, Trushin N, Agarwai S, et al. 1999. Evaluation of butylated hydroxyanisole, myo-inositol, curcumin, esculetin, resveratrol and lycopene as inhibitors of benzo[a]pyrene plus 4-(methylnitrosamino)-1-(3–pyridyl)-1-butanone-induced lung tumorigenesis in A/J mice. *Cancer Lett.* 137:123–30

27. Hertog MGL, Hollman PCH, Katan MB, Kromhout D. 1993. Intake of potentially anticarcinogenic flavonoids and their determinants in adults in the Netherlands. *Nutr. Cancer* 20:21–29

28. Hollman PC, Bijsman MN, van Gameren Y, Cnossen EP, de Vries JH, Katan MB. 1999. The sugar moiety is a major determinant of the absorption of dietary flavonid glycosides in man. *Free Radic. Res.* 31:569–73

29. Hollman PCH, deVries JHM, van Leeuwen SD, Mengelers MJB, Katan MB. 1995. Absorption of dietary quercetin in healthy ileostomy volunteers. *Am. J. Clin. Nutr.* 62:1276–82

30. Hollman PCH, Tiojburg LBM, Yang CS. 1997. Bioavailability of flavonoids from tea. *Crit. Rev. Food Sci. Nutr.* 37:719–38

31. Hsieh TC, Wu JM. 2000. Grape-derived chemopreventive agent resveratrol decreases prostate-specific antigen (PSA) expression in LNCaP cells by an androgen receptor (AR)-independent mechanism. *Anticancer Res.* 20:225–28

32. Huang C, Ma W-Y, Goranson A, Dong Z. 1999. Resveratrol suppresses cell transformation and induces apoptosis through a p53-dependent pathway. *Carcinogenesis* 20:237–42

33. Huang M-T, Lou Y-R, Ma W, Newmark HL, Reuhl KR, Conney AH. 1994. Inhibitory effects of dietary curcumin on forestomach, duodenal, and colon carcinogenesis in mice. *Cancer Res.* 54:5841–47

34. Huang M-T, Smart RC, Wong C-Q, Conney AH. 1988. Inhibitory effect of curcumin, chlorogenic acid, caffeic acid, and ferulic acid on tumor promotion in mouse skin by 12-O tetradecanoylphorbol-13-acetate. *Cancer Res.* 48:5941–46

35. Huang M-T, Lou Y-R, Xie JG, Ma W, Lu YP, et al. 1998. Effect of dietary curcumin and dibenzoylmethane on formation of

7, 12-dimethylbenz [a]anthracene-induced mammary tumors and lymphomas/leukemias in Sencar mice. *Carcinogenesis* 19: 1697–700

36. Huang M-T, Newmark HL, Frenkel K. 1997. Inhibitory effects of curcumin on tumorigenesis in mice. *J. Cell Biochem. Suppl.* 27:26–34

37. Huang M-T, Xie J-G, Wang Z-Y, Ho C-T, Lou Y-R, et al. 1997. Effects of tea, decaffeinated tea, and caffeine on UVB light induced complete carcinogenesis in SKH-1 mice: demonstration of caffeine as a biologically important constituent of tea. *Cancer Res.* 57:2623–29

38. Huang YT, Hwang JJ, Lee PP, Ke FC, Huang JH, et al. 1999. Effects of luteolin and quercetin, inhibitors of tyrosine kinase, on cell growth and metastasis-associated properties in A431 cells overexpressing epidermal growth factor receptor. *Br. J. Pharmacol.* 128:999–1010

39. Imai K, Suga K, Nakachi K. 1997. Cancer-preventive effects of drinking green tea among a Japanese population. *Prev. Med.* 26:769–75

40. Inano H, Onoda M, Inafuku N, Kubota M, Kamada Y, et al. 1999. Chemoprevention by curcumin during the promotion stage of tumorigenesis of mammary gland in rats irradiated with $\gamma$-rays. *Carcinogenesis* 20:1011–18

41. Jacobsen BK, Knutsen SF, Fraser GE. 1998. Does high soy milk intake reduce prostate cancer incidence? The Adventist health study (United States). *Cancer Causes Control* 9:553–57

42. Jang M, Cai L, Udeani GO, Slowing KV, Thomas CF, et al. 1997. Cancer chemopreventive activity of resveratrol, a natural product derived from grapes. *Science* 275:218–20

43. Jang M, Pezzuto JM. 1999. Cancer chemopreventive activity of resveratrol. *Drugs Exp. Clin. Res.* 25:65–77

44. Jenab M, Thompson LU. 1996. The influence of flaxseed and lignans on colon carcinogenesis and beta-glucuronidase activity. *Carcinogenesis* 17:1343–48

45. Katiyar SK, Mukhtar H. 1996. Tea in chemoprevention of cancer: epidemiologic and experimental studies (review). *Int. J. Oncol.* 8:221–38

46. Kawamori T, Lubet R, Steele VE, Kelloff GJ, Kaskey RB, et al. 1999. Chemopreventive effect of curcumin, a naturally occurring anti-inflammatory agent, during the promotion/progression stages of colon cancer. *Cancer Res.* 59:597–601

47. Kelloff GJ, Crowell JA, Steele VE, Lubet RA, Malone WA, et al. 2000. Progress in cancer chemoprevention: development of diet-derived chemopreventive agents. *J. Nutr.* 130:467–71

48. Khanduja KL, Gandhi RK, Pathania V, Syal N. 1999. Prevention of *N*-nitrosodiethylamine-induced lung tumorigenesis by ellagic acid and quercetin in mice. *Food Chem. Toxicol.* 37:313–18

49. Knekt P, Järvinen R, Seppänen R, Heliövaara M, Teppo L, et al. 1997. Dietary flavonoids and the risk of lung cancer and other malignant neoplasms. *Am. J. Epidemiol.* 146:223–30

50. Kohlmeier L, Weterings KGC, Steck S, Kok FJ. 1997. Tea and cancer prevention: an evaluation of the epidemiologic literature. *Nutr. Cancer* 27:1–13

51. Kurzer MS, Xu X. 1997. Dietary phytoestrogens. *Annu. Rev. Nutr.* 17:353–81

52. Lamartiniere CA, Murrill WB, Manzolillo PA, Zhang JX, Garnes S, et al. 1998. Genistein alters the ontogeny of mammary gland development and protects against chemically-induced mammary cancer in rats. *Proc. Soc. Exp. Biol. Med.* 217:358–64

53. Landau JM, Wang Z-Y, Yang G-Y, Ding W, Yang CS. 1998. Inhibition of spontaneous formation of lung tumors and rhabdomyosarcomas in A/J mice by black and green tea. *Carcinogenesis* 19:501–7

54. Leth T, Justesen U. 1998. Analysis of

flavonoids in fruits, vegetables and beverages by HPLC-UV and LC-MS and estimation of the total daily flavonoid intake in Denmark. In *Polyphenols in Food*, ed. R Amado, H Andersson, S Bardocz, F Serra, pp. 39–40. Luxembourg: Off. Off. Publ. Eur. Commun.

55. Li C, Lee M-J, Sheng S, Prabhu S, Winnik B, et al. 2000. Structural identification and characterization of two metabolites of catechins in human urine and blood after tea ingestion. *Chem. Res. Toxicol.* 13:177–84

56. Liao S, Umekita Y, Guo J, Kokontis JM, Hiipakka RA. 1995. Growth inhibition and regression of human prostate and breast tumors in athymic mice by tea epigallocatechin gallate. *Cancer Lett.* 96:239–43

57. Lou Y-R, Lu Y-P, Xie J-G, Huang M-T, Conney AH. 1999. Effects of oral administration of tea, decaffeinated tea, and caffeine on the formation and growth of tumors in high-risk SKH-1 mice previously treated with ultraviolet B light. *Nutr. Cancer* 33:146–53

58. Lu LJ, Anderson KE, Grady JJ, Kohen F, Nagamani M. 2000. Decreased ovarian homones during a soy diet: implications for breast cancer prevention. *Cancer Res.* 60:4112–21

59. Lu LJ, Cree M, Josyula S, Nagamani M, Grady JJ, Anderson KE. 2000. Increased urinary excretion of 2-hydroxyestrone but not 16α-hydroxyestrone in premenopausal women during a soy diet containing isoflavones. *Cancer Res.* 60:1299–305

60. Mahmoud NN, Carothers AM, Grunberger D, Bilinski RT, Churchill MR, et al. 2000. Plant phenolics decrease intestinal tumors in an animal model of familial adenomatous polyposis. *Carcinogenesis* 21:921–27

61. Makita H, Tanaka T, Fujitsuka H, Tatematsu N, Satoh K, et al. 1996. Chemoprevention of 4-nitroquinoline 1-oxide-induced rat oral carcinogenesis by the dietary flavonoids chalcone, 2-hydroxychalcone, and quercetin. *Cancer Res.* 56:4904–9

62. Marchand LL, Murphy SP, Hankin JH,

Wilkens LR, Kolonel LN. 2000. Intake of flavonoids and lung cancer. *J. Natl. Cancer Inst.* 92:154–60

63. Menon LG, Kuttan R, Nair MG, Chang YC, Kuttam G. 1998. Effect of isoflavones genistein and daidzein in the inhibition of lung metastasis in mice induced by B16F-10 melanoma cells. *Nutr. Cancer* 30:74–77

64. Messina MJ, Persky V, Setchell KD, Barnes S. 1994. Soy intake and cancer risk: a review of the *in vitro* and *in vivo* data. *Nutr. Cancer* 21:113–31

65. Mitchell SH, Zhu W, Young CYF. 1999. Resveratrol inhibits the expression and function of the androgen receptor in LNCaP prostate cancer cells. *Cancer Res.* 59:5892–95

66. Miyazawa T, Nakagawa K, Kudo M, Muraishi K, Someya K. 1999. Direct intestinal absorption of red fruit anthocyanins, cyanidin-3-glucoside and cyanidin-3,5-diglucoside, into rats and humans. *J. Agric. Food Chem.* 47:1083–91

67. Morand C, Manach C, Drespy V, Demingne C, Remesy C. 1999. Respective bioavailability of quercetin aglycon and of its glycoside in a rat model. In *Int. Conf. Food Factors: Chem. Health Promot., Kyoto, Jpn.* Abstr. no. S05-1

68. Morse MA, Kresty LA, Steele VE, Kelloff GJ, Boone CW, et al. 1997. Effects of theaflavins on N-nitrosomethylbenzylamine-induced esophageal tumorigenesis. *Nutr. Cancer* 29:7–12

69. Mutoh M, Takahashi M, Fukuda K, Matsushima-Hibiya Y, Mutoh H, et al. 2000. Suppression of cyclooxygenase-2 promoter-dependent transcriptional activity in colon cancer cells by chemopreventive agents with a resorch-type structure. *Carcinogenesis* 21:959–63

70. Nakachi K, Suemasu K, Suga K, Takeo T, Imai K, Higashi Y. 1998. Influence of drinking green tea on breast cancer malignancy among Japanese patients. *Jpn. J. Cancer Res.* 89:254–61

71. Nesbitt PD, Lam Y, Thompson LU. 1999. Human metabolism of mammalian lignan precursors in raw and processed flaxseed. *Am. J. Clin. Nutr.* 69:549–55

72. Ohta T, Nakatsugi S, Watanabe K, Kawamori T, Ishikawa F, et al. 2000. Inhibitory effects of bifidobacterium-fermented soy milk on 2-amino-1-methyl-6-phenylimidaz[4,5-b]pyridine-induced rat mammary carcinogenesis, with a partial contribution of its component isoflavones. *Carcinogenesis* 21:937–41

73. Olthol MR, Hollman PCH, Vree TB, Katan MB. 2000. Bioavailabilities of quercetin-3-glucoside and quercetin-4′-glucoside do not differ in humans. *J. Nutr.* 130:1200–3

74. Onozawa M, Fukuda K, Ohtani M, Akaza H, Sugimura T, Wakabavashi K. 1998. Effects of soybean isoflavones on cell growth and apoptosis of the human prostatic cancer cell line LNCaP. *Jpn. J. Clin. Oncol.* 28:360–63

75. Pereira MA, Grubbs CJ, Barnes LH, Li H, Olson GR, et al. 1996. Effects of the phytochemicals, curcumin and quercetin, upon azoxymethane-induced colon cancer and 7,12-dimethylbanz[a]anthracene-induced mammary cancer in rats. *Carcinogenesis* 17:1305–11

76. Plummer SM, Holloway KA, Manson MM, Munks RJ, Kaptein A, et al. 1999. Inhibition of cyclooxygenase 2 expression in colon cells by the chemopreventive agent curcumin involves inhibition of NF-κB activation via the NIK/IKK signalling complex. *Oncogene* 18:6013–20

77. Pollard M, Luckert PH. 1997. Influence of isoflavones in soy protein isolate on development of induced prostate-related cancer in L-W rats. *Nutr. Cancer* 28:41–45

78. Rao CV, Wang CX, Sim B, Lubet R, Kelloff G, et al. 1997. Enhancement of experimental colon cancer by genistein. *Cancer Res.* 57:3717–22

79. Richter M, Ebermann R, Marian B. 1999. Quercetin-induced apoptosis in colorectal tumor cells: possible role of EGF receptor signaling. *Nutr. Cancer* 34:88–99

80. Rogers AE, Hafer LJ, Iskander YS, Yang S. 1998. Black tea and mammary gland carcinogenesis by 7,12-dimethylbenz[a]anthracene in rats fed control or high fat diets. *Carcinogenesis* 19:1269–73

80a. Santos-Buelga C, Scalbert A. 2000. Proanthocyanidins and tannins-like compounds—nature, occurrence, dietary intake and effects on nutrition and health. *J. Sci. Food Agri.* 80:1094–117

81. Scalbert A, Williamson G. 2000. Dietary intake and bioavailability of polyphenols. *J. Nutr.* 130:2073S–85S

82. Serraino M, Thompson LU. 1992. Flaxseed supplementation and early markers of colon carcinogenesis. *Cancer Lett.* 63:159–65

83. Shoba G, Joy D, Joseph T, Majeed M, Rajendran R, Srinivas PS. 1998. Influence of piperine on the pharmacokinetics of curcumin in animals and human volunteers. *Plant Med.* 64:353–56

84. Singletary K, MacDonald C, Iovinelli M, Fisher C, Wallig M. 1998. Effect of the beta-diketones diferuloylmethane (curcumin) and dibenzoylmethane on rat mammary DNA adducts and tumors induced by 7,12-dimethylbenz[a]anthracene. *Carcinogenesis* 19:1039–43

85. So FV, Guthrie N, Chambers AF, Moussa M, Carroll KK. 1996. Inhibition of human breast cancer cell proliferation and delay of mammary tumorigenesis by flavonoids and citrus juices. *Nutr. Cancer* 26:167–81

86. Sorensen IK, Kristiansen E, Mortensen A, Nicolaisen GM, Wijnands JA, et al. 1998. The effect of soy isoflavones on the development of intestinal neoplasia in ApcMin mouse. *Cancer Lett.* 130:217–25

87. Steerenberg PA, Garssen J, Dortant PM, van der Vliet H, Geerse E. 1997. The effect of oral quercetin on UVB-induced tumor growth and local immunosuppression in SKH-1. *Cancer Lett.* 114:187–89

88. Strack D. 1997. Phenolic metabolism. In

*Plant Biochemistry*, ed. PM Dey, JB Harbourne, pp. 387–416. San Diego, CA: Academic

89. Strick R, Strissel PL, Borgers S, Smith SL, Rowley JD. 2000. Dietary bioflavonoids induce cleavage in the MLL gene and may contribute to infant leukemia. *Proc. Natl. Acad. Sci. USA* 97:4790–95

90. Su LJ, Arab L. 2000. Tea consumption and the reduced risk of colon cancer: results from a national prospective cohort study. *Proc. Ann. Meet. Am. Assoc. Cancer Res., 91st.* 41:Abstr. no. 5141

91. Su S-J, Yeh T-M, Lei H-Y, Chow N-H. 2000. The potential of soybean foods as a chemoprevention approach for human urinary tract cancer. *Clin. Cancer Res.* 6:230–36

92. Subbaramaiah K, Michaluart P, Chung WJ, Tanabe T, Telang N, Dannenberg AJ. 1999. Resveratrol inhibits cyclooxygenase-2 transcription in human mammary epithelial cells. *Ann. NY Acad. Sci.* 889:214–23

93. Tanaka T, Kojima T, Kawamori T, Wang A, Suzui M, et al. 1993. Inhibition of 4-nitroquinoline-1-oxide-induced rat tongue carcinogenesis by the naturally occurring plant phenolics caffeic, ellagic, chlorogenic and ferulic acids. *Carcinogenesis* 14:1321–25

94. Tessitore L, Davit A, Sarotto I, Caderni G. 2000. Resveratrol depresses the growth of colorectal aberrant crypt foci by affecting *bax* and *p21*[CIP] expression. *Carcinogenesis* 21:1619–22

95. Thompson LU. 2000. Lignans and isoflavones. In *Carcinogenic/Anticarcinogenic Factors in Food*, ed. G Eisenbrand, AD Dayan, PS Elias, W Grunow, J Schlatter, pp. 334–47. Dtsch. Forsch.gem., Ger.: Wiley-VCH

96. Thompson LU, Rickard SE, Orcheson LJ, Seidl MM. 1996. Flaxseed and its lignan and oil components reduce mammary tumor growth at a late stage of carcinogenesis. *Carcinogenesis* 17:1373–76

97. Tou JCL, Thompson LU. 1999. Exposure to flaxseed or its lignan component during different developmental stages influences rat mammary gland structures. *Carcinogenesis* 20:1831–35

98. Tsan MF, White JE, Maheshwari JG, Bremner TA, Sacco J. 2000. Resveratrol induces Fas signalling-independent apoptosis in THP-1 human monocytic leukemia cells. *Br. J. Haematol.* 109:405–12

99. Turner RT, Evans GL, Zhang M, Maran A, Sibonga JD. 1999. Is resveratrol and estrogen agonist in growing rats? *Endocrinology* 140:50–54

100. Verma AK. 1992. Modulation of mouse skin carcinogenesis and epidermal phospholipid biosynthesis by the flavonol quercetin. In *Phenolic Compounds in Food and Health II*, ed. M-T Huang, C-T Ho, CY Lee, pp. 250–64. Washington, DC: ACS Books Ser. 507

101. Verma AK, Johnson JA, Gould MN, Tanner MA. 1988. Inhibition of 7,12 dimethylbenz(a)anthracene and N-nitrosomethylurea induced rat mammary cancer by dietary flavonol quercetin. *Cancer Res.* 48:5754–58

102. Vinson JA, Hao Y, Su X, Zubik L. 1998. Phenol antioxidant quantity and quality in foods: vegetables. *J. Agric. Food Chem.* 46:3630–34

103. Watanabe S, Arai Y, Haba R, Uehara M, Adlercruetz H, et al. 2000. Dietary intake of flavonoids and isoflavonoids by Japanese and their pharmacokinetics and bioactivities. In *Phytochemicals and Phytopharmaceuticals*, ed. F Shahidi, CT Ho, pp. 164–74. Champaign, IL: AOCS Press

104. Wolffram S, Weber T, Grenacher B, Scharrer E. 1995. A $Na^+$-dependent mechanism is involved in mucosal uptake of cinnamic acid across the jejunal brush border in rats. *J. Nutr.* 125:1300–8

105. Wu AH. 1999. Diet and breast carcinoma in multiethnic populations. *Cancer* 88S:1239–44

106. Xu Y, Ho C-T, Amin SG, Han C, Chung F-L. 1992. Inhibition of tobacco-specific nitrosamine-induced lung tumorigenesis in A/J mice by green tea and its major polyphenol as antioxidants. *Cancer Res.* 52:3875–79

107. Yamanaka N, Oda O, Nagao S. 1997. Pro-oxidant activity of caffeic acid, dietary non-flavonoid phenolic acid, on $Cu^{2+}$-induced low density lipoprotein oxidation. *FEBS Lett.* 405:186–90

108. Yamane T, Takahashi T, Kuwata K, Oya K, Inagake M, et al. 1995. Inhibition of N-methyl-N'-nitro-N-nitrosogua-nidine-induced carcinogenesis by (−)-epigallocatechin gallate in the rat glandular stomach. *Cancer Res.* 55:2081–84

109. Yan L, Yee JA, Li D, McGuire MH, Thompson LU. 1998. Dietary flaxseed supplementation and experimental metastasis of melanoma cells in mice. *Cancer Lett.* 124:181–86

110. Yang CS, Chen L, Lee M-J, Balentine D, Kuo MC, Schantz SP. 1998. Blood and urine levels of tea catechins after ingestion of different amounts of green tea by human volunteers. *Cancer Epidemiol. Biomark. Prev.* 7:351–54

111. Yang CS, Chen L, Lee M-J, Landau JM. 1996. Effects of tea on carcinogenesis in animal models and humans. In *Dietary Phytochemicals in Cancer Prevention and Treatment*, ed. Am. Inst. Cancer Res., pp. 51–61. New York: Plenum

112. Yang CS, Chung JY, Yang G-Y, Chhabra SK, Lee M-J. 2000. Tea and tea polyphe-nols in cancer prevention. *J. Nutr.* 130:472S–78S

113. Yang CS, Kim S, Yang G-Y, Lee M-J, Liao J, et al. 1999. Inhibition of carcinogenesis by tea: bioavailability of tea polyphenols and mechanisms of actions. *Proc. Soc. Exp. Biol. Med.* 220:213–17

114. Yang CS, Landau JM. 2000. Effects of tea consumption on nutrition and health. *J. Nutr.* 130:2409–12

115. Yang CS, Wang Z-Y. 1993. Tea and cancer: a review. *J. Natl. Cancer Inst.* 58:1038–49

116. Yang G-Y, Wang Z-Y, Kim S, Liao J, Seril D, et al. 1997. Characterization of early pulmonary hyperproliferation, tumor progression and their inhibition by black tea in a 4-(methylnitrosamino)-1-(3-pyridyl)-1 butanone (NNK)-induced lung tumorigenesis model with A/J mice. *Cancer Res.* 57:1889–94

117. Zhao J, Wang J, Chen Y, Agarwal R. 1999. Anti-tumor-promoting activity of a polyphenolic fraction isolated from grape seeds in the mouse skin two-stage initiation-promotion protocol and identification of procyanidin B5-3'-gallate as the most effective antioxidant constituent. *Carcinogenesis* 20:1737–45

118. Zhou JR, Mukherjee P, Gugger ET, Tanaka T, Blackburn GL, Clinton SK. 1998. Inhibition of murine bladder tumorigenesis by soy isoflavones via alterations in the cell cycle, apoptosis, and angiogenesis. *Cancer Res.* 58:5231–38

Annu. Rev. Nutr. 2001. 21:407–28

# MEGALIN- AND CUBILIN-MEDIATED ENDOCYTOSIS OF PROTEIN-BOUND VITAMINS, LIPIDS, AND HORMONES IN POLARIZED EPITHELIA

## Søren K Moestrup[1] and Pierre J Verroust[2]

[1]Department of Medical Biochemistry, University of Aarhus, 8000 Århus C, Denmark, and [2]Inserm U538, CHU St. Antoine, 75012 Paris, France; e-mail: skm@biobase.dk, verroust@infobiogen.fr

**Key Words**   vitamin A, vitamin $B_{12}$, vitamin D, HDL

■ **Abstract**   Polarized epithelia have several functional and morphological similarities, including a high capacity for uptake of various substances present in the fluids facing the apical epithelial surfaces. Studies during the past decade have shown that receptor-mediated endocytosis, rather than nonspecific pinocytosis, accounts for the apical epithelial uptake of many carrier-bound nutrients and hormones. The two interacting receptors of distinct evolutionary origin, megalin and cubilin, are main receptors in this process. Both receptors are apically expressed in polarized epithelia, in which they function as biological affinity matrices for overlapping repertoires of ligands. The ability to bind multiple ligands is accounted for by a high number of replicated low-density lipoprotein receptor type-A repeats in megalin and CUB (complement C1r/C1s, Uegf, and bone morphogenic protein-1) domains in cubilin. Here we summarize and discuss the structural, genetic, and functional aspects of megalin and cubilin, with emphasis on their function as receptors for uptake of protein-associated vitamins, lipids, and hormones.

## CONTENTS

0199-9885/01/0715-0407$14.00

# INTRODUCTION

Uptake of nutrients is a main function of polarized epithelia facing such transcellular fluids as the gastrointestinal fluid, renal ultrafiltrate, cerebrospinal fluid, and various secretes. The transport of the substances occurs by nonspecific fluid-phase transfer and by means of specific channels, transporters, and receptors present in the apical membrane of the polarized epithelium. Whereas channels and transporters preferably account for the uptake of small substances (e.g. ions, amino acids, and monosaccharides), larger particles (proteins and lipoproteins) are pinocytosed or specifically endocytosed.

The concept of receptor-mediated endocytosis was established by Brown & Goldstein (12) on the basis of their studies of the uptake of low-density lipoprotein (LDL) and the identification of the LDL receptor. Later, many other endocytic receptors of different classes were identified and the molecular mechanism of endocytosis was characterized in more detail (65). In the plasma membrane, most endocytic receptors are clustered in the clathrin-coated regions, where the internalization is initiated (65). Clathrin heavy and light chains are organized in basket-like structures of the plasma membrane that pinch off the cytosolic side as clathrin-coated vesicles (35). The vesicles, which contain the receptors and their ligands, are subsequently uncoated and delivered to early endosomes that are acidified by ATP-dependent proton pumps. The low pH ($<5$) causes most ligands and receptors to segregate. The membrane-bound receptors recycle back to the membrane in small vesicular or tubular compartments, whereas the bulk of the volumen containing the ligands fuses with lysosomes. In this late stage of endocytosis, the ligands are degraded into their subcomponents (e.g. amino acids, fatty acids, cholesterol, vitamins, and hormones). Some receptor-ligand pairs deviate from this general scheme of receptor-mediated endocytosis (65). Endocytosis may, for instance, also occur in non–clathrin-coated regions of the plasma membrane (30), and the transport of ligands and receptors may follow other routes after internalization. Transferrin is an example of a ligand not released from its receptor after internalization (65). It recycles back to the membrane after delivery of iron in the endosome. The cation-independent mannose-6-phosphate receptor is an example of a receptor not only recycling back to the membrane but also trafficking between the endocytic apparatus (65) and the *trans*-Golgi network.

Receptor-mediated endocytosis in polarized epithelia (Figure 1) is, in principle, the same as in nonepithelial cells. However, some receptor-ligand systems in

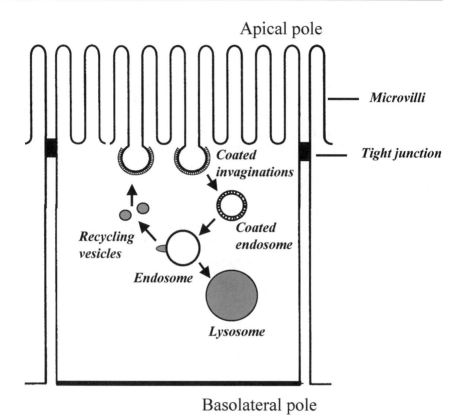

**Figure 1**  A schematic presentation of the polarized epithelial cell. Megalin and cubilin are apically expressed receptors in the invaginating coated intermicrovillar areas where they mediate uptake of ligands in the tissue fluid facing the apical pole. The receptors recycle via recycling vesicles, which pinch off the endosomes. The bulk of ligands are degraded in the lysosomes.

polarized cells are strictly allocated to either of the two functionally and biochemically distinct areas: the apical and basolateral membranes. The transferrin receptor (3) and the immunoglobulin A receptor (64) are examples of basolaterally expressed receptors, which pick up their ligands on the basolateral surface. Megalin (synonymous with gp330) and cubilin (synonymous with gp280 and IFCR) (59) are examples of membrane receptors expressed in the apical membrane, particularly in the invaginating clathrin-coated regions of the intermicrovillar surfaces (Figure 1).

In this review, we focus on the role of megalin- and cubilin-mediated endocytosis for the epithelial uptake of vitamins, hormones, and lipids bound to protein carriers.

## STRUCTURE OF CUBILIN AND MEGALIN

### Megalin

Megalin is a 600-kDa transmembrane protein (Figure 2) and the largest known mammalian single-chain receptor (~4600 amino acids) (32, 80). Megalin belongs to the LDL receptor family, which constitutes a small group of receptors that share common structural features (26). The 600-kDa, LDL receptor-related protein is the closest relative to megalin. cDNA cloning of the LDL receptor family proteins in humans and various species has disclosed a very high conservation of the receptors throughout evolution. For instance, a protein with a similar primary structure and almost identical composition of protein modules has been described in the nematode *C. elegans* (94). One common feature of receptors of the LDL receptor family is the presence of a least one ligand-binding region, represented by a cluster of LDL receptor type A repeats flanked by epidermal growth factor (EGF)-type repeats. Ligand interactions occur within the type A repeats, which are ~40–amino acid negatively charged calcium-binding (23) protein modules. Megalin is heterogenously glycosylated with various forms of N-glycans (63). Furthermore,

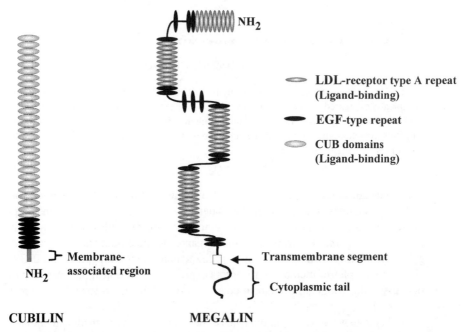

**Figure 2**  Schematic presentation of the modular structure of the 600-kDa megalin (32, 80) and the 460-kDa cubilin molecules (41, 59). LDL, low-density lipoprotein; EGF, epidermal growth factor; CUB, complement C1r/C1s, Uegf, and bone morphogenic protein-1.

megalin has a rare posttranslational modificationg by carrying the oligo/poly-$\alpha$2,8-deaminoneuraminic acid (97).

Megalin has a single transmembrane segment, a short cytoplasmic tail, and a large ectodomain containing four ligand-binding regions connected by YWTD propeller repeats and EGF repeats. The cytoplasmic tail of megalin contains three conserved Scr-homology binding regions, three proteinase kinase C phoshorylation sites, seven casein kinase II sites, and three $\Psi$XNPXY motifs (in which $\Psi$ represents a hydrophobic residue) mediating binding to adaptor proteins and the clustering in coated pits. Disabled protein-2, a mitogen-responsive phosphoprotein thought to be an adaptor protein involved in signal transduction, has been shown to bind to the cytoplasmic tail of megalin (68). Whether megalin is signal-transducing is unknown but other receptors of the LDL receptor family have been shown to mediate signal transduction (90).

## Cubilin

Cubilin is a 460-kDa glycoprotein (Figure 2) comprising $\sim$3600 amino acids. cDNA cloning of cubilin from rat (59), dog (93), and humans (41) has shown similarity in primary structure and an identical organization of 35 protein modules—eight EGF repeats followed by 27 CUB (complement C1r/C1s, Uegf, and bone morphogenic protein-1) domains. Cubilin has no classical membrane-spanning segment, but the amino-terminal region contains a $\sim$100–amino acid stretch of importance for membrane association (43). A putative amphipatic helix motif (43) and a potentially palmitoylated cysteine (M Kristiansen & SK Moestrup, unpublished data) in the amino-terminal region might be involved in the membrane attachment. The amino-terminal region also has a cleavage site (positioned between residue 10 and 11) for the Golgi proteinase furin (41).

The CUB domain region, which accounts for 85% of the entire protein, represents a region for ligand binding. CUB domains 5–8 and 13–14 have been disclosed as the regions responsible for binding intrinsic factor (IF)–vitamin $B_{12}$ (IF-$B_{12}$) and receptor-associated protein (RAP) (43). Genetic studies have identified mutations in CUB domains 5–8 as a cause of $B_{12}$ malabsorption (see below) (1, 42). Structural analysis of CUB domains of spermadhesins has shown that the domains consist of two layers of five-stranded $\beta$-sheets (77). The crystal structure of dimeric spermadhesin consisting of two CUB domains has revealed that the $\beta$-sheet layers from the two CUB domains can face each other (77). If the continuous 27 CUB domains of cubilin are connected with the $\beta$-sheet layers facing, the less-conserved $\beta$-turn regions may be surface-exposed like the antigen binding hypervariable $\beta$-turns in the Fab regions of immunoglobulins. From a structural point of view, the CUB domain region therefore seems to be a well-designed biological matrix for multiple protein interactions.

No other known receptors have close homology to cubilin, which has some structural relationship (59) to a number of EGF and CUB domain-containing proteins (e.g. the bone morphogenic proteins) involved in development.

**TABLE 1**   Main expression sites of cubilin and megalin[a]

| Site | Cubilin | Megalin |
|---|---|---|
| Kidney proximal tubule | + | + |
| Kidney glomerulus[b] | − | + |
| Ileum | + | + |
| Lung | + | + |
| Thyroid | ? | + |
| Thymus | + | + |
| Parathyroid | ? | + |
| Ependyma | ? | + |
| Eye, ciliary body | ? | + |
| Inner ear epithelium | ? | + |
| Choroid plexus | ? | + |
| Oviduct and uterus | + | + |
| Epididymis | ? | + |
| Yolk sac | + | + |
| Syncytiotrophoblast | + | + |
| Trophectoderm | ? | + |

[a]From References 28, 38, 50, 78, 81, 95.
[b]Only in rats.

# EXPRESSION OF CUBILIN AND MEGALIN

## Tissue Distribution

The main tissue expression sites of megalin and cubilin (79) are listed in Table 1. For both proteins, the expression is most abundant in the visceral yolk sac and in the renal proximal tubule cells, in particular the initial segments of the proximal tubule (19). These absorptive epithelia are characterized by high endocytic activity and degradation of the internalized components (14). Their apical poles are exposed to a wide panel of cubilin and megalin ligands. In the remaining tissues, cubilin and megalin is generally less abundant.

## Cellular Expression

The subcellular localization of cubilin and megalin has been studied in detail in the proximal tubule cell and the yolk sac (14, 19, 45, 46). The two receptors are strikingly colocalized (59) in the apical endocytic apparatus of the cells.

On the plasma membrane of renal proximal tubule and yolk sac, cubilin and megalin are mainly detected in intermicrovillar areas (19) (Figure 1). Within the cell, they are present in small and large endocytic vesicles, as well as in specialized electron-dense tubular-vesicular structures, which account for the recycling of internalized plasma membrane and receptors (19).

## Processing and Trafficking

The biosynthesis of megalin and cubilin has been described in visceral yolk sac and renal epithelial cells (4, 6, 52, 73–75). As expected for the two high-molecular-weight proteins, the maturation and membrane association are slow, the $t_{1/2}$ being 90 min for megalin and several hours for cubilin. The biosynthesis of megalin is marked by its suggested rapid association (within 30 min) with RAP, the endoplasmic reticulum protein important for the processing of megalin and LDL receptor-related protein (9, 91), another 600-kDa member of the LDL receptor family. RAP binds to multiple sites in the ligand-binding regions of LDL receptor-related protein (LRP) (2) and probably also in megalin (69).

The biosynthesis of cubilin is complex and deviates from that of megalin. Association with RAP during biosynthesis has not been demonstrated, and it is possible (93) that RAP has no importance for cubilin processing because RAP-deficient mice have normal cubilin expression (9). However, genetic analysis of dogs with an inherited lack of functional cubilin indicates that some sort of accessory activity is required for proper cubilin expression. In these dogs, the receptor accumulates in the endoplasmic reticulum, or the early Golgi (24, 25), instead of being processed to the plasma membrane. Genetic analysis has shown no linkage between the processing failure and the cubilin gene.

Pulse-chase studies in yolk sac epithelial cells have suggested that newly synthesized cubilin initially reaches the cell membrane in an immature (endo H sensitive) form, which has not been terminally glycosylated in the Golgi apparatus. Immature cubilin is then presumably recycled by as-yet-unknown pathways through the Golgi before its final expression on the cell surface (4). In the same cells, megalin is addressed to the plasma membrane in a mature endo H–resistant form. Recent studies (92) based on PNGase F and endo H digestion suggest that terminal glycosylation of cubilin may be less extensive in the kidney than in the ileum, indicating an organ-specific process. The posttranslational modification of cubilin may involve cleavage by furin, as suggested by the finding (41) that affinity-purified human cubilin is truncated at the furin cleavage site. Studies in opossum kidney cells suggest that cubilin may be palmitoylated (73).

Little is known about the mechanisms regulating the expression of cubilin and megalin. In vitro up-regulation of megalin by retinoids, vitamin D, or cAMP has been demonstrated in cultured rat kidney proximal tubule cells, human JEG-3 cells, and the mouse embryonic cell line F9 (21, 47). A comparative analysis has shown that cubilin and megalin are expressed at similar levels in F9 cells differentiated by retinoic acid (28).

Although cubilin clearly functions as an endocytic receptor, its primary structure, does not predict any classical transmembrane segment or signals for endocytosis. It is therefore tempting to suggest that cubilin trafficking is assisted by other structures. The following findings now indicate that megalin has such a function. (*a*) Megalin and cubilin coexpress at the cellular and subcellular level in several epithelia (59) and cell lines (21, 28). (*b*) Cubilin binds in vitro to megalin (59). (*c*) Megalin antibodies inhibit uptake of cubilin ligands (28, 40). (*d*) Megalin-deficient mice have an internalization defect of cubilin (R Kozyraki, J Fyfe, PJ Verroust, C Jacobsen, A Dautry-Varsat, TE Willnow, EI Christensen, SK Moestrup, manuscript in preparation).

## LIGANDS FOR CUBILIN AND MEGALIN

Table 2 lists the many ligands reported to bind to megalin and cubilin. This section deals with some general features of ligand binding to the two receptors. More specific aspects of individual ligands relating to ligands specific for various tissues are described in the next section, on the role of the receptors in various epithelia.

The ligands of both receptors are substances of different structure and function. A predominant group is represented by proteins having a carrier function for vitamins, lipids, hormones, and minerals. This group of ligands indicates a broad nutritional function of the receptors. Binding of other proteins, such as albumin and immunoglobulin G light chains, may merely reflect a general protein-rescuing function of the receptors for reuse of the amino acids. The nutritional perspective of this protein uptake applies to the kidney and, in particular, the yolk sac, where the receptors seem to account for a high protein reabsorption. Enzymes, enzyme-protein complexes, and toxins make up other groups of ligands. By scavenging these types of endogenous and exogenous substances, the receptors may indirectly regulate the toxicity of substances in the tissue fluids lining the polarized epithelia.

The ligands of megalin and cubilin bind with a wide range of affinities to the receptors. A high affinity may have a physiological rationale when the receptor density is low in certain tissues. For instance, IF-$B_{12}$ is an intestinal ligand binding with high affinity ($K_d = 1$–2 nM) to cubilin (8, 41). The high affinity is necessary for effective recognition by cubilin, which has a relatively low expression in the terminal ileum (92). Decreased affinity of the binding of IF-$B_{12}$ is known as a cause of $B_{12}$ deficiency disease (1, 42). On the other hand, a high capacity for uptake may compensate for the low affinity of a ligand-receptor interaction. Albumin reabsorption in the proximal tubules exemplifies such a situation. Cubilin/megalin–mediated albumin uptake (7, 20) accounts for a major part of the protein uptake in the proximal tubule, which has a dense expression of both receptors. Furthermore, the low affinity may cause a more even distribution of albumin uptake along the entire proximal tubule.

Megalin- and cubilin-mediated uptake of receptor-bound ligand ultimately leads to delivery of the bulk of ligand in lysosomes and degradation of the protein components. Nonprotein substances such as vitamins, hormones, drugs, and toxins escape degradation and will either accumulate or be transported out of the lysosomes to the cytosol.

**TABLE 2** Megalin and cubilin ligands[a]

| | **Megalin** | **Cubilin** |
|---|---|---|
| Vitamin-carrier complexes | $TC$-$B_{12}$<br>Vitamin D–binding protein, vitamin D<br>Retinol-binding protein, vitamin A | $IF$-$B_{12}$ |
| Lipid-binding proteins | Apo B<br>Apo E<br>Apo J/clusterin<br>Apo H/$\beta_2$-glycoprotein-I<br>Apo(a) | Apo A-I |
| Hormone/hormone-binding proteins | PTH<br>Transthyretin<br>Thyroglobulin<br>Insulin | |
| Mineral-binding protein | | Transferrin[b] |
| Drugs | Aminoglycosides<br>Polymyxin B<br>Aprotinin | |
| Toxins | Trichosantin | |
| Enzymes and enzyme inhibitors | PAI-1<br>PAI-1-urokinase<br>PAI-1-tPA<br>Pro-urokinase<br>Lipoprotein lipase<br>$\alpha$-Amylase | |
| Other | Albumin<br>RAP<br>Ig light chains[c]<br>$Ca^{2+}$<br>C1q<br>Lactoferrin<br>$\beta_2$-Microglobulin<br>EGF<br>Prolactin<br>Lysozyme<br>Cytochrome $c$<br>$\beta_1$-Microglobulin<br>PAP-1<br>Odorant-binding protein<br>Seminal vesicle secretory protein II | Albumin<br>RAP<br>Ig light chains<br>$Ca^{2+}$ |

[a]From References 5, 7–9, 13, 16, 17, 20, 29, 36, 37, 39, 40, 46, 56, 57, 60, 61, 66, 67, 70, 71, 76, 81, 83–86, 88, 96. TC, Transcobalamin; $B_{12}$, vitamin $B_{12}$; IF, intrinsic factor; Apo, apolipoprotein; PTH, parathyroid hormone; PAI, plasminogen activator inhibitor; tPA, tissue plasminogen activator; RAP, receptor-associated protein; Ig, immunoglobulin; EGF, epidermal growth factor; PAP, pancreatitis-associated protein.

[b]From unpublished data, R Kozyraki, J Fyfe, PJ Verroust, C Jacobsen, A Dautry-Varsat, TE Willnow, EI Christensen, SK Moestrup.

[c]From unpublished data (H Birn, M Leboulleux, SK Moestrup, PM Ronco, P Aucoutner, EI Christensen).

The binding of all megalin and cubilin ligands is dependent on calcium, which binds to the type A repeats of LDL receptor family protein (23) and probably also to the CUB domains of cubilin. Whether calcium is an integrated part of the receptor during the entire endocytic and recycling pathway or whether it is delivered in cells as a ligand is unknown. If a receptor-mediated net transport into the cell of calcium takes place, it might be a part of the nonregulated calcium transport system in the kidney (16). Furthermore, a megalin-mediated calcium transport might explain previous data indicating that megalin is a putative sensor for calcium in the parathyroid gland (32, 51).

The presence of basic motifs (e.g. heparin-binding sites) is a common feature of most ligands binding to megalin, and there is structural and functional evidence that electrostatic interactions between acidic regions of the type A repeats and the basic regions of the ligands are essential for the ligand-receptor recognition (57). Electrostatic interactions are probably also important for the pH-dependent binding of ligands to cubilin.

## MEGALIN AND CUBILIN FUNCTION IN VARIOUS EPITHELIA

### Intestine

Both megalin and cubilin are expressed in the intestinal epithelium, but only one physiological ligand is known so far—the IF-$B_{12}$ complex (8, 82).

The daily supply of vitamin $B_{12}$ (cobalamin) in food is limited to a few micrograms, which are transported and absorbed by means of specific carriers and receptors (Figure 3). Vitamin $B_{12}$ is initially bound to another vitamin $B_{12}$ binder, haptocorrin, which is degraded in the upper small intestine. Vitamin $B_{12}$ subsequently binds to IF, which is taken up in the terminal ileum by cubilin-mediated endocytosis. Only the vitamin $B_{12}$-bound form of IF is effectively recognized (8). The importance of IF for vitamin $B_{12}$ absorption is evident from the vitamin $B_{12}$ deficiency state (causing megaloblastic anemia and neurological symptoms) in patients with decreased production of IF. Uptake of IF-$B_{12}$ in the enterocyte is followed by degradation of IF, modification of the cobalamin and transport to the basolateral membrane, where the vitamin is released into plasma in complex with a third vitamin $B_{12}$ binder, transcobalamin (TC). The TC-$B_{12}$ complex is essential for transport and uptake in the organism. Megalin functions as a receptor for TC-$B_{12}$ uptake in the kidney (56), whereas another as-yet-unidentified protein functions as the receptor for TC-$B_{12}$ uptake in the nonepithelial tissues.

In agreement with the terminal ileum being the principal site for cubilin-mediated uptake of IF-$B_{12}$, a recent study of the segmental distribution of cubilin in the canine intestine has shown that the varied expression of cubilin parallels the IF-$B_{12}$ binding activity (92). Furthermore, the crucial role of cubilin for the

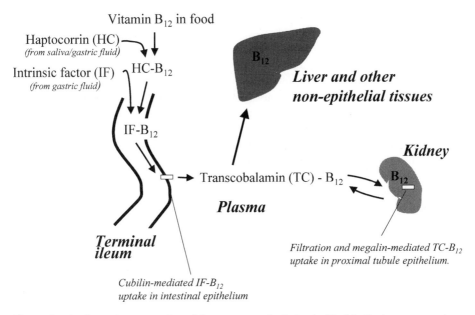

**Figure 3**   A schematic presentation of the transport of cobalamin ($B_{12}$) in the human organism. Cubilin accounts for the uptake of IF-$B_{12}$ in the terminal ileum. The vitamin is subsequently secreted into plasma in complex with TC. The TC-$B_{12}$ is essential for the general distribution of $B_{12}$ in the body. Megalin accounts for the uptake of TC-$B_{12}$ complex in the renale proximal tubule, which may function as a short-term storage site for $B_{12}$.

uptake of IF-$B_{12}$ in the intestine has been settled by the identification of mutations in patients with Imerslund-Gräsbecks disease, a rare condition (~200 cases reported worldwide) characterized by malabsorption of vitamin $B_{12}$ (27, 33). In many, but not all, cases, the vitamin $B_{12}$ deficiency is accompanied by a vitamin $B_{12}$–resistant proteinuria (27, 33). Two mutations in the cubilin gene [localized on chromosome 10p (41)] have been characterized in the Finnish population (1). The most prevalent mutation, designated FM1, is a point mutation in the coding region that causes the substitution of Pro$_{1297}$ to Leu in CUB domain 8. This substitution is located within the IF-$B_{12}$ binding region (CUB domains 5–8) of cubilin, and a recent mutagenesis study (42) of the IF-$B_{12}$ binding region of recombinant cubilin has shown that the mutation strongly decreases the affinity of the binding of cubilin to IF-$B_{12}$. Most of the patients with the FM1 mutation have only a modest proteinuria, indicating that the genetic defect mainly affects the binding of IF-$B_{12}$. It has been suggested that the other known disease-causing cubilin mutation (FM2), an intronic mutation, results in the in-frame insertion of multiple stop codons in CUB domain 6. One patient and one carrier are known to have the FM2 mutation. Concordant with the suggested truncation of cubilin in CUB domain 6 by the FM2 mutation, the FM2 patient has a strong proteinuria and excretion of cubilin ligands (40) (SK Moestrup, A de la Chapelle, R Krahe, unpublished data).

Genetic defects in genes other than cubilin may also account for the Imerslund-Gräsbeck disease. There are two lines of evidence for this. (*a*) Genetic analysis of Imerslund-Gräsbeck patients in Norway has not disclosed any mutations in the cubilin gene (1). (*b*) Genetic analysis of a dog model of human Imerslund-Gräsbeck disease (including strong proteinuria) has shown no linkage to the cubilin gene and no mutations in the coding region of the gene (93). However, the affected dogs have an abnormal processing of cubilin, leading to intracellular accumulation and abnormal glycosylation of the protein (25, 92). This finding combined with the genetic findings has led to the conclusion that the dogs are affected by an as-yet-unknown defect in a gene encoding an accessory activity required for cubilin brush-border expression (93).

## Kidney

Under normal conditions, the proteins in the glomerular tiltrate are reabsorbed in the proximal tubule (18). Transcellular transport of intact protein is minimal, and it is now well established that the main part of protein undergo internalization and degradation by proximal tubule cells. A number of biochemical and in vivo studies [for a review, see Christensen et al (15)], including analysis of megalin-deficient mice (44) or analysis of dogs with functional cubilin deficiency (7, 43), have provided strong evidence that cubilin and megalin act as key receptors for protein endocytosis by the tubule cells. The spectrum of proteins excreted is not completely defined, but it is evident that cubilin (7) and megalin (44) deficiency lead to excretion of a different but overlapping set of proteins also seen in the urine of patients with renal tubular deficiency (Fanconi syndrome). This observation combined with experimental data on the receptor binding of single ligands suggests three types of binding/uptake properties of the reabsorbed protein. (*a*) Megalin is the main binder. This is the case, for instance, for retinol-binding protein (17), transcobalamin (56), and $\beta_2$-glycoprotein-I (61), which are internalized and degraded as described for other ligands of the LDL receptor family. (*b*) Cubilin is the main binder. The most studied examples in this group are transferrin (R Kozyraki, J Fyfe, PJ Verroust, C Jacobsen, A Dautry-Varsat, TE Willnow, EI Christensen, SK Moestrup, manuscript in preparation) and apolipoprotein (apo) A-I (40), the main protein of high-density lipoprotein (HDL). For these ligands, the internalization of the cubilin ligand complex requires megalin. (*c*) Both cubilin and megalin may be able to bind the ligand, as reported for albumin (7, 20).

In conclusion, the megalin- and cubilin-mediated endocytosis in the proximal tubule may be regarded as a highly efficient mechanism for rescuing various nutrients present in the renal ultrafiltrate. Although several grams of filtered protein are reabsorbed, and degraded daily by this mechanism, the rescue of protein-bound components as vitamins may be physiologically more important than the protein itself.

Megalin-mediated uptake of carrier-bound vitamins A, $B_{12}$ (cobalamin), and D is followed by lysosomal degradation of the protein carrier. Vitamin D, which is endocytosed as the 25-OH $D_3$ form, undergoes a second hydroxylation in the proximal tubule, leading to the active 1,25-$(OH)_2$ vitamin $D_3$. In addition, the kidney seems to function as a storage organ for $B_{12}$. The intracellular pathways by which the vitamins, internalized along with their carrier proteins, reenter the circulation are largely unknown, but the transport probably involves vesicular transport. Whatever the exact mechanism, the importance of the megalin-mediated uptake is evidenced by studies of megalin-deficient mice, which in addition to developmental defects (see section on embryonic tissues) have bone malformation (67), loss of the three vitamins in the urine, and no storage of $B_{12}$ in the kidney (10, 17, 67).

The receptors may also rescue lipid by internalizing various apolipoproteins, such as the megalin ligand $\beta_2$-glycoprotein-1 (binder of acidic phospholipids) and the cubilin ligand apo A-1 (40, 61), which constitute the major protein of HDL. However, although the kidney is the main catabolic site of apo A-1, it probably represents uptake of lipid-poor apo A-1 rather than lipid-loaded HDL particles (58). In the nonparticle form, apo-A1 has a size, which readily may pass the glomerular filtration barrier. The smallest HDL particles might also to a limited extent pass the barrier, but the physiological significance of this is unclear (58).

The endocytic properties of megalin and cubilin may also have inexpedient consequences, by mediating uptake of various exogenous components, such as drugs and toxins. Some polybasic drugs, for instance the aminoglycosides, are known to bind to the negatively charged megalin (57). Aminoglycosides accumulate in the lysosomes and can in elevated concentrations cause damage of the proximal tubules. Trichosanthin is an example of a plant toxin binding to LDL receptor family proteins, including megalin (13). It inactivates type I ribosomes and is strongly nephrotoxic, probably because of renal filtration and megalin-mediated uptake in the proximal tubules. Although not reported, it seems conceivable that other drugs and toxins may use megalin as a gate for cellular uptake.

Megalin (37) and cubilin (40) can be detected in the normal urine by immunoblotting. The excretion of the receptors is probably due to shedding of the proximal tubule epithelial cells. Detection of the receptors and estimation of their size might show to have diagnostic relevance, for instance for analysis of cubilin defects in Imerslund-Gräsbeck patients (40).

## Yolk Sac

The yolk sac is an organ found in all species, although it has markedly different structures and functions. In rodents, it is derived, around embryonic day 7, from the very first endodermal cells that migrate from the inner cell mass to line the blastocoelic cavity. By embryonic day 9 (Figure 4), the yolk sac completely surrounds the embryo in such a manner that its absorptive surface faces the

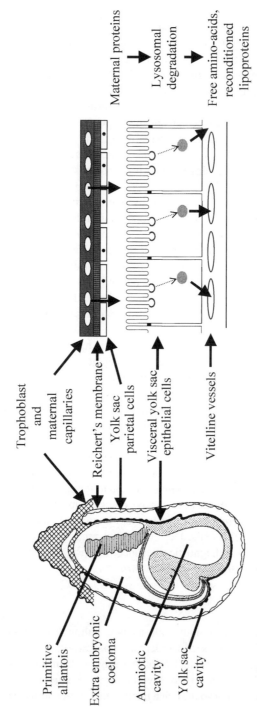

**Figure 4** Anatomy and function of the murine yolk sac. (*Left*) Around day 10 of gestation, the yolk sac completely surrounds the embryo and constitutes the sole interface between the fetus and the mother. The parietal epithelium is permeable to maternal proteins. In the current hypothetical model of yolk sac function, megalin and cubilin, expressed at the apical pole of the visceral epithelial cells, can endocytose the proteins, which are present in the yolk sac cavity. Cholesterol freed by degradation of lipoproteins is reconditioned into nascent lipoproteins synthesized by yolk sac epithelial cells and transferred to the embryo.

surrounding decidual tissue in contact with the maternal circulation. The yolk sac remains functional during the entire pregnancy and constitutes the only maternal-fetal interface during organogenesis until establishment of the allantoic placenta around embryonic day 10. There is little, if any, transcellular transport across the yolk sac, and the key exchanges involve receptor-mediated internalization and degradation of proteins present in the maternal plasma(34).

Cubilin and megalin (79) are expressed in the apical yolk sac very early and remain expressed at a high level throughout gestation. As previously suggested by the deleterious effects of anti-cubilin antibodies on fetal development in rats (78), cubilin probably plays a crucial role in the initial phase of this process, i.e. in the uptake of maternal components. Cubilin, in association with megalin, can bind and internalize a variety of plasma proteins, including the most abundant, albumin. It may thus be important for the supply of amino acids used by the embryo, which, as shown elsewhere (11, 48, 49), are produced by degradation of maternal protein. The cubilin-megalin system can also internalize HDL (40) and LDL (85), which suggests that cubilin and megalin may be involved in the transfer to the fetus of maternal cholesterol and other lipids. The as-yet-incompletely defined pathway (31) involves internalization of maternal lipoproteins—largely HDL in rodents—at the apical pole of the visceral yolk sac followed by lysosomal degradation of the protein component (Figure 4). The internalized cholesterol is reloaded into apo B–containing particles secreted into fetal vessels at the basal pole of the visceral yolk sac (22, 72, 87).

Disruption of the megalin gene causes serious defects, including holoprosen-cephaly, and most megalin-deficient mice die shortly after birth (89). The patho-genesis of the holoproencephaly in megalin-deficient mice is unknown, and it has not been elucidated whether the malformation relates to defective megalin-mediated transport in the yolk sac or in the embryonic tissue, e.g. the megalin-expressing neuroepithelium or kidney epithelium. However, there are many causes of holoprosencephaly (including vitamin A and cholesterol deficiency), the patho-genic mechanisms underlying the neurological malformations in the megalin-deficient mice may be complex.

## Thyroid Gland

The polarized epithelium of the thyroid gland has a specialized function. It digests thyroglobulin harboring the thyroid hormones thyroxine (T4) and triodothyronine (T3) [for a review, see Marino & McCluskey (53)]. Thyroglobulin is synthesized by thyrocytes and secreted into the lumen of the thyroid follicles, where it represents the major component of colloid. Here, the thyroglobulin undergoes iodination of tyrosyl residues, leading to the formation of T3 and T4 in the thyroglobulin molecule. Subsequent uptake of iodinated thyroglobulin in the epithelial cells is followed by lysosomal degradation of the major pool of the protein leading to release of T3 and T4. Some thyroglobulin is also transcytosed to the basolateral sur-face without being degraded, and some thyroglobulin is recycled back to the colloid fluid. This has suggested the existence of distinct pathways for thyroglobulin—a lysosomal pathway, a transcytosis pathway, and a recycling pathway (53).

Recent work by Marino and coworkers (53–55) has shown that megalin, which is expressed in the apical membrane of the thyroid epithelial cells, binds and mediates endocytosis of thyroglobulin. It has been suggested that in addition to the megalin-mediated endocytosis, nonspecific fluid-phase pinocytosis and endocytosis mediated by a thyroid asioglycoprotein receptor account for uptake of thyroglobulin from the apical surface. The quantitative importance in vivo of each of these uptake pathways remains to be defined (53).

Megalin may play other roles in relation to the thyroid hormones by mediating uptake of transthyretin (84), a carrier of T4. Transthyretin is filtered and reabsorped in the kidney, which is a major organ for conversion of T4 to the active form T3. No renal reabsorption of transthyretin is seen in megalin-deficient mice, and it is therefore conceivable that these mice have a lower renal supply of T4 for conversion to T3.

Cubilin expression and/or function in the thyroid gland has not been investigated.

## Other Tissues Expressing Megalin and Cubilin

Megalin and/or cubilin is expressed in a number of polarized epithelia, e.g. type II pneumocytes in the lung, the choroid plexus, the ependyma of the brain, the parathyroid, and the epithelia of the reproductive system (Table 1). Little is known about physiological ligands for the receptors in these tissues. Current knowledge mostly relates to the reproductive system: Apo J (clusterin) has been shown to bind to megalin in the efferent duct and epididymal epithelia rat seminal vesicle (62), and seminal vesicle secretory protein II has been demonstrated as a ligand for megalin expressed by epithelial cells lining the ductal region and the ampulla of the rat seminal vesicle (76). However, the expression of megalin and cubilin in several reproductive organs may suggest other ligands. Interesting candidates are the sex hormone–binding proteins, which have been proposed (90) because megalin is known to bind another steroid carrier, the vitamin D–binding protein (67).

## CONCLUSIONS AND FUTURE PERSPECTIVES

Megalin and cubilin are mutually interacting, high-molecular-weight receptors expressed in polarized epithelia. So far, a number of nutritionally important ligands for cubilin and megalin have been identified in various epithelia. In the intestine, cubilin functions as the essential receptor for uptake of vitamin $B_{12}$ in complex with IF. Mutations in the cubilin gene are now known to explain some cases of disease-causing malabsorption of vitamin $B_{12}$ (Imerslund-Gräsbeck's disease). In the kidney, both receptors are involved in the reabsorption of several proteins in the glomerular ultrafiltrate. The kidney ligands include carrier proteins for vitamins (A, $B_{12}$, and D) and lipids. A similar multiligand role is suggested for the receptors in the yolk sac epithelium of rodents. Furthermore, cubilin and megalin may account for a substantial uptake of LDL and HDL holoparticles in the yolk sac. In the thyroid, megalin functions as a receptor for uptake of thyroglobulin, which harbors the thyroid hormones.

Future directions of research on the two receptors will probably lead to a more comprehensive and complete ligand list. This may provide new information on the function of the receptors in those epithelia, where their role presently remains obscure. At the molecular level, it will be intriguing to further characterize the processing and trafficking of cubilin and megalin. It might reveal novel basic knowledge on receptor transport and provide new insight into pathogenic mechanisms of diseases with affected cubilin and/or megalin function.

**Visit the Annual Reviews home page at www.AnnualReviews.org**

## LITERATURE CITED

1. Aminoff M, Carter JE, Chadwick RB, Johnson C, Grasbeck R, et al. 1999. Mutations in CUBN, encoding the intrinsic factor-vitamin B12 receptor, cubilin, cause hereditary megaloblastic anaemia 1. *Nat. Genet.* 21:309–13

2. Andersen OM, Christensen LL, Christensen PA, Sorensen ES, Jacobsen C, et al. 2000. Identification of the minimal functional unit in the low density lipoprotein receptor-related protein for binding the receptor-associated protein (RAP). A conserved acidic residue in the complement-type repeats is important for recognition of RAP. *J. Biol. Chem.* 275:21017–24

3. Anderson GJ, Powell LW, Halliday JW. 1990. Transferrin receptor distribution and regulation in the rat small intestine. Effect of iron stores and erythropoiesis. *Gastroenterology* 98:576–85

4. Baricault L, Galceran M, Ronco PM, Trugnan G, Verroust PJ. 1995. Unusual processing of GP280, a protein associated with the intermicrovillar areas of yolk sac epithelial cells: plasma membrane delivery of immature protein. *Biochem. Biophys. Res. Commun.* 212:353–59

5. Batuman V, Verroust PJ, Navar GL, Kaysen JH, Goda FO, et al. 1998. Myeloma light chains are ligands for cubilin (gp280). *Am. J. Physiol.* 275:F246–54

6. Biemesderfer D, Dekan G, Aronson PS, Farquhar MG. 1993. Biosynthesis of the gp330/44-kDa Heymann nephritis antigenic complex: assembly takes place in the ER. *Am. J. Physiol.* 264:F1011–20

7. Birn H, Fyfe JC, Jacobsen C, Mounier F, Verroust PJ, et al. 2000. Cubilin is an albumin binding protein important for renal tubular albumin reabsorption. *J. Clin. Invest.* 105:1353–61

8. Birn H, Verroust PJ, Nexo E, Hager H, Jacobsen C, et al. 1997. Characterization of an epithelial approximately 460-kDa protein that facilitates endocytosis of intrinsic factor-vitamin B12 and binds receptor-associated protein. *J. Biol. Chem.* 272:26497–504

9. Birn H, Vorum H, Verroust PJ, Moestrup SK, Christensen EI. 2000. Receptor-associated protein is important for normal processing of megalin in kidney proximal tubules. *J. Am. Soc. Nephrol.* 11:191–202

10. Birn H, Willnow TE, Nielsen R, Norden

AG, Moestrup SK, et al. 2001. Megalin-mediated endocytosis of transcobalamin-B$_{12}$ and lysosomal accumulation of vitamin B12 in rat kidney proximal tubule. *Am. J. Phys.* In press

11. Brent RL, Beckman DA, Jensen M, Koszalka TR. 1990. Experimental yolk sac dysfunction as a model for studying nutritional disturbances in the embryo during early organogenesis. *Teratology* 41:405–13

12. Brown MS, Goldstein JL. 1986. A receptor-mediated pathway for cholesterol homeostasis. *Science* 232:34–47

13. Chan WL, Shaw PC, Tam SC, Jacobsen C, Gliemann J, Nielsen MS. 2000. Trichosanthin interacts with and enters cells via LDL receptor family members. *Biochem. Biophys. Res. Commun.* 270:453–57

14. Christensen EI, Birn H, Verroust P, Moestrup SK. 1998. Megalin-mediated endocytosis in renal proximal tubule. *Ren. Fail.* 20:191–99

15. Christensen EI, Birn H, Verroust P, Moestrup SK. 1998. Membrane receptors for endocytosis in the renal proximal tubule. *Int. Rev. Cytol.* 180:237–84

16. Christensen EI, Gliemann J, Moestrup SK. 1992. Renal tubule gp330 is a calcium binding receptor for endocytic uptake of protein. *J. Histochem. Cytochem.* 40:1481–90

17. Christensen EI, Moskaug JO, Vorum H, Jacobsen C, Gundersen TE, et al. 1999. Evidence for an essential role of megalin in transepithelial transport of retinol. *J. Am. Soc. Nephrol.* 10:685–95

18. Christensen EI, Nielsen S. 1991. Structural and functional features of protein handling in the kidney proximal tubule. *Semin. Nephrol.* 11:414–39

19. Christensen EI, Nielsen S, Moestrup SK, Borre C, Maunsbach AB, et al. 1995. Segmental distribution of the endocytosis receptor gp330 in renal proximal tubules. *Eur. J. Cell Biol.* 66:349–64

20. Cui S, Verroust PJ, Moestrup SK, Christensen EI. 1996. Megalin/gp330 mediates uptake of albumin in renal proximal tubule. *Am. J. Physiol.* 271:F900–7

21. Czekay RP, Orlando RA, Woodward L, Adamson ED, Farquhar MG. 1995. The expression of megalin (gp330) and LRP diverges during F9 cell differentiation. *J. Cell Sci.* 108(4):1433–41

22. Farese RV Jr, Cases S, Ruland SL, Kayden HJ, Wong JS, et al. 1996. A novel function for apolipoprotein B: Lipoprotein synthesis in the yolk sac is critical for maternal-fetal lipid transport in mice. *J. Lipid Res.* 37:347–60

23. Fass D, Blacklow S, Kim PS, Berger JM. 1997. Molecular basis of familial hypercholesterolaemia from structure of LDL receptor module. *Nature* 388:691–93

24. Fyfe JC, Giger U, Hall CA, Jezyk PF, Klumpp SA, et al. 1991. Inherited selective intestinal cobalamin malabsorption and cobalamin deficiency in dogs. *Pediatr. Res.* 29:24–31

25. Fyfe JC, Ramanujam KS, Ramaswamy K, Patterson DF, Seetharam B. 1991. Defective brush-border expression of intrinsic factor-cobalamin receptor in canine inherited intestinal cobalamin malabsorption. *J. Biol. Chem.* 266:4489–94

26. Gliemann J. 1998. Receptors of the low density lipoprotein (LDL) receptor family in man. Multiple functions of the large family members via interaction with complex ligands. *Biol. Chem.* 379:951–64

27. Gräsbeck R, Gordin RKI, Kuhlbäck B. 1960. Selective vitamin B12 malabsorption and proteinuria in young people. *Acta Med. Scand.* 167:289–96

28. Hammad SM, Barth JL, Knaak C, Argraves WS. 2000. Megalin acts in concert with cubilin to mediate endocytosis of high density lipoproteins. *J. Biol. Chem.* 275:12003–8

29. Hammad SM, Stefansson S, Twal WO, Drake CJ, Fleming P, et al. 1999. Cubilin, the endocytic receptor for intrinsic factor-vitamin B(12) complex, mediates high-density lipoprotein holoparticle

endocytosis. *Proc. Natl. Acad. Sci. USA* 96:10158–63

30. Hansen SH, Sandvig K, van Deurs B. 1991. The preendosomal compartment comprises distinct coated and noncoated endocytic vesicle populations. *J. Cell Biol.* 113:731–41

31. Herz J, Willnow TE, Farese RV Jr. 1997. Cholesterol, hedgehog and embryogenesis. *Nat. Genet.* 15:123–24

32. Hjalm G, Murray E, Crumley G, Harazim W, Lundgren S, et al. 1996. Cloning and sequencing of human gp330, a $Ca^{2+}$-binding receptor with potential intracellular signaling properties. *Eur. J. Biochem.* 239:132–37

33. Imerslund O. 1960. Idiophatic chronic megaloblastic anemia in children. *Acta. Paediatr. Scan.* 49:1–115

34. Jollie WP. 1990. Development, morphology, and function of the yolk-sac placenta of laboratory rodents. *Teratology* 41:361–81

35. Kirchhausen T. 2000. Clathrin. *Annu. Rev. Biochem.* 69:699–727

36. Kounnas MZ, Argraves WS, Strickland DK. 1992. The 39-kDa receptor-associated protein interacts with two members of the low density lipoprotein receptor family, alpha-2-macroglobulin receptor and glycoprotein 330. *J. Biol. Chem.* 267:21162–66

37. Kounnas MZ, Chappell DA, Strickland DK, Argraves WS. 1993. Glycoprotein 330, a member of the low density lipoprotein receptor family, binds lipoprotein lipase in vitro. *J. Biol. Chem.* 268:14176–81

38. Kounnas MZ, Haudenschild CC, Strickland DK, Argraves WS. 1994. Immunological localization of glycoprotein 330, low density lipoprotein receptor related protein and 39-kDa receptor associated protein in embryonic mouse tissues. *In Vivo* 8:343–51

39. Kounnas MZ, Loukinova EB, Stefansson S, Harmony JA, Brewer BH, et al. 1995. Identification of glycoprotein 330 as an endocytic receptor for apolipoprotein J/clusterin. *J. Biol. Chem.* 270:13070–75; Erratum. 1995. *J. Biol. Chem.* 270(39): 23234

40. Kozyraki R, Fyfe J, Kristiansen M, Gerdes C, Jacobsen C, et al. 1999. The intrinsic factor-vitamin B12 receptor, cubilin, is a high-affinity apolipoprotein A-I receptor facilitating endocytosis of high-density lipoprotein. *Nat. Med.* 5:656–61

41. Kozyraki R, Kristiansen M, Silahtaroglu A, Hansen C, Jacobsen C, et al. 1998. The human intrinsic factor-vitamin B12 receptor, cubilin: molecular characterization and chromosomal mapping of the gene to 10p within the autosomal recessive megaloblastic anemia (MGA1) region. *Blood* 91:3593–600; Erratum. 1998. *Blood* 92(7):2608

42. Kristiansen M, Aminoff M, Jacobsen C, de la Chapelle A, Krahe R, et al. 2000. Cubilin P1297L mutation associated with hereditary megaloblastic anemia 1 causes impaired recognition of intrinsic factor-vitamin $B_{12}$ by cubilin. *Blood* 96:405–9

43. Kristiansen M, Kozyraki R, Jacobsen C, Nexo E, Verroust PJ, Moestrup SK. 1999. Molecular dissection of the intrinsic factor-vitamin B12 receptor, cubilin, discloses regions important for membrane association and ligand binding. *J. Biol. Chem.* 274:20540–44

44. Leheste JR, Rolinski B, Vorum H, Hilpert J, Nykjaer A, et al. 1999. Megalin knockout mice as an animal model of low molecular weight proteinuria. *Am. J. Pathol.* 155:1361–70

45. Le Panse S, Ayani E, Nielsen S, Ronco P, Verroust P, Christensen EI. 1997. Internalization and recycling of glycoprotein 280 in epithelial cells of yolk sac. *Eur. J. Cell Biol.* 72:257–67

46. Le Panse S, Verroust P, Christensen EI. 1997. Internalization and recycling of glycoprotein 280 in BN/MSV yolk sac epithelial cells: a model system of relevance to receptor-mediated endocytosis in the renal proximal tubule. *Exp. Nephrol.* 5:375–83

47. Liu W, Yu WR, Carling T, Juhlin C, Rastad J, et al. 1998. Regulation of gp330/megalin expression by vitamins A and D. *Eur. J. Clin. Invest.* 28:100–7

48. Lloyd JB. 1990. Cell physiology of the rat visceral yolk sac: a study of pinocytosis and lysosome function. *Teratology* 41:383–93

49. Lloyd JB, Beckman DA, Brent RL. 1998. Nutritional role of the visceral yolk sac in organogenesis-stage rat embryos. *Reprod. Toxicol.* 12:193–95

50. Lundgren S, Carling T, Hjalm G, Juhlin C, Rastad J, et al. 1997. Tissue distribution of human gp330/megalin, a putative $Ca^{2+}$-sensing protein. *J. Histochem. Cytochem.* 45:383–92

51. Lundgren S, Hjalm G, Hellman P, Ek B, Juhlin C, et al. 1994. A protein involved in calcium sensing of the human parathyroid and placental cytotrophoblast cells belongs to the LDL-receptor protein superfamily. *Exp. Cell Res.* 212:344–50

52. Lundstrom M, Orlando RA, Saedi MS, Woodward L, Kurihara H, Farquhar MG. 1993. Immunocytochemical and biochemical characterization of the Heymann nephritis antigenic complex in rat L2 yolk sac cells. *Am. J. Pathol.* 143:1423–35

53. Marino M, McCluskey RT. 2000. Role of thyroglobulin endocytic pathways in the control of thyroid hormone release. *Am. J. Physiol.* 279:C1295–306

54. Marino M, Zheng G, Chiovato L, Pinchera A, Brown D, et al. 2000. Role of megalin (gp330) in transcytosis of thyroglobulin by thyroid cells. A novel function in the control of thyroid hormone release. *J. Biol. Chem.* 275:7125–37

55. Marino M, Zheng G, McCluskey RT. 1999. Megalin (gp330) is an endocytic receptor for thyroglobulin on cultured fisher rat thyroid cells. *J. Biol. Chem.* 274:12898–904

56. Moestrup SK, Birn H, Fischer PB, Petersen CM, Verroust PJ, et al. 1996. Megalin-mediated endocytosis of transcobalamin-vitamin-B12 complexes suggests a role of the receptor in vitamin-B12 homeostasis. *Proc. Natl. Acad. Sci. USA* 93:8612–17

57. Moestrup SK, Cui S, Vorum H, Bregengard C, Bjorn SE, et al. 1995. Evidence that epithelial glycoprotein 330/megalin mediates uptake of polybasic drugs. *J. Clin. Invest.* 96:1404–13

58. Moestrup SK, Kozyraki R. 2000. Cubilin, a high-density lipoprotein receptor. *Curr. Opin. Lipidol.* 11:133–40

59. Moestrup SK, Kozyraki R, Kristiansen M, Kaysen JH, Rasmussen HH, et al. 1998. The intrinsic factor-vitamin B12 receptor and target of teratogenic antibodies is a megalin-binding peripheral membrane protein with homology to developmental proteins. *J. Biol. Chem.* 273:5235–42

60. Moestrup SK, Nielsen S, Andreasen P, Jorgensen KE, Nykjaer A, et al. 1993. Epithelial glycoprotein-330 mediates endocytosis of plasminogen activator-plasminogen activator inhibitor type-1 complexes. *J. Biol. Chem.* 268:16564–70

61. Moestrup SK, Schousboe I, Jacobsen C, Leheste JR, Christensen EI, Willnow TE. 1998. $\beta$2-Glycoprotein-I (apolipoprotein H) and $\beta$2-glycoprotein-I-phospholipid complex harbor a recognition site for the endocytic receptor megalin. *J. Clin. Invest.* 102:902–9

62. Morales CR, Igdoura SA, Wosu UA, Boman J, Argraves WS. 1996. Low density lipoprotein receptor-related protein-2 expression in efferent duct and epididymal epithelia: evidence in rats for its in vivo role in endocytosis of apolipoprotein J/clusterin. *Biol. Reprod.* 55:676–83

63. Morelle W, Haslam SM, Ziak M, Roth J, Morris HR, Dell A. 2000. Characterization of the N-linked oligosaccharides of megalin (gp330) from rat kidney. *Glycobiology* 10:295–304

64. Mostov KE. 1994. Transepithelial transport of immunoglobulins. *Annu. Rev. Immunol.* 12:63–84

65. Mukherjee S, Ghosh RN, Maxfield FR.

1997. Endocytosis. *Physiol. Rev.* 77:759–803

66. Niemeier A, Willnow T, Dieplinger H, Jacobsen C, Meyer N, et al. 1999. Identification of megalin/gp330 as a receptor for lipoprotein(a) in vitro. *Arterioscler. Thromb. Vasc. Biol.* 19:552–61

67. Nykjaer A, Dragun D, Walther D, Vorum H, Jacobsen C, et al. 1999. An endocytic pathway essential for renal uptake and activation of the steroid 25-(OH) vitamin D3. *Cell* 96:507–15

68. Oleinikov AV, Zhao J, Makker SP. 2000. Cytosolic adaptor protein Dab2 is an intracellular ligand of endocytic receptor gp600/megalin. *Biochem. J.* 347(3):613–21

69. Orlando RA, Exner M, Czekay RP, Yamazaki H, Saito A, et al. 1997. Identification of the second cluster of ligand-binding repeats in megalin as a site for receptor-ligand interactions. *Proc. Natl. Acad. Sci. USA* 94:2368–73

70. Orlando RA, Kerjaschki D, Kurihara H, Biemesderfer D, Farquhar MG. 1992. gp330 associates with a 44-kDa protein in the rat kidney to form the Heymann nephritis antigenic complex. *Proc. Natl. Acad. Sci. USA* 89:6698–702

71. Orlando RA, Rader K, Authier F, Yamazaki H, Posner BI, et al. 1998. Megalin is an endocytic receptor for insulin. *J. Am. Soc. Nephrol.* 9:1759–66

72. Raabe M, Flynn LM, Zlot CH, Wong JS, Veniant MM, et al. 1998. Knockout of the abetalipoproteinemia gene in mice: reduced lipoprotein secretion in heterozygotes and embryonic lethality in homozygotes. *Proc. Natl. Acad. Sci. USA* 95:8686–91

73. Ramanujam KS, Seetharam S, Dahms NM, Seetharam B. 1994. Effect of processing inhibitors on cobalamin (vitamin B12) transcytosis in polarized opossum kidney cells. *Arch. Biochem. Biophys.* 315:8–15

74. Ramanujam KS, Seetharam S, Seetharam B. 1991. Synthesis and secretion of cobal-

amin binding proteins by opossum kidney cells. *Biochem. Biophys. Res. Commun.* 179:543–50

75. Ramanujam KS, Seetharam S, Seetharam B. 1992. Leupeptin and ammonium chloride inhibit intrinsic factor mediated transcytosis of [57Co]cobalamin across polarized renal epithelial cells. *Biochem. Biophys. Res. Commun.* 182:439–46

76. Ranganathan S, Knaak C, Morales CR, Argraves WS. 1999. Identification of low density lipoprotein receptor-related protein-2/megalin as an endocytic receptor for seminal vesicle secretory protein II. *J. Biol. Chem.* 274:5557–63

77. Romero A, Romao MJ, Varela PF, Kolln I, Dias JM, et al. 1997. The crystal structures of two spermadhesins reveal the CUB domain fold. *Nat. Struct. Biol.* 4:783–88

78. Sahali D, Mulliez N, Chatelet F, Dupuis R, Ronco P, Verroust P. 1988. Characterization of a 280-kD protein restricted to the coated pits of the renal brush border and the epithelial cells of the yolk sac. Teratogenic effect of the specific monoclonal antibodies. *J. Exp. Med.* 167:213–18

79. Sahali D, Mulliez N, Chatelet F, Laurent-Winter C, Citadelle D, et al. 1992. Coexpression in humans by kidney and fetal envelopes of a 280-kDa-coated pit-restricted protein. Similarity with the murine target of teratogenic antibodies. *Am. J. Pathol.* 140:33–44

80. Saito A, Pietromonaco S, Loo AK, Farquhar MG. 1994. Complete cloning and sequencing of rat gp330/"megalin," a distinctive member of the low density lipoprotein receptor gene family. *Proc. Natl. Acad. Sci. USA* 91:9725–29

81. Seetharam B, Christensen EI, Moestrup SK, Hammond TG, Verroust PJ. 1997. Identification of rat yolk sac target protein of teratogenic antibodies, gp280, as intrinsic factor-cobalamin receptor. *J. Clin. Invest.* 99:2317–22

82. Seetharam B, Levine JS, Ramasamy M, Alpers DH. 1988. Purification, properties,

and immunochemical localization of a receptor for intrinsic factor-cobalamin complex in the rat kidney. *J. Biol. Chem.* 263:4443–49

83. Sim RB, Moestrup SK, Stuart GR, Lynch NJ, Lu J, et al. 1998. Interaction of C1q and the collectins with the potential receptors calreticulin (C1qR/collectin receptor) and megalin. *Immunobiology* 199:208–24

84. Sousa MM, Norden AG, Jacobsen C, Willnow TE, Christensen EI, et al. 2000. Evidence for the role of megalin in renal uptake of transthyretin. *J. Biol. Chem.* 275:88176–81

85. Stefansson S, Chappell DA, Argraves KM, Strickland DK, Argraves WS. 1995. Glycoprotein 330/low density lipoprotein receptor-related protein-2 mediates endocytosis of low density lipoproteins via interaction with apolipoprotein B100. *J. Biol. Chem.* 270:19417–21

86. Stefansson S, Kounnas MZ, Henkin J, Mallampalli RK, Chappell DA, et al. 1995. gp330 on type II pneumocytes mediates endocytosis leading to degradation of pro-urokinase, plasminogen activator inhibitor-1 and urokinase-plasminogen activator inhibitor-1 complex. *J. Cell Sci.* 108(6):2361–68

87. Terasawa Y, Cases SJ, Wong JS, Jamil H, Jothi S, et al. 1999. Apolipoprotein B-related gene expression and ultrastructural characteristics of lipoprotein secretion in mouse yolk sac during embryonic development. *J. Lipid Res.* 40:1967–77

88. Willnow TE, Goldstein JL, Orth K, Brown MS, Herz J. 1992. Low density lipoprotein receptor-related protein and gp330 bind similar ligands, including plasminogen activator-inhibitor complexes and lactoferrin, an inhibitor of chylomicron remnant clearance. *J. Biol. Chem.* 267:26172–80

89. Willnow TE, Hilpert J, Armstrong SA, Rohlmann A, Hammer RE, et al. 1996.

Defective forebrain development in mice lacking gp330/megalin. *Proc. Natl. Acad. Sci. USA* 93:8460–64

90. Willnow TE, Nykjaer A, Herz J. 1999. Lipoprotein receptors: new roles for ancient proteins. *Nat. Cell Biol.* 1:E157–62

91. Willnow TE, Rohlmann A, Horton J, Otani H, Braun JR, et al. 1996. RAP, a specialized chaperone, prevents ligand-induced ER retention and degradation of LDL receptor-related endocytic receptors. *EMBO J.* 15:2632–39

92. Xu D, Fyfe JC. 2000. Cubilin expression and posttranslational modification in the canine gastrointestinal tract. *Am. J. Physiol. Gastrointest. Liver Physiol.* 279:G748–56

93. Xu D, Kozyraki R, Newman TC, Fyfe JC. 1999. Genetic evidence of an accessory activity required specifically for cubilin brush-border expression and intrinsic factor-cobalamin absorption. *Blood* 94:3604–6

94. Yochem J, Greenwald I. 1993. A gene for a low density lipoprotein receptor-related protein in the nematode *Caenorhabditis elegans. Proc. Natl. Acad. Sci. USA* 90:4572–76

95. Zheng G, Bachinsky DR, Stamenkovic I, Strickland DK, Brown D, et al. 1994. Organ distribution in rats of two members of the low-density lipoprotein receptor gene family, gp330 and LRP/alpa 2MR, and the receptor-associated protein (RAP). *J. Histochem. Cytochem.* 42:531–42

96. Zheng G, Marino M, Zhao J, McCluskey RT. 1998. Megalin (gp330): a putative endocytic receptor for thyroglobulin (Tg). *Endocrinology* 139:1462–65

97. Ziak M, Meier M, Roth J. 1999. Megalin in normal tissues and carcinoma cells carries oligo/poly alpha2,8 deaminoneuraminic acid as a unique posttranslational modification. *Glycoconjugation J.* 16:185–88

Annu. Rev. Nutr. 2001. 21:429–52

# Interrelationships of Key Variables of Human Zinc Homeostasis: Relevance to Dietary Zinc Requirements

## Michael Hambidge and Nancy F Krebs

*Section of Nutrition, Department of Pediatrics, University of Colorado Health Sciences Center, Denver, Colorado 80262; e-mail: michael.hambidge@uchsc.edu, nancy.krebs@uchsc.edu*

**Key Words** factorial, endogenous, excretion, absorption, stable isotopes

■ **Abstract** Currently, estimates of human zinc requirements depend primarily on a factorial approach. The availability of tracer techniques employing zinc stable isotopes has facilitated the acquisition of data on major variables of zinc homeostasis in addition to those that can be measured with careful metabolic balance techniques. These data have promising potential to facilitate and improve the factorial approach. The thesis proposed in this paper is that realistic estimations of dietary zinc requirements by a factorial approach require attention to the dynamic interrelationships between major variables of zinc homeostasis. This applies especially to the positive relationship between endogenous fecal zinc and total absorbed zinc, which is the essential starting point in estimating physiologic and, from there, dietary requirements.

## CONTENTS

0199-9885/01/0715-0429$14.00

# INTRODUCTION

The considerable incentive for giving priority to refining our concepts and knowledge of human dietary zinc requirements is attributable to several factors. First is our increasing awareness that not only does human zinc deficiency occur in a variety of circumstances, it also appears to be a public health problem of global proportions (17, 19). Second, in contrast to earlier concepts, the optimal physiologic range for zinc intake and absorption may be limited, with even moderate excess causing previously unexpected and undesirable disruption of normal physiology (54). An obvious corollary to this concern is that it is more prudent to determine requirements as reliably as possible than to simply err on the side of excess in order to minimize the risk of deficiency. Third, zinc deficiency has been well documented in populations in North America (11, 12, 15, 53) whose zinc intake, although not matching earlier recommended daily allowances from the National Academy of Sciences (51), appears to be adequate when compared with standards published more recently (10, 69). Thus, there is an unresolved paradox. On the one hand is the well-documented occurrence of human zinc deficiency in apparently healthy subjects. On the other is evidence, or what appears to be reasonable interpretation of data, from studies of zinc balance (28) or homeostasis/metabolism (59) that zinc requirements are extraordinarily small. If true, this would appear to preclude any practical risk of zinc deficiency except in very special circumstances, for example poor bioavailability.

A first step in addressing this paradox is to achieve a more precise understanding of human zinc requirements in healthy adults whose dietary zinc is of good bioavailability. This chapter focuses on an evaluation of recent data and reevaluation of less recent data on aspects of human zinc homeostasis that are pertinent to estimating human dietary zinc requirements. These data include information utilized by the Standing Committee on the Scientific Evaluation of Dietary Reference Intakes of the Food and Nutrition Board of the Institute of Medicine, as well as its Panel on Vitamin A, Vitamin K, Boron, Chromium, Copper, Iodine, Iron, Manganese, Molybdenum, Nickel, Silicon, Vanadium and Zinc (10). This recent report included estimated average requirements (EARs) for zinc. From these figures, calculations were also derived for corresponding figures for recommended dietary allowances for individuals and for mean requirements for populations. The purpose of this review is not to derive a specific set of figures but to take a fresh look at the principles underlying the factorial approach to the derivation of EARs for zinc. Any extent to which our examples of estimates of physiologic requirements differ from those published recently by the Food and Nutrition Board reflects differences in the databases utilized. This also serves as a timely reminder of the current need for more extensive experimental data.

# OVERVIEW OF ZINC HOMEOSTASIS AND THE ROLE OF ZINC STABLE ISOTOPE TECHNIQUES

This paper is written at a time of real progress in our understanding of zinc metabolism at a subcellular and molecular level, including the identification of several zinc transporters (8) and progress in elucidation of the role(s) of metallothionein in zinc metabolism (45). These advances are leading to better understanding of the complexities of zinc metabolism and homeostasis in each organ and system, with the promise of further progress in the immediate future. At the same time, tracer kinetic studies combined with model-based compartmental analyses are advancing our broad understanding of whole-body zinc metabolism and especially of those pools of zinc that exchange rapidly with zinc in plasma (48, 64). To continue to advance our understanding of human zinc homeostasis and, thence, of human zinc dietary requirements, there is a special need for a clearer understanding of the regulation of zinc metabolism in the gastrointestinal tract. This can be achieved with a combination of molecular/cellular and human tracer/metabolic techniques.

One of the vital variables of zinc homeostasis, and the principal focus of this paper, is endogenous fecal zinc and its interrelationships with total absorbed zinc and with rapidly exchanging zinc pools (EZP). These measurements cannot be achieved simply by measuring total zinc, as is done in the balance technique; they depend on tracer methodology. In this paper, stable isotope techniques are emphasized not only because of our own experience with them, but also because, although still in an early stage of their potential application, these techniques have yielded the information pertinent to the thrust of this paper. The use of stable isotopes for exploring human zinc metabolism is not without potential pitfalls and technical challenges (16). However, it also has advantages, perhaps the most important of which is that three of the five naturally occurring stable isotopes of zinc are in low enough natural abundance to be employed as tracers in studies of human zinc metabolism. In other words, it is feasible to administer three different zinc tracers simultaneously. This means, for example, that different zinc tracers can be administered intravenously and orally on the same day. Within the past decade, as we have gained more experience in their application, zinc stable isotope techniques have been refined considerably. However, the majority of the studies we refer to are first-generation studies, which have depended on the simultaneous acquisition of precise balance data to determine one of the core variables of zinc homeostasis, namely endogenous fecal zinc. It is because of the ability tracer techniques confer to derive simultaneously determinations of zinc absorption and intestinal excretion of endogenous zinc that stable isotope data figure so prominently in this paper. Yet, we need to be sensitive to the limited amount of data, in terms of both number of studies reported and number of subjects per report. We also should be cognizant of the fact that none of the studies have been directed specifically to exploring the interrelationships of key variables of zinc homeostasis as a means of advancing knowledge of dietary zinc requirements. Moreover, in general, individual data are no longer available from several of these studies, which limits their potential to contribute to the goals of this paper.

## ALTERNATIVE STRATEGIES FOR ESTIMATING AVERAGE DIETARY ZINC REQUIREMENTS

The importance of efforts to improve knowledge of dietary zinc requirements through refinement of our knowledge of pertinent core features of zinc homeostasis is highlighted by reflecting on the dearth of alternative viable strategies. In particular there is a lack of adequate epidemiological data, including laboratory, functional, and clinical biomarkers of zinc nutritional status (17, 18, 67). Current knowledge of human zinc deficiency is dependent primarily on the results of careful intervention studies, using physiologic rather than pharmacologic quantities of zinc (3, 4, 17, 19). In theory, such studies could yield useful information on dietary zinc requirements, but the extent to which this is possible has been limited by the paucity of dietary data collected. No epidemiologic data can provide information on dietary requirements unless it includes information on dietary zinc intake, including baseline dietary data in intervention studies. Currently, epidemiologic data of one type or another can provide only limited supportive data for estimates of dietary zinc requirements derived from experimental metabolic data, and this is unlikely to change in the near future. Although zinc is by no means unique among the micronutrients in this regard, these limitations of epidemiologic data assume progressively greater importance in parallel with the growing recognition of the extraordinarily exciting biology and of the public health importance of this nutritionally essential element.

# FACTORIAL APPROACH

Inevitably, therefore, committees charged with developing estimates of dietary zinc requirements rely primarily on experimental data pertaining to zinc homeostasis (68, 69). Although whole-body turnover rates have been proposed as one means of assessing requirements (30), the information they yield is really limited to a long-term measure of zinc absorption, which, alone, does not define zinc requirements. To achieve reliable estimates of zinc requirements experimentally requires accurate measurements/calculations of the parameters that are required in the factorial equation.

Assuming there is no physiologic need to have positive zinc balance (as in a growing child), physiologic requirements are limited to the absorption of zinc necessary to replace total obligatory endogenous zinc excretion. Dietary zinc requirements can then be calculated by dividing this value for physiologic requirement by the fraction of dietary zinc absorbed. This is the essence of the factorial approach (31). Other strategies for progressing from physiologic requirement, i.e. the amount of required absorbed zinc, to an EAR are also available, especially with the wealth of data that can be derived from zinc stable isotope studies.

# INTESTINAL EXCRETION OF ENDOGENOUS ZINC

Substantial quantities of endogenous zinc are secreted into the lumen of the small intestine postprandially (40, 46). This secretion is believed to be primarily via the pancreatic exocrine secretions and possibly the intestinal mucosa (50, 52). A percentage of this endogenous zinc is reabsorbed, which is essential to maintain homeostasis; the remainder is excreted in the feces, where it can be measured with tracer techniques (34).

The feces are the major route of excretion of endogenous zinc, typically approximately twofold that of all other routes combined, but with much variation. This variation results from the regulation, by as-yet-unidentified mechanisms, of the quantity of endogenous zinc excreted by the intestine, in sensitive and rapid response to changes in zinc absorption (26) and status (29). These changes are sustained. Habitually low zinc intakes are associated with impressive evidence of intestinal conservation of endogenous zinc (42). Endogenous fecal zinc varies by as much as an order of magnitude in response to these mechanisms to maintain zinc homeostasis.

The outstanding importance of the regulation of endogenous fecal zinc in the maintenance of zinc homeostasis is apparent when it is considered that this is the only variable of zinc homeostasis known to be regulated by changes in zinc homeostasis. Rates of excretion of endogenous zinc via other organ systems involved with the excretion of endogenous zinc appear to change only with severe dietary zinc restriction (1, 20, 28, 49). Fractional absorption of zinc varies inversely with dietary intake of bioavailable zinc, which has the effect of modulating changes in total absorbed zinc. However, this effect is insufficient to totally stabilize total absorbed zinc at an optimal level, and evidence is not conclusive for a role of zinc status in regulating zinc absorption (9).

Endogenous fecal zinc is the largest and most elusive variable in the determination of physiologic zinc requirements. Endogenous fecal zinc is at the core of the interrelationships between variables of zinc homeostasis that we need to unravel.

## NON-INTESTINAL EXCRETION OF ENDOGENOUS ZINC

Although non-intestinal routes of excretion of endogenous zinc are not the primary focus of this paper, they are essential for estimation of physiologic requirements and, therefore, of dietary requirements by the factorial approach.

### Kidneys

Current thinking is that the quantity of zinc excreted via the kidney in healthy humans is not affected by dietary zinc intake and absorption except in extreme situations, e.g. zinc deprivation. Therefore, assuming that zinc intake is not very low, the kidneys do not have a discernible regulatory role in the maintenance of zinc homeostasis in normal circumstances. There are, however, unexplained inter-laboratory/investigator differences in the quantities of zinc excreted in the urine, and a more thorough evaluation of this route of excretion over the range of dietary zinc intake and absorption typical for North America and elsewhere is justified before any final conclusion is reached. Meanwhile, the average 24-h urine zinc excretion for 18 studies of young adult males is $0.63 \pm 0.15$ mg of Zn day$^{-1}$ (1, 2, 7, 14, 21, 25–28, 41, 44, 49, 55, 56, 59, 60, 62, 63). The corresponding figure for 11 studies of young adult females outside the reproductive cycle is $0.44 \pm 0.12$ mg of Zn day$^{-1}$ (6, 13, 14, 24, 25, 42, 48, 57, 58, 61, 66).

### Integument

Data are, understandably, much more limited for zinc excretion via the integument. For current purposes, we rely on two sets of data from the US Department of Agriculture, Agricultural Research Service Grand Forks Human Nutrition Research Center in North Dakota (28, 49), for young adult males whose average excretion was 0.54 mg of Zn day$^{-1}$. Extrapolation to adult women on a body surface basis gives a corresponding figure of 0.46 mg of Zn day$^{-1}$. Though cumbersome and fraught with the potential for contamination or incomplete collections, additional data are desirable.

### Semen and Menses

Excretion of zinc in semen has been reported to average 0.1 mg day$^{-1}$ (28) but can presumably vary widely depending on the frequency of ejaculation. Higher losses

**TABLE 1**   Nonintestinal excretion of endogenous Zn

| Excretory Route | Men | Women |
|---|---|---|
| Urine | 0.63 | 0.44 |
| Integument | 0.54 | 0.46[a] |
| Semen/menses | 0.1 | — |
| Total | 1.3 | 0.9 |

[a]Extrapolated from male data (28) on basis of surface area. Results are in milligrams of zinc per day.

via this route have been reported (1). Losses in menses, when averaged over the entire month, are negligible, 0.005 mg day$^{-1}$ (20). Excretion of endogenous zinc via nonintestinal routes when zinc intake is restricted is considered below.

Altogether, the nonintestinal losses of endogenous zinc are substantial and may approximate the intestinal endogenous losses when zinc intake and absorption are relatively low. Current knowledge, however, indicates that they do not have the same vital regulatory role and, indeed, may be regarded as a constant over a substantial range of zinc intake and absorption. This probably encompasses the value for absorption that is necessary to match physiologic requirements. Subject to further information, approximate values are given in Table 1.

## METABOLIC BALANCE

Data for each of the nonintestinal routes of excretion of endogenous zinc are acquired as part of a comprehensive approach to determining zinc balance. The factorial method for estimating zinc requirements is obviously dependent on information derived from complete, as opposed to the more typical crude, balance studies, in which the only endogenous losses measured are those in feces and urine. Because endogenous fecal zinc is not measured with the metabolic balance technique, it is not possible to determine the physiologic requirement for zinc by this means. Despite this limitation, it is theoretically possible to estimate an average dietary requirement by plotting either crude balance or net (apparent) absorption vs dietary zinc for subjects consuming their habitual diets or who have had adequate time to adapt to a change in diet prior to the balance study. In the case of crude balance, it is necessary to adjust for endogenous losses other than feces and urine; it is also necessary to adjust balance in the case of net absorption for zinc excretion in urine. The limited application of this approach to the estimation of dietary zinc requirements, despite a wealth of literature data, appears to stem from awareness of the propensity for errors. These do not need to be of great magnitude, compared with that of the overall measurements of intake and excretion, to provide substantially different results and, thus, different interpretations.

Mean results of zinc balance studies for men and women are illustrated in Figures 1*a* and *b*, respectively. These results are for crude balance, i.e. dietary zinc − (fecal zinc + urine zinc). The calculated adjustments required for other endogenous zinc losses for men and women are indicated. For men, there was no discernible relationship between balance and diet zinc over a range of intake from less than 2 up to 20 mg day$^{-1}$, a circumstance that first received attention several years ago (31). For women, there is, as would be expected for both genders, a significant positive linear regression for balance vs dietary zinc, but with a wide confidence interval.

Figure 1*a* suggests that zinc balance is maintained over a wide range, including a remarkably low intake (28), of zinc. This is in contrast to a theoretical pattern of continuing variation in body zinc (5) over a low-to-high normal range of intake, the evidence for which is discussed later.

## ADAPTATION

Adaptation has received considerable attention in discussion and interpretation of metabolic studies designed to explore aspects of whole-body zinc homeostasis with or without a goal of estimating dietary zinc requirements. This attention has been driven, in part, by the goal of understanding to what extent humans can adapt to dietary restriction. The ability to adapt has been evaluated primarily on the basis of zinc metabolic balance. Whether this yardstick is adequate, even if all sources of loss are considered, is questionable. One example of why we regard the restoration of balance following introduction of a zinc-restricted diet as inadequate evidence of satisfactory adaptation is the positive association between habitual dietary zinc intake (47) or absorbed zinc (42) and the total quantity of zinc in those combined pools of zinc that exchange readily (within 3 days) with zinc in plasma (EZP). "Adaptation" to a restricted intake is, therefore, not without a cost, which may be limited to diminution of short-term zinc stores as hepatic metallothionein (43), but which could also involve impairment of zinc-dependent physiology. Thus, even if, when dietary zinc is restricted, balance is eventually fully restored, this does not necessarily imply that this level of intake is optimal. At the very least, the individual may be ill-equipped to deal with those stress situations that may require more zinc.

Another reason adaptation has attracted attention is that most experimental metabolic studies of humans on low zinc intakes have depended on a period of experimental zinc depletion in closely supervised metabolic units. Dietary restriction

$\longrightarrow$

**Figures 1*a* and 1*b***    Zn balance vs dietary Zn. Means for young adult men (*a*) and women (*b*). (Solid lines) Crude zero balance (excretion in feces and urine only); (dotted lines) adjusted zero balances accounting for estimated losses via integument/semen/menses. Data from extensive, but not exhaustive, literature search (high phytate diets excluded). Numbers denote references.

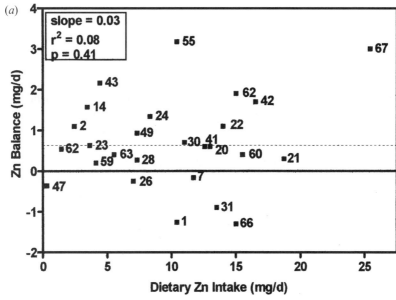

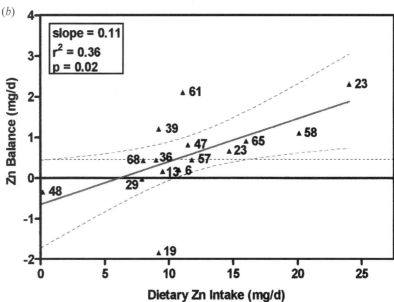

has been of variable duration, and there has been, and continues to be, considerable discussion and uncertainty on how long it takes to fully "adapt" to the zinc-restricted diet.

An aspect of adaptation that is especially pertinent to the theme of this paper relates to the strategy that has been used to derive a value for endogenous fecal zinc for the factorial approach to estimating physiologic requirements. Specifically, the excretion of endogenous zinc on a nearly zinc-free diet has been extrapolated back to zero time to derive an estimate of obligatory intestinal excretion of endogenous zinc in the nonadapted state (1). This figure, however, presumably depends on initial zinc status prior to introduction of the severely zinc-restricted diet. The World Health Organization (WHO) (69) proposed two numbers for endogenous fecal zinc to use in the calculation of physiologic requirements: one for the fully adapted individual ("basal") and one for the nonadapted ("normative"). Although it is not entirely clear how the precise numbers were derived, they were based on the same concept of adapted and nonadapted on a zinc-free or low-zinc diet. The differences in the critical value for endogenous fecal zinc derived from this approach are in sharp contrast to those derived from the approach developed in this paper, as is illustrated below (see Figure 6).

## INTERRELATIONSHIP BETWEEN ENDOGENOUS FECAL ZINC AND TOTAL ABSORBED ZINC

This section considers the evidence for a strong positive interrelationship between the quantity of exogenous dietary zinc absorbed and the quantity of endogenous zinc excreted via the intestine. Physiologically, this may not be a direct cause-effect relationship. Rather, it is assumed that total absorbed zinc affects zinc "status," which, in turn, rapidly affects endogenous fecal zinc. The positive correlations we have observed between total absorbed zinc and EZP (the size of the combined pools of zinc that exchange with zinc in plasma within 3 days) (36, 39, 42) and between EZP and endogenous fecal zinc (36, 39, 42) are consistent with this viewpoint.

The relationship between endogenous fecal zinc and total absorbed zinc, although indirect and of uncertain variability, offers new insight into strategies for improving the factorial approach to the estimation of human zinc dietary requirements and is the principal focus of this paper. Before considering the paradigm that we propose and the experimental evidence in support of this paradigm, it is useful to contrast alternative paradigms for the relationship between endogenous fecal zinc and total absorbed zinc and their implications.

The line of equality in Figure 2, for example, depicts the theoretical relationship between total endogenous losses and total absorbed zinc if zinc requirements are zero (i.e. if no endogenous losses occur) at zero intake absorption and if there is no accumulation of body zinc as total absorbed zinc increases progressively from zero. In this model, endogenous zinc excretion is matched by total absorbed zinc at

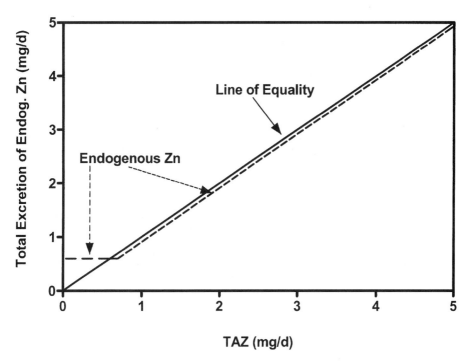

**Figure 2** Theoretical models for relationship between total excretion of endogenous Zn and total absorbed Zn that do not fit experimental data. See text for description. TAZ, total absorbed zinc.

all levels of absorption. It is generally accepted, however, that there is an obligatory loss of endogenous zinc at zero absorption. Although the experimental evidence for this is still limited, it is also physiologically likely. The most useful information we have on this topic is provided by two carefully conducted and detailed balance studies on almost zinc-free diets that were undertaken by Baer & King (1) and Hess et al (20) in the 1970s and 1980s. One of these studies involved women fed a diet providing 0.15 mg of Zn day$^{-1}$. The other involved young men fed a diet providing 0.28 mg of Zn day$^{-1}$. Although tracer studies were not included, the windows for possible total absorbed zinc and endogenous fecal zinc values were extremely narrow, and it needed only minor extrapolation back to the $y$-axis (zero total absorbed zinc) for endogenous fecal zinc or for urine zinc calculations at zero intake/absorption. Depending, to a small extent, on the precise FAZ and the slope of endogenous fecal zinc vs total absorbed zinc used to extrapolate to the $y$-axis, the figure for endogenous fecal zinc at zero total absorbed zinc is approximately 0.25 mg of Zn day$^{-1}$. The mean urine loss was 0.14 mg of Zn day$^{-1}$. There are conflicting data on whether integumental losses decrease at very restricted zinc intakes (28, 49). Assuming they remain about the same as for urine (28), for obligatory losses at zero intake these would add another 0.14 mg of Zn day$^{-1}$, giving a total of 0.53 mg of Zn day$^{-1}$. Losses in semen have been reported to account for 9% of total endogenous zinc excretion at an intake of 1.4 mg of Zn day$^{-1}$ (22), increasing the calculated total obligatory excretion of zinc at zero total absorbed zinc to 0.6 mg of Zn day$^{-1}$. Figures for females are a little lower. If we accept these figures, we require a different model than the line of equality, one hypothetical example of which is depicted in Figure 2.

An assumption that appears to have been made, if not explicitly stated, in estimating physiologic requirements is that endogenous losses calculated at zero intake/absorption do not change until total absorbed zinc has increased sufficiently to meet physiologic requirements. This model is also depicted in Figure 2, which also assumes that, once total absorbed zinc is sufficient to meet physiologic requirements, any further increases are paralleled by identical increases in endogenous excretion in order to maintain balance. The implications of this assumption with respect to the resulting extremely low estimate of requirements has been "softened" considerably by two factors. One has been the use of generous figures, in view of the data just discussed, for endogenous zinc excretion at zero intake. The second has been to calculate a figure for endogenous fecal zinc at zero intake for nonadapted individuals (1), as discussed earlier. This has provided the basis for the "normative" figures of the WHO (69). Before leaving Figure 2, it should be noted that there is no experimental data to support this model, however appealing theoretically.

# EXPERIMENTAL DATA ON THE INTERRELATIONSHIP BETWEEN ENDOGENOUS FECAL ZINC AND TOTAL ABSORBED ZINC

The general pattern of the interrelationship between endogenous fecal zinc and total absorbed zinc has been elucidated in animal models, including research by Weigand & Kirchgessner (65). This work clearly demonstrated that both total absorbed zinc and endogenous fecal zinc increased as dietary zinc increased. Replotting the data indicates that the slope of the regression of endogenous fecal zinc and total absorbed zinc was similar to that discussed below for human studies. Moreover, endogenous fecal zinc progressively increased with increasing total absorbed zinc at total absorbed zinc levels lower than those required for maximal growth in young rats, i.e. lower than physiologic requirements. The significance of this observation is discussed below.

In our experience with zinc stable isotope studies of healthy subjects (not consuming a high phytate diet), a strongly positive correlation between endogenous fecal zinc and total absorbed zinc has been consistent both in infants (33, 35–38) and in adults (42). This is illustrated in Figure 3, which depicts data from young nulliparous Chinese women consuming their habitual diet (42). One of the

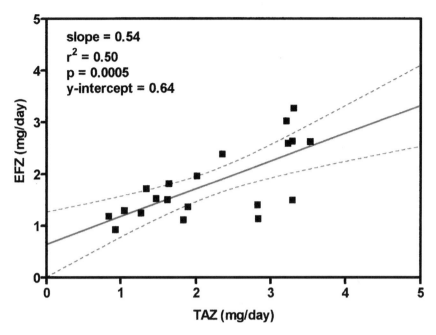

**Figure 3** Endogenous fecal Zn (EFZ) vs total absorbed Zn (TAZ) for young Chinese women (42). Linear regression with 95% confidence intervals shown.

valuable features of this plot is that it includes numerous unusually low values for total absorbed zinc, the result of the habitually low-zinc diet of the rural Chinese women included in this study. The importance of these low total absorbed zinc values and several features of this plot are discussed further below.

Although in the 1980s, a positive correlation between endogenous fecal zinc and total absorbed zinc was proposed for humans, this was not backed by experimental data and, moreover, was only thought likely at levels of total absorbed zinc above those required to maintain balance (31). However, a number of zinc stable isotope studies in the 1980s and 1990s (Table 2) have provided a new perspective. These have included the following: measurements of FAZ; information on dietary zinc, allowing calculation of total absorbed zinc; and either measurement of (26) or information that allowed calculation of endogenous fecal zinc in the same week as for total absorbed zinc (22–25, 32, 41, 48, 59–63). In no instance was the relationship between endogenous fecal zinc and total absorbed zinc a specified and major objective of the study. In most instances individual data are not available. However, plotting of the means for these studies has proved to be an interesting and informative exercise. The duration ranged from 1 week to 6 months (Table 2), with one study being undertaken while subjects were on their habitual diet. Although the briefer studies left some question about the completeness of adaptation to the

**TABLE 2**  Summary of zinc stable isotopes studies included in Figure 4

| Reference | Year | Gender | Diet Zn (mg/day) | Duration | Type of Diet[a] | No. |
|---|---|---|---|---|---|---|
| 26 | 1984 | M | 7.1 | 1 week | Food | 1 |
| 62 | 1984 | M | 15.0 | 7 weeks | LF/Zn++ | 4 |
| 63 | 1985 | M | 16.5 | 3 weeks | Food | 6 |
| 63 | 1985 | M | 5.5 | 7 weeks | Food | 6 |
| 60 | 1986 | M | 15.5 | 2 months | SP/Zn++ | 6 |
| 59 | 1991 | M | 5.7 | 1 week | SP/Zn++ | 5 |
| 59 | 1991 | M | 0.9 | 5 weeks | SP | 5 |
| 25 | 1992 | M | 14.0 | 2 weeks | Food | 14 |
| 41 | 1993 | M | 12.6 | 4 weeks | Food | 8 |
| 41 | 1993 | M | 4.1 | 6 months | SP | 8 |
| 61 | 1991 | F | 11.8 | 9 weeks | SP | 4 |
| 61 | 1991 | F | 9.0 | 9 weeks | SP | 4 |
| 25 | 1992 | F | 7.8 | 9 weeks | Food | 14 |
| 24 | 1998 | F | 11.1 | 8 weeks | Food | 21 |
| 24 | 1998 | F | 9.2 | 8 weeks | Food | 21 |
| 32 | 1996 | M/F | 10.7 | 3 weeks | Food | 8 |
| 48 | 2000 | M/F | 9.2 | Habitual | Food | 4 |
| 60 | 1986 | Elderly M | 15.5 | 12 weeks | SP | 6 |
| 23 | 1995 | Elderly F | 13.0 | 7 weeks | Food | 14 |
| 23 | 1995 | Elderly F | 6.7 | 7 weeks | Food | 14 |

[a]LF, liquid formula; SP, semipurified; Zn++, Zn supplement added.

experimental diet, for the shorter intervals in Table 2, the diet in these studies did not differ much in zinc content from the subjects' habitual diet. Diet zinc ranged from 0.9 to 16.5 mg day$^{-1}$, i.e. very low to high "normal" and the bioavailability of zinc from all diets is judged to be average to high.

The plot of mean endogenous fecal zincs vs mean total absorbed zincs for these studies is given in Figure 4. The similarities between this plot and that for individual Chinese women is noted. The data for young males, which comprise the single largest subgroup of studies, are identical to those utilized by the Food and Nutrition Board, Institute of Medicine (10). The linear regression for this group had a slope of 0.60, $r^2 = 0.73$, $y$-intercept = 0.27, and $P = 0.002$. The salient features of these plots of endogenous fecal zinc vs total absorbed zinc are discussed below.

Together, these data provide substantial support for a positive linear relationship between endogenous fecal zinc and total absorbed zinc. This raises a number of questions and also invites a new and quantitatively important concept in the

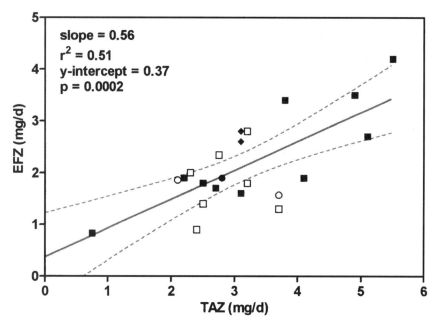

**Figure 4**  Linear regression of mean endogenous fecal Zn (EFZ) vs mean total absorbed Zn (TAZ) for adults. Regression includes means for young males (solid squares), young females (open squares), elderly males (solid circles), elderly females (open circles), and young mixed gender (solid diamonds).

calculation of physiologic requirements for zinc. These issues are addressed in the following sections.

## SALIENT FEATURES OF THE REGRESSION EQUATIONS FOR ENDOGENOUS FECAL ZINC VS TOTAL ABSORBED ZINC

Several features of the experimental plots of endogenous fecal zinc vs total absorbed zinc, including those illustrated in Figures 3 and 4, are relevant to the theme of this paper.

### Linearity

These plots are linear, with no suggestion that any other regression would provide a better fit and no indication of an inflexion point over the range of total absorbed zinc included in the experimental data.

## The Same Linear Relationship Between Endogenous Fecal Zinc and Total Absorbed Zinc is Maintained at Low Levels of Total Absorbed Zinc

The study with an animal model (65) demonstrated that endogenous fecal zinc increased with increases in zinc intake and in total absorbed zinc at levels of intake that were lower than those required to maintain maximal growth. In other words, endogenous fecal zinc increased progressively with increases in total absorbed zinc at levels of total absorbed zinc that were less than those required for matching physiologic requirements. These data are not supportive of the model depicted in Figure 2 but are supportive of the strategy proposed in this paper for estimating physiologic requirements.

The human data are a little more difficult to interpret because there is no general agreement for figures for physiologic requirements. Our calculations of these are discussed below, but we will assume an extremely conservative theoretical figure of 2.0 mg of Zn day$^{-1}$ for young adult women. Figures 3 and 4 between them include a substantial number of points below this number that appear to fit well with the overall linear regressions. These observations are consistent with those in the study of the animal model discussed above (65). Together they provide support for the hypothesis that endogenous fecal zinc increases with increasing total absorbed zinc at levels of total absorbed zinc that are lower than those needed to match physiologic requirements. Considered from another viewpoint, these observations indicate that not only is there an obligatory excretion of zinc by the intestine on zinc-free diets, there is also an obligatory increase in endogenous fecal zinc in tandem with total absorbed zinc, even at levels of total absorbed zinc that are less than those needed to match physiologic requirements. Once again, they are not consistent with the model in Figure 2.

### Y-Axis Intercept

Without putting weight on an observation obtained by extrapolating linear regressions of endogenous fecal zinc vs total absorbed zinc beyond measured data points, it is not without interest that the y-intercepts derived from these extrapolations were in good agreement with the calculations of endogenous fecal zinc at zero absorption already discussed. These intercepts are, therefore, supportive of the legitimacy of these calculations and are also consistent with the hypothesis that the linear regression between endogenous fecal zinc and total absorbed zinc holds even to the very lowest levels of absorption.

### Slope of Linear Regression of Endogenous Fecal Zinc on Total Absorbed Zinc

A feature of the linear regression of endogenous fecal zinc on total absorbed zinc in our infant studies and in Figures 3 and 4 has been the consistency of the slope between 0.5 and 0.6. Considering that the relationship between these two key variables is presumably indirect rather than direct, this consistency is perhaps unexpected and requires further careful research. Further research is also a priority because of the implications of this slope, which contrasts notably with the model depicted in Figure 2 for values of total absorbed zinc both below and above those that correspond to physiologic requirements and, therefore, which contrasts with current published concepts of zinc homeostasis. These implications are discussed in the next section.

# IMPLICATIONS OF EXPERIMENTAL DATA ON THE RELATIONSHIP BETWEEN ENDOGENOUS FECAL ZINC AND TOTAL ABSORBED ZINC

Current data on urine zinc excretion (which merit further research) reveal no evidence to suggest that the kidneys have any role in maintaining zinc homeostasis except at extremely high and low intakes. The same applies to the integument and testes, and indeed, it is difficult to envisage that these organs, zinc excretion via which is subject to so much individual and environmental variation, have a serious regulatory role rather than an incidental impact on zinc homeostasis. Given these circumstances, a slope for the regression of endogenous fecal zinc on total absorbed zinc of <1 implies a positive zinc balance when the total absorbed zinc exceeds the physiologic requirement. It also implies a negative balance when total absorbed zinc is insufficient to match physiologic requirements. In other words, these data suggest that there is a very narrow range at which balance is truly achieved, rather than a plateau over a wide range of intake and absorption.

This concept of an optimal point is illustrated in Figure 5, which is based on the endogenous fecal zinc and total absorbed zinc data depicted in Figure 4, together with a calculated constant (Table 1) for nonintestinal endogenous losses for women.

The line of equality between endogenous losses and total absorbed zinc in Figure 5 is identical to the line depicted in Figure 2. Except at low levels of zinc intake, which are associated with diminution of nonintestinal excretion of endogenous zinc (indicated by interrupted line in Figure 5), these nonintestinal losses are added as a constant, giving a line parallel to the linear regression for endogenous fecal zinc on total absorbed zinc, and 0.9 mg of Zn day$^{-1}$ (Table 1) above this regression. This plot indicates that the physiologic requirement is one specific number that is the value for total absorbed zinc at which the line of equality intersects the line depicting total endogenous zinc losses. This particular set of data indicates a calculated physiologic requirement for young women of 2.8 mg of Zn day$^{-1}$. This figure is obviously considerably higher than that which would be derived from the model depicted in Figure 2, unless the value for endogenous zinc losses at zero absorption were to be set arbitrarily high.

The mixed-gender endogenous fecal zinc vs total absorbed zinc regression was used in Figure 5 because of the lack of adequate female data apart from the data

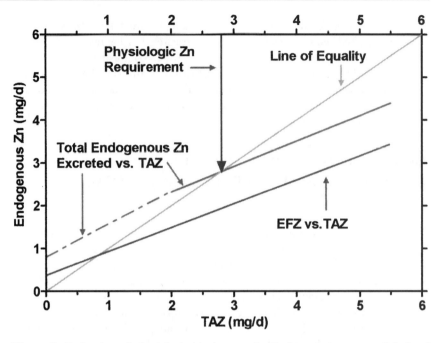

**Figure 5** Estimation of physiologic requirement for Zn for young women: Calculated nonintestinal excretion of endogenous Zn for women added to linear regression for endogenous fecal zinc (EFZ) vs total absorbed zinc (TAZ) (Figure 3) to give calculated total endogenous Zn excretion. Intercept of that line with the line of equality is the estimated physiologic requirement (2.8 mg of Zn day$^{-1}$).

from the China study (42). Substituting the latter regression gives an estimated physiologic requirement of 3.4 mg of Zn day$^{-1}$. These differences are likely to reflect the limitations of available data rather than being related to gender. For the experimental data available at this time, total absorbed zinc explains only about 50% of variance in endogenous fecal zinc. It will require high-quality prospective studies to determine how much higher this figure might be if experimental limitations are minimized.

## ALTERNATIVE SCENARIOS THAT WOULD RESULT IN MUCH LOWER ESTIMATES OF PHYSIOLOGIC REQUIREMENTS

Two alternative scenarios merit consideration. The first is related to the reduced urine zinc excretion (1, 20, 28), the reduced zinc per ejaculation (22), and the probable reduction in integumental zinc (28) at very low levels of zinc intake (i.e. <3–4 mg day$^{-1}$ with further reduction at <0.3 mg day$^{-1}$). Given this lower excretion of zinc via nonintestinal routes, does the line of equality intersect the line for total endogenous zinc losses at a level of total absorbed zinc much lower than that suggested in Figure 5, even if the positive linear regression of endogenous fecal zinc on total absorbed zinc does extend to the *y*-axis? After all, there is evidence that crude balance is not far from being achieved with a zinc intake as low as 0.28 mg day$^{-1}$ (1). Is it not, therefore, reasonable to anticipate that just a little more zinc intake would be sufficient to achieve balance? Currently, there are insufficient experimental data to totally exclude this possibility. However, given the data that are available, and making some estimates in converting data related to dietary intake into data related to absorption, it appears that this does not occur. Approximate calculated total endogenous zinc losses at low intakes of zinc are depicted by the interrupted line in Figure 5.

The second scenario that could give lower figures for calculated physiologic requirements is to utilize the model depicted in Figure 2. This, in fact, has been the "standard" approach to factorial calculations, even if not necessarily explicitly stated in these terms. A standard figure has been used for endogenous fecal zinc and, therefore, for total endogenous excretion of zinc (30, 31, 69). As illustrated in Figure 6, if the dynamic interrelationship between endogenous fecal zinc and total absorbed zinc is not considered, the calculated obligatory loss of endogenous zinc via the intestine is much lower. A conceptual difference in the approach described in this paper is that there is no attempt to determine a number for obligatory endogenous fecal zinc, which is then used as part of a sum to estimate physiologic requirements. Rather, this figure for endogenous fecal zinc is only apparent retrospectively from the plot (Figures 5 and 6). Instead of being a static number, endogenous fecal zinc will be found to vary substantially with physiologic requirements and, therefore, with several factors, including gender, that affect physiologic requirement.

## ESTIMATED AVERAGE REQUIREMENTS

With the information already in hand from the same zinc stable isotope/metabolic studies, it is straightforward to progress from the calculated physiologic requirement to derive the estimated average requirement (EAR). The simplest and most direct route is to plot total absorbed zinc vs dietary zinc intake using data from the same study. From this plot, the dietary zinc that corresponds to the total absorbed zinc that matches the physiologic requirement is the EAR. Alternatively, fractional absorption can be plotted vs total absorbed zinc, and the "critical" figure for fractional absorption that corresponds to the total absorbed zinc matching physiologic requirement can be determined. The physiologic requirement divided by this figure for fractional absorption gives the EAR.

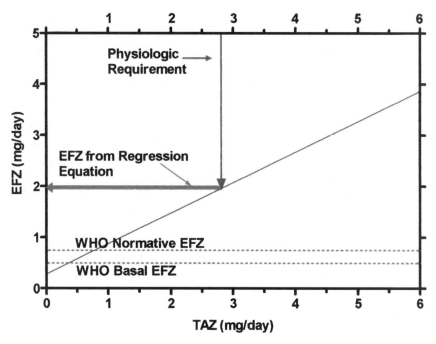

**Figure 6**    Comparison of endogenous fecal zinc (EFZ) at level of physiologic requirement determined by method described in paper with basal and normative EFZ figures for the World Health Organization (WHO) (69).

## CONCLUDING REMARKS

Well-designed zinc stable isotope tracer/metabolic studies can provide a wealth of information on zinc homeostasis, which is invaluable in refining estimates of physiologic and dietary requirements. To derive optimal value from such studies, data analyses should include a special focus on the interrelationships between major variables of zinc homeostasis. These include, especially, the interrelationship between endogenous fecal zinc and total absorbed zinc. Maximal use should be made of individual data, rather than limiting data analyses to comparisons of means, and more research is needed that includes individuals on a range of zinc intake and absorption, including the challenging task of achieving this at low levels of diet zinc. Prospective studies are essential to confirm the validity of utilizing the interrelationship between endogenous fecal zinc and total absorbed zinc in factorial calculations of dietary zinc requirements and to explore if and how we might improve further on the approach proposed in this paper. Meanwhile, we conclude that although the numbers are not yet definite, they represent a distinct advance conceptually in tackling the enigma of intestinal excretion of endogenous zinc in factorial calculations of dietary zinc requirements.

**Visit the Annual Reviews home page at www.AnnualReviews.org**

## LITERATURE CITED

1. Baer MT, King JC. 1984. Tissue zinc levels and zinc excretion during experimental zinc depletion in young men. *Am. J. Clin. Nutr.* 39:556–70
2. Behall KM, Scholfield DJ, Lee K, Powell AS, Moser PB. 1987. Mineral balance in adult men: effect of four refined fibers. *Am. J. Clin. Nutr.* 46:307–14
3. Bhutta ZA, Black RE, Brown KH, Gardner JM, Gore S, et al. 1999. Prevention of diarrhea and pneumonia by zinc supplementation in children in developing countries: pooled analysis of randomized controlled trials. *J. Pediatr.* 135:689–97
4. Brown KH, Peerson JM, Allen LH. 1998. Effect of zinc supplementation on children's growth: a meta-analysis of intervention trials. *Bibl. Nutr. Diet.* 54:76–83
5. Buckley WT. 1996. Application of compartmental modeling to determination of trace element requirements in humans. *J. Nutr.* 126:2312–19S
6. Colin MA, Taper LJ, Ritchey SJ. 1983. Effect of dietary zinc and protein levels on the utilization of zinc and copper by adult females. *J. Nutr.* 113:1480–88
7. Coudray C, Bellanger J, Castiglia-Delavaud C, Remesy C, Vermorel M, Rayssignuier Y. 1997. Effect of soluble or partly soluble dietary fibres supplementation on absorption and balance of calcium, magnesium, iron and zinc in healthy young men. *Eur. J. Clin. Nutr.* 51:375–80
8. Cousins RJ, McMahon RJ. 2000. Integrative aspects of zinc transporters. *J. Nutr.* 130:1384–87S
9. Evans GW, Johnson EC, Johnson PE. 1979. Zinc absorption in the rat determined by radioisotope dilution. *J. Nutr.* 109:1258–64
10. Food Nutr. Board, Inst. Med. 2001. *Dietary Reference Intakes for Vitamin A, Vitamin K, Boron, Chromium, Copper, Iodine, Iron, Manganese, Molybdenum, Nickel, Silicon, Vanadium and Zinc.* Washington, DC: Natl. Acad. In press
11. Gibson RS, Vanderkooy PD, MacDonald AC, Goldman A, Ryan BA, Berry M. 1989. A growth-limiting, mild zinc-deficiency syndrome in some southern Ontario boys with low height percentiles. *Am. J. Clin. Nutr.* 49:1266–73
12. Goldenberg RL, Tamura T, Neggers Y, Copper RL, Johnston KE, et al. 1995. The effect of zinc supplementation on pregnancy outcome. *JAMA* 274:463–68
13. Greger JL, Abernathy RP, Bennett OA. 1978. Zinc and nitrogen balance in adolescent females fed varying levels of zinc and soy protein. *Am. J. Clin. Nutr.* 31:112–16
14. Hallfrisch J, Powell A, Carafelli C, Reiser S, Prather ES. 1987. Mineral balances of men and women consuming high fiber diets with complex or simple carbohydrate. *J. Nutr.* 117:48–55
15. Hambidge K. 1989. Mild zinc deficiency in human subjects. In *Zinc in Human Biology*, ed C Mills. London: Springer-Verlag
16. Hambidge KM, Krebs NF, Miller L. 1998. Evaluation of zinc metabolism with use of stable-isotope techniques: implications for the assessment of zinc status. *Am. J. Clin. Nutr.* 68:410–13S
17. Hambidge M. 2000. Human zinc deficiency. *J. Nutr.* 130:1344–49S
18. Hambidge M, Krebs N. 1995. Assessment of zinc status in man. *Indian J. Pediatr.* 62X:169–80
19. Hambidge M, Krebs N. 1999. Zinc, diarrhea, and pneumonia. *J. Pediatr.* 135:661–64
20. Hess FM, King JC, Margen S. 1977. Zinc excretion in young women on low zinc intakes and oral contraceptive agents. *J. Nutr.* 107:1610–20
21. Holbrook JT, Smith JC Jr, Reiser S. 1989. Dietary fructose or starch: effects on

copper, zinc, iron, manganese, calcium, and magnesium balances in humans. *Am. J. Clin. Nutr.* 49:1290–94

22. Hunt CD, Johnson PE, Herbel J, Mullen LK. 1992. Effects of dietary zinc depletion on seminal volume and zinc loss, serum testosterone concentrations, and sperm morphology in young men. *Am. J. Clin. Nutr.* 56:148–57

23. Hunt JR, Gallagher SK, Johnson LK, Lykken GI. 1995. High-versus low-meat diets: effects on zinc absorption, iron status, and calcium, copper, iron, magnesium, manganese, nitrogen, phosphorus, and zinc balance in postmenopausal women. *Am. J. Clin. Nutr.* 62:621–32

24. Hunt JR, Matthys LA, Johnson LK. 1998. Zinc absorption, mineral balance, and blood lipids in women consuming controlled lactoovovegetarian and omnivorous diets for 8 wk. *Am. J. Clin. Nutr.* 67:421–30

25. Hunt JR, Mullen LK, Lykken GI. 1992. Zinc retention from an experimental diet based on the US FDA Total Diet Study. *Nutr. Res.* 126:2345–53S

26. Jackson MJ, Jones DA, Edwards RH, Swainbank IG, Coleman ML. 1984. Zinc homeostasis in man: studies using a new stable isotope-dilution technique. *Br. J. Nutr.* 51:199–208

27. Johnson MA, Baier MJ, Greger JL. 1982. Effects of dietary tin on zinc, copper, iron, manganese, and magnesium metabolism of adult males. *Am. J. Clin. Nutr.* 35:1332–38

28. Johnson PE, Hunt CD, Milne DB, Mullen LK. 1993. Homeostatic control of zinc metabolism in men: zinc excretion and balance in men fed diets low in zinc. *Am. J. Clin. Nutr.* 57:557–65

29. Johnson PE, Hunt JR, Ralston NV. 1988. The effect of past and current dietary Zn intake on Zn absorption and endogenous excretion in the rat. *J. Nutr.* 118:1205–9

30. King J, Turnlund J. 1989. Human zinc requirements. In *Kinetic Models of Trace Element and Mineral Metabolism during Development*, ed. KN Siva Subramanian, ME Wastney. Boca Raton: CRC

31. King JC. 1986. Assessment of techniques for determining human zinc requirements. *J. Am. Diet. Assoc.* 86:1523–28

32. Knudsen E, Jensen M, Solgaard P, Sorensen SS, Sandstrom B. 1995. Zinc absorption estimated by fecal monitoring of zinc stable isotopes validated by comparison with whole-body retention of zinc radioisotopes in humans. *J. Nutr.* 125:1274–82

33. Krebs N, Reidinger CJ, Miller LV, Borschel M. 2000. Zinc Homeostasis in normal infants fed a casein hydrolysate formula. *J. Pediatr. Gastroenterol. Nutr.* 30:29–33

34. Krebs N, Miller LV, Naake VL, Lei S, Westcott JE, et al. 1995. The use of stable isotope techniques to assess zinc metabolism. *J. Nutr. Biochem.* 6:292–307

35. Krebs N, Reidinger C, Westcott JE, Miller LV, Fennessey PV, Hambidge KM. 1995. *Stable Isotope Studies of Zinc Metabolism in Infants.* In *Kinetic Models of Trace Element and Mineral Metabolism during Development*, ed. KN Siva Subramanian, ME Wastney pp. 65–72. Boca Raton: CRC

36. Krebs N, Westcott J, Miller L, Herrmann T, Hambidge K. 2000. Exchangeable zinc pool (EZP) in normal infants: correlates with parameters of zinc homeostasis. *FASEB J.* 14:A205

37. Krebs NF, Reidinger C, Westcott J, Miller LV, Fennessey PV, Hambidge KM. 1994. Whole body zinc metabolism in full-term breastfed and formula fed infants. *Adv. Exp. Med. Biol.* 352:223–26

38. Krebs NF, Reidinger CJ, Miller LV, Hambidge KM. 1996. Zinc homeostasis in breast-fed infants. *Pediatr. Res.* 39:661–65

39. Krebs NF, Westcott J. 2001. Zinc and breastfed infants: if and when is there a risk of deficiency? *Proc. 10th Int. Conf., Int. Soc. Res. Hum. Milk Lactation.* New York: Plenum. In press

40. Krebs NF, Westcott J, Miller LV. 1999.

Localization of secretion and reabsorption of endogenous zinc by compartmental modeling of intestinal data. *FASEB J.* 13:A214

41. Lee DY, Prasad AS, Hydrick-Adair C, Brewer G, Johnson PE. 1993. Homeostasis of zinc in marginal human zinc deficiency: role of absorption and endogenous excretion of zinc. *J. Lab. Clin. Med.* 122:549–56

42. Lei S, Mingyan X, Miller LV, Tong L, Krebs NF, Hambidge KM. 1996. Zinc absorption and intestinal losses of endogenous zinc in young Chinese women with marginal zinc intakes. *Am. J. Clin. Nutr.* 63:348–53

43. Lowe NM, Bremner I, Jackson MJ. 1991. Plasma 65Zn kinetics in the rat. *Br. J. Nutr.* 65:445–55

44. Mahalko JR, Sandstead HH, Johnson LK, Milne DB. 1983. Effect of a moderate increase in dietary protein on the retention and excretion of Ca, Cu, Fe, Mg, P, and Zn by adult males. *Am. J. Clin. Nutr.* 37:8–14

45. Maret W. 2000. The function of zinc metallothionein: a link between cellular zinc and redox state. *J. Nutr.* 130:1455–58S

46. Matseshe JW, Phillips SF, Malagelada JR, McCall JT. 1980. Recovery of dietary iron and zinc from the proximal intestine of healthy man: studies of different meals and supplements. *Am. J. Clin. Nutr.* 33:1946–53

47. Miller LV, Hambidge KM, Naake VL, Hong Z, Westcott JL, Fennessey PV. 1994. Size of the zinc pools that exchange rapidly with plasma zinc in humans: alternative techniques for measuring and relation to dietary zinc intake. *J. Nutr.* 124:268–76

48. Miller LV, Krebs NF, Hambidge KM. 2000. Development of a compartmental model of human zinc metabolism: identifiability and multiple studies analyses. *Am. J. Physiol. Regul. Integr. Comp. Physiol.* 279:R1681–84

49. Milne DB, Canfield WK, Mahalko JR, Sandstead HH. 1983. Effect of dietary zinc on whole body surface loss of zinc: impact on estimation of zinc retention by balance method. *Am. J. Clin. Nutr.* 38:181–86

50. Montgomery ML, Sheline GE, Chaikoff IL. 1943. The elimination of administered zinc in pancreatic juice, duodenal juice, and bile of the dog as measured by its radioactive isotope ($Zn^{65}$). *J. Exp. Med.* 78:151–59

51. Natl. Res. Counc. 1989. *Recommended Dietary Allowances.* Washington, DC: Natl. Acad. 10th ed.

52. Pekas JC. 1966. Zinc 65 metabolism: gastrointestinal secretion by the pig. *Am. J. Physiol.* 211:407–13

53. Penland JG. 2000. Behavioral data and methodology issues in studies of zinc nutrition in humans. *J. Nutr.* 130:361–64S

54. Schlesinger L, Arevalo M, Arredondo S, Lonnerdal B, Stekel A. 1993. Zinc supplementation impairs monocyte function. *Acta Paediatr.* 82:734–38

55. Snedeker SM, Smith SA, Greger JL. 1982. Effect of dietary calcium and phosphorus levels on the utilization of iron, copper, and zinc by adult males. *J. Nutr.* 112:136–43

56. Spencer H, Asmussen CR, Holtzman RB, Kramer L. 1979. Metabolic balances of cadmium, copper, manganese, and zinc in man. *Am. J. Clin. Nutr.* 32:1867–75

57. Swanson CA, King JC. 1982. Zinc utilization in pregnant and nonpregnant women fed controlled diets providing the zinc RDA. *J. Nutr.* 112:697–707

58. Taper LJ, Hinners ML, Ritchey SJ. 1980. Effects of zinc intake on copper balance in adult females. *Am. J. Clin. Nutr.* 33:1077–82

59. Taylor CM, Bacon JR, Aggett PJ, Bremner I. 1991. Homeostatic regulation of zinc absorption and endogenous losses in zinc-deprived men. *Am. J. Clin. Nutr.* 53:755–63; Erratum. 1992. *Am. J. Clin. Nutr.* 56(2):462

60. Turnlund JR, Durkin N, Costa F, Margen S. 1986. Stable isotope studies of zinc absorption and retention in young and elderly men. *J. Nutr.* 116:1239–47

61. Turnlund JR, Keyes WR, Hudson CA, Betschart AA, Kretsch MJ, Sauberlich HE. 1991. A stable-isotope study of zinc, copper, and iron absorption and retention by young women fed vitamin B-6-deficient diets. *Am. J. Clin. Nutr.* 54:1059–64

62. Turnlund JR, King JC, Keyes WR, Gong B, Michel MC. 1984. A stable isotope study of zinc absorption in young men: effects of phytate and alpha-cellulose. *Am. J. Clin. Nutr.* 40:1071–77

63. Wada L, Turnlund JR, King JC. 1985. Zinc utilization in young men fed adequate and low zinc intakes. *J. Nutr.* 115:1345–54

64. Wastney ME, Aamodt RL, Rumble WF, Henkin RI. 1986. Kinetic analysis of zinc metabolism and its regulation in normal humans. *Am. J. Physiol. Regul. Integr. Comp. Physiol.* 251:R398–408

65. Weigand E, Kirchgessner M. 1980. Total true efficiency of zinc utilization: determination and homeostatic dependence upon the zinc supply status in young rats. *J. Nutr.* 110:469–80

66. Wisker E, Nagel R, Tanudjaja TK, Feldheim W. 1991. Calcium, magnesium, zinc, and iron balances in young women: effects of a low-phytate barley-fiber concentrate. *Am. J. Clin. Nutr.* 54:553–59

67. Wood RJ. 2000. Assessment of marginal zinc status in humans. *J. Nutr.* 130:1350–54S

68. World Health Org. 1973. *Trace Elements in Human Nutrition. Rep. WHO Expert Comm. WHO Tech. Rep. Ser. No. 532:9–15.* Geneva, Switzerland: WHO

69. World Health Org. 1996. *Trace Elements in Human Nutrition and Health.* Geneva, Switzerland: WHO

Annu. Rev. Nutr. 2001. 21:453–73

# MAMMALIAN SELENIUM-CONTAINING PROTEINS

## Dietrich Behne and Antonios Kyriakopoulos

*Hahn-Meitner-Institut Berlin, Department Molecular Trace Element Research in the Life Sciences, Glienicker Strasse 100, D-14109 Berlin, Germany; e-mail: behne@hmi.de; kyriakopoulos@hmi.de*

**Key Words**   selenoproteins, glutathione peroxidases, iodothyronine deiodinases, thioredoxin reductases, novel selenium compounds

■ **Abstract**   Mammalian selenium-containing proteins can be divided into three groups: proteins containing nonspecifically incorporated selenium, specific selenium-binding proteins, and specific selenocysteine-containing selenoproteins. Selenoproteins with known functions identified so far include five glutathione peroxidases, two deiodinases, several thioredoxin reductases, and selenophosphate synthetase 2. Alternative splicing leads to a greater variety of selenoproteins, as was shown in the cases of a specific sperm nuclei glutathione peroxidase and some thioredoxin reductases. Selenoprotein P, selenoprotein W, a 15-kDa selenoprotein, an 18-kDa selenoprotein, and several selenoproteins identified in silico from nucleotide sequence databases were found to contain selenocysteine but their functions are not known. Gel electrophoretic separation of tissue samples from rats labeled in vivo with $^{75}$Se showed the existence of further selenium-containing proteins.

## CONTENTS

0199-9885/01/0715-0453$14.00                                                     **453**

# INTRODUCTION

As early as 1916, selenium was detected in normal human tissue samples, and it was suggested that "it may have a position in the organism which will without doubt be of the utmost significance in the study of the life processes" (49). However, this finding remained without any impact, as was emphasized in 1953 in the following statement (52): "[T]he data of T. Gassmann, who claimed to have found small amounts of selenium in normal human bone and tooth tissue and who attributes an essential importance to selenium, may be the result of an error." Four years later, Schwarz & Foltz showed that liver necrosis induced in rats by feeding them a purified vitamin E–deficient diet could be prevented by adding selenium (88). Subsequent studies of animals and humans proved that selenium is an essential element necessary for growth and fertility, and that selenium deficiency or a combined low selenium and low vitamin E status may lead to various disorders (37). Tissues that in animals were found to be affected include cardiac muscle, erythrocytes, eye, liver, kidney, pancreas, skeletal muscle, skin, smooth muscle, spermatozoa, and testis. In humans, selenium was shown to have a protective effect against Keshan disease, an endemic cardiomyopathy that occurred in selenium-deficient areas in China. Selenium deficiency also seems to be a pathogenic factor in Kaschin-Beck disease, an osteoarthropathy endemic in selenium-deficient regions in Northeast Asia, and cardiomyopathy and muscular disorders have been observed in patients on parenteral nutrition with a very low selenium intake.

Ever since the discovery of its essentiality, in 1957, the question of the chemical form in which selenium is biologically active has been of great interest. This question seemed to be settled in 1973, when glutathione peroxidase (GPx) was identified as a selenoenzyme (81). It catalyzes the reduction of peroxides and is thus part of the cellular antioxidant defense system.

The biological role of selenium in the form of GPx could explain several, but not all, effects of selenium deficiency. This indication that there might be further biologically active forms of selenium was supported by the finding that about two thirds of selenium present in the organism is not bound to this enzyme but is contained in other compounds (18). The discovery of a codon responsible for the incorporation of selenium in the form of selenocysteine into specific proteins in bacteria as well as in mammalian cells (30, 106) suggested that various selenoproteins are expressed in this way.

Information on the presence of a larger number of selenium-containing proteins was then obtained from experiments in which rats and mice were labeled in vivo by administration of $^{75}$Se-selenite and the selenium-containing proteins identified from the tracer distribution after chromatographic or gel electrophoretic separation (10, 29, 40, 45, 56). These compounds differed in their distribution among tissues (10) and subcellular fractions (17). This suggested that they are part of several metabolic pathways of the element and might be involved in different intracellular processes. The discovery of a hierarchy among the selenoproteins that, with insufficient selenium intake, results in the preferential supply of the element to certain selenium-containing proteins, with GPx being last in the ranking order (10), likewise indicated the existence of further biologically important selenoproteins.

Following these findings, numerous studies have been carried out that led to the identification of several selenoenzymes with key roles in the physiological processes. However, although with the advanced methods in molecular biology and protein biochemistry our knowledge in this field has rapidly increased, this work is still far from being completed. In this review, the state of research on the mammalian selenium-containing proteins is presented and discussed.

## CLASSIFICATION OF THE SELENIUM-CONTAINING PROTEINS

The selenium-containing proteins known so far can be divided into three groups: proteins into which the element is incorporated nonspecifically, specific selenium-binding proteins, and specific proteins that contain selenium in the form of genetically encoded selenocysteine and that have been defined as selenoproteins. In addition there are proteins in which selenium has been detected but for which no information on its binding form is as yet available. The incorporation of dietary selenium into the different types of selenium-containing proteins is shown schematically in Figure 1.

In several distribution studies, of which only a few are mentioned here as examples, the retention of selenium in the tissues was found to be much higher when given as selenomethionine than when given as selenocystine, selenite, or selenate (42, 85, 104). In the investigation of the selenium-containing proteins in rat tissues after labeling with normal and large doses of selenite and selenomethionine, it was shown that the higher tissue selenium contents were due to nonspecific incorporation into a large number of proteins (14). The studies carried out in this field indicated that the distribution of the element among the different selenium-containing proteins depends to a certain extent on the chemical form and dosage of dietary selenium, as is summarized in the schematic diagram in Figure 1.

### Specific Selenoproteins

After ingestion of normal amounts of selenite, selenate, or selenocysteine, nearly all of the element is transported via an intermediary pool into specific selenocysteine-containing selenoproteins, which are responsible for its biological

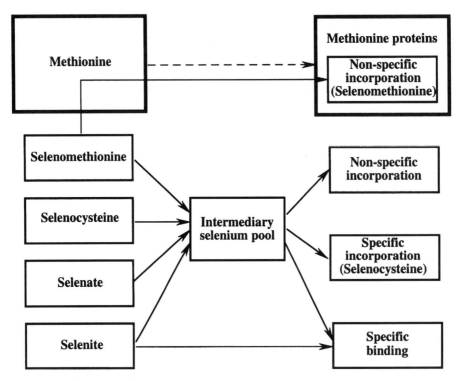

**Figure 1**   Types of selenium-containing proteins present in the mammalian organism and effects of the chemical forms of dietary selenium on the uptake of the element by these proteins. (For details see text.)

effects. Their levels are homeostatically controlled and cannot be increased by additional selenium supplementation.

## Nonspecific Selenium-Containing Proteins

In the case of dietary selenomethionine, a part of the element is metabolized in the same way as the other selenium compounds. A certain percentage, however, is deposited directly nonspecifically into proteins in place of methionine and is therefore mainly found in methionine-rich proteins present in the organism in higher concentrations. This part that follows the metabolic pathways of methionine appears to be dependent only on the ratio of selenomethionine and methionine. It can therefore be influenced by changing the selenomethionine concentration as well as by changing the methionine concentration in the diet. This means that the amount of selenium incorporated nonspecifically increases with increased intake of selenomethionine (14, 42, 85, 104), but also with diets with low methionine levels (27, 102). In the latter case, however, with normal selenomethionine supply, the increase in nonspecific incorporation results in a decrease in the concentrations and effects of the specific selenoproteins (102).

## Selenium-Binding Proteins

The third group of selenium-containing proteins comprises the specific proteins in which selenium is only attached to the molecules. So far they include two proteins of 14 kDa (5) and 56 kDa (6), which have been detected in mouse liver. The chemical form of selenium in these compounds is not known, but from the findings that the TGA codon responsible for selenocysteine incorporation is not present in the coding regions of the genes and that the levels of the two proteins are not dependent on dietary selenium supply, it could be concluded that the element is only firmly bound to these compounds. No information is available on the function of the 56-kDa protein, but it has been suggested that the 14-kDa protein may act as a growth regulatory molecule and that by modulating its function selenium may inhibit cell growth.

In mouse tissues, a protein of about 17 kDa has been found that specifically binds selenite administered either in vitro or in vivo (87). Its function is not known, but it has been suggested that it may be active in the intracellular transport of the element.

## MAMMALIAN SELENOPROTEINS: General Points

The biological effects of selenium in mammals are due to certain proteins that contain the element in the form of covalently bound selenocysteine. For the specific uptake of selenium by these proteins, several factors are necessary. They prevent the substitution of selenium by sulfur, which has similar chemical and physical properties and is present in the biosphere in much higher concentrations. One of the unique features in the incorporation of selenocysteine is the use of the UGA codon, which normally serves as a termination signal and needs an mRNA stem-loop structure located in the 3' untranslated region and specific translation factors to be recognized as the codon for selenocysteine insertion (70). Another one is the biosynthesis of selenocysteine, which takes place on its tRNA and is achieved by serine being first loaded onto this tRNA and then transformed into the selenoamino acid by reaction with selenophosphate. However, the knowledge of the different stages of selenoprotein expression in mammals (21, 70) is less complete than in the case of the bacterial systems (23, 24).

A further interesting aspect in the formation of mammalian selenoproteins is the existence of a hierarchy in selenoprotein expression, which ensures that in periods of insufficient dietary selenium intake, the selenium levels in certain tissues are maintained and within each tissue the levels of certain selenoproteins (10). Recent studies of rats showed that even after extreme experimental selenium depletion over six generations, which led to a drastic decrease in the selenium concentrations in liver, skeletal muscle, and blood below 1% of normal levels, the brain still contained 60% of the concentration found in control animals. In this hierarchy the brain is followed by spinal marrow, pituitary, thyroid, ovaries, and adrenals (16). Within most of the tissues, the phospholipid hydroperoxide GPx (PHGPx) and an 18-kDa selenoprotein were most preferentially supplied with the element whereas the cellular GPx and the plasma GPx (pGPx) were supplied last (D Behne & A Kyriakopoulos, submitted for publication). The intracellular hierarchy in the expression of the selenoproteins may be regulated mainly by differences in the stability of their mRNAs in selenium deficiency (19, 32, 94). The ranking order among tissues and selenoproteins with regard to the incorporation of the element may supply information on the sites that are likely to be affected in selenium deficiency, and on the selenoproteins involved in selenium-related diseases. The preferential supply of selenium to certain high-priority selenoproteins may also explain the fact that the total disruption of selenoprotein synthesis achieved by knocking out the selenocysteyl-tRNA gene in mice resulted in early embryonal lethality (25), whereas in rats fed a selenium-deficient diet for 16 generations no increased mortality could be observed (D Behne, unpublished data).

## SELENOPROTEINS WITH KNOWN FUNCTIONS

All the selenoproteins identified so far are enzymes, with the selenocysteine residue responsible for their catalytic functions. Their metabolic importance is based on the fact that in contrast to the thiol in the cysteine-containing enzymes, the selenol is fully ionized at normal physiological pH and that under comparable conditions it is of much higher reactivity than the thiol group (89). The selenoenzymes known so far are listed in Table 1. They include the GPxs, the iodothyronine deiodinases, the thioredoxin reductases, and a selenophosphate synthetase. With the exception of the latter, they are catalytically active in redox processes by using thiols as electron donors. Although enzymatic functions have been established, for most of them information on metabolic role and biological significance is far from complete.

## Glutathione Peroxidases

GPxs catalyze the reduction of hydrogen peroxide and organic hydroperoxides and thus protect the cells from oxidative damage. As the name indicates, glutathione normally serves as the electron donor, but there are cases where other thiols are oxidized in order to fulfill a specific biological role. So far, five selenocysteine-containing GPxs have been detected: the cytosolic or classical GPx, a GPx found in the gastrointestinal tract, pGPx, PHGPx, and, as the most recent member of this family, another tissue-specific GPx, which is only present in the sperm nuclei.

***Cytosolic or Classical Glutathione Peroxidase***    The cytosolic GPx (cGPx) was the first identified selenoprotein (46, 81). It is present in nearly all tissues but is unevenly distributed. In rats, the measurement of GPx activity in the tissue cytosols, which almost completely stems from cGPx, showed the highest values

**TABLE 1**    Mammalian selenoproteins with known functions

| Selenoprotein | Abbreviations used | Significant studies |
|---|---|---|
| Glutathione peroxidases | GPxs | |
|   Cytosolic or classical GPx | cGPx, GPx1 | 46, 81 |
|   Gastrointestinal GPX | GI-GPx, GPx-GI, GPx2 | 33 |
|   Plasma GPx | pGPx GPx3 | 95 |
|   Phospholipid hydroperoxide GPx | PHGPx, GPx4 | 99 |
|   Sperm nuclei GPx | snGPx | 78 |
| Iodothyronine deiodinases | | |
|   Type 1 deiodinase | D1, 5'DI | 3, 13 |
|   Type 2 deiodinase? | D2, 5'DII | |
|   Type 3 deiodinase | D3, 5'DIII | 39 |
| Thioredoxin reductases | TrxRs | |
|   Thioredoxin reductase 1 | TrxR1 | 96 |
|   Thioredoxin reductase 2 | TrxR2 | 47, 67, 74, 103 |
|   Thioredoxin reductase 3 | TrxR3 | 90 |
| Selenophosphate synthetase 2 | SPS2 | 55 |

in the liver and erythrocytes whereas at the other end of the scale the levels in the skeletal muscle and the brain were lower by about two orders of magnitude (18). The enzyme, which consists of four identical selenocysteine-containing subunits of about 22 kDa, catalyzes the reduction of hydrogen peroxide and various soluble organic peroxides. In this way it contributes to the antioxidant defense against reactive molecules and free radicals and complements the effects of vitamin E, which acts as a free radical scavenger. However, the losses in cGPx activity in selenium-deficient animals did not lead to pathological changes (94). Even after drastic selenium depletion in rats fed a selenium-deficient diet for 16 generations, with a decrease in liver cGPx activity below the detection limit, no lesions were observed that could be attributed to the loss in cGPx activity (D Behne, unpublished data). The same was true with cGPx knockout mice, which showed normal development (59). Effects were observed, however, after application of relatively high doses of paraquat in the knockout mice, which were affected to a much greater extent than the control animals (31, 43). The fact that the mutation of a benign strain of coxsackie virus into a virulent myocarditis-inducing genotype, previously observed in selenium-deficient mice (7), also occurred in the knockout mice indicated that this mutation was due to the lack in cGPx (8). These effects, together with the pathological changes observed in animals with combined selenium and vitamin E deficiency (37), suggest that under normal physiological conditions a low cGPx activity may be compensated for by other components of the antioxidative system, but that the protective effects of cGPx are of particular importance when the organism is exposed to additional stress factors.

*Gastrointestinal Glutathione Peroxidase*    The gastrointestinal GPx (GI-GPx) is similar to cGPx in that it is a cytosolic selenoenzyme that consists of four identical selenocysteine-containing subunits slightly below 22 kDa and catalyzes the reduction of various peroxides (33). Unlike cGPx, however, it is a tissue-specific enzyme that was found in rats only in the GI tract and in humans only in the GI tract and the liver. In the epithelium of the rodent GI tract it contributes to about half the total GPx activity (44). Because of its tissue specificity, GI-GPx may be a major component in the defense system against ingested lipid hydroperoxides (44) and may be of importance in the prevention of colon cancer (35).

*Plasma Glutathione Peroxidase*    Plasma GPx (pGPx) was identified as a tetrameric GPx with subunits of approximately 23 kDa. It differs from cGPx and GI-GPx in that it is a glycoprotein and is present in the extracellular fluids (95). It is expressed in various tissues, from where it is secreted into the extracellular fluids, but the kidney has the highest concentration of pGPx mRNA and is the main site of production for this enzyme (4, 34, 105). In vitro experiments showed that like the other tetrameric GPxs, it catalyzes the reduction of hydrogen peroxide and various organic peroxides when glutathione is used as a substrate. However, its specific enzymatic activity is only 10% that of cGPx (95). Although it was identified more than 10 years ago, its biological significance is still not clear. This is mainly due to the fact that the glutathione concentration in blood plasma is too low to serve as a suitable substrate for this enzyme. However, it has been shown that in this catalytic reaction, thioredoxin and glutaredoxin are better suited as electron donors than is glutathione (22), and this finding might stimulate research on the biological role of pGPx.

*Phospholipid Hydroperoxide Glutathione Peroxidase*    Phospholipid hydroperoxide GPx (PHGPx) was the second mammalian selenoenzyme to be identified (99). Unlike the three GPxs described above, it is a monomer of 19.7 kDa. It is found in the tissues in both cytosolic and membrane-associated forms (83). In vitro translation of the full-length PHGPx mRNA showed the existence of a PHGPx precursor with an additional N-terminal leader sequence responsible for the specific import of the enzyme into the mitochondria (1, 79). Unlike the other tetrameric GPxs, PHGPx can directly reduce phospholipid and cholesterol hydroperoxides (97, 99) and was thus considered primarily as a factor in the protective system against the oxidative destruction of biomembranes. In the meantime, the results of numerous studies suggest that the enzyme may have important functions in the redox regulation of a variety of processes, such as inflammation and apoptosis, although in most of these cases it is not yet known to what extent the other GPxs may also be involved in these reactions. A significant role of PHGPx, only fulfilled by this enzyme, has, however, been found in spermatogenesis.

Earlier findings that selenium is highly enriched in the spermatozoa in the form of a selenoprotein located in the outer mitochondrial membrane (28), that the testicular selenium concentration rises sharply after the onset of puberty (9) and changes considerably by gonadotropin-related interruption and reconstitution of spermatogenesis (11), and that a 19.7-kDa selenoprotein, present not only in the testis but also in all the other tissues, is by far the most prominent selenium compound in the spermatozoa (10) were explained when it was shown that the sperm mitochondrial membrane selenoprotein is in fact PHGPx (98) and that the increase in testis selenium during pubertal maturation is due to the abundant expression of this enzyme in the round spermatids (72). However, while in the rat testis PHGPx activity is very high (82), it is below the limit of detection in the epididymal spermatozoa (98). Here the enzyme constitutes at least 50% of the proteins present in the mitochondrial capsule, but it is present in an inactive, oxidatively cross-linked form. These findings indicate a change in the biological role of PHGPx from that of an enzyme protecting against peroxide-induced damage to that of an inactive, but still important, matrix component.

*Sperm Nuclei Glutathione Peroxidase*     After labeling rats in vivo with $^{75}$Se and separating the tissue homogenates by sodium dodecyl sulfate–polyacrylamide gel electrophoresis (SDS-PAGE), a 34-kDa selenoprotein was detected that was present only in testis and spermatozoa (10). It appeared after the onset of puberty and was localized in the nuclei of the late spermatids (12). During these stages of sperm development, the nuclei undergo considerable changes characterized by the replacement of the histones by the protamines and the reorganization and condensation of the DNA, which result in compact, very tightly packed nuclei stabilized by cross-linking of the protamine thiols. The protein was identified as a specific sperm nuclei GPx (snGPx), which differs from PHGPx in its N-terminal sequence (78). This sequence, which is encoded for by an alternative exon in the first intron of the PHGPx gene, is responsible for the specific biological role of snGPx. It contains a signal for the localization of the enzyme within the nuclei, where it is the only selenoprotein present, and a polyarginine-rich region by which it is attached to the DNA. In selenium-depleted rats where the concentration of snGPx had decreased to one third of normal, chromatin condensation was severely disturbed. We were able to show that the enzyme acts as a protamine thiol peroxidase responsible for disulfide cross-linking and thus is necessary for sperm maturation and male fertility.

# Iodothyronine Deiodinases

The iodothyronine deiodinases have major physiological roles in that they catalyze the activation and inactivation of the thyroid hormones that regulate various metabolic processes and are indispensable for the normal development of fetal brain. The family of the deiodinases consists of three members that differ with regard to their tissue distribution and their role in the deiodination of thyroxine and its metabolites. With the numerous reviews available on this subject, only a few main findings are presented.

*Type 1 Deiodinase*     A second important enzymatic function of selenium was detected in 1990, when two groups showed that a membrane-bound, selenium-containing 27-kDa protein, which had been found in the thyroid, liver, and kidney of rats (10), was identical to the subunit of type 1 deiodinase (D1) and in this way identified this enzyme as a selenoenzyme (3, 13). It was also shown that it contains one covalently bound selenium atom per molecule in its active center (13). Cloning of rat D1 cDNA proved the existence of an in-frame UGA codon responsible for the incorporation of selenocysteine into this enzyme (20). D1 is located mainly in the thyroid, liver, kidney, and pituitary. It can catalyze monodeiodination of the iodothyronines at the 5′-position of the phenolic ring or at the 5-position of the tyrosyl ring. 5′-Deiodination of thyroxine ($T_4$) results in the formation of the biologically active hormone 3,3′,5-triiodothyronine ($T_3$), whereas by means of 5-deiodination, the inactive isomer 3,3′,5′-triiodothyronine (reverse $T_3$) is produced. 5-Deiodination of $T_3$ and 5′-deiodination of reverse $T_3$ then lead to the inactive 3,3′-diiodothyronine ($T_2$). The biological role of D1 is to provide $T_3$ to the plasma, to inactivate $T_4$ and $T_3$, and to eliminate reverse $T_3$ from the circulation. The decrease in $T_3$ production from $T_4$ found in the liver of selenium-deficient rats (3, 13) shows the importance of an adequate selenium supply with regard to thyroid hormone metabolism.

*Type 2 Deiodinase*    Although cDNA cloning has shown that type 2 deiodinase (D2) in amphibian tissue is a selenoenzyme (41) and evidence has been provided that the same is true with the mammalian D2 (38, 86), final proof is still not available, as in the clones assumed to code for selenocysteine-containing D2 in mammals, the structures responsible for the incorporation of this amino acid have not been identified. A nonselenocysteine-containing, biologically active D2 subunit has recently been found (68). Further studies are therefore needed to solve the question of the role of selenium in the enzymatic D2 activity. D2 is membrane bound, has subunits of about 30 kDa, and is expressed predominantly in brain, brown adipose tissue, pituitary, and placenta. It only catalyzes 5′-monodeiodination and converts $T_4$ to $T_3$ and reverse $T_3$ to $T_2$. Its main biological role is the local intracellular production of $T_3$ from circulating plasma $T_4$ in the tissues that express this enzyme and is thus a major factor in tissue-specific regulation.

*Type 3 Deiodinase*    Cloning of the type 3 deiodinase (D3) cDNA from rat established that D3 is a selenoenzyme (39). It is a 32-kDa selenoprotein mainly located in the central nervous system, placenta, and skin. D3 catalyzes the deiodination of the tyrosyl ring and is thus able to inactivate the thyroid hormones by producing reverse $T_3$ from $T_4$ and $T_2$ from $T_3$. In this way it protects the developing mammalian brain from exposure to excessive amounts of $T_3$ (62) and regulates the supply of $T_4$ and $T_3$ from the mother to the fetus (75).

## Thioredoxin Reductases

Mammalian thioredoxin reductases are a family of homodimeric flavoenzymes present in various tissues. In addition to the flavin and the active site of the prokaryotic homologs with their redox-active disulfide, they also contain selenocysteine as the penultimate C-terminal amino acid residue (50), which is indispensable for their enzymatic activity (53). Thioredoxin reductases are named for their ability to catalyze the NADPH-dependent reduction of oxidized thioredoxin. Reduced thioredoxin is a central factor in cellular redox regulation. It provides reducing equivalents for various redox-dependent systems, e.g. for ribonucleotide reductase essential for DNA synthesis and for the redox regulation of transcription factors, and has important functions in regulating cell growth and inhibiting apoptosis (77). The significance of thioredoxin for the mammalian organism was shown in an experiment in which the disruption of the thioredoxin gene resulted in early embryonic lethality (73). In addition to thioredoxin, mammalian thioredoxin reductases are able to use other substrates, including hydroperoxides, dehydroascorbate, and various enzymes and proteins (60). This broad substrate specificity has been attributed to the presence of selenocysteine situated in the flexible C-terminal extension (53).

***Thioredoxin Reductase 1***    A selenium-containing 56-kDa protein, purified from [75]Se-labeled human lung cancer cells, was the first thioredoxin reductase to be identified as a mammalian selenocysteine-containing thioredoxin reductase (96). This cytosolic enzyme, later named thioredoxin reductase 1 (TrxR1), is a dimer with two identical 56-kDa subunits. The sequence of the TrxR1 cDNA, obtained from a human placental library, was found to have 44% identity with that of the eukaryotic and prokaryotic glutathione reductases, but only 31% with that of the prokaryotic thioredoxin reductases (48).

***Thioredoxin Reductase 2***    A second selenocysteine-containing thioredoxin reductase, the mitochondrial thioredoxin reductase 2 (TrxR2), was described by four groups in 1999, when either its cDNA was cloned from human tissues (47), human adrenal (74), and rat liver (67), or its sequence was determined after purification of the protein from bovine adrenal cortex (103). They were around 56 kDa for the human and bovine proteins and about 53 kDa for the rat enzyme. The sequence identity between the mitochondrial TrxR2 and the cytosolic TrxR1 of the same species was found to be 54% (47), 56% (74), 54% (67), and 57% (103). TrxR2 differs from TrxR1 by an N-terminal extension identified as a mitochondrial leader sequence (74). The biological role of TrxR2 in the mitochondria is not known, but it may be mainly involved in the protection against mitochondria-mediated oxidative stress.

***Further Thioredoxin Reductases***    A third selenocysteine-containing thioredoxin reductase, listed here as thioredoxin reductase 3 (TrxR3), was purified from [75]Se-labeled mouse testis, where it is preferentially expressed (90). The deduced sequence of the human enzyme shows 70% identity to that of TrxR1. It contains a long N-terminal extension and, at about 65 kDa, has a higher molecular mass than the other two isozymes.

It has recently been observed that TrxR1 isolated from mouse liver, mouse liver tumor, and a human T-cell line exhibited considerable heterogeneity, which, as with the production of snGPx (78), is due to alternative splicing of the first exons of the TrxR1 gene. By means of homology analyses, three isoforms of mouse and rat TrxR1 mRNA could be distinguished. Expression of multiple mRNA forms was also observed for human TrxR2 (91). By means of an algorithm that scans nucleotide sequence databases for mammalian selenocysteine insertion elements, two selenoproteins, SelZf1 and SelZf2, were identified that share a common domain with TrxR2 and probably are produced by alternative splicing (69). The findings of the two studies suggest the existence of further thioredoxin reductase species, which may differ with regard to their distribution among tissues and subcellular compartments and may have specific biological roles.

## Selenophosphate Synthetase 2

Selenophosphate synthetase catalyzes the reaction of selenide with AMP. The product, selenophosphate, acts as the selenium donor for the biosynthesis of selenocysteine. In addition to selenophosphate synthetase 1, which contains threonine in its active center (71), a selenocysteine-containing homolog of about 50 kDa has been identified in various human and mouse tissues (55). Information on the differences in the functions of the two enzymes in the biosynthesis of the mammalian selenoproteins is not yet available. The detection of a selenoenzyme that is involved in the production of the selenoproteins is of special interest with regard to the regulation of the mammalian selenium metabolism.

# SELENOPROTEINS WITH UNKNOWN FUNCTIONS

## Selenoprotein P

A selenium-containing protein not related to GPx was found in rat plasma in 1977 (57) and was then shown to contain selenium in the form of selenocysteine (76). Selenoprotein P (SelP) (see Table 2 for a list of all selenoproteins with unknown functions) is a glycoprotein of 43 kDa and constitutes more than 60% of the plasma selenium (80). Cloning of rat liver cDNA showed that SelP contains 10 selenocysteines (58) and thus is different from all other selenoproteins so far identified, which have only one selenocysteine residue per molecule or subunit. A cDNA obtained from bovine brain suggested the existence of a second SelP with 12 selenocysteine residues (84). SelP is mainly expressed in liver but is also present in other tissues. Although it was the second selenoprotein to be detected, its function is still unknown. Because of its extracellular location and its high selenium content, it was thought to act as a selenium transport protein (76). On the other hand, the fact that protection against diquat-induced liver lesions found after administration of selenium to selenium-deficient rats coincided with the appearance of SelP, suggested that it may act as an antioxidant (26). This hypothesis is supported by the finding that in human plasma, it contributes to the destruction

**TABLE 2**   Mammalian selenoproteins with unknown functions

| Selenoprotein | Abbreviations used | Significant studies |
|---|---|---|
| Selenoprotein P | SelP | 58, 76 |
| Selenoprotein W | SelW | 100, 101 |
| 15-kDa selenoprotein | Sel15 | 51, 61 |
| 18-kDa selenoprotein | Sel18 | 65 |
| Selenoprotein R | SelR | 63 |
| Selenoprotein T | SelT | 63 |
| Selenoprotein N | SelN | 69 |
| Selenoprotein X | SelX | 69 |
| Selenoprotein Zf1 | SelZf1 | 69 |
| Selenoprotein Zf2 | SelZf2 | 69 |

of peroxynitrite, thought to be an important factor in inflammatory toxicity (2). Further studies are needed to find out more about its significance and biological role.

## Selenoprotein W

Selenoprotein W (SelW) was first purified from rat skeletal muscle and was shown to be a cytosolic selenoprotein of slightly less than 10 kDa (100). Cloning of its cDNA indicated that it contains one selenocysteine residue per molecule (101). It is enriched in skeletal and heart muscle, brain, testis, and spleen but was also found in a large number of other tissues (93). Its biochemical and physiological role is not known. However, the protein isolated from muscle tissue was found to contain glutathione, which may have been bound as a reactant in an enzymatic redox cycle (54). The finding that glial cells with overexpressed levels of SelW were more resistant to peroxidation than normal cells (92) could likewise suggest a redox function.

## 15-kDa Selenoprotein

By labeling rats with [75]Se, isolating a 15-kDa selenium compound, and analyzing its amino acids, a selenocysteine-containing protein was identified. It is an acid protein with a pI value of 4.5 and stems from a cytosolic selenoprotein of 240 kDa. It is present in various tissues but is highly expressed in the epithelial cells of the prostate gland (61). A 15-kDa selenoprotein was then found in [75]Se-labeled human T cells and was shown to contain a selenocysteine residue encoded by TGA. It, too, has a native form of 200–240 kDa and is likewise highly expressed in the prostatic tissue (51). We have recently been able to show that the 15-kDa selenoprotein detected in rats and the human 15-kDa selenoprotein are the same protein in two different mammalian species (D Röthlein, A Kyriakopoulos, D Behne, submitted for publication), and therefore we refer to both as the 15-kDa selenoprotein (Sel15). Its function and biological significance are not known; however, further investigation of it is of special interest because of the decreased incidence of prostatic cancer with selenium supplementation (36). The recent finding that the gene for Sel15 is located on a chromosome often affected in cancer (64) supports the hypothesis that this protein might play a role in the observed relationship between selenium and this disease.

## 18-kDa Selenoprotein

An 18-kDa selenium-containing protein was detected in various tissues of rats (10). It was identified as a selenocysteine-containing selenoprotein with a pI of about 4.6–4.8, which is mainly present in the mitochondrial membranes (65). Its biological function is still unknown. However, an interesting characteristic is the fact that in the hierarchy of selenium distribution, it was found to be one of the most preferentially supplied proteins (D Behne & A Kyriakopoulos, submitted for publication), which can be taken as an indication of its biological significance.

## Further Selenoproteins Identified in Silico

Two computer programs have been developed that allow the identification of mammalian selenoprotein genes by scanning the nucleotide sequence databases for the selenocysteine insertion sequence elements necessary for decoding UGA as selenocysteine (63, 69). Nucleotide sequences corresponding to two novel selenoproteins, SelR and SelT, have been found in one of the studies (63). Calculated from their cDNA sequences, the human proteins are 12.6 kDa and 18.8 kDa for SelR and SelT, respectively. The other study describes four novel selenoproteins, SelN, SelX, SelZf1, and SelZf2, the latter two of which, both TrxR2 homologs, were mentioned above (69). SelN, SelX, and SelZ are calculated to be 58, 16, and 48 kDa, respectively. By means of Northern blot hybridization of human tissues, SelN mRNA was found to be ubiquitously expressed, but was enriched in pancreas, ovary, prostate and spleen. SelX mRNA was mainly present in liver and leukocytes and was low in lung, placenta, and brain. SelZ mRNA was enriched in kidney, liver, testis, and prostate and was low in thymus. With the exception of the TrxR2 homologs, no information on the functions of these selenoproteins is available.

## SELENIUM-CONTAINING PROTEINS NOT YET IDENTIFIED

Labeling experiments with $^{75}$Se in combination with electrophoretic and chromatographic methods of protein separation (10, 29, 40, 45, 56) have been valuable tools in selenium research, which, with most of the mammalian selenoproteins identified so far, gave a first indication of their existence and their distribution in the organism. After further improvement of these labeling techniques, mainly by using severely selenium-depleted rats and [75]Se-selenite with a very high specific activity, we were able to determine selenium compounds present in the organism at very low concentrations. After separation by SDS-PAGE and autoradiography of the labeled compounds, 28 selenium-containing bands ranging from 116 to 8 kDa could be distinguished (15). This range was extended by applying a modified tricine-SDS-PAGE, which allows the determination of smaller proteins. Using this method, four additional selenium-containing proteins of approximately 7, 5, 4, and 3 kDa were detected (66). By applying two-dimensional SDS-PAGE/isoelectric focusing, some of the selenium-containing bands could be further resolved into several spots with different isoelectric points. Although a few of these compounds may be precursors or metabolic products of the same selenoprotein, and selenium-binding proteins also have to be taken into account, these findings suggest that in addition to the selenocysteine-containing proteins detected so far, there are further mammalian selenoproteins awaiting identification.

## OUTLOOK

Considerable progress has recently been made in selenium research and particularly in the identification of novel selenocysteine-containing proteins. The findings that selenoproteins are produced by alternative splicing (78, 91) and that there are several additional selenium-containing proteins present in the tissues (15, 66) suggest that further mammalian selenoproteins exist. With the advanced methods now available in molecular biology, protein biochemistry, and protein analysis, it may be assumed that most of these compounds will be identified in the near future.

The more difficult task, however, is the functional characterization of novel selenoproteins that do not belong to one of the selenoenzyme families already known. Selenoprotein P, which was detected more than 20 years ago, is an example of this difficulty.

An even greater challenge is presented by studies carried out to clarify the biological roles of the mammalian selenoproteins. With the exception either of specific tasks, such as the regulation of thyroid hormone metabolism by the deiodinases and the production of selenophosphate by selenophosphate synthetase 2 (55), or of tasks restricted to a certain site of action, as with PHGPx in the sperm mitochondrial membrane (98) and snGPx in the sperm nuclei (78), relatively little evidence is available concerning the physiological roles of the selenoproteins. This is mainly due to the fact that because of the similarities in the enzymatic functions of the different members of one selenoenzyme family and the metabolic links between these families, it is often difficult to allocate a certain selenium-mediated effect to a single selenoprotein among all the others present in the tissues.

Another difficulty arises from the hierarchy in the selenium distribution between tissues and selenoproteins (10, 16). It is not possible to study pathological changes in relation to the concentration of a preferentially supplied selenoprotein in a high-priority tissue, as its level cannot be decreased sufficiently, even in severe selenium depletion.

In these cases gene knockout studies of experimental animals will therefore be valuable tools to investigate the selenoproteins to clarify their roles in reproduction, development, stress management and the maintenance of various metabolic processes.

Another important task for the near future is the investigation of the regulatory mechanisms responsible for selenium distribution and homeostasis and the study of the protective effects of additional selenium supplementation. In this way it will be possible to answer the question regarding the optimal selenium intake for achieving the most beneficial effects.

**Visit the Annual Reviews home page at www.AnnualReviews.org**

## LITERATURE CITED

1. Arai M, Imai H, Sumi D, Imanaka T, Takano T, et al. 1996. Import into mitochondria of phospholipid hydroperoxide glutathione peroxidase requires a leader sequence. *Biochem. Biophys. Res. Commun.* 227:433–39

2. Arteel GE, Mostert V, Oubrahim H, Briviba K, Abel J, Sies H. 1998. Protection by selenoprotein P in human plasma against peroxynitrite-mediated oxidation and nitration. *Biol. Chem.* 379:1201–5

3. Arthur JR, Nicol F, Beckett GJ. 1990. Hepatic iodothyronine 5'-deiodinase. The role of selenium. *Biochem. J.* 272:537–40

4. Avissar N, Ornt DB, Yagil Y, Horowitz S, Watkins RH, et al. 1994. Human kidney proximal tubules are the main source of plasma glutathione peroxidase. *Am. J. Physiol.* 266:C367–75

5. Bansal MP, Cook RG, Danielson KG, Medina D. 1989. A 14 kilodalton selenium-binding protein in mouse liver is fatty acid-binding protein. *J. Biol. Chem.* 264:13780–84

6. Bansal MP, Mukhopadhyay T, Scott J, Cook RG, Medina D. 1990. DNA sequencing of a mouse liver protein that binds selenium: implications for selenium's mechanism of action in cancer prevention. *Carcinogenesis* 11:2071–73

7. Beck MA, Esworthy RS, Ho YS, Chu FF. 1998. Glutathione peroxidase protects mice from viral-induced myocarditis. *FASEB J.* 12:1143–49

8. Beck MA, Kolbeck PC, Shi Q, Rohr LH, Morris VC, Levander OA. 1994. Increased virulence of a human enterovirus (coxsackievirus B3) in selenium-deficient mice. *J. Infect. Dis.* 170:351–57

9. Behne D, Duk M, Elger W. 1986. Selenium content and glutathione peroxidase activity in the testis of the maturing rat. *J. Nutr.* 116:1442–47

10. Behne D, Hilmert H, Scheid S, Gessner H, Elger W. 1988. Evidence for specific selenium target tissues and new biologically important selenoproteins. *Biochim. Biophys. Acta* 966:12–21

11. Behne D, Höfer H, von Berswordt-Wallrabe R, Elger W. 1982. Selenium in the testis of the rat: studies on its regulation and its importance for the organism. *J. Nutr.* 112:1682–87

12. Behne D, Kyriakopoulos A, Kalcklösch M, Weiss-Nowak C, Pfeifer H, et al. 1997. Two new selenoproteins found in the prostatic glandular epithelium and in the spermatid

nuclei. *Biomed. Environ. Sci.* 10:340–45

13. Behne D, Kyriakopoulos A, Meinhold H, Köhrle J. 1990. Identification of type I iodothyronine 5'-deiodinase as a selenoenzyme. *Biochem. Biophys. Res. Commun.* 173:1143–49

14. Behne D, Kyriakopoulos A, Scheid S, Gessner H. 1991. Effects of chemical form and dosage on the incorporation of selenium into tissue proteins in rats. *J. Nutr.* 121:806–14

15. Behne D, Kyriakopoulos A, Weiss-Nowak C, Kalcklösch M, Westphal C, Gessner H. 1996. Newly found selenium-containing proteins in the tissues of the rat. *Biol. Trace Elem. Res.* 55:99–110

16. Behne D, Pfeifer H, Röthlein D, Kyriakopoulos A. 2000. Cellular and subcellular distribution of selenium and selenium-containing proteins in the rat. In *Trace Elements in Man and Animals* 10, ed. AM Roussel, AE Favier, RA Anderson, pp. 29–34. New York: Kluwer/Plenum

17. Behne D, Scheid S, Kyriakopoulos A, Hilmert H. 1990. Subcellular distribution of selenoproteins in the liver of the rat. *Biochim. Biophys. Acta* 1033:219–25

18. Behne D, Wolters W. 1983. Distribution of selenium and glutathione peroxidase in the rat. *J. Nutr.* 113:456–61

19. Bermano G, Arthur JR, Hesketh JE. 1996. Selective control of cytosolic glutathione peroxidase and phospholipid hydroperoxide glutathione peroxidase mRNA stability by selenium supply. *FEBS Lett.* 387:157–60

20. Berry MJ, Banu L, Larsen PR. 1991. Type I iodothyronine deiodinase is a selenocysteine-containing enzyme. *Nature* 349:438–40

21. Berry MJ, Martin GW III, Low SC. 1997. RNA and protein requirements for eukaryotic selenoprotein synthesis. *Biomed. Environ. Sci.* 10:182–89

22. Björnstedt M, Xue J, Huang W, Akesson B, Holmgren A. 1994. The thioredoxin and glutaredoxin systems are efficient electron donors to human plasma glutathione peroxidase. *J. Biol. Chem.* 269:29382–84

23. Böck A. 1994. Incorporation of selenium into bacterial selenoproteins. In *Selenium in Biology and Human Health*, ed. RF Burk, pp. 9–24. New York: Springer

24. Böck A. 2000. Biosynthesis of selenoproteins—an overview. *BioFactors* 11:77–78

25. Bösl MR, Takaku K, Oshima M, Nishimura S, Taketo MM. 1997. Early embryonic lethality caused by targeted disruption of the mouse selenocysteine tRNA gene (Trsp). *Proc. Natl. Acad. Sci. USA* 94:5531–34

26. Burk RF, Hill KE, Awad JA, Morrow JD, Kato T, et al. 1995. Pathogenesis of diquat-induced liver necrosis in selenium-deficient rats. Assessment of the roles of lipid peroxidation by measurement of $F_2$ isoprostanes. *Hepatology* 21:561–69

27. Butler JA, Beilstein MA, Whanger PD. 1989. Influence of dietary methionine on the metabolism of selenomethionine in rats. *J. Nutr.* 119:1001–9

28. Calvin HI, Cooper GW, Wallace E. 1981. Evidence that selenium in rat sperm is associated with a cysteine-rich structural protein of the mitochondrial capsules. *Gamete Res.* 4:139–49

29. Calvin HI, Grosshans K, Musicant-Shikora SR, Turner SI. 1987. A developmental study of rat sperm and testis selenoproteins. *J. Reprod. Fertil.* 81:1–11

30. Chambers I, Frampton J, Goldfarb P, Affara N, McBain W, Harrison PR. 1986. The structure of the mouse glutathione peroxidase gene: the selenocysteine in the active site is encoded by the "termination codon," TGA. *EMBO J.* 5:1221–27

31. Cheng WH, Ho Y-S, Valentine BA, Ross DA, Combs GF, Lei XG. 1998. Cellular glutathione peroxidase is the mediator of body selenium to protect against paraquat lethality in transgenic mice. *J. Nutr.* 128:1070–76

32. Christensen MJ, Burgener KW. 1992. Dietary selenium stabilizes glutathione

peroxidase mRNA in rat liver. *J. Nutr.* 122:1620–26

33. Chu FF, Doroshow JH, Esworthy RS. 1993. Expression, characterization, and tissue distribution of a new cellular selenium-dependent glutathione peroxidase, GSHPx-GI. *J. Biol. Chem.* 268:2571–76

34. Chu FF, Esworthy RS, Doroshow JH, Doan K, Liu X-F. 1992. Expression of plasma glutathione peroxidase in human liver in addition to kidney, heart, lung, and breast in humans and rodents. *Blood* 79:3233–38

35. Chu FF, Esworthy RS, Ho Y-S, Swiderek K, Elliiot RW. 1997. Expression and chromosomal mapping of mouse Gpx2 gene encoding the gastrointestinal form of glutathione peroxidase, GPX-GI. *Biomed. Environ. Sci.* 10:156–62

36. Clark LC, Dalkin B, Krongrad A, Combs GF Jr, Turnbull BW, et al. 1998. Decreased incidence of prostate cancer with selenium supplementation: results of a double-blind cancer prevention trial. *Br. J. Urol.* 81:730–34

37. Combs GF Jr, Combs SB. 1986. *The Role of Selenium in Nutrition.* Orlando, FL: Academic. 525 pp.

38. Croteau W, Davey JC, Galton VA, St Germain DL. 1996. Cloning of the mammalian type II iodothyronine deiodinase. *J. Clin. Invest.* 98:405–17

39. Croteau W, Whittemore SL, Schneider MJ, St Germain DL. 1995. Cloning and expression of a cDNA for a mammalian type III iodothyronine deiodinase. *J. Biol. Chem.* 270:16569–75

40. Danielson KG, Medina D. 1986. Distribution of selenoproteins in mouse mammary epithelial cells in vitro and in vivo. *Cancer Res.* 46:4582–89

41. Davey JC, Becker KB, Schneider MJ, St. Germain DL, Galton VA. 1995. Cloning of a cDNA for the type II iodothyronine deiodinase. *J. Biol. Chem.* 270:26786–89

42. Deagen JT, Butler JA, Beilstein MA, Whanger PD. 1987. Effects of dietary se-

lenite, selenocystine and selenomethionine on selenocysteine lyase and glutathione peroxidase activities and on selenium levels in rat tissues. *J. Nutr.* 117:91–98

43. de Haan JB, Bladier C, Griffiths P, Kelner M, O'Shea RD, et al. 1998. Mice with a homozygous null mutation for the most abundant glutathione peroxidase, Gpx1, show increased susceptibility to the oxidative stress-inducing agents paraquat and hydrogen peroxide. *J. Biol. Chem.* 273:22528–36

44. Esworthy RS, Swiderek KM, Ho YS, Chu FF. 1998. Selenium-dependent glutathione peroxidase-GI is a major glutathione peroxidase activity in the mucosal epithelium of rodent intestine. *Biochim. Biophys. Acta* 1381:213–26

45. Evenson JK, Sunde RA. 1988. Selenium incorporation into selenoproteins in the Se-adequate and Se-deficient rat. *Proc. Soc. Exp. Biol. Med.* 187:169–80

46. Flohé L, Günzler WA, Schock HH. 1973. Glutathione peroxidase: a selenoenzyme. *FEBS Lett.* 32:132–34

47. Gasdaska PY, Berggren MM, Berry ML, Powis G. 1999. Cloning, sequencing and functional expression of a novel human thioredoxin reductase. *FEBS Lett.* 442:105–11

48. Gasdaska PY, Gasdaska JR, Cochran S, Powis G. 1995. Cloning and sequencing of a human thioredoxin reductase. *FEBS Lett.* 373:5–9

49. Gassmann T. 1916. Der Nachweis des Selens im Knochen- und Zahngewebe. *Hoppe-Seyler's Z. Physiol. Chem.* 97:307–10

50. Gladyshev VN, Jeang K-T, Stadtman TC. 1996. Selenocysteine, identified as the penultimate C-terminal residue in human T-cell thioredoxin reductase, corresponds to TGA in the human placental gene. *Proc. Natl. Acad. Sci. USA* 93:6146–51

51. Gladyshev VN, Jeang KT, Wootton JC, Hatfield DL. 1998. A new human selenium-containing protein. Purification,

characterization, and cDNA sequence. *J. Biol. Chem.* 273:8910–15

52. Gmelin-Inst. Anorgan. Chem., ed. 1953. *Gmelins Handbuch der Anorganischen Chemie, Selen,* Vol. 1, Part A, p. 24. Weinheim/Bergstr., Ger.: Verlag Chemie. 8th ed.

53. Gromer S, Wissing J, Behne D, Ashman K, Schirmer H, et al. 1998. A hypothesis on the catalytic mechanism of the selenoenzyme thioredoxin reductase. *Biochem. J.* 332:591–92

54. Gu Q-P, Beilstein MA, Barofsky E, Ream W, Whanger PD. 1999. Purification, characterization and glutathione binding to selenoprotein W from monkey muscle. *Arch. Biochem. Biophys.* 361:25–33

55. Guimaraes MJ, Peterson D, Vicari A, Cocks BG, Copeland NG, et al. 1996. Identification of a novel SelD homolog from eukaryotes, bacteria, and archea: Is there an autoregulatory mechanism in selenocysteine metabolism? *Proc. Natl. Acad. Sci. USA* 93:15086–91

56. Hawkes WC, Wilhelmsen EC, Tappel A. 1985. Abundance and tissue distribution of selenocysteine-containing proteins in the rat. *J. Nutr.* 113:456–61

57. Herrman JL. 1977. The properties of a rat serum protein labelled by the injection of sodium selenite. *Biochim. Biophys. Acta* 500:61–70

58. Hill KE, Lloyd RS, Yang J-G, Read R, Burk RF. 1991. The cDNA for rat selenoprotein P contains 10 TGA codons in the open reading frame. *J. Biol. Chem.* 266:10050–53

59. Ho Y-S, Magnenat J-L, Bronson RT, Cao J, Gargano M, et al. 1997. Mice deficient in cellular glutathione peroxidase develop normally and show no increase sensitivity to hyperoxia. *J. Biol. Chem.* 272:16644–51

60. Holmgren A, Björnstedt M. 1995. Thioredoxin and thioredoxin reductase. *Methods Enzymol.* 252B:199–208

61. Kalcklösch M, Kyriakopoulos A, Hammel C, Behne D. 1995. A new selenoprotein found in the glandular epithelial cells of the rat prostate. *Biochem. Biophys. Res. Commun.* 217:162–70

62. Kaplan MM. 1986. Regulatory influences on iodothyronine deiodination in animal tissues. In *Thyroid Hormone Metabolism,* ed. G Hennemann, pp. 231–53. New York: Dekker

63. Kryukov GV, Kryukov VM, Gladyshev VN. 1999. New mammalian selenocysteine-containing proteins identified with an algorithm that searches for selenocysteine insertion sequence elements. *J. Biol. Chem.* 274:33888–97

64. Kumaraswamy E, Malykh A, Korotkov KV, Kozyavkin S, Hu Y, et al. 2000. Structure-expression relationships of the 15-kDa selenoprotein gene. Possible role of the protein in cancer etiology. *J. Biol. Chem.* 275:35540–47

65. Kyriakopoulos A, Hammel C, Gessner H, Behne D. 1996. Characterization of an 18 kDa-selenium-containing protein in several tissues of the rat. *Am. Biotech. Lab.* 14:22

66. Kyriakopoulos A, Röthlein D, Pfeifer H, Bertelsmann H, Kappler S, Behne D. 2000. Detection of small selenium-containing proteins in tissues of the rat. *J. Trace Elem. Med. Biol.* 14:170–83

67. Lee SR, Kim JR, Kwon KS, Yoon HW, Levine RL, et al. 1999. Molecular cloning and characterization of a mitochondrial selenocysteine-containing thioredoxin reductase from rat liver. *J. Biol. Chem.* 274:4722–34

68. Leonard DM, Stachelek SJ, Safran M, Farwell AP, Kowalik TF, Leonard JL. 2000. Cloning, expression, and functional characterization of the substrate binding subunit of rat type II iodothyronine 5′-deiodinase. *J. Biol. Chem.* 275:25194–201

69. Lescure A, Gautheret D, Carbon P, Krol A. 1999. Novel selenoproteins identified in silico and in vivo by using a conserved RNA structural motif. *J. Biol. Chem.* 274:38147–54

70. Low SC, Berry MJ. 1996. Knowing when

not to stop. Selenocysteine incorporation in eukaryotes. *Trends Biochem. Sci.* 21:203–8

71. Low SC, Harney JW, Berry MJ. 1995. Cloning and functional characterization of human selenophosphate synthetase, an essential component of selenoprotein synthesis. *J. Biol. Chem.* 270:21659–64

72. Maiorino M, Wissing JB, Brigelius-Flohé R, Calabrese F, Roveri A, et al. 1998. Testosterone mediates expression of the selenoprotein PHGPx by induction of spermatogenesis and not by direct transcriptional gene activation. *FASEB J.* 12:1359–70

73. Matsui M, Oshima M, Oshima H, Takaku K, Maruyama T, et al. 1996. Early embryonic lethality caused by targeted disruption of the mouse thioredoxin gene. *Dev. Biol.* 178:179–85

74. Miranda-Vizuete A, Damdimopoulos AE, Pedrajas JR, Gustafsson JA, Spyrou G. 1999. Human mitochondrial thioredoxin reductase. *Eur. J. Biochem.* 261:405–12

75. Mortimer RH, Galligan JP, Cannell GR, Addison RS, Roberts MS. 1996. Maternal to fetal thyroxine transmission in the human term placenta is limited by inner ring deiodination. *J. Clin. Endocrinol. Metab.* 81:2247–49

76. Motsenbocker MA, Tappel AL. 1982. A selenocysteine-containing selenium-transport protein in rat plasma. *Biochim. Biophys. Acta* 719:147–53

77. Mustacich D, Powis G. 2000. Thioredoxin reductase. *Biochem. J.* 346:1–8

78. Pfeifer H, Conrad M, Roethlein D, Kyriakopoulos A, Brielmeier M, et al. 2001. Identification of a specific sperm nuclei selenoenzyme necessary for protamine thiol cross-linking during sperm maturation. *FASEB J.* 10.1096/fj.00-0655fje

79. Pushpa-Rekha TR, Burdsall AL, Oleksa LM, Chisolm GM, Driscoll DM. 1995. Rat phospholipid-hydroperoxide glutathione peroxidase. cDNA cloning and identi-fication of multiple transcription and translation start sites. *J. Biol. Chem.* 270:26993–99

80. Read R, Bellow T, Yang J-G, Hill KE, Palmer IS, Burk RF. 1990. Selenium and amino acid composition of selenoprotein P, the major selenoprotein in rat serum. *J. Biol. Chem.* 265:17899–905

81. Rotruck JT, Pope AL, Ganther HE, Swanson AB, Hafeman DG, Hoekstra WG. 1973. Selenium: biochemical role as a component of glutathione peroxidase. *Science* 179:588–90

82. Roveri A, Casaco A, Maiorino M, Dalan P, Calligaro A, Ursini F. 1992. Phopholipid hydroperoxide glutathione peroxidase of rat testis: gonadotropin dependency and immunocytochemical identification. *J. Biol. Chem.* 267:6142–46

83. Roveri A, Maiorino M, Ursini F. 1994. Enzymatic and immunological measurements of soluble and membrane-bound PHGPx. *Methods Enzymol.* 233:202–12

84. Saijoh K, Saito N, Lee MJ, Fujii M, Kobayashi T, Sumino K. 1995. Molecular cloning of cDNA encoding a bovine selenoprotein P-like protein containing 12 selenocysteines and a (His-Pro) rich domain insertion, and its regional expression. *Mol. Brain Res.* 30:301–11

85. Salbe AD, Levander OA. 1990. Effect of various dietary factors on the deposition of selenium in the hair and nails of rats. *J. Nutr.* 120:200–6

86. Salvatore D, Bartha T, Harney JW, Larsen PR. 1996. Molecular biological and biochemical characterization of the human type 2 selenodeiodinase. *Endocrinology* 137:3308–15

87. Sani BP, Woodard JL, Pierson MC, Allen RD. 1988. Specific binding proteins for selenium in rat tissues. *Carcinogenesis* 9:277–84

88. Schwarz K, Foltz TM. 1957. Selenium as an integral part of factor 3 against dietary liver degeneration. *J. Am. Chem. Soc.* 79:3292–93

89. Stadtman TC. 1996. Selenocysteine. *Annu. Rev. Biochem.* 65:83–100

90. Sun Q-A, Wu Y, Zappacosta F, Jeang K-T, Lee BJ, et al. 1999. Redox regulation of cell signaling by selenocysteine in mammalian thioredoxin reductases. *J. Biol. Chem.* 274:24522–30

91. Sun Q-A, Zappacosta F, Factor VM, Wirth PJ, Hatfield DL, Gladyshev VN. 2001. Heterogeneity within animal thioredoxin reductases: evidence for alternative first exon splicing. *J. Biol. Chem.* 276:3106–14

92. Sun Y, Gu G-P, Whanger PD. 1998. Antioxidant function of selenoprotein W using overexpressed and underexpressed cultured rat glial cells. *FASEB J.* 12:A824

93. Sun Y, Ha P-C, Butler JA, Ou B-R, Yeh J-Y, Whanger P. 1998. Effect of dietary selenium on selenoprotein W and glutathione peroxidase in 28 tissues of the rat. *J. Nutr. Biochem.* 9:23–27

94. Sunde RA, Thompson RM, Palm MD, Weiss SL, Thompson KM, Evenson JK. 1997. Selenium regulation of selenium-dependent glutathione peroxidases in animals and transfected CHO cells. *Biomed. Environ. Sci.* 10:346–55

95. Takahashi K, Avissar N, Whitin J, Cohen H. 1987. Purification and characterization of human plasma glutathione peroxidase: a selenoglycoprotein distinct from the known cellular enzyme. *Arch. Biochem. Biophys.* 256:677–86

96. Tamura T, Stadtman TC. 1996. A new selenoprotein from human lung adenocarcinoma cells: purification, properties, and thioredoxin activity. *Proc. Natl. Acad. Sci. USA* 93:1006–11

97. Thomas JP, Maiorino M, Ursini F, Girotti AW. 1990. Protective action of phospholipid hydroperoxide glutathione peroxidase against membrane-damaging lipid peroxidation. In situ reduction of phospholipid and cholesterol hydroperoxides. *J. Biol. Chem.* 265:454–61

98. Ursini F, Heim S, Kiess M, Maiorino M, Roveri A, et al. 1999. Dual function of the selenoprotein PHGPx during sperm maturation. *Science* 285:1393–96

99. Ursini F, Maiorino M, Gregolin C. 1985. The selenoenzyme phospholipid hydroperoxide glutathione peroxidase. *Biochim. Biophys. Acta* 839:62–70

100. Vendeland SC, Beilstein MA, Chen CL, Jensen ON, Barofsky E, Whanger PD. 1993. Purification and properties of selenoprotein-W from rat muscle. *J. Biol. Chem.* 268:17103–7

101. Vendeland SC, Beilstein MA, Yeh JY, Ream W, Whanger PD. 1995. Rat skeletal muscle selenoprotein W: cDNA clone and mRNA modulation by dietary selenium. *Proc. Natl. Acad. Sci. USA* 92:8749–53

102. Waschulewski IH, Sunde RA. 1988. Effect of dietary methionine on tissue selenium and glutathione peroxidase (EC 1.11.1.9) activity in rats given selenomethionine. *Br. J. Nutr.* 60:57–68

103. Watabe S, Makino Y, Ogawa K, Hiroi T, Yamamoto Y, Takahashi SY. 1999. Mitochondrial thioredoxin reductase in bovine adrenal cortex. Its purification, nucleotide/amino acid sequence, and identification of selenocysteine. *Eur. J. Biochem.* 264:74–84

104. Whanger PD, Butler JA. 1988. Effects of various dietary levels of selenium as selenite or selenomethionine on tissue selenium levels and glutathione peroxidase activity in rats. *J. Nutr.* 118:846–52

105. Yoshimura S, Watanabe K, Suemizu H, Onozawa T, Mizoguchi J, et al. 1991. Tissue specific expression of the plasma glutathione peroxidase gene in rat kidney. *J. Biochem.* 109:918–23

106. Zinoni F, Birkmann A, Stadtman TC, Böck A. 1986. Nucleotide sequence and expression of the selenocysteine-containing polypeptide of formate dehydrogenase (formate-hydrogen-lyase-linked) from *Escherichia coli. Proc. Natl. Acad. Sci. USA* 83:4650–54

Annu. Rev. Nutr. 2001. 21:475–98

# WHAT ARE PRESCHOOL CHILDREN EATING? A REVIEW OF DIETARY ASSESSMENT[1]

## Mary K Serdula, Maria P Alexander, Kelley S Scanlon, and Barbara A Bowman

*Division of Nutrition and Physical Activity, Centers for Disease Control and Prevention, Atlanta, Georgia 30341-3717; e-mail: mserdula@cdc.gov, kscanlon@cdc.gov, bbowman@cdc.gov*

**Key Words** validity, reproducibility, reliability, child, diet assessment, nutrient intake, food intake

■ **Abstract** Accurate assessment of dietary intake among preschool-aged children is important for clinical care and research, for nutrition monitoring and evaluating nutrition interventions, and for epidemiologic research. We identified 25 studies published between January 1976 and August 2000 that evaluated the validity of food recalls ($n = 12$), food frequency questionnaires ($n = 9$), food records ($n = 2$), or other methods ($n = 2$). We identified four studies that evaluated the reproducibility of food frequency questionnaires. Validity studies varied in validation standard and study design, making comparisons between studies difficult. In general, food frequency questionnaires overestimated total energy intake and were better at ranking, than quantifying, nutrient intake. Compared with the validation standard, food recalls both overestimated and underestimated energy intake. When choosing a method to estimate diet, both purpose of the assessment and practicality of the method must be considered, in addition to the validity and reproducibility reported in the scientific literature.

## CONTENTS

---

[1]The US Government has the right to retain a nonexclusive, royalty-free license in and to any copyright covering this paper.

## INTRODUCTION

Assessment of dietary intake among preschool-aged children ($\leq$5 years old) is essential for monitoring the nutritional status of the population as well as for conducting epidemiologic research on the link between diet and health. In addition, dietary assessment is important for pediatric clinical care and research. Dietary behaviors of particular interest are those emphasized in national dietary guidelines (37), in the nutrition objectives of Healthy People 2010 (38), in specific nutrient intake recommendations, such as *Dietary Reference Intakes* (19), and in clinical guidelines (6). Every evaluation of compliance with dietary guidelines or recommendations is limited, however, by the validity and reproducibility of the dietary assessment tool used for measuring intake. In addition, monitoring of trends in dietary intake is limited by changes in dietary assessment methods because caution must be used in comparing across surveys where dietary assessments were conducted differently.

Rapid change characterizes the diet of young children. Early on, most infants consume small quantities of milk at frequent intervals; older infants and toddlers consume larger quantities of milk and weaning foods or table foods. By age 2–3 years, most children consume foods eaten by the rest of the family. Assessment of dietary intake is also affected by social factors, such as day care, which can limit a parent's ability to report what a child actually consumed.

Techniques commonly used to assess the diets of preschool-aged children include respondent-based methods, such as dietary recalls, dietary records, and food frequency questionnaires (FFQs), investigator-based techniques, such as direct observation and collection of duplicate portions, and physiologic measures, such as doubly labeled water, or biomarkers of dietary intake, such as serum carotenoids (13). To measure dietary intakes of preschool children, valid, reliable, and age-appropriate assessment techniques are required that are both practical and suited to the needs of the researcher or clinician. In this paper, we review the methods currently used to measure dietary intake of preschool-aged children and the challenges of using such methods. Because the assessment of milk intake has been reviewed separately (KS Scanlon, manuscript in preparation), we did not include studies of this behavior.

## METHODOLOGY

In the absence of an absolute gold standard for dietary assessment (39), measurement of the validity of a dietary assessment technique is based on comparison with a second technique. In this report, validity is defined as the degree to which results from one dietary assessment technique match the results obtained through the validity technique, in this report referred to as the validation standard. Reproducibility is the extent to which the questionnaire measurements are consistent across administrations at different times (39).

The studies we include were selected from those of preschool-aged children conducted in developed or developing countries and published in English between January 1976 and August 2000. Studies were identified through MEDLINE and POPLINE literature searches using the following key words: diet, nutrition assessment, infant food, infant nutrition, child nutrition, validity, reproducibility, comparability, and accuracy. Additional articles were identified using the references in the identified studies.

We included studies with children over age 5 only when they had a substantial number of preschool children. We excluded studies where the referent period (time period when the diet was measured by the dietary technique being evaluated) did not coincide or overlap with the referent period for the validation standard (15, 23, 29). We also excluded studies that evaluated dietary assessment measures for populations rather than individual children (32). Finally, we excluded studies of breastfeeding or infant formula feeding. Two reports (9, 24) were based on the same study; we counted them as a single study.

In all, we selected 29 studies from 23 published reports that assessed the validity or reproducibility of dietary intake methods. For clarity of presentation, when more than one validity or reproducibility study was included in the same publication that evaluated separate dietary methods, we discuss them as separate studies. We identified 25 studies that evaluated the validity of food recalls, food records, FFQs, and other methods. We identified an additional four studies that evaluated the reproducibility of FFQs.

We briefly describe each of these dietary assessment methods, discuss the results of the validity and reproducibility studies for that method, and present summary tables with details of each study.

# FOOD RECALLS

Trained interviewers administer food recalls to collect information on everything a subject consumes during a specified period (35), most often the previous 24 h or less. Because of day-to-day variability, multiple recalls are required to estimate the usual nutrient intakes of individual children. A single recall can be used to calculate the group mean nutrient intake in a population, but multiple recalls are needed to estimate the prevalence of low or high intakes (39). How many recall days are needed to calculate usual intake depends on the nutrient (28). When the required recall days are not available, statistical methods can be used to estimate usual intake adjusting for predicted within-person and between-person variability (14). For preschoolers, caregivers may be asked to provide detailed information about dietary intake, such as brand names, ingredients of mixed dishes, and food preparation methods, and to estimate amounts consumed. Visual prompts for quantifying portion size, such as food models, pictures of foods, or standard household utensils, are often used. Once the recall data are collected, they are coded by skilled personnel, often by direct data entry into a software program for calculating nutrient intake.

## Validity

Of the 12 food recall validity studies we reviewed (Table 1), most assessed a complete 24-h recall (2, 8, 11, 12, 17, 18, 21, 25, 30, 31). Two studies assessed a single meal (3, 9). The referent periods of the food recall and the validation standard coincided in all except one study, in which the referent period was not specified and was assumed to be the same (30).

The validation standard varied widely, making comparisons difficult. Food recalls were compared with direct observation in four studies, with food records in six, and total energy expenditure as measured by doubly labeled water, collection of duplicate portions, and serum lipid concentrations in one each. Recalls of dietary intake typically were obtained from parents or the primary caretaker without input from the child. The exception was the study by Eck et al (9), which evaluated recalls completed by the mother alone, the father alone, and the mother and father with input from the child (consensus). Studies used different strategies where the mother was unable to provide a complete recall because the child attended day care. In the studies that addressed this issue, one conducted separate recall interviews of day care personnel (18) whereas another excluded segments of both the recall and the validation standard when the mother was not with the child and unable to report (2).

In the studies that compared recalled with observed intake (2, 3, 8, 9), the relative difference in mean energy intake was within 10%. In the comparison using doubly labeled water (21), 24-h recalls underestimated mean energy intake by 3%. In the study using duplicate portions (17), recalls overestimated intake of energy by 10%. Similar results for energy and nutrient intake were reported in studies that used respondent-based measures (such as food records) as the validation standard (8, 11, 12, 18, 25, 30), with recalled energy intake within 15% of measured energy.

Among the nine studies that reported correlations for energy and macronutrients, in seven (3, 8, 9, 11, 17, 18, 25) the correlation coefficients were always ≥0.45. In the remaining two studies, correlations were usually much lower (12, 21). In the doubly labeled water study, the Pearson correlation coefficient was 0.25 for energy (21). In another study (12) that compared repeated 24-h recalls with weighed food records, correlations were 0.06–0.25 for energy and 0.30–0.48 for protein.

Agreement on food items between the food recalls and the validation standard varied by food group. Typically, main meal items were more likely to be recalled than snack foods and desserts (9, 11, 12). In general, respondents were more likely to omit than to add food items (2, 3, 8, 12, 25). There was no consistent pattern in the ability of respondents to estimate portion sizes, with studies reporting both overestimation and underestimation of various foods in the recalls. In their study of Senegalese weanling children (age 11–18 months), Dop et al (8) reported that mothers had more difficulty estimating portion sizes of foods served from the common household pot than of food served separately.

Only a few studies examined the effect of sex, ethnicity, or weight status on recall validity, and none examined the effect of age. No significant differences in validity by sex or by body mass index of the child or parents were found when doubly labeled water was used as the validation standard (21). When observation was used as the standard, Caucasian and Mexican-American mothers more likely to underreport energy and nutrient intakes and African-American mothers more likely to overreport (2). In this study, mothers who were with their preschool children most of the day ("at-home") were significantly more likely to be able to report intake for all of the day than were mothers whose preschoolers were in daycare more than 4.5 h per day ("not-at-home"). Among mothers able to report intake, however, not-at-home and at-home mothers demonstrated similar accuracy in estimating energy and nutrient intake.

## FOOD RECORDS

With food records, caregivers record detailed information about all food and beverages (including preparation method) consumed during a specified time period (35). Methods used to quantify the amount consumed have included weighing or measuring food and visual estimation. Ideally, information is recorded at consumption, improving estimation of portion size and eliminating the problem of forgetting. Recording detailed information on food intake, which necessitates the immediate quantification of portion size, is labor intensive, however, and carries a higher respondent burden than do food recalls or FFQs. As with food recalls, multiple sample days are required to estimate usual intake, and the data must be coded by skilled personnel.

### Validity

The only two studies that evaluated the validity of weighed food records for preschool-aged children (7, 16) used 4–5 days of records and were conducted in industrialized countries (Table 2). Population demographics and referent periods differed, however, as did the validation standard. The doubly labeled water method was the validation standard in one study (7), with diet history the method in the other (16).

Mean energy intake calculated from food records underestimated total energy expenditure from the doubly labeled water method by 3%, with a correlation of 0.41 between food records and doubly labeled water (7). Similarly, when compared with diet history, food records underestimated mean energy intake by approximately 7% (16).

**TABLE 1**  Validity of food recall[a]

| Reference | Population | Instrument | Validation standard | Referent period[b] | Macronutrient correlations | Range of correlations (all nutrients and energy) | Mean energy difference[c] | Nutrient and energy differences[d] | Quantitative/ qualitative and other differences |
|---|---|---|---|---|---|---|---|---|---|
| Baranowski et al (2) | 3–5 years, 29 M/27 F, 48% Caucasian, 41% African-American, 11% Hispanic, US | 24-h recall | 12-h observation | Same day | — | — | −7% (1053 vs 1138 kcal) | Recall underestimated 2 of 9 nutrients and overestimated 2 (significance testing not shown) | Excluded from analysis times when mothers and/or observers were not with child and could not report Food items: 65% mean precise agreement, 7% mean partial agreement; mothers were more likely to underreport (18%) than overreport (10%) Regression analysis on differences in nutrient scores showed no effects for amount of time mother and child were together during the day or for socioeconomic status. Caucasion and Mexican-American mothers more likely to underreport intake and African-Americans more likely to overreport |

| Basch et al (3) | 4–7 years, 18 M/28 F, Latino, US | Evening meal recall excerpted from 24-h recall | Evening meal observation | Same day | Adjusted (energy) Pearson: 0.71 energy, 0.50 protein, 0.52 fat | Adjusted (energy) Pearson: −0.10 phosphorous to 0.82 iron (18 nutrients) | +9% (507 vs 465 kcal) | Recall significantly overestimated 7 of 18 nutrients | Food items: For 9 of 10 most frequently eaten food groups, observed and recalled frequencies were identical; mothers' recalls tended to omit foods more often than add them Portion sizes: 51% of recalled portion sizes were equivalent to observed, 16% were underestimated; 34% were overestimated |
|---|---|---|---|---|---|---|---|---|---|
| | | | | | | | | | Mothers in the not-at-home group were less likely to be able to report on their child's intake for a whole or part of the day compared with at-home mothers; however, when not-at-home mothers reported, they were as accurate as at-home mothers |
| Dop et al (8) | 11–18 months, 24 M/21 F, Senegal | 24-h recall | 12-h observation | Same day | — | — | — | — | Food items: Among consumers, millet-sorghum was omitted on 16% of recalls and fish on 24%. Mothers tend to omit foods rather than add them |
| | | 24-h recall, mean of 2 consecutive days | 12-h weighed food records w/observation | Same day | Spearman: 0.75 energy, 0.75 protein, 0.70 fat | Spearman: 0.70 fat to 0.80 carbohydrate (4 nutrients) | +1% (413 vs 407 kcal) | No significant differences for 4 of 4 nutrients | Food items: Spearman correlations for 7 food groups ranged from 0.43 for fish |

(*Continued*)

481

TABLE 1  (Continued)

| Reference | Population | Instrument | Validation standard | Referent period[b] | Macronutrient correlations | Range of correlations (all nutrients and energy) | Mean energy difference[c] | Nutrient and energy differences[d] | Quantitative/ qualitative and other differences |
|---|---|---|---|---|---|---|---|---|---|
| | | (breast milk not included) | and test weighing (precise weighing technique), mean of 2 consecutive days (breast milk not included) | | | | | | to 0.91 for millet-sorghum; among consumers, millet-sorghum was omitted in 11% of recalls and fish in 13% among nonconsumers, fish was added in 31% of recalls. Portion sizes: Mothers had more difficulty estimating portion sizes of foods from the "common household pot" (e.g. rice, oil, & fish) than foods served in common household measures as standard portions (e.g. wheat products, beverages, gruel, dairy, etc) |
| Eck et al (9) [also Klesges et al (24)] | 4–9.5 years, 34 M & F, US | Lunch recall interview of fathers, mothers, and consensus recall of mother, father, and child | Lunch observation | Same day | Unadjusted Pearson: fathers −0.83 energy, 0.79 protein[e], 0.72 fat[e], mothers −0.64 energy, 0.56 protein[e], 0.65 fat[e]; | Unadjusted Pearson: mothers− 0.56 protein[e]; consensus −0.91 protein[e] (9 nutrients) | Fathers, −5% (545 vs 572 kcal); mothers, −4% (550 vs 572 kcal); consensus, −2% (558 vs 572 kcal) | No significant differences for 9 of 9 nutrients. | Food items: Only fathers' recalls of number of nondairy beverage items and snacks/dessert items were significantly different from number of items observed; only mothers' recalls of calories from dairy foods/beverages and snacks/desserts were significantly different from observed; however, overestimation/underestimation ranged greatly—from 27% |

(Continued)

| Study | Subjects | Method | Reference method | Interval | Correlations (energy, protein) | Correlations (nutrients) | Difference | Significance | Food items |
|---|---|---|---|---|---|---|---|---|---|
| | | | | | | | | | under for breads (fathers) to 50% over for fruits (fathers); obesity status of parents and child did not significantly affect accuracy of recall (24) |
| Ferguson et al (11) | 4–6 years, 29 M & F, Malawi | 24-h food recall | Weighed food record | Same day | consensus −0.87 energy, 0.91 protein[e], 0.85 fat[e] Unadjusted Spearman: 0.47 energy, 0.50 protein | Unadjusted Spearman: 0.28 vitamin C to 0.55 zinc (6 nutrients) | −14% (1133 vs 1314 kcal) (medians) | No significant differences for 6 of 6 nutrients | Food items: Consumption of main meal dishes was more accurately recalled than snack foods; 44% of fruits to 90% of cakes were omitted by the recalls; fruit consumption was also recalled when not consumed; average grams recalled were significantly higher than recorded for fruit and lower for porridge; no significant differences for other food groups |
| Ferguson et al (12) | 56 ± 9.4 months (mean ± SD), 33 M/39 F, Ghana (2 villages—Slepor and Gidantuba) | 24-h recall, median of 2 consecutive days | Weighed food records, median of 2 consecutive days | Same day | Intraclass: Slepor—0.06 energy, 0.30 protein; Gidantuba—0.25 energy, 0.48 protein | Intraclass: Slepor—0.06 energy to 0.78 vitamin A (5 nutrients) | Slepor;—15% (1025 vs 1207 kcal) (medians); Gidantuba: +1% (1160 vs 1146 kcal) (medians) | Slepor: recall significantly underestimated 4 of 5 nutrients; Gidantuba: recall significantly underestimated 1 of 5 nutrients | Food items: Intraclass correlations for percentage of energy obtained from selected food groups ranged from 0.29 for meat, poultry, and fish (Slepor) to 0.79 for cereals (Slepor); less than 15% of main meal foods and purchased meals to over 60% of fruits and snacks were omitted; less than 20% of all food types were added when not consumed. Portion sizes: In Slepor, recall significantly underestimated banku (a staple) and stew and overestimated soup portions; in Gidantuba, recall significantly overestimated banku |

**TABLE 1** (*Continued*)

| Reference | Population | Instrument | Validation standard | Referent period[b] | Macronutrient correlations | Range of correlations (all nutrients and energy) | Mean energy difference[c] | Nutrient and energy differences[d] | Quantitative/ qualitative and other differences |
|---|---|---|---|---|---|---|---|---|---|
| Horst et al (17) | 6 months, 41 M & F (nonbreastfed), Netherlands | 24-h recall | 24-h duplicate portion method | Same day | Unadjusted Spearman: 0.77 energy, 0.90 protein, 0.84 fat | Unadjusted Spearman: 0.69 potassium to 0.96 phosphorous (9 nutrients) | +10% (747 vs 680 kcal) | Recall significantly overestimated 7 of 9 nutrients | Food groups: Recall significantly overestimated amount (weight) of infant formula, fruit, and cooked dishes such as meat, potatoes, eggs, vegetables |
| Iannotti et al (18) | 2–4 years, 17 M & F, US | 24-h recall, mean of 3 days | Measured food records, mean of 3 days | Same day | Unadjusted Pearson: 0.45 energy | Unadjusted Pearson: 0.43 sodium to 0.79 cholesterol (5 nutrients) | −4% (1053 vs 1095 kcal) | No significant mean differences for 5 of 5 nutrients | Both usual caregivers and day caregivers provided recall information |
| Johnson et al (21) | 4–7 years, 12 M/12 F, US | 24-h recall, mean of 3 days | TEE with doubly labeled water over 14 days | Overlapping days—TEE encompassed 3 days of recall | Unadjusted Pearson: 0.25 energy | — | −3% (1553 vs 1607 kcal) | — | No difference in misreporting by BMI/obesity status of child or parent; misreporting of energy intake not statistically different between boys and girls |
| Klesges et al (25) | 2–4 years, 17 M/13 F, US | 24-h recall | 24-h weighed food record | Same day | Unadjusted Pearson: 0.48 energy, 0.63 protein | Unadjusted Pearson: 0.48 energy to 0.75 saturated fat and cholesterol (7 nutrients) | +1% (1132 vs 1122 kcal) | No significant differences for 7 of 7 nutrients | Food items: Correct recall of 96% of foods eaten; 4% underreporting (not identifying foods eaten); 0% overreporting (identifying food not eaten) |

| Persson & Calgren (30) | 4 & 8 years, 477 M & F, Sweden | 24-h recall | 7-day food records | — | — | — | −0.2% (1780 vs 1784 kcal) | Recall overestimated 1 of 8 nutrients and underestimated 2 of 8 nutrients (significance testing not shown) | — |
|---|---|---|---|---|---|---|---|---|---|
| Shea et al (31) | 4-5 years, 57 M/51 F, Hispanic, US | 24-h recall, mean of 4 administered 4 times over 1 year | Serum lipid concentration | Overlapping | — | — | — | — | Total serum cholesterol and LDL cholesterol increased significantly across tertiles of total fat, saturated fat, calorie-adjusted saturated fat intake, and calorie-adjusted total fat (LDL cholesterol only); after adjusting for age, sex, and BMI, association remained significant |

[a]M, male; F, female; TEE, total energy expenditure; FFQ, food frequency questionnaire; BMI, body mass index; LDL, low-density lipoprotein; SD, standard deviation of the mean.

[b]Correspondence of referent period of validation standard and instrument. The referent period is the time period of the diet, as measured by the dietary assessment technique.

[c]Mean energy difference, {[instrument (mean) − validation (mean) standard]/validation (mean) standard}.

[d]Differences in mean energy and nutrient intake; underestimation/overestimation indicates statistically significant difference or >5% difference when significance testing not shown.

[e]As percentage of kilocalories.

**TABLE 2**  Validity of food records[a]

| Reference | Population | Instrument | Validation standard | Referent period[b] | Macronutrient correlations | Range of correlations (all nutrients and energy) | Mean energy difference[c] | Nutrient and energy differences[d] | Quantitative/ qualitative and other differences |
|---|---|---|---|---|---|---|---|---|---|
| Davies et al (7) | 1.5–4.5 years, 42 M/39 F, UK | Weighed food records from 4 days | TEE with doubly labeled water assessed over 10 days | Overlapping days—TEE encompassed 4 days of records | 0.41 energy[e] | — | −3% (1141 vs 1178 kcal) | — | Mean energy difference was greatest for 1.0– 2.5 year olds (6% underestimation) and smallest for 3.5–4.5 year olds (1% overestimation) |
| Harbottle & Duggan (16) | 4–40 months, 117 M & F, Indo-Asians, UK | Weighed food records/ inventories from 4 days (children <12 months) to 5 days (children >12 months) | Diet history | — | — | — | −7% (778 vs 838 kcal) | Records significantly underestimated 2 of 5 nutrients | Mean differences varied by age group and were significant for energy at 12 to <18 months, for iron at 6 to <12 months and 12 to <18 months, and for vitamin C at <6 months |

[a]M, male; F, female; TEE, total energy expenditure; FFQ, food frequency questionnaire; BMI, body mass index; LDL, low-density lipoprotein.

[b]Correspondence of referent period of validation standard and instrument. The referent period is the time of the diet, as measured by the dietary assessment technique.

[c]Mean energy difference, ([instrument (mean)—validation (mean) standard]/validation (mean) standard).

[d]Differences in mean energy and nutrient intake; underestimation/overestimation indicates statistically significant difference or >5% difference when significance testing not shown.

[e]Type of correlation not specified.

486

## FOOD FREQUENCY QUESTIONNAIRES

On an FFQ, which typically includes a long list of foods and beverages, respondents are asked to report frequency of consumption and, on some instruments, portion size (35). For preschoolers, the usual referent period is the past month to the past year. Because of the longer referent period, usual individual intake may be inferred from a single FFQ. With quantitative FFQs, portion size is collected for all foods; on semiquantitative FFQs, this information is collected only for foods that are consumed in typical portion sizes (e.g. bread slices, milk glasses). On the nonquantitative FFQs, portion size is not collected; nutrient intakes are calculated based on standard portion sizes.

### Validity

The validity of FFQs for measuring the intake of preschool children was examined in nine studies (5, 10, 18, 22, 30, 31, 33, 34, 36) (Table 3). All these studies used FFQs to assess general dietary intake, with one exception (34). This study investigated the validity of an abbreviated FFQ to measure intakes of calcium (34) and is discussed separately.

Frequency of food consumption was assessed for usual current intake (30) and for intake over the preceding week (18), month (5), 3 months (36), 6 months (33), or 1 year (10, 22). One study did not provide information on the referent period (31). Except for one study (30), all used an FFQ based on the Willett FFQ. Among the eight studies, 24-h recalls (5, 33, 36) and food records (18, 30) were most commonly used as the validation standard. FFQs were also compared with physiological measures—energy expenditure as measured by doubly labeled water (22) and serum lipid levels (31). Finally, one study (10) compared a 1-year FFQ with the mean of three 4-month FFQs administered at 4-month intervals.

When compared with multiple 24-h recalls, the FFQ overestimated mean energy intake by 0.2% (5), 41% (36), and 73% (33). The high percentage of overestimation in the latter study may be partially explained by the study design—foods consumed in the absence of the mother were deleted from food recalls, which was the validation standard. The percentage energy difference between the FFQ and the doubly labeled water study was 59% (22). In that study, the FFQ used adult portion sizes, which were 25%–33% greater than the typical serving suggested for preschoolers.

The correlations between FFQs and other methods of dietary assessment varied by the validation standard, the nutrients assessed, and how the correlations were adjusted. Unadjusted correlations between a 1-year FFQ and the mean of three consecutive 4-month FFQs were the highest: 0.61 for energy, 0.67 for protein, and 0.63 for fat (10). Two studies adjusted both for energy intake and for the effect of intraindividual variability in intake (5, 33). Stein et al reported adjusted correlations of 0.29 for protein and 0.28 for fat for boys and 0.51 and 0.39 for

**TABLE 3** Validity of food frequency questionnaires[a]

| Reference | Population | Instrument | Validation standard | Referent period[b] | Macronutrient correlations | Range of correlations (all nutrients and energy) | Mean energy difference[c] | Nutrient and energy differences[d] | Quantitative/ qualitative and other differences |
|---|---|---|---|---|---|---|---|---|---|
| Standard/modified FFQ | | | | | | | | | |
| Blum et al (5) | 1–5 years old, 233 M & F, 56% Native American, 44% Caucasian, US | Mean of two 1-month FFQs; administered 1 month apart | Mean of three 24-h recalls administered over 1 month | 3 days of recall encompassed within 1-month FFQ | Adjusted[e] Pearson: 0.43 protein, 0.62 fat | Adjusted[e] Pearson: 0.26 fiber to 0.63 magnesium (20 nutrients) | +0.2% (1688 vs 1684 kcal) | FFQ overestimated 12 of 20 nutrients and underestimated 3 (significance testing not shown) | Average correlations were similar in younger and older children— 0.51 for 1–2 years and 0.49 for 3–5 years; average nutrient correlations not were similar between Native American (0.51) and Caucasian children (0.49) |
| Eck et al (10) | 5.2 ± 0.6 years (mean ± SD), 108 M & F, US | 1-year FFQ | Mean of three 4-month FFQ administered 4 months apart | Same 1-year period | 0.61 energy, 0.67 protein, 0.63 fat[f] | 0.53 carbohydrates to 0.74 calcium[e] (7 nutrients) | +0.9% (1967 vs 1949 kcal) | No differences for 7 of 7 nutrients (significance testing not shown) | — |
| Iannotti et al (18) | 2–4 years, 17 M & F, US | 1-week FFQ | Mean of 3 days of measured food records | 3 days of food records encompassed within 1 week FFQ | Unadjusted Pearson: 0.37 energy | Unadjusted Pearson: 0.15 for fatty acid (% kilocalories) to 0.40 colsterol (5 nutrients) | — | — | — |
| C Kaskoun et al (22) | 4–7 years, 22 M/23 F, 80% Caucasian, 20% Native | 1-year FFQ | TEE with doubly labeled water assessed | Overlapping TEE within 1-year FFQ | — | — | +59% (2180 vs 1372 kcal) | — | FFQ serving sizes based on adult portions; no significant differences by sex or ethnicity; no difference by body composition of child |

| | | | | | | | | |
|---|---|---|---|---|---|---|---|---|
| | American, US | | over 14 days | | | | | or mother; paternal percent body fat significantly correlated with misreporting |
| Persson & Calgren (30) | 4 & 8 years, 477 M & F, Sweden | FFQ of "current" intake | 7-day food records | — | — | — | — | Food items: FFQ significantly overestimated 14 of 27 food items and underestimated 9 of 27 food items for 4 year olds |
| Shea et al (31) | 4–5 years, 57 M/51 F, Hispanic, US | Mean of two FFQs[g] administered 6 months apart | Serum lipid concentration | Overlapping | — | — | — | Total serum cholesterol and LDL cholesterol increased significantly across tertiles of total fat, saturated fat, calorie-adjusted total fat, and calorie-adjusted saturated fat. These associations remained significant after adjusting for age, sex, and BMI |
| | | | Mean of four 24-h recall interviews administered over 1 year | Same 1 year period | — | — | — | FFQ overestimated intake of total fat, saturated fat, and cholesterol; when mean intakes from the FFQ were compared with recalls, children in the highest tertile had values of 137.7 vs 79.3 g for total fat, 53.7 vs 31.4 g for saturated fat, and 578.9 vs 438.9 mg for cholesterol; overall mean intakes of percent calories from fat were 33.2% vs 33.0%, respectively |
| Stein et al (33) | 44–60 months, 112 M/112 F, 91% Hispanic, 8% African- | Two 6-month FFQs adminis- | Four 24-h recall interviews admini- | Same 1-year period | Adjusted Pearson[e]: boys—0.34 energy, 0.29 | Adjusted Pearson[e]: boys— 0.05 poly- | Boys— +66% (2667 vs 1604 kcal); girls—+73% | Boys—FFQ significantly overestimated 10 of 10 | Excluded from analysis of recall data times when food was consumed outside of parents' supervision; |

*(Continued)*

**TABLE 3** (*Continued*)

| Reference | Population | Instrument | Validation standard | Referent period[b] | Macronutrient correlations | Range of correlations (all nutrients and energy) | Mean energy difference[c] | Nutrient and energy differences[d] | Quantitative/ qualitative and other differences |
|---|---|---|---|---|---|---|---|---|---|
| | American, 1% Caucasian, US | tered 6 months apart | stered over 1 year | | protein, 0.28 fat; girls— 0.59 energy, 0.59 protein, 0.39 fat | unsaturated fat to 0.71 potassium; girls— −0.14 sodium to 0.78 potassium (10 nutrients) | (2586 vs 1492 kcal) | nutrients; girls—FFQ significantly overestimated 10 of 10 nutrients | correlations were generally higher among girls than boys Food items: FFQ overestimated frequency of consumption of items such as dairy products, meat, fruits, and vegetables |
| Treiber et al (36) | 3–5 years, 33 M & F, US | 3-month FFQ (n = 51) | Mean of two 24-h recalls administered 1 week apart (N = 33) | Recall encompassed within 3-month FFQ | Unadjusted Pearson: 0.41 protein | Unadjusted Pearson: 0.40 potassium to 0.62 cholesterol (4 nutrients) | +41% (2309 vs 1635 kcal) | FFQ overestimated 10 of 11 nutrients and underestimated 1 (significance testing) | Recall was administered only to parents who directly observed all food intake |
| Abbreviated FFQ | | | | | | | | | |
| Taylor & Goulding (34) | 3–6 years 63 M & F New Zealand | 1-year FFQ Specific to calcium intake | 4-day estimated food records | — | — | 0.52[f] calcium | — | +18.0% (942 mg vs 798 mg calcium) | — |

aM, male, F, female, TEE, total energy expenditure; FFQ, food frequency questionnaire; BMI, body mass index; LDL, low-density lipoprotein; SD, standard deviation.

bCorrespondence of referent period of validation standard and instrument. The referent period is the time of the diet as measured by the dietary assessment technique.

cMean difference = [(instrument (mean) − validation (mean))/validation (mean) standard].

dDifferences in mean energy and nutrient intake; underestimation/overestimation indicates statistically significant difference or >5% difference when significance testing not shown.

eCorrelation coefficients adjusted for energy intake and within person variation. Energy correlations were adjusted for within person variability only.

fType of correlation not specified.

gReferent period not specified.

girls (33). Blum et al reported adjusted correlations of 0.43 for protein and 0.62 for total fat (5).

Stein et al found that the FFQ consistently overestimated the frequency of intake of food servings such as meat, dairy products, and fruits and vegetables when compared with the mean of four 24-h recalls (33). In a similar analysis, when Persson & Carlgren compared FFQs with 7-day food records, the FFQ significantly overestimated 14 of 27 food items and underestimated 9 of 27 items (30).

Three studies examined the effect of demographic factors on FFQ validity. In one study, correlations between FFQs and recalls were generally higher among girls than boys (33). In another study, average correlations between the FFQ and multiple recalls were similar across age and ethnicity (5). Finally, correlations between the FFQ and doubly labeled water showed no significant differences between energy intake and energy expenditure by sex, ethnicity, or body composition of the child or mother (22).

One study evaluated the validity of using abbreviated FFQs for preschool children to estimate calcium intake (34). In this study, the FFQ and a 4-day food record were used to categorize children into quartiles of mean calcium intake. "Correct classification" was defined as the proportion of children placed by the FFQ in the same or adjacent quartile in which they were classified by the food record. "Gross misclassification" was defined as placing children in the lowest quartile by one method and the highest quartile by the other. The FFQ overestimated mean calcium intake by an average of 18%, but it correctly classified 84% of children and "grossly misclassified" only 3%.

## Reproducibility

Of the four studies that measured the reproducibility of FFQs in estimating dietary intake of preschool children (Table 4), one study evaluated reproducibility of instruments administered 1 week apart (36), one at 4 months apart (10), and two at 6 months (31, 33). Treiber et al (36) found no differences in energy intake between the first and second FFQ administration. Pearson correlations between the first and second FFQ were 0.46 for energy, 0.55 for protein, and 0.67 for fat. Correlations for energy and 10 nutrients ranged from 0.42 for carbohydrates to 0.74 for sodium. Eck et al administered a FFQ three times at 4-month intervals (10). No significant differences were found in the mean intake of energy or six nutrients between the first and second or second and third administration. Of the two studies that evaluated FFQs administered 6 months apart, Shea et al noted intraclass correlations of 0.39 for energy and 0.38 for fat (31). Correlations among energy and three nutrients ranged from 0.19 to 0.39. On the other hand, Stein et al found a wider range of correlations (33). Values of Cronbach's coefficient alpha, a special case of the intraclass correlation coefficient, ranged from 0.40 for protein to 0.73 for energy among boys and from 0.17 for sodium to 0.71 for energy among girls.

**TABLE 4** Reproducibility of food frequency questionaires[a]

| Reference | Population | Instrument | Time difference[b] | Macronutrient correlations | Range of correlations (all nutrients and energy) | Mean energy difference[c] | Nutrient and energy differences[d] | Quantitative/ qualitative and other differences |
|---|---|---|---|---|---|---|---|---|
| Eck et al (10) | 5.2 ± 0.6 years (mean ± SD), 108 M & F, US | 4-month FFQ | 4-month intervals (4 months, 8 months, 12 months) | — | — | 4 vs 8 months + 2% (1964 vs 1924), 8 vs 12 months − 2% (1924 vs 1959) | No differences between assessments for 7 of 7 nutrients, between assessments at 4 months and 8 months or 8 months and 12 months (significance testing not shown) | — |
| Shea et al (31) | 4–5 years, 57 M/51 F, Hispanic, US | FFQ | 6 months | Intraclass: 0.39 energy, 0.38 fat | Intraclass: 0.19 cholesterol to 0.39 energy (4 nutrients) | — | — | — |
| Stein et al (33) | 44–60 months, 112 M/112 F, 91% Hispanic, 8% African-American, 1% Caucasian, US | 6-month FFQ | 6 months | Cronbach alpha: boys—0.73 energy, 0.40 protein, 0.48 fat; girls—0.71 energy, 0.30 protein, 0.32 fat | Cronbach alpha: boys—0.40 protein to 0.73 energy (10 nutrients); girls—0.17 sodium to 0.71 energy | — | — | — |
| Treiber et al (36) | 3–5 years, 51 M & F, US | 3-months FFQ | 1 week | Unadjusted Pearson: 0.46 energy, 0.55 protein, 0.67 fat | Unadjusted Pearson: 0.42 carbohydrates to 0.74 sodium (11 nutrients) | +4% (2350 vs 2269 kcal) | Of 11 nutrients, no significant differences in mean intake between first and second FFQ | — |

[a]M, male; F, female; TEE, total energy expenditure; FFQ, food frequency questionnaire; BMI, body mass index; LDL, low-density lipoprotein; SD, standard deviation.
[b]Time interval between first and second administration of the instrument.
[c]Mean energy difference, [(first administration—second administration)/first administration].
[d]Differences in mean energy and nutrient intake; underestimation/overestimation indicates statistically significant difference or >5% difference when significance testing not shown.
[e]Referent period not specified.

## OTHER STUDIES

Two studies investigate the validity of other methods for assessing preschool diets (Table 5). In one, estimated energy intake from diet histories was compared with energy expenditure measured from the doubly labeled water method (26). Diet histories assess usual meal patterns, food intake, and other information in an extensive 1- to 2-h interview or questionnaire (35). In contrast to other diet assessment methods, a diet history is both qualitative and quantitative, allowing detailed information about food preparation, eating habits, and food consumption to be collected. In this study, diet history overestimated total energy expenditure by 12% in 3-year-old children and 8% in 5-year-olds (26).

Finally, the usefulness of an abbreviated questionnaire to measure intake of vitamin A was examined (1). Using the recommendations of the International Vitamin A Consultative Group, a food checklist was created using commonly eaten foods high in vitamin A, and mothers were asked about foods consumed in the previous 24 h. The Consumption Index, a simplified scoring system based on the vitamin A content of the food and standard portion size, was used to classify children into low, moderate, or high risk of vitamin A deficiency based on 6 days of 24-h food checklists and weighed food records. Although there were some differences in the mean scores on individual days, there were no significant differences in mean scores for all days combined for children classified at high risk.

## DISCUSSION

The preschool years are critical for growth and development, with more rapid and frequent transitions in dietary patterns occurring than in other age groups. Although the importance of preschool diet has been well established, measuring dietary intake in children younger than 5 years remains a challenging area of study. We identified studies that examined the validity of food recalls, food records, FFQs, and diet history and also identified studies that examined the reproducibility of FFQs. The heterogeneity of study designs, the relatively small study populations, and the limited number of studies examined restrict our ability to draw general conclusions. Even among studies using the same dietary assessment method, there were differences in how the assessment was conducted. For example, FFQs varied as to whether portion-size information was collected, and if so, how portion sizes were assessed. The length and type of food lists also varied among FFQs. Both food recall and records varied in how many days of intake were collected. Food recalls also varied on how much probing was done and how portion-size information was collected.

The validation standard chosen is an important consideration in interpreting study findings. We found a variety of validation standards, including two physiologic measures (doubly labeled water and serum lipids), investigator-based measurements, such as collection of duplicate portions or direct observation, and

**TABLE 5** Other validity studies[a]

| Reference | Population | Instrument | Validation standard | Referent period[b] | Macronutrient correlations | Range of correlations (all nutrients and energy) | Mean energy difference[c] | Nutrient and energy differences[d] | Quantitative/ qualitative and other differences |
|---|---|---|---|---|---|---|---|---|---|
| Abdullah Ahmed (1) | 2–5 years, 121 M & F, Bangladesh | 6 simplified 24-food check-lists (foods containing vitamin A) | 6-day weighed food record | Same days | — | — | — | — | Consumption index, a simplified score based on vitamin A content of food and portion size, was calculated based on vitamin A content of food serving size for both the food checklists and the weighed food records. Matched pair analysis showed some differences between methods in the mean consumption index on individual days; however, no significant differences in the mean consumption index value for all days among children categorized at high risk |
| Livingstone et al (26) | 3 & 5 years, 12 M/8 F, UK | Diet history | TEE with doubly labeled water; assessed over 10–14 days | Overlapping | — | — | 3 years, +12% (1412 vs 1257 kcal); 5 years, +8% (1565 vs 1455 kcal) | — | No significant difference between estimates by sex |

[a]M, male; F, female; TEE, total energy expenditure; FFQ, food frequency questionnaire; BMI, body mass index; LDL, low-density lipoprotein.

[b]Correspondence of referent period of validation standard and instrument. The referent period is the time of the diet, as measured by the dietary assessment technique.

[c]Mean energy difference, {[instrument (mean)−validation (mean) standard]/validation (mean) standard}.

[d]Differences in mean energy and nutrient intake; under/overestimation indicates statistically significant difference or >5% difference when significance testing not shown.

494

respondent-based measures, such as food recalls, FFQs, and food records. Because dietary intake cannot be measured with absolute precision in free-living populations, there is no true validation standard. Thus, validation studies are best seen as comparative studies, with the validity of the dietary method being assessed established by how well it compares with a second method of dietary assessment. Ideally, the errors inherent in the validation standard are independent of those in the method being assessed; to the extent that errors in the two methods are related, the comparison of the two methods will lead to artificially inflated correlations (39). To illustrate, related errors would be expected if both methods are respondent based (food recalls, food records, and FFQs). Most of the studies in this review used respondent-based methods for both the method being assessed and the validation standard. In contrast, errors in physiologic measures (biochemical markers or doubly labeled water) are independent of errors in respondent-based measures (4). Still, although biochemical markers such as serum nutrient concentrations provide an independent measure of nutrient intake, many are also influenced by nondietary factors and thus cannot be used as markers of intake. Some nutrient concentrations (e.g. calcium and vitamin A) are under tight physiologic regulation and thus respond less to diet, whereas others (e.g. carotenoids) vary with dietary intake and would be more appropriate markers.

Other factors to consider in interpreting validation studies are the effects of the dietary assessment method on dietary behaviors and the congruence of referent periods. The dietary assessment method itself may alter behavior; caregivers who are being observed may alter their child's diet to make it more socially acceptable. In addition, caregivers who are recording a diet may simplify it to make recording easier. A large difference in referent periods may influence results as well, but we could not gauge such effects. We found that multiple 24-h food recalls were commonly used to assess the validity of FFQs whose referent period was 3 months to 1 year, and that two or three 24-h periods were usually collected to assess dietary intake during that referent period.

Despite the key role of diet in the growth and development of young children, relatively few studies were available, especially in children under 3 years of age. Most of the studies investigated the validity of food recalls and full FFQs. Only two studies investigated abbreviated methods that assessed a single nutrient; future studies should further investigate the feasibility of abbreviated methods in young children. There were no consistent differences in the validity or reproducibility of the dietary assessment measures with regard to age or ethnicity, but few studies had adequate sample size to examine these factors. Future studies of dietary assessment techniques need to evaluate patterns of misreporting, particularly with regard to the maternal factors (e.g. education, stay-at-home status), age of the child, and ethnicity.

In conclusion, this review can serve as a guide to researchers and clinicians for selecting dietary methods for their work with preschool children. When choosing a method to estimate dietary intake, the intended purpose of the assessment, as well as its practicality, must first be considered. The FFQ is relatively easy to administer and is unlikely to affect dietary intake. In general, FFQs overestimate total energy intake and are better at ranking, rather than quantifying, usual intake. The differences in energy intake between the FFQ and other methods of assessment are greater than those required to determine precisely the energy balance parameters needed in the context of energy balance or obesity studies. In contrast, food records and recalls can be used to both rank and quantify nutrient intakes. Because of day-to-day variability in intake, however, food records and recalls require multiple days of collection to measure usual intakes of individual persons. Nevertheless, mean nutrient intakes of a population can be calculated from a single dietary recall or record. Compared with FFQs, food recalls and food records (in particular) require more effort on the part of the researcher/clinician and the respondent. On the other hand, methods for collecting food record or recall information require little adaptation for different population or age groups. In contrast, the FFQ requires the food list and portion sizes to be appropriate to the population under investigation. Once a method is selected, after considering the intended purpose of the assessment as well as the constraints of the setting, researchers and clinicians can use the results of published studies included here as a guide to evaluate and possibly adopt the chosen dietary method.

## ACKNOWLEDGMENTS

We thank Cathleen Gillespie for her statistical input and Peter Taylor and Carol Ballew for their editorial input.

**Visit the Annual Reviews home page at www.AnnualReviews.org**

## LITERATURE CITED

1. Abdullah M, Ahmed L. 1993. Validating a simplified approach to the dietary assessment of vitamin A intake in preschool children. *Eur. J. Clin. Nutr.* 47:115–22
2. Baranowski T, Sprague D, Baranowski JH, Harrison JA. 1991. Accuracy of maternal dietary recall for preschool children. *J. Am. Diet. Assoc.* 91:669–74
3. Basch CE, Shea S, Arliss R, Contento IR, Rips J, et al. 1990. Validation of mothers' reports of dietary intake by 4 to 7 year-old children. *Am. J. Public Health* 80:1314–17
4. Bingham SA. 1994. The use of 24-h urine samples and energy expenditure to validate dietary assessments. *Am. J. Clin. Nutr.* 59:227–31S
5. Blum RE, Wei EK, Rockett HR, Lange-

liers JD, Leppert J, et al. 1999. Validation of a food frequency questionnaire in Native American and Caucasian children 1 to 5 years of age. *Mat. Child Health J.* 3:167–72
6. Comm. Nutr. 1998. *Pediatric Nutrition Handbook*. Elk Grove Village, IL: Am. Acad. Pediatr. 4th ed.
7. Davies PS, Coward WA, Gregory J, White A, Mills A. 1994. Total energy expenditure and energy intake in the preschool child: a comparison. *Br. J. Nutr.* 72:13–20
8. Dop MC, Milan C, Milan C, N'Diaye AM. 1994. The 24-h recall for Senegalese weanlings: a validation exercise. *Eur. J. Clin. Nutr.* 48:643–53
9. Eck LH, Klesges RC, Hanson CL. 1989.

Recall of a child's intake from one meal: Are parents accurate? *J. Am. Diet. Assoc.* 89:784–89

10. Eck LH, Klesges RC, Hanson CL, White J. 1991. Reporting retrospective dietary intake by food frequency questionnaire in a pediatric population. *J. Am. Diet. Assoc.* 91:606–8

11. Ferguson EL, Gibson RS, Onupuu S, Sabry JH. 1989. The validity of the 24-h recall for estimating the energy and selected nutrient intakes of a group of rural Malawian preschool children. *Ecol. Food Nutr.* 23:273–85

12. Ferguson EL, Gibson RS, Opare-Obisaw C. 1994. The relative validity of the repeated 24-h recall for estimating energy and selected nutrient intakes of rural Ghanian children. *Eur. J. Clin. Nutr.* 48:241–52

13. Gibson AS. 1990. *Principles of Individual Assessment.* New York: Oxford Univ. Press

14. Guenther PM, Kott PS, Carriquiry AL. 1997. Development of an approach for estimating usual nutrient intake distributions at the population level. *J. Nutr.* 127:1106–12

15. Hagman U, Bruce A, Persson LA, Samuelson G, Sjolin S. 1986. Food habits and nutrient intake in childhood in relation to health and socio-economic conditions. A Swedish Multicentre Study 1980–81. *Acta Paediatr. Scand. Suppl.* 328:1–56

16. Harbottle L, Duggan MB. 1993. Dietary assessment in Asian children—a comparison of the weighed inventory and diet history methods. *Eur. J. Clin. Nutr.* 47:666–72

17. Horst CH, Obermann-De Boer GL, Kromhout D. 1988. Validity of the 24-h recall method in infancy: the Leiden Pre-School Children Study. *Int. J. Epidemiol.* 17:217–21

18. Iannotti RJ, Zuckerman AE, Blyer EM, O'Brien RW, Finn J, Spillman DM. 1994. Comparison of dietary intake methods with young children. *Psychol. Rep.* 74:883–89

19. Inst. Med. 2000. *Dietary Reference Intakes: Applications in Dietary Assessment.* Washington, DC: Natl. Acad. Sci.

20. Int. Vitamin A Consult. Group. 1989. *Guidelines for the Development of Simplified Dietary Assessment to Identify Groups at Risk for Inadequate Intake of Vitamin A.* Rep. Int. Vitamin A Consult. Group. Washington, DC: Nutr. Found.

21. Johnson RK, Driscoll P, Goran MI. 1996. Comparison of multiple-pass 24-h recall estimates of energy intake with total energy expenditure determined by the doubly labeled water method in young children. *J. Am. Diet. Assoc.* 96:1140–44

22. Kaskoun MC, Johnson RK, Goran MI. 1994. Comparison of energy intake by semiquantitative food-frequency questionnaire with total energy expenditure by the doubly labeled water method in young children. *Am. J. Clin. Nutr.* 60:43–47

23. Kigutha HN. 1997. Assessment of dietary intake in rural communities: experiences in Kenya. *Am. J. Clin. Nutr.* 65 (Suppl.):1168–72S

24. Klesges RC, Hanson CL, Eck LH, Durff AC. 1988. Accuracy of self-reports of food intake in obese and normal-weight individuals: effects of parental obesity on reports of children's dietary intake. *Am. J. Clin. Nutr.* 48:1252–56

25. Klesges RC, Klesges LM, Brown G, Frank GC. 1987. Validation of the 24-h dietary recall in preschool children. *J. Am. Diet. Assoc.* 87:1383–85

26. Livingstone MB, Prentice AM, Coward WA, Strain JJ, Black AE. 1992. Validation of estimates of energy intake by weighed dietary record and diet history in children and adolescents. *Am. J. Clin. Nutr.* 56:29–35

27. McPherson RS, Hoelscher D, Alexander M, Scanlon KS, Serdula MK. 2000. Dietary assessment methods among school-aged children: validity and reliability. *Prev. Med.* 31:S11–33

28. Nelson M, Black AE, Morris JA, Cole TJ.

1989. Between- and within-subject variation in nutrient intake from infancy to old age: estimating the number of days required to rank dietary intakes with desired precision. *Am. J. Clin. Nutr.* 50:115–67

29. Olinto MT, Victora CG, Barros FC, Gigante DP. 1995. Twenty-four-hour recall overestimates the dietary intake of malnourished children. *J. Nutr.* 125:880–84

30. Persson LA, Carlgren G. 1984. Measuring children's diets: evaluation of dietary assessment techniques in infancy and childhood. *Int. J. Epidemiol.* 13:506–17

31. Shea S, Basch CE, Irigoyen M, Zybert P, Rips JL, et al. 1991. Relationships of dietary fat consumption to serum total and low-density lipoprotein cholesterol in Hispanic pre-school children. *Prev. Med.* 20:237–49

32. Sloan NL, Rosen D, de la Paz T, Arita M, Temalilwa C, Solomons NW. 1997. Identifying areas with vitamin A deficiency: the validity of a semiquantitative food frequency method. *Am. J. Public Health* 87:186–91

33. Stein AD, Shea S, Basch CE, Contento I, Zybert P. 1992. Consistency of the Willett semiquantitative food frequency questionnaire and 24-h dietary recalls in estimating nutrient intakes of preschool children. *Am. J. Epidemiol.* 135:667–77

34. Taylor RW, Goulding A. 1998. Validation of a short food frequency questionnaire to assess calcium intake in children aged 3 to 6 years. *Eur. J. Clin. Nutr.* 52:464–65

35. Thompson FE, Byers T. 1994. Dietary assessment resource manual. *J. Nutr.* 124(Suppl.):2245–317S

36. Treiber FA, Leonard SB, Frank G, Musante L, Davis H, et al. 1990. Dietary assessment instruments for preschool children: reliability of parental responses to the 24-h recall and a food frequency questionnaire. *J. Am. Diet. Assoc.* 90:814–20

37. US Dep. Agric., US Dep. Health Hum. Serv. 2000. *Nutrition and Your Health: Dietary Guidelines for Americans. Home and Garden Bull. No. 232.* Washington, DC: Gov. Print. Off. 5th Ed.

38. US Dep. Health Hum. Serv. 2000. *Tracking Healthy People 2010.* Washington, DC: US Gov. Print. Off.

39. Willett W. 1998. *Nutritional Epidemiology.* New York: Oxford Univ. Press. 2nd ed.

# SUBJECT INDEX

## A

Absorption
  apolipoprotein A-IV in
    regulation of food intake
    and, 231, 237–38
  fat metabolism in insects
    and, 23, 32–33
  nutritional iron deficiency
    and, 1, 4–11
  polyphenols and cancer,
    386–88
  zinc homeostasis and, 429,
    438–46
*ACC1* gene
  *Saccharomyces cerevisiae*
    fatty acid metabolism
    and, 108–9
Accessory factors
  C/EBP regulation of gene
    expression and, 141,
    152–54
Accumulation
  folate catabolism and, 260,
    261–62
*Acheta domesticus*
  fat metabolism in insects
    and, 27–28, 36
Activation
  peroxisomal β-oxidation
    and PPARα, 201–2,
    216–17
  *Saccharomyces cerevisiae*
    fatty acid metabolism
    and, 100–1
Acute phase response
  vitamin A and, 167,
    172–74
Acyl-CoA-binding protein
  peroxisomal β-oxidation
    and PPARα, 209
Adaptive metabolic system

peroxisomal β-oxidation
  and PPARα, 193–224
Adolescents
  nutritional iron deficiency
    and, 4, 14, 17
*Aedes aegypti*
  fat metabolism in insects
    and, 28–29
*Aeschna cyanea*
  fat metabolism in insects
    and, 33
Africa
  "fetal origins" hypothesis
    and, 80–81
  vitamin A and, 183
African Americans
  African diaspora and
    nutritional consequences,
    47–65
African diaspora
  nutritional consequences of
    adult anthropometrics,
    56–59
  childhood
    undernutrition,
    54–56
  diabetes, 59–61
  diet in Africa and the
    diaspora, 52
  historical background,
    48–51
  hypertension, 61–63
  introduction, 48
  miscellaneous
    nutrition-related
    outcomes, 63–65
  nutrition transition,
    53–54
  obesity, 56–59
  summary, 65
Alcohol

folate catabolism and, 273
*p*-Aminobenzoylglutamate
  folate catabolism and, 264
*Ancylostoma duodenale*
  gastrointestinal nematodes,
    nutrition, and immunity,
    298
Anemia
  "fetal origins" hypothesis
    and, 78
  nutritional iron deficiency
    and, 4, 10, 11–14
Anorexia
  maintenance dialysis
    patients and, 343, 352–56
Anthopometrics
  adult
    African diaspora and
    nutritional
    consequences, 56–59
Anticonvulsant drugs
  folate catabolism and, 255,
    272
Antihelminthics
  gastrointestinal nematodes,
    nutrition, and immunity,
    311
Antioxidants
  polyphenols and cancer,
    381, 385–86
AOX deficiency
  peroxisomal β-oxidation
    and PPARα, 216–19
*APA1* gene
  *Saccharomyces cerevisiae*
    fatty acid metabolism
    and, 110
Apical epithelial surfaces
  megalin- and
    cubilin-mediated
    endocytosis, 407–23

**499**

# CUMULATIVE INDEXES

## CONTRIBUTING AUTHORS, VOLUMES 17–21

# CHAPTER TITLES, VOLUMES 17–21

## Proteins, Peptides, and Amino Acids

## Vitamins

## Nutrition and Metabolic Regulation